SCIENCE AND PSEUDOSCIENCE
IN CLINICAL PSYCHOLOGY

Science and Pseudoscience in Clinical Psychology

Edited by
SCOTT O. LILIENFELD
STEVEN JAY LYNN
JEFFREY M. LOHR

Foreword by
CAROL TAVRIS

THE GUILFORD PRESS
New York   London

© 2003 The Guilford Press
A Division of Guilford Publications, Inc.
72 Spring Street, New York, NY 10012
www.guilford.com

Printed in the United States of America

This book is printed on acid-free paper.

Last digit is print number: 9 8 7 6 5 4 3 2 1

Library of Congress Cataloging-in-Publication Data

Science and pseudoscience in clinical psychology / edited by Scott O.
  Lilienfeld, Steven Jay Lynn, Jeffrey M. Lohr.
       p.   cm.
    Includes bibliographical references and index.
    ISBN 1-57230-828-1 (hbk.)
    1. Clinical psychology. 2. Psychotherapy. 3. Medical misconceptions.
  4. Psychiatry—Research. I. Lilienfeld, Scott O., 1960– II. Lynn,
  Steven J. III. Lohr, Jeffrey M.
  RC467 .S432 2003
  616.89—dc21   2002014071

About the Editors

Scott O. Lilienfeld, PhD, is Associate Professor of Psychology at Emory University in Atlanta. He has authored or coauthored approximately 100 articles and book chapters on such topics as the assessment and causes of personality disorders, the relation of personality traits to anxiety disorders, conceptual issues in psychiatric classification and diagnosis, projective testing, multiple personality disorder, and the problem of pseudoscience in clinical psychology. He is founder and editor of the new journal *The Scientific Review of Mental Health Practice*. Dr. Lilienfeld also serves on the editorial boards of several major journals, including the *Journal of Abnormal Psychology, Psychological Assessment, Clinical Psychology: Science and Practice, Clinical Psychology Review,* the *Journal of Clinical Psychology, Skeptical Inquirer,* and *The Scientific Review of Alternative Medicine.* He is past president of the Society for a Science of Clinical Psychology, and he was the recipient of the 1998 David Shakow Award for Early Career Contributions to Clinical Psychology from Division 12 (Society for Clinical Psychology) of the American Psychological Association.

Steven Jay Lynn, PhD, ABPP (Clinical, Forensic), is a licensed clinical psychologist and Professor of Psychology at the State University of New York at Binghamton. A former president of American Psychological Association's Division 30 (Psychological Hypnosis), he is a recipient of the division's award for distinguished contributions to scientific hypnosis. Dr. Lynn is a fellow of many professional organizations and an advisory editor to many professional journals, including the *Journal of Abnormal Psychology.* He is also the author of 11 books and more than 200 articles and chapters on hypnosis, memory, fantasy, victimization, and psychotherapy.

Jeffrey M. Lohr, PhD, is Professor of Psychology at the University of Arkansas–Fayetteville. He has been a licensed psychologist in Arkansas with a part-time independent practice since 1976. Dr. Lohr's research interests focus on anxiety disorders, domestic violence, and the efficacy of psychosocial treatments. His teaching interests include abnormal psychology, behavior modification and therapy, research methods, and professional issues in mental health practice.

Contributors

Timothy Anderson, PhD, Department of Psychology, Ohio University, Athens, Ohio

Laura Arnstein, MA, Department of Psychology, State University of New York at Binghamton, Binghamton, New York

Patricia A. Boyle, PhD, Department of Psychiatry and Human Behavior, Brown University, Providence, Rhode Island

Howard N. Garb, PhD, Behavioral Health, VA Pittsburgh Healthcare System, Pittsburgh, Pennsylvania

John P. Garske, PhD, Department of Psychology, Ohio University, Athens, Ohio

Jennifer Gillis, MA, Department of Psychology, State University of New York at Binghamton, Binghamton, New York

Richard Gist, PhD, Department of Psychology, Johnson County Community College, Overland Park, Kansas

Russell E. Glasgow, PhD, AMC Cancer Research Center, Denver, Colorado

Tammy R. Hammond, MS, Department of Psychology, State University of New York at Binghamton, Binghamton, New York

G. Perry Hill, PhD, School of Allied Health Professionals, Louisiana State University Medical Center, Shreveport, Louisiana

Wayne Hooke, MA, private practice, Vancouver, Washington, and Department of Psychology, Portland Community College, Portland, Oregon

John Hunsley, PhD, School of Psychology, University of Ottawa, Ottawa, Ontario, Canada

Irving Kirsch, PhD, Department of Psychology, University of Connecticut, Storrs, Connecticut

Elisa Krackow, MS, Department of Psychology, State University of New York at Binghamton, Binghamton, New York

Catherine M. Lee, PhD, School of Psychology, University of Ottawa, Ottawa, Ontario, Canada

Scott O. Lilienfeld, PhD, Department of Psychology, Emory University, Atlanta, Georgia

Stephen A. Lisman, PhD, Department of Psychology, State University of New York at Binghamton, Binghamton, New York

Timothy Lock, PhD, Department of Psychology, State University of New York at Binghamton, Binghamton, New York

Elizabeth F. Loftus, PhD, Department of Psychology, University of Washington, Seattle, Washington

Jeffrey M. Lohr, PhD, Department of Psychology, University of Arkansas, Fayetteville, Arkansas

Steven Jay Lynn, PhD, Department of Psychology, State University of New York at Binghamton, Binghamton, New York

James MacKillop, MA, Department of Psychology, State University of New York at Binghamton, Binghamton, New York

Joseph T. McCann, PsyD, JD, United Health Services Hospitals and State University of New York Upstate Medical University–Clinical Campus, Binghamton, New York

Timothy E. Moore, PhD, Department of Psychology, Glendon College/ York University, Toronto, Ontario, Canada

Abraham Nievod, PhD, JD, private practice, Berkeley, California

Raymond G. Romanczyk, PhD, BCBA, Department of Psychology, State University of New York at Binghamton, Binghamton, New York

Gerald M. Rosen, PhD, private practice, Seattle, Washington

Deborah Rosenbaum, MA, Department of Psychology, State University of New York at Binghamton, Binghamton, New York

Kelley L. Shindler, BA, Department of Psychology, State University of New York at Binghamton, Binghamton, New York

Margaret Thaler Singer, PhD, Department of Psychology, University of California, Berkeley, California

Latha V. Soorya, MA, Department of Psychology, State University of New York at Binghamton, Binghamton, New York

David F. Tolin, PhD, Anxiety Disorders Center, The Institute of Living, Hartford, Connecticut

Harald Walach, PhD, Institute of Environmental Medicine and Department of Epidemiology, University Hospital, Freiburg, Germany

Daniel A. Waschbusch, PhD, Department of Psychology, Dalhousie University, Halifax, Nova Scotia, Canada

Allison Weinstein, MA, Department of Psychology, State University of New York at Binghamton, Binghamton, New York

Nona Wilson, PhD, Department of Counselor Education, University of Wisconsin, Oshkosh, Wisconsin

James M. Wood, PhD, Department of Psychology, University of Texas, El Paso, Texas

The Widening Scientist–Practitioner Gap

A View from the Bridge

CAROL TAVRIS

I was sitting in a courtroom, watching the title of this book—*Science and Pseudoscience in Clinical Psychology*—in action. A pediatric psychologist, a woman with a PhD in clinical psychology from a prestigious university, was testifying about the reasons for her sure and certain diagnosis that the defendant was a "Munchausen by proxy" mother, and that the woman's teenage son was not in fact ill with an immune disorder but rather was "in collusion" with his disturbed mother to produce his symptoms.

No one disputes that some mothers have induced physical symptoms in their children and subjected them to repeated hospitalizations; some cases have been captured on hospital video cameras. There is a term for this cruel behavior; we call it child abuse. When the child dies at the hands of an abusive parent, we have a term for that, too; we call it murder. But many clinicians suffer from syndromophilia. They have never met a behavior they can't label as a mental disorder. One case is an oddity, two is a coincidence, and three is an epidemic.

Once a syndrome is labeled, it spawns experts who are ready and willing to identify it, treat it, and train others to be ever alert for signs of it. No new disorder is "rare" to these experts; it is "mistaken" for something else or "underdiagnosed." Munchausen by proxy (MBP; factitious disorder by proxy in the appendix to DSM-IV) is the latest trendy disorder to capture clinical and media attention (Mart, 1999; see also Chapter 4). Experts all over the country are training nurses, physicians, and clinicians to be on the lookout for Munchausen mothers, and here was one of them. I watched as this clinical psychologist—I'll call her Dr. X—revealed the pseudoscientific assumptions, methods, and ways of thinking that have become common in clinical practice, as this volume will consider in depth:

• Dr. X relied on projective tests to determine that the mother had psychological problems. Quite apart from the problems of reliability and validity with these tests (see Chapter 3), no one has any idea whether real MBP mothers have any characteristic mental disorder, any more than we know whether child-abusing fathers do. Moreover, evidence of a "mental disorder" in this defendant would not reliably indicate that she *was* an MBP mother anyway.

• Dr. X knew nothing about the importance of testing clinical assumptions empirically, let alone of operationally defining her terms. What does "in collusion" mean? How does a MBP mother's behavior differ from that of any mother of a chronically sick child, or, for that matter, from that of any loving mother?

• Dr. X knew nothing about confirmation bias (see Chapter 2) or the principle of falsifiability, and how these might affect clinical diagnosis. Once she decided this mother was a "classic Munch.," as she wrote in her notes, that was that. Nothing the mother did or said could change her mind. This is because, she testified, Munchausen mothers are so deceptively charming, educated, and persuasive. Nothing the child said could change her mind. This is because, she said, he naturally wants to remain with his mother, in spite of her abusiveness. No testimony from immunologists that the child really did have an immune disorder could change her mind. This is because, she explained, Munchausen mothers force doctors to impose treatments on their children by interpreting "borderline" medical conditions as problems needing intervention.

• Dr. X understood nothing about the social psychology of diagnosis: for example, how a rare problem, such as "dissociative identity disorder" (see Chapter 5) or "Munchausen by proxy" syndrome, becomes overreported when clinicians start looking for it everywhere and are rewarded with fame, acclaim, and income when they find it (Acocella, 1999).

• Dr. X understood nothing about the problem of error rates (Mart, 1999): that in their zeal to avoid false negatives (failing to identify mothers who are harming their children), clinicians might significantly boost the rate of false positives (mistakenly labeling mothers as having MBP syndrome). "This disorder destroys families," she said, apparently without pausing to consider that mistaken diagnoses do the same.

In short, this clinical psychologist received a PhD without having acquired a core understanding of the basic principles of critical and scientific thinking. Many teachers lament the woeful lack of science education of their undergraduate students, who are expected to digest a vast assortment of facts and bits of knowledge but rarely have learned how to think about them. But this problem is also widespread in graduate clinical psychology programs and psychiatric residencies, where students can earn a PhD or an MD without ever having considered the basic epistemological assumptions and methods of their profession (see also Chapter 16): What kinds of evidence are needed before we can draw strong conclusions? Are there alternative hypotheses that I have not considered? Why are so many diagnoses of mental illness based on consensus—a group vote—rather than on empirical evidence, and what does this process reveal about problems of reliability and validity in diagnosis? An ethnographic study of the training of psychiatrists showed that psychiatric residents learn how to make quick diagnoses, prescribe medication, and, in a dwindling number of locations, do psychodynamic talk therapy, but rarely do they learn to be skeptical, ask questions, analyze research, or consider alternative explanations or treatments (Luhrmann, 2000).

I am neither an academic nor a clinician, but as a social psychologist by training and a writer by profession, I have long been interested in the influence of psychological theories on society (and in the influence of societal events on psychological theories). Because psychotherapists of all kinds are the ones who get public attention—they tend to be the ones who are writing advice columns, writing pop-psych books, going on talk shows, and testifying as experts in court cases—the public is largely ignorant of the kind of research done by psychological scientists on clinical issues or any other psychological topic. Thus, I have been especially interested in the schism between psychological science and much of clinical practice, and its implications for individuals and for the larger culture.[1]

And what a schism it has become. I have been keeping a list of the widely held beliefs, promoted by many clinicians and other psychotherapists, that have been discredited by empirical evidence. Here is just a sampling:

- Almost all abused children become abusive parents.
- Almost all children of alcoholics become alcoholic.
- Children never lie about sexual abuse.
- Childhood trauma invariably produces emotional symptoms that carry on into adulthood.
- Memory works like a tape recorder, clicking on at the moment of birth.

---

[1]Of course, there are many clinical psychologists who are also scientists, and who do both clinical work and research with equal skill; the other contributors to this volume are examples. However, the very reason for this book is that scientifically minded clinicians are becoming a rapidly dwindling minority within their profession.

- Hypnosis can reliably uncover buried memories.
- Traumatic experiences are usually repressed.
- Hypnosis reliably uncovers accurate memories.
- Subliminal messages strongly influence behavior.
- Children who masturbate or "play doctor" have probably been sexually molested.
- If left unexpressed, anger builds up like steam in a teapot until it explodes.
- Projective tests like the Rorschach validly diagnose personality disorders, most forms of psychopathology, and sexual abuse.

All of these mistaken ideas can have, and have had, devastating consequences in people's lives. In that same courtroom, I heard a social worker explain why she had decided to remove a child from her mother's custody: The mother had been abused as a child, and "we all know" that this is a major risk factor for the mother's abuse of her own child one day. Obviously no one had taught this social worker about disconfirming cases. In fact, longitudinal studies find that although being abused as a child increases the risk of becoming an abusive parent, the large majority of abused children—about two thirds—do not become abusive parents (Kaufman & Zigler, 1987).

Of course, there has always been a gap between psychological science and clinical practice. In many ways, it is no different from the natural tensions that exist between researchers and practitioners in any field—medicine, engineering, education, psychiatry, physics—when one side is doing research and the other is working in an applied domain: their goals and training are inherently quite different. The goal of psychotherapy, for example, is to help the suffering individual who is sitting there; the goal of psychological research is to explain and predict the behavior of people in general. That is why many therapists maintain that research methods and findings capture only a small, shriveled image of the real person (Edelson, 1994). Therapy, they note, was helping people long before science or psychology were invented. Professional training, therefore, should teach students how to do therapy, not how to do science.

In psychology, this divergence in goals and training was present at the conception. Empirical psychology and psychoanalysis were born of different fathers in the late 19th century, and never got along. Throughout the 20th century, they quarreled endlessly over fundamental assumptions about the meaning of science and truth. How do we know what is true? What kind of evidence is required to support a hypothesis? To early psychoanalysts, "science" had nothing to do with controlled experiments, interviews, or statistics (Hornstein, 1992). In constructing what they saw as a "science of the mind," psychoanalysts relied solely on their own interpretations of cases they saw in therapy, of myths and literature, and of people's behavior. To empirically minded psychologists, the idea that analysts could claim to be doing science while chucking out the cardinal rules of the scientific method—replicable findings, verifiable data, objective confirmation of evidence, and the concerted effort to control prejudices and any other possible sources of bias—was alarming. When psychoanalysis first became popular in the United States in the 1920s, many scientific psychologists regarded it as a popular craze, something on a par with mind reading or phrenology, which would blow over. John Watson called it "voodooism." "Psychoanalysis attempts to creep in wearing the uniform of science," wrote another critic at the time, "and to strangle it from the inside" (quoted in Hornstein, 1992). Replace *psychoanalysis* in that sentence with eye movement desensitization and reprocessing (EMDR) or thought field therapy (TFT), and the attitude is just as prevalent today among psychological scientists.

By the 1960s and 1970s, as the popularity of psychoanalysis was waning, new therapies were emerging. It was easy to tell how pseudoscientific *they* were. Unlike the Freudians, who said you needed to be in treatment for 5 years, these new guys were offering miracle therapies that promised to cure you in 5 days, 5 minutes, or 5 orgasms.

In the heyday of the countercultural revolution, these therapies multiplied like rabbits. Martin Gross's book *The Psychological Society* (1978) included marathon therapy, encounter therapy, nude therapy, crisis therapy, primal-scream therapy, electric sleep therapy, body-image therapy, deprivation therapy, expectation therapy, alpha-wave therapy, "art of living" therapy, "art of loving" therapy, and "do it now" therapy. In the 1980s, pop therapy had gone high-tech. Electrical gizmos promised to get both halves of your brain working at their peak (Chance, 1989): the Graham Potentializer, the Tranquilite, the Floatarium, the Transcutaneous Electro-Neural Stimulator, the Brain SuperCharger, and the Whole Brain Wave Form Synchro-Energizer.

At first, most psychological scientists paid as little heed to the explosion of post-Freudian pop therapies and technologies as they had to psychoanalysis. These therapies were a blot on the landscape of psychology, perhaps, but a benign nuisance; the worst thing that consumers might suffer was a loss of money and dignity.

But by the mid-1980s North America was in the midst of three social contagions, which some call hysterical epidemics or moral panics (Jenkins, 1998; Showalter, 1997): recovered-memory therapy (see Chapter 8), the daycare sex-abuse scandals, and multiple personality disorder (now officially called dissociative identity disorder in DSM-IV; see Chapter 5). All three phenomena had been fomented by the erroneous and scientifically unvalidated claims of psychotherapists, using subjective and unreliable methods. Moreover, many of the people making these claims were psychiatrists and clinical psychologists, along with social workers and generic "psychotherapists" who had taken a weekend course somewhere on child abuse. Hadn't they taken Psychology 101? Had no one taught them about control groups, memory, child development, the limitations of hypnosis?

Apparently not. Poole, Lindsay, Memon, and Bull (1995) found that large minorities of registered psychotherapists in the United States and England were using subjective, highly influential techniques such as hypnosis, dream analysis, and guided imagery related to abuse situations to "uncover" repressed memories of childhood sexual abuse. Replications of this study in the United States and Canada have found that the percentages have not declined appreciably in recent years (Katz, 2001; Nunez, Poole, & Memon, in press; Polusny & Follette, 1996; see also Chapter 8).

And when Michael Yapko (1994) surveyed nearly 1,000 members of the American Association of Marriage and Family Therapists, he found that more than half believed that "hypnosis can be used to recover memories from as far back as birth"; one third agreed that "the mind is like a computer, accurately recording events that actually occurred"; and one fourth of them—this is scary—agreed that "someone's feeling certain about a memory means the memory is likely to be correct." None of these statements is true; on the contrary, they are belied by extensive research on the normal processes of memory confabulation, distortion, and error (Brainerd, Reyna, & Brandse, 1995; Garry, Manning, & Loftus, 1996; Loftus & Ketcham, 1994; Schacter, 1996). There was no difference between MAs and PhDs in their endorsement of these items.

The recovered-memory movement showed in glaring lights how far apart empirical psychology and clinical psychology had grown. After World War II, the two sides had tried forging an alliance: The "scientist-practitioner model" would govern the training of clinical psychologists, who would draw on the most relevant findings of research psychology in diagnosing and treating clients. This harmonious ideal is still in place in a number of clinical psychology programs across the United States and Canada, where students learn research methods, the empirical findings on cognitive processes as well as on mental disorders and psychopathology, and the data on the assessment of therapeutic methods and outcomes. But like the Ten Commandments, the scientist-practitioner model has been easier to preach than to obey. The inherent tensions between the two sides grew, and by the early 1990s, researchers and clinicians were speaking openly of the "scientist–practitioner gap" (Persons, 1991).

Today, however, calling it a "gap" is like saying there is an Israeli–Arab "gap" in the Middle East. It is a war, involving deeply held beliefs, political passions, views of human nature and the nature of knowledge, and—as all wars ultimately involve—money, territory, and livelihoods. Anyone who has disputed the accuracy of recovered memories of sex abuse or who has publicly questioned any of the many popular but unvalidated therapies (e.g., EMDR, facilitated communication [FC], critical incident stress debriefing [CISD], or "rebirthing") or projective tests (e.g., the Ror-schach) knows the inflammatory nature of such criticism and the invective with which it will be received. In 1993, I wrote an essay for the *New York Times Book Review*, pointing out the scientifically unfounded, indeed of-ten preposterous, claims about memory and trauma that characterized popular books on recovered memories of incest, such as *The Courage to Heal* and *Secret Survivors*. I didn't say anything that you wouldn't learn in Psych 101, yet the *Book Review* received dozens of irate letters from psy-chiatrists, social workers, and clinical psychologists. One feminist psychia-trist accused me of writing a "malicious screed," while another clinician, representing the consensus of the letter writers, said my essay placed me "directly on the side of the molesters, rapists, pedophiles and other misogy-nists."

The current war between psychological scientists and clinicians—as opposed to the normal squabbling between researchers and practitioners that had been going on for decades—stems from several economic and cul-tural forces. One has been the rapid proliferation of psychotherapists of all kinds. Many are graduated from "freestanding" schools, unconnected to university psychology departments, where they typically learn only to do therapy—and sometimes only a vague kind of psychodynamic therapy at that. Others take brief certification courses in hypnotherapy or various counseling programs, and then promote themselves as experts in a particu-lar method. Because so many kinds of therapy are now competing in the marketplace of treatments, and because of the economic challenges posed by managed care, these specialties have become precious sources of income to many therapists. People who earn their living from giving Rorschach workshops, TFT training, setting up crisis-intervention programs, adminis-tering projective tests, or diagnosing sexual abuse are not going to be re-ceptive to evidence questioning the validity of their methods or assump-tions.

In North America today, entire industries sail under the flags of pseudoscience, and there is a cultural reason for their popularity as well as an economic one. Cross-cultural psychologists have studied how cultures differ in their need for certainty and tolerance of ambiguity, and hence, for example, whether they are willing to try to live with life's inherent uncer-tainties or pass laws to try to reduce or eliminate them (Cvetkovich & Earle, 1994; Hofstede & Bond, 1988). The United States is a culture that has a low tolerance for uncertainty; hence our attraction to "zero toler-ance" policies that fruitlessly attempt to eradicate drug abuse and to "ab-stinence only" sex-education programs that fruitlessly attempt to eradicate sex among teenagers.

In such a culture pseudoscience is particularly attractive, because pseudoscience by definition promises certainty, whereas science gives us probability and doubt. Pseudoscience is popular because it confirms what we believe; science is unpopular because it makes us question what we believe. Good science, like good art, often upsets our established ways of seeing the world. Bruce Rind and his colleagues discovered this to their dismay when they published their meta-analysis suggesting that child sexual abuse, carefully defined, does not inevitably produce severe psychopathology in adulthood (Rind, Tromovitch, & Bauserman, 1998). Did the public rise as one to praise them for this scientific "reassurance" that most people survive terrible experiences? Hardly. Instead, Congress passed a resolution condemning their research, and an odd consortium of religious conservatives and recovered-memory psychotherapists mobilized an attack on the researchers' motives, methods, and findings (Rind, Tromovitch, & Bauserman, 2000).

Longing for certainty about difficult problems, the public turns to psychologists who will give them *the* answer: Which parent should get custody? Is this rapist cured? Is this child's terrible accusation accurate? What therapy can make me better, fast? Scientists speak in the exasperating language of probability: "It is likely that. . . ." How much more appealing are the answers of clinicians who are prepared to say, with certainty: "This mother is paranoid, believing that her husband is out to get her," "This rapist is definitely cured," "Children never lie about sexual abuse," or "Thought field therapy can fix you in 5 minutes."

Pseudoscientific programs, potions, and therapies have always been an entrenched part of American culture, along with moonshine and Puritanism. The cultural mix of pragmatism, an optimistic belief that anything can be changed and improved, and impatience with anything that takes much time has created a long-standing market for instant solutions. All a clever entrepreneur has to do is apply a formula historically guaranteed to be successful: (Quick Fix + Pseudoscientific Gloss) × Credulous Public = High Income. That is why, when TFT, FC, neurolinguistic programming, and rebirthing have traveled the route of electric sleep therapy and the Transcutaneous Electro-Neural Stimulator, new miracle therapies with different acronyms will rise to take their place. It's the American way.

Pseudoscientific therapies will always remain with us, because there are so many economic and cultural interests promoting them. But their potential for harm to individuals and society is growing, which is why it is more important than ever for psychological scientists to expose their pretensions and dangers. As Richard McNally says, the best way to combat pseudoscience is to do good science. Indeed, good psychological science has already helped slow, if not yet overturn, the hysterical epidemics of our recent history that wrought so much harm. Psychological science has given us a better understanding of memory, of the processes of influence and suggestibility in therapy that create such iatrogenic disorders as "multiple personalities," and of better ways of interviewing children and assessing their accounts and memories (Poole & Lamb, 1998). Good psychological science has helped clinicians develop the most effective interventions for specific problems. Research has distinguished therapeutic techniques that are merely ineffective from those that are harmful—such as rebirthing, in which therapists in Colorado smothered a 10-year-old girl to death as they supposedly helped her to be "reborn" (see Chapter 7), and CISD programs, which can actually delay a victim's recovery from disasters and traumas (see Chapter 9, this volume).

Yet the essential difference between scientific psychology and psychotherapy will always remain, too. "In therapy, the trick is to tell stories that satisfy; in science the trick is to tell stories that predict," says Michael Nash (personal communication). "A story that is satisfying—a compelling narrative that makes our lives meaningful—need not be true in some objective sense. So therapists are right when they say that research can't help individuals learn to live with suffering, resolve moral dilemmas, or make sense of their lives. But they must be disabused of the notion that their clients' stories are literally true, or that they have no part in shaping them."

The scientist–practitioner gap, then, may not matter much in the subjective, immeasurable process of helping a client find wisdom and a story that satisfies. But it does matter in the practice of incompetent, coercive, or harmful therapy. And it matters profoundly when therapists step outside their bounds, claiming expertise and *certainty* in domains in which unverified clinical opinion can ruin lives, and where knowledge of good psychological science can save them.

REFERENCES

Acocella, J. (1999). *Creating hysteria: Women and multiple personality disorder.* San Francisco: Jossey-Bass.

Brainerd, C. J., Reyna, V. F., & Brandse, E. (1995). Are children's false memories more persistent than their true memories? *Psychological Science, 6,* 359–364.

Chance, P. (1989, November). The other 90%. *Psychology Today,* pp. 20–21.

Cvetkovich, G. T., & Earle, T. C. (1994). Risk and culture. In W. J. Lonner & R. Malpass (Eds.), *Psychology and culture* (pp. 217–224). Boston: Allyn & Bacon.

Edelson, M. (1994). Can psychotherapy research answer this psychotherapist's questions? In P. F. Talley, H. H. Strupp, & S. F. Butler (Eds.), *Psychotherapy research and practice: Bridging the gap* (pp. 60–87). New York: Basic Books.

Garry, M., Manning, C. G., & Loftus, E. F. (1996). Imagination inflation: Imagining a childhood event inflates confidence that it occurred. *Psychonomic Bulletin and Review, 3,* 208–214.

Gross, M. (1978). *The psychological society.* New York: Random House.

Hofstede, G., & Bond, M. H. (1988). The Confucius connection: From cultural roots to economic growth. *Organizational Dynamics, 18,* 5–21.

Hornstein, G. (1992). The return of the repressed: Psychology's problematic relations with psychoanalysis, 1909–1960. *American Psychologist, 47,* 254–263.

Jenkins, P. (1998). *Moral panic: Changing concepts of the child molester in modern America*. New Haven, CT: Yale University Press.

Katz, Z. (2001). Canadian psychologists' education, trauma history, and the recovery of memories of childhood sexual abuse (Doctoral dissertation, Simon Fraser University, 2001). *Dissertations Abstracts International, 61*, 3848.

Kaufman, J., & Zigler, E. (1987). Do abused children become abusive parents? *American Journal of Orthopsychiatry, 57*, 186–192.

Loftus, E. F., & Ketcham, K. (1994). *The myth of repressed memory*. New York: St. Martin's Press.

Luhrmann, T. M. (2000). *Of two minds: The growing disorder in American psychiatry*. New York: Knopf.

Mart, E. (1999). Problems with the diagnosis of factitious disorder by proxy in forensic settings. *American Journal of Forensic Psychology, 17*, 69–82.

Nunez, N., Poole, D. A., & Memon, A. (in press). Psychology's two cultures revisited: Implications for the integration of science with practice. *Scientific Review of Mental Health Practice*.

Persons, J. B. (1991). Psychotherapy outcome studies do not accurately represent current models of psychotherapy: A proposed remedy. *American Psychologist, 46*, 99–106.

Polusny, M. A., & Follette, V. M. (1996). Remembering childhood sexual abuse: A national survey of psychologists' clinical practices, beliefs, and personal experiences. *Professional Psychology: Research and Practice, 27*, 41–52.

Poole, D. A., & Lamb, M. E. (1998). *Investigative interviews of children*. Washington, DC: American Psychological Association.

Poole, D. A., Lindsay, D. S., Memon, A., & Bull, R. (1995). Psychotherapy and the recovery of memories of childhood sexual abuse: U.S. and British practitioners' opinions, practices, and experiences. *Journal of Consulting and Clinical Psychology, 63*, 426–437.

Rind, B., Tromovitch, P., & Bauserman, R. (1998). A meta-analytic examination of assumed properties of child sexual abuse using college samples. *Psychological Bulletin, 124*, 22–53.

Rind, B., Tromovitch, P., & Bauserman, R. (2000). Condemnation of a scientific article: A chronology and refutation of the attacks and a discussion of threats to the integrity of science. *Sexuality and Culture, 4*, 1–62.

Schacter, D. L. (1996). *Searching for memory: The brain, the mind, and the past*. New York: Basic Books.

Showalter, E. (1997). *Hystories: Hysterical epidemics and modern culture*. New York: Columbia University Press.

Tavris, C. (1993, January 3). Beware the incest-survivor machine. *The New York Times Book Review*, pp. 1, 16–18.

Yapko, M. (1994). *Suggestions of abuse: True and false memories of childhood sexual trauma*. New York: Simon & Schuster.

Preface

This book is likely to make a number of readers angry. Some readers will probably object to portions of the book on the grounds that their cherished clinical techniques or brands of psychotherapy have been targeted for critical examination. For them, this book may be a bitter pill to swallow. Other readers will probably be deeply disturbed, even incensed, by the growing proliferation of questionable and unvalidated techniques in clinical psychology. For them, this will be a book that is long overdue. If we manage to leave readers in both camps at least a bit distressed, we will have been successful, because we will have gotten their attention.

Our purpose in this edited volume is to subject a variety of therapeutic, assessment, and diagnostic techniques in clinical psychology to incisive but impartial scientific scrutiny. We have elected to focus on techniques that are novel, controversial, or even questionable, but that are currently influential and widely used. By providing thoughtful evaluations of clinical techniques on the boundaries of present scientific knowledge, we intend to assist readers with the crucial goal of distinguishing science from pseudoscience in mental health practice.

As will become clear throughout the book, unscientific and otherwise questionable techniques have increasingly come to dominate the landscape of clinical psychology and allied fields. Survey data suggest that for many psychological conditions, including mood and anxiety disorders, patients are more likely to seek out and receive scientifically unsupported than supported interventions. Yet no book exists to help readers differentiate techniques within clinical psychology that are ineffective, undemonstrated, or harmful from those that are grounded solidly in scientific evidence.

This book is the first major volume devoted exclusively to distinguishing scientifically unsupported from scientifically supported practices in modern clinical psychology. Many readers may find this fact surprising. Nevertheless, as we point out later in the book (Chapter 16), the field of clinical psychology has traditionally been reluctant to subject novel and controversial methods to careful scientific evaluation. This reluctance has left a major gap, and to a substantial extent our book will fill it.

We have urged the authors of each chapter to be as objective and dispassionate as possible. In addition, we have encouraged them to be not only appropriately critical when necessary, but constructive. To this end, each chapter features both a discussion of which clinical techniques are ineffective, unvalidated, or undemonstrated, and also a discussion of which techniques are empirically supported or promising. Our mission is not merely to debunk—although in certain cases debunking is a needed activity in science—but to enlighten. Not all methods that are novel or superficially implausible are necessarily worthless or ineffective. Reflexive dismissal of the new and untested is as ill advised as is blind acceptance. We have tried to ensure that our authors avoid both errors.

This book should be of considerable interest to several audiences: (1) practicing clinicians across the spectrum of mental health professions, including clinical psychology, psychiatry, social work, counseling, and psychiatric nursing; (2) academicians and researchers whose work focuses on psychopathology and its diagnosis and treatment; (3) current and would-be consumers of mental health treatment techniques; (4) educated laypersons interested in mental illness; and (5) graduate students and advanced undergraduates wishing to learn more about the science and pseudoscience of clinical psychology. With respect to the latter group, this book is suitable as either a primary or supplemental text for graduate and advanced undergraduate courses in clinical psychology, psychotherapy, and assessment. In addition, this book should be of interest to lawyers, educators, physicians, nurses, and others whose work bears on clinical psychology and allied mental health disciplines.

Although many of the chapters deal with conceptually and methodologically challenging issues, we have tried to keep technical language to a minimum. In addition, each of the major chapters of the book contains a glossary of key concepts and terms that should prove useful to readers unfamiliar with each major content area.

We are grateful to a number of individuals who have helped to bring this book to fruition. In particular, we thank Jim Nageotte and Kitty Moore at The Guilford Press, whose advice, assistance, and moral support throughout the project have been invaluable. We also thank Richard McNally, David Tolin, James Herbert, Jerry Davison, Jerry Rosen, Richard Gist, Grant Devilly, Robert Montgomery, John W. Bush, Liz Roemer, Ron Kleinknecht, Carol Tavris, and a host of other colleagues and friends whose ideas have helped to inform and shape this book. Finally, we thank our spouses, Lori, Fern, and Mary Beth, for their support, patience, and forbearance—which at times bordered on the irrational—throughout the writing and production of this book. We dedicate this book to them.

SCOTT O. LILIENFELD
STEVEN JAY LYNN
JEFFREY M. LOHR

Contents

Science and Pseudoscience in Clinical Psychology

Initial Thoughts, Reflections, and Considerations

SCOTT O. LILIENFELD
STEVEN JAY LYNN
JEFFREY M. LOHR

As Bob Dylan wrote, "The times they are a-changin'." Over the past several decades, clinical psychology and allied disciplines (e.g., psychiatry, social work, counseling) have borne witness to a virtual sea-change in the relation between science and practice. A growing minority of clinicians appear to be basing their therapeutic and assessment practices primarily on clinical experience and intuition rather than on research evidence. As a consequence, the term "scientist–practitioner gap" is being invoked with heightened frequency (see foreword to this volume by Carol Tavris; Fox, 1996), and concerns that the scientific foundations of clinical psychology are steadily eroding are being voiced increasingly in many quarters (Dawes, 1994; Kalal, 1999; McFall, 1991). It is largely these concerns that have prompted us to compile this edited volume, which features chapters by distinguished experts across a broad spectrum of areas within clinical psychology. Given the markedly changing landscape of clinical psychology, we believe this book to be both timely and important.

Some might contend that the problem of unsubstantiated treatment techniques is not new and has in fact dogged the field of clinical psychology virtually since its inception. To a certain extent, they would be correct. Nevertheless, the growing availability of information resources (some of which have also become misinformation resources), including popular psychology books and the Internet, the dramatic upsurge in the number of mental health training programs that do not emphasize scientific training (Beyerstein, 2001), and the burgeoning industry of fringe psychotherapies, have magnified the gulf between scientist and practitioner to a problem of critical proportions.

THE SCIENTIST–PRACTITIONER GAP AND ITS SOURCES

What are the primary sources of the growing scientist–practitioner gap? As many authors have noted (see Lilienfeld, 1998, 2001, for a discussion), some practitioners in clinical psychology and related mental health disciplines appear to making increased use of unsubstantiated, untested, and otherwise questionable treatment and assessment methods. Moreover, psychotherapeutic methods of unknown or doubtful validity are proliferating on an almost weekly basis. For example, a recent and highly selective sampling of fringe psychotherapeutic practices (Eisner, 2000; see also Singer & Lalich, 1996) included neurolinguistic programming, eye movement desensitization and reprocessing, Thought Field Therapy, Emotional Freedom Technique, rage reduction therapy, primal scream therapy, feeling therapy, Buddha psychotherapy, past lives therapy, future lives therapy, alien abduction therapy, angel therapy, rebirthing, Sedona method, Silva method, entity depossession therapy, vegetotherapy, palm therapy, and a plethora of other methods (see also Chapter 7).

Moreover, a great deal of academic and media coverage of such fringe treatments is accompanied by scant critical evaluation. For example, a recent edited volume (Shannon, 2002) features 23 chapters on largely unsubstantiated psychological techniques, including music therapy, homeopathy, breath work, therapeutic touch, aromatherapy, medical intuition, acupuncture, and body-centered psychotherapies. Nevertheless, in most chapters these techniques receive minimal scientific scrutiny (see Corsini, 2001, for a similar example).

Additional threats to the scientific foundations of clinical psychology and allied fields stem from the thriving self-help industry. This industry produces hundreds of new books, manuals, and audiotapes each year (see Chapter 14), many of which promise rapid or straightforward solutions to complex life problems. Although some of these self-help materials may be efficacious, the overwhelming majority of them have never been subjected to empirical scrutiny. In addition, an ever-increasing contingent of self-help "gurus" on television and radio talk shows routinely offer advice of questionable scientific validity to a receptive, but often vulnerable, audience of troubled individuals (see Chapter 15).

Similarly questionable practices can be found in the domains of psychological assessment and diagnosis. Despite well-replicated evidence that statistical (actuarial) formulas are superior to clinical judgment for a broad range of judgmental and predictive tasks (Grove, Zald, Lebow, Snitz, & Nelson, 2000), most clinicians continue to rely on clinical judgment even in cases in which it has been shown to be ill advised. There is also evidence that many practitioners tend to be overconfident in their judgments and predictions, and to fall prey to basic errors in reasoning (e.g., confirmatory bias, illusory correlation) in the process of case formulation (Chapter 2). Moreover, many practitioners base their interpretations on assessment instruments (e.g., human figure drawing tests, Rorschach Inkblot Test, Myers–Briggs Type Indicator, anatomically detailed dolls) that are either highly controversial or questionable from a scientific standpoint (see Chapter 3).

Still other clinicians render confident diagnoses of psychiatric conditions, such as dissociative identity disorder (known formerly as multiple personality disorder), whose validity remains in dispute (see Chapter 5, but see also Gleaves, May, & Cardena, 2001, for a different perspective). The problem of questionable diagnostic labels is especially acute in courtroom settings, where psychiatric labels of unknown or doubtful validity (e.g., road rage syndrome, sexual addiction, premenstrual dysphoric disorder) are sometimes invoked as exculpatory defenses (see Chapter 4).

STRIKING A BALANCE BETWEEN EXCESSIVE OPEN-MINDEDNESS AND EXCESSIVE SKEPTICISM

It is critical to emphasize that at least some of the largely or entirely untested psychotherapeutic, assessment, and diagnostic methods reviewed in this volume may ultimately prove to be efficacious or valid. It would be a serious error to dismiss any untested techniques out of hand or antecedent to prior critical scrutiny. Such closed-mindedness has sometimes characterized debates concerning the efficacy of novel psychotherapies (Beutler & Harwood, 2001). Nevertheless, a basic tenet of science is that the burden of proof always falls squarely on the claimant, not the critic (see Shermer, 1997). Consequently, it is up to the proponents of these techniques to demonstrate that they work, not up to the critics of these techniques to demonstrate the converse.

As Carl Sagan (1995b) eloquently pointed out, scientific inquiry demands a unique mix of open-mindedness and penetrating skepticism (see also Shermer, 2001). We must remain open to novel and untested claims, regardless of how superficially implausible they might appear at first blush.

At the same time, we must subject these claims to incisive scrutiny to ensure that they withstand the crucible of rigorous scientific testing. As space scientist James Oberg observed, keeping an open mind is a virtue but this mind cannot be so open that one's brains fall out (Sagan, 1995a; see also Chapter 9). Although the requirement to hold all claims to high levels of critical scrutiny applies to all domains of science, such scrutiny is especially crucial in applied areas, such as clinical psychology, in which erroneous claims or ineffective practices have the potential to produce harm.

WHY POTENTIALLY PSEUDOSCIENTIFIC TECHNIQUES CAN BE HARMFUL

Some might respond to our arguments by contending that although many of the techniques reviewed in this book are either untested or ineffective, most are likely to prove either efficacious or innocuous. From this perspective, our emphasis on the dangers posed by such techniques is misplaced, because unresearched mental health practices are at worst inert.

Nevertheless, this counterargument overlooks several important considerations. Specifically, there are at least three major ways in which unsubstantiated mental health techniques can be problematic (Lilienfeld, 2002; see also Beyerstein, 2001). First, some of these techniques may be harmful per se. The tragic case of Candace Newmaker, the 10-year-old Colorado girl who was smothered to death in 2000 by therapists practicing a variant of rebirthing therapy (see Chapter 7), attests to the dangers of implementing untested therapeutic techniques (see Mercer, in press). There is also increasing reason to suspect that certain suggestive techniques (e.g., hypnosis, guided imagery) for unearthing purportedly repressed memories of childhood trauma may exacerbate or even produce psychopathology by inadvertently implanting false memories of past events (see Chapters 7 and 8). Even the use of facilitated communication for infantile autism (see Chapter 13) has resulted in erroneous accusations of child abuse against family members. Moreover, there is accumulating evidence that certain widely used treatment techniques, such as critical incident stress debriefing (see Chapter 9), peer group interventions for adolescents with conduct disorders (Dishion, McCord, & Poulin, 1999), and certain self-help programs (Rosen, 1987; see Chapter 14) can be harmful. Consequently, the oft-held assumption that "doing something is always better than doing nothing" in the domain of psychotherapy is likely to be mistaken. As psychologist Richard Gist reminds us, doing something is not license to do anything.

Second, even psychotherapies that are by themselves innocuous can indirectly produce harm by depriving individuals of scarce time, financial resources, or both. Economists refer to this side effect as "opportunity cost." As a consequence of opportunity cost, individuals who would otherwise use their time and money to seek out demonstrably efficacious treatments may be left with precious little of either. Such individuals may therefore be less likely to obtain interventions that could prove beneficial.

Third, the use of unsubstantiated techniques eats away at the scientific foundations of the profession of clinical psychology (Lilienfeld, 1998; McFall, 1991). As one of us (Lilienfeld, 2002) recently observed:

> Once we abdicate our responsibility to uphold high scientific standards in administering treatments, our scientific credibility and influence are badly damaged. Moreover, by continuing to ignore the imminent dangers posed by questionable mental health techniques, we send an implicit message to our students that we are not deeply committed to anchoring our discipline in scientific evidence or to combating potentially unscientific practices. Our students will most likely follow in our footsteps and continue to turn a blind eye to the widening gap between scientist and practitioner, and between research evidence and clinical work. (p. 9)

In addition, the promulgation of treatment and assessment techniques of questionable validity can undermine the general public's faith in the profession of clinical psychology, and lead citizens to place less trust in the assertions of clinical researchers and practitioners.

THE DIFFERENCES BETWEEN SCIENCE AND PSEUDOSCIENCE: A PRIMER

One of the major goals of this book is to distinguish scientific from pseudoscientific claims in clinical psychology. To accomplish this goal, however, we must first delineate the principal differences between scientific and pseudoscientific research programs. As one of us has noted elsewhere (Lilienfeld, 1998), science probably differs from pseudoscience in degree rather than in kind. Science and pseudoscience can be thought of as Roschian (Rosch, 1973) or open (Meehl & Golden, 1982; Pap, 1953) concepts, which possess intrinsically fuzzy boundaries and an indefinitely extendable list of indicators. Nevertheless, the fuzziness of such categories does not mean that distinctions between science and pseudoscience are fictional or entirely arbitrary. As psychophysicist S. S. Stevens observed, the fact that the precise boundary between day and night is indistinct does not imply that day and night cannot be meaningfully differentiated (see Leahey & Leahey, 1983). From this perspective, pseudosciences can be conceptualized as possessing a fallible, but nevertheless useful, list of indicators or "warning signs." The more such warning signs a discipline exhibits, the more it begins to cross the murky dividing line separating science from pseudoscience (see also Herbert et al., 2000). A number of philosophers of science (e.g., Bunge, 1984) and psychologists (e.g., Ruscio, 2001) have outlined some of the most frequent features of pseudoscience. Among these features are the following (for further discussions, see Herbert et al., 2000; Hines, 1988; Lilienfeld, 1998):

1. *An overuse of ad hoc hypotheses designed to immunize claims from falsification.* From a Popperian or neo-Popperian standpoint (see Popper, 1959) assertions that could never in principle be falsified are unscientific (but see McNally, in press, for a critique of Popperian notions). The repeated invocation of ad hoc hypotheses to explain away negative findings is a common tactic among proponents of pseudoscientific claims. Moreover, in most pseudosciences, ad hoc hypotheses are simply "pasted on" to plug holes in the theory in question. When taken to an extreme, ad hoc hypotheses can provide an impenetrable barrier against potential refutation. For example, some proponents of eye movement desensitization and reprocessing (EMDR) have argued that negative findings concerning EMDR are almost certainly attributable to low levels of fidelity to the treatment procedure (see Chapter 9). But they have typically been inconsistent in their application of the treatment fidelity concept (Rosen, 1999).

It is crucial to emphasize that the invocation of ad hoc hypotheses in the face of negative evidence is sometimes a legitimate strategy in science. In scientific research programs, however, such maneuvers tend to enhance the theory's content, predictive power, or both (see Lakatos, 1978).

2. *Absence of self-correction.* Scientific research programs are not necessarily distinguished from pseudoscientific research programs in the verisimilitude of their claims, because proponents of both programs frequently advance incorrect assertions. Nevertheless, in the long run most scientific research programs tend to eliminate these errors, whereas most pseudoscientific research programs do not. Consequently, intellectual stagnation is a hallmark of most pseudoscientific research programs (Ruscio, 2001). For example, astrology has changed remarkably little in the past 2,500 years (Hines, 1988).

3. *Evasion of peer review.* On a related note, many proponents of pseudoscience avoid subjecting their work to the often ego-bruising process of peer review (Ruscio, 2001; see also Gardner, 1957, for illustrations). In some cases, they may do so on the grounds that the peer review process is inherently biased against findings or claims that contradict well-established paradigms (e.g., see Callahan, 2001a, for an illustration involving Thought Field Therapy; see also Chapter 9). In other cases, they may avoid the peer review process on the grounds that their assertions cannot be evaluated adequately using standard scientific methods. Although the peer review process is far from flawless (see Peters & Ceci, 1982, for a striking example), it remains the best mechanism for self-correction in sci-

ence, and assists investigators in identifying errors in their reasoning, methodology, and analyses. By remaining largely insulated from the peer review process, some proponents of pseudoscience forfeit an invaluable opportunity to obtain corrective feedback from informed colleagues.

4. *Emphasis on confirmation rather refutation.* The brilliant physicist Richard Feynman (1985) maintained that the essence of science is a bending over backwards to prove oneself wrong. Bartley (1962) similarly maintained that science at its best involves the maximization of constructive criticism. Ideally, scientists subject their cherished claims to grave risk of refutation (Meehl, 1978; see also Ruscio, 2001). In contrast, pseudoscientists tend to seek only confirming evidence for their claims. Because a determined advocate can find at least some supportive evidence for virtually any claim (Popper, 1959), this confirmatory hypothesis-testing strategy is not an efficient means of rooting out error in one's web of beliefs.

Moreover, as Bunge (1967) observed, most pseudosciences manage to reinterpret negative or anomalous findings as corroborations of their claims (see Herbert et al., 2000). For example, proponents of extrasensory perception (ESP) have sometimes interpreted isolated cases of worse than chance performance on parapsychological tasks (known as "psi missing") as evidence of ESP (Gilovich, 1991; Hines, 1988).

5. *Reversed burden of proof.* As noted earlier, the burden of proof in science rests invariably on the individual making a claim, not on the critic. Proponents of pseudoscience frequently neglect this principle and instead demand that skeptics demonstrate beyond a reasonable doubt that a claim (e.g., an assertion regarding the efficacy of a novel therapeutic technique) is false. This error is similar to the logician's ad ignorantium fallacy (i.e., the argument from ignorance), the mistake of assuming that a claim is likely to be correct merely because there is no compelling evidence against it (Shermer, 1997). For example, some proponents of unidentified flying objects (UFOs) have insisted that skeptics account for every unexplained report of an anomalous event in the sky (Hines, 1988; Sagan, 1995a). But because it is essentially impossible to prove a universal negative, this tactic incorrectly places the burden of proof on the skeptic rather than the claimant.

6. *Absence of connectivity.* In contrast to most scientific research programs, pseudoscientific research programs tend to lack "connectivity" with other scientific disciplines (Bunge, 1983; Stanovich, 2001). In other words, pseudosciences often purport to create entirely new paradigms out of whole cloth rather than to build on extant paradigms. In so doing, they often neglect well-established scientific principles or hard-won scientific knowledge. For example, many proponents of ESP argue that it is a genuine (although heretofore undetected) physical process of perception, even though reported cases of ESP violate almost every major law of physical signals (e.g., ESP purportedly operates just as strongly from thousands of

miles away as it does from a few feet away). Although scientists should always remain open to the possibility that an entirely novel paradigm has successfully overturned all preexisting paradigms, they must insist on very high standards of evidence before drawing such a conclusion.

7. *Overreliance on testimonial and anecdotal evidence.* Testimonial and anecdotal evidence can be quite useful in the early stages of scientific investigation. Nevertheless, such evidence is typically much more helpful in the context of discovery (i.e., hypothesis generation) than in the context of justification (i.e., hypothesis testing; see Reichenbach, 1938). Proponents of pseudoscientific claims frequently invoke reports from selected cases (e.g., "This treatment clearly worked for Person X, because Person X improved markedly following the treatment") as a means of furnishing dispositive evidence for these claims. For example, proponents of certain treatments (e.g., secretin) for autistic disorder (see Chapter 13) have often pointed to uncontrolled case reports of improvement as supportive evidence.

As Gilovich (1991) observed, however, case reports almost never provide sufficient evidence for a claim, although they often provide necessary evidence for this claim. For example, if a new form of psychotherapy is efficacious, one should certainly expect at least some positive case reports of improvement. But such case reports do not provide adequate evidence that the improvement was attributable to the psychotherapy, because this improvement could have been produced by a host of other influences (e.g., placebo effects, regression to the mean, spontaneous remission, maturation; see Cook & Campbell, 1979).

8. *Use of obscurantist language.* Many proponents of pseudoscience use impressive sounding or highly technical jargon in an effort to provide their disciplines with the superficial trappings of science (see van Rillaer, 1991, for a discussion of "strategies of dissimulation" in pseudoscience). Such language may be convincing to individuals unfamiliar with the scientific underpinnings of the claims in question, and may therefore lend these claims an unwarranted imprimatur of scientific legitimacy.

For example, the developer of EMDR explained the efficacy of this treatment as follows (see also Chapter 9):

> [The] valences of the neural receptors (synaptic potential) of the respective neuro networks, which separately store various information plateaus and levels of adaptive information, are represented by the letters Z through A. It is hypothesized that the high-valence target network (Z) cannot link up with the more adaptive information, which is stored in networks with a lower valence. That is, the synaptic potential is different for each level of affect held in the various neuro networks. . . . The theory is that when the processing system is catalyzed in EMDR, the valence of the receptors is shifted downward so that they are capable of linking with the receptors of

the neuro networks with progressively lower valences. . . . (Shapiro, 1995, pp. 317–318)

9. *Absence of boundary conditions.* Most well-supported scientific theories possess boundary conditions, that is, well-articulated limits under which predicted phenomena do and do not apply. In contrast, many or most pseudoscientific phenomena are purported to operate across an exceedingly wide range of conditions. As Hines (1988, 2001) noted, one frequent characteristic of fringe psychotherapies is that they are ostensibly efficacious for almost all disorders regardless of their etiology. For example, some proponents of Thought Field Therapy (see Chapter 9) have proposed that this treatment is beneficial for virtually all mental disorders. Moreover, the developer of this treatment has posited that it is efficacious not only for adults but for "horses, dogs, cats, infants, and very young children" (Callahan, 2001b, p. 1255).

10. *The mantra of holism.* Proponents of pseudoscientific claims, especially in organic medicine and mental health, often resort to the "mantra of holism" (Ruscio, 2001) to explain away negative findings. When invoking this mantra, they typically maintain that scientific claims can be evaluated only within the context of broader claims and therefore cannot be judged in isolation. For example, some proponents of the Rorschach Inkblot Test have responded to criticisms of this technique (see Chapter 3) by asserting that clinicians virtually never interpret results from a Rorschach in isolation. Instead, in actual practice clinicians consider numerous pieces of information, only one of which may be a Rorschach protocol. There are two major difficulties with this line of reasoning. First, it implies that clinicians can effectively integrate in their heads a great deal of complex psychometric information from diverse sources, a claim that is doubtful given the research literature on clinical judgment (see Chapter 2). Second, by invoking the mantra of holism, proponents of the Rorschach and other techniques can readily avoid subjecting their claims to the risk of falsification. In other words, if research findings corroborate the validity of a specific Rorschach index, Rorschach proponents can point to these findings as supportive evidence, but if these findings are negative, Rorschach proponents can explain them away by maintaining that "clinicians never interpret this index in isolation anyway" (see Merlo & Barnett, 2001, for an example). This "heads I win, tails you lose" reasoning places the claims of these proponents largely outside of the boundaries of science.

We encourage readers to bear in mind the aforementioned list of pseudoscience indicators (see Ruscio, 2001, for other useful indicators) when evaluating the claims presented in this volume. At the same time, we remind readers that these indicators are only probabilistically linked to pseudoscientific research programs. Scientists, even those who are well trained, are not immune from such practices. In scientific research programs, however, such practices tend to be weeded out eventually through the slow but steady process of self-correction. In contrast to sciences, in which erroneous claims tend to be gradually ferreted out by a process akin to natural selection (e.g., see Campbell's [1974] discussion of evolutionary epistemology), pseudosciences tend to remain stagnant in the face of contradictory evidence.

CONSTRUCTIVE EFFORTS TO ADDRESS THE PROBLEM

Until fairly recently the field of clinical psychology has shown relatively little interest in addressing the threats posed by pseudoscientific or otherwise questionable practices. Paul Meehl (1993), perhaps the foremost clinical psychologist of the latter half of the 20th century, observes,

> It is absurd, as well as arrogant, to pretend that acquiring a Ph.D. somehow immunizes me from the errors of sampling, perception, recording, retention, retrieval, and inference to which the human mind is suspect. In earlier times, all introductory psychology courses devoted a lecture or two to the classic studies in the psychology of testimony, and one mark of a psychologist was hard-nosed skepticism about folk beliefs. It seems that quite a few clinical psychologists never got exposed to this basic feature of critical thinking. My teachers at [the University of] Minnesota . . . shared what Bertrand Russell called the dominant passion of the true scientist—the passion not to be fooled and not to fool anybody else . . . all of them asked the two searching questions of positivism: "What do you mean?" "How do you know?" If we clinicians lose that passion and forget those questions, we are little more than be-doctored, well-paid soothsayers. I see disturbing signs that this is happening and I predict that, if we do not clean up our clinical act and provide our students with role models of scientific thinking, outsiders will do it for us. (pp. 728–729)

Nevertheless, the past decade has witnessed a number of constructive efforts to address the problems posed by questionable and potentially pseudoscientific methods in clinical psychology. Two of these efforts have originated within the American Psychological Association (APA), an organization that has been chastised for turning a blind eye to the festering problem of pseudoscience within clinical psychology (Lilienfeld, 1998). First, Division 12 of the APA has advanced a set of criteria for empirically supported treatments (ESTs) for adult and childhood disorders, along with provisional lists of therapeutic techniques that satisfy these criteria (see Chambless & Ollendick, 2001, for a thoughtful review). Vigorous and healthy debate surrounds the criteria established for identifying ESTs as well as the current list of ESTs (Herbert, 2000; see also Chapter 6 for a critique of the current status of ESTs). Despite this controversy, it seems clear that the increasing push toward ESTs reflects a heightened emphasis on distinguishing interventions that are scientifically supported from those whose support is negligible or nonexistent. Second, there is suggestive evidence that certain APA committees have begun to move in the direction of addressing the threats posed by unsubstantiated psychotherapies. For example, several years ago, the APA Continuing Education (CE) Committee turned down workshops on Thought Field Therapy for CE credit on the grounds that the scientific evidence for this treatment was not sufficiently compelling (or even suggestive) to warrant its dissemination to practitioners (Lilienfeld & Lohr, 2000; see also Chapters 7 and 9).

In addition, the Committee for the Scientific Investigation of Claims of the Paranormal recently established a new subcommittee dedicated to evaluating the validity of questionable or untested mental health claims. Finally, Prometheus Books recently launched an interdisciplinary journal, *The Scientific Review of Mental Health Practice*, which is devoted to distinguishing scientifically supported from scientifically unsupported claims in clinical psychology, psychiatry, social work, and allied disciplines. These and other recent developments (see Lilienfeld, 2002) suggest that careful attention is at long last being accorded to questionable and potentially pseudoscientific practices in clinical psychology and to distinguishing them from practices with stronger evidentiary support. We hope that readers will find this edited volume to represent another constructive step in this direction.

THE GOALS OF THIS VOLUME

With the aforementioned considerations in mind, the primary goal of this edited volume is to assist readers—whom we hope will include clinical researchers, practicing psychologists, psychiatrists, social workers, counselors, and psychiatric nurses, graduate students in clinical psychology and allied disciplines (e.g., social work, counseling), medical students, lawyers, educators, and educated laypersons—with the important task of distinguishing techniques in clinical psychology that are scientifically supported or promising from those that are scientifically unsupported or untested. To assist readers with this task, we have asked the authors of each chapter to delineate not only which techniques and claims are devoid of empirical support, but also which are either empirically supported or promising. In this way, we expect readers to emerge with an enhanced understanding and appreciation of the differences between mental health techniques that are and are not grounded in solid scientific evidence. In addition, as noted earlier, we intend to assist readers with the task of identifying research programs in clinical psychology that embody many of the features of pseudoscience and to distinguish them from research programs that exemplify the core features of scientific epistemology (e.g., self-correction).

We have organized this volume into five major sections. First, we begin with an examination of questionable or untested practices and assumptions in the domains of psychological assessment and diagnosis. Second, we examine general controversies in psychotherapy that cut across multiple psychological disorders. Third, we turn to largely untested or unsubstantiated treatment techniques (both psychotherapeutic and psychopharmacological) for various adult psychological conditions, including posttraumatic stress disorder, alcoholism, and depression. Fourth, we examine similarly untested and unsubstantiated treatments for childhood disorders, with a particular focus on attention-deficit/hyperactivity disorder and infantile autism. Fifth, we examine the modern self-help movement in its various incarnations. We conclude the volume with a brief set of constructive remedies for narrowing the gap between scientist and practitioner.

By concluding this volume on a relatively optimistic note, we intend to leave readers with the impression that the problem of pseudoscience in contemporary clinical psychology, although formidable in severity and scope, may not be intractable. If our sanguine assessment is correct, a future generation of clinical psychologists may perceive this volume as a mere historical curiosity, a legacy of a bygone era when clinical practices were often unsubstantiated and not routinely grounded in the best available scientific evidence. Nothing would please us more.

REFERENCES

Bartley, W. W. (1962). *The retreat to commitment*. New York: Knopf.

Beutler, L. E., & Harwood, T. M. (2001). Antiscientific attitudes: What happens when scientists are unscientific? *Journal of Clinical Psychology, 57*, 43–51.

Beyerstein, B. L. (2001). Fringe psychotherapies: The public at risk. *The Scientific Review of Alternative Medicine, 5*, 70–79.

Bunge, M. (1967). *Scientific research*. New York: Springer.

Bunge, M. (1983). Speculation: Wild and sound. *New Ideas in Psychology, 1*, 3–6.

Bunge, M. (1984, Fall). What is pseudoscience? *Skeptical Inquirer, 9*, 36–46.

Callahan, R. J. (2001a). The impact of Thought Field Therapy on heart rate variability. *Journal of Clinical Psychology, 57*, 1154–1170.

Callahan, R. J. (2001b). Thought Field Therapy: Response to our critics and a scrutiny of some old ideas of science. *Journal of Clinical Psychology, 57*, 1251–1260.

Campbell, D. T. (1974). Evolutionary epistemology. In P. A. Schilpp (Ed.), *The philosophy of Karl R. Popper* (pp. 412–463). LaSalle, IL: Open Court.

Chambless, D. L., & Ollendick, T. H. (2001). Empirically supported psychological interventions: Controversies and evidence. *Annual Review of Psychology, 52*, 685–716.

Cook, T. D., & Campbell, D. T. (1979). *Quasi-experimentation: Design and analysis issues for field settings*. Boston: Houghton Mifflin.

Corsini, R. J. (Ed.). (2001). *Handbook of innovative therapy* (2nd ed.). New York: Wiley.

Dawes, R. M. (1994). *House of cards: Psychology and psychotherapy built on myth*. New York: Free Press.

Dishion, T., McCord, J., & Poulin, F (1999). When interventions harm: Peer groups and problem behavior. *American Psychologist, 54*, 755–764.

Eisner, D. A. (2000). *The death of psychotherapy: From Freud to alien abductions*. Westport, CT: Praeger.

Feynman, R. P. (with R. Leighton). (1985). *Surely you're joking, Mr. Feynman: Adventures of a curious character*. New York: Norton.

Fox, R. E. (1996). Charlatanism, scientism, and psychology's social contract. *American Psychologist, 51*, 777–784.

Gardner, M. (1957). *Fads and fallacies in the name of science*. New York: Dover.

Gilovich, T. (1991). *How we know what isn't so: The fallibility of human reason in everyday life*. New York: Free Press.

Gleaves, D. H., May, M. C., & Cardena, E. (2001). An examination of the diagnostic validity of dissociative identity disorder. *Clinical Psychology Review, 21*, 577–608.

Grove, W. M., Zald, D. H., Lebow, B. S., Snitz, B. E., & Nelson, C. (2000). Clinical versus mechanical prediction: A meta-analysis. *Psychological Assessment, 12*, 19–30.

Herbert, J. D. (2000). Defining empirically supported treatments: Pitfalls and possible solutions. *Behavior Therapist, 23*, 113–134.

Herbert, J. D., Lilienfeld, S. O., Lohr, J. M., Montgomery, R. W., O'Donohue, W. T, Rosen, G. M., & Tolin, D. F. (2000). Science and pseudoscience in the development of eye movement desensitization and reprocessing. *Clinical Psychology Review, 20*, 945–971.

Hines, T. (1988). *Pseudoscience and the paranormal: A critical examination of the evidence*. Buffalo, NY: Prometheus Books.

Hines, T. M. (2001). The Doman–Delcato patterning treatment for brain damage. *Scientific Review of Alternative Medicine, 5*, 80–89.

Kalal, D. M. (1990, April). Critical thinking in clinical practice: Pseudoscience, fad psychology, and the behavior therapist. *The Behavior Therapist*, 81–84.

Lakatos, I. (1978). *Philosophical papers: Vol. 1. The methodology of scientific research programmes* (J. Worrall & G. Currie, Eds.). New York: Cambridge University Press.

Leahey, T. H., & Leahey, G. E. (1983). *Psychology's occult doubles: Psychology and the problem of pseudoscience*. Chicago: Nelson–Hall.

Lilienfeld, S. O. (1998). Pseudoscience in contemporary clinical psychology: What it is and what we can do about it. *Clinical Psychologist, 51*, 3–9.

Lilienfeld, S. O. (2001, August 25). *Fringe psychotherapies: Scientific and ethical implications for clinical psychology*. Paper presented at the Annual Meeting of the American Psychological Association, San Francisco.

Lilienfeld, S. O. (2002). The Scientific Review of Mental Health Practice: Our raison d'être. *Scientific Review of Mental Health Practice, 1*, 5–10.

Lilienfeld, S. O., & Lohr, J. M. (2000). News and comment: Thought Field Therapy educators and practitioners sanctioned. *Skeptical Inquirer, 24*, 5.

McFall, R. M. (1991). Manifesto for a science of clinical psychology. *Clinical Psychologist, 44*, 75–88.

McNally, R. J. (in press). The demise of pseudoscience. *Scientific Review of Mental Health Practice*.

Meehl, P. E. (1978). Theoretical risks or tabular asterisks: Sir Karl, Sir Ronald, and the slow progress of soft psychology. *Journal of Consulting and Clinical Psychology, 46*, 816–834.

Meehl, P. E. (1993). Philosophy of science: Help or hindrance? *Psychological Reports, 72*, 707–733.

Meehl, P. E., & Golden, R. R. (1982). Taxometric methods. In P. C. Kendall & J. N. Butcher (Eds.), *Handbook of research methods in clinical psychology* (pp. 127–181). New York: Wiley.

Mercer, J. (in press). Attachment therapy: A treatment without empirical support. *Scientific Review of Mental Health Practice*.

Merlo, L., & Barnett, D. (2001, September). All about inkblots. *Scientific American, 285*, 13.

Pap, A. (1953). Reduction sentences and open concepts. *Methodos, 5*, 3–30.

Peters, D. P., & Ceci, S. J. (1982). Peer-review practices of psychological journals: The fate of published articles, submitted again. *Behavioral and Brain Sciences, 5*, 187–255.

Popper, K. R. (1959). *The logic of scientific discovery.* New York: Basic Books.

Reichenbach, H. (1938). *Experience and prediction.* Chicago: University of Illinois Press.

Rosch, E. (1973). Natural categories. *Cognitive Psychology, 4*, 328–350.

Rosen, G. M. (1987). Self-help treatment books and the commercialization of psychotherapy. *American Psychologist, 42*, 46–51.

Rosen, G. M. (1999). Treatment fidelity and research on eye movement desensitization and reprocessing. *Journal of Anxiety Disorders, 13*, 173–184.

Ruscio, J. (2001). *Clear thinking with psychology: Separating sense from nonsense.* Pacific Grove, CA: Wadsworth.

Sagan, C. (1995a). *The demon-haunted world: Science as a candle in the dark.* New York: Random House.

Sagan, C. (1995b, January/February). Wonder and skepticism. *Skeptical Inquirer, 19*, 24–30.

Shannon, S. (Ed.). (2002). *Handbook of complementary and alternative therapies in mental health.* San Diego, CA: Academic Press.

Shapiro, F. (1995). *Eye movement desensitization and reprocessing: Basic protocols, principles, and procedures.* New York: Guilford Press.

Shermer, M. (1997). *Why people believe weird things: Pseudoscience, superstition, and other confusions of our time.* New York: Freeman.

Shermer, M. (2001). *The borderlands of science: Where sense meets nonsense.* New York: Oxford University Press.

Singer, M. T., & Lalich, J. (1996). *Crazy therapies: What are they? Do they work?* San Francisco: Jossey-Bass.

Stanovich, K. (2001). *How to think straight about psychology* (6th ed.). New York: HarperCollins.

van Rillaer, J. (1991). Strategies of dissimulation in the pseudosciences. *New Ideas in Psychology, 9*, 235–244.

PART I

CONTROVERSIES IN ASSESSMENT AND DIAGNOSIS

2

Understanding Why Some Clinicians Use Pseudoscientific Methods

Findings from Research on Clinical Judgment

HOWARD N. GARB
PATRICIA A. BOYLE

Grand claims are frequently made for pseudoscientific methods, and many clinicians honestly believe that they can help clients by using them. The question arises, "If pseudoscientific methods are not valid, then why are grand claims made for them and why do some clinicians think that they are valid?" There are many reasons, and some reasons may apply to some clinicians but not to others. Obviously, if one develops a new assessment instrument or treatment intervention, there are personal and financial reasons for believing in, and overstating, the value of one's product. Once grand claims have been made, clinicians may use an assessment instrument or treatment intervention to see if it works. After all, if it really is a great assessment instrument or treatment intervention, then it would be irresponsible not to use it. However, once clinicians use pseudoscientific methods with clients, why do they not see that they are invalid and ineffective?

The purpose of this chapter is to explain why it can be difficult to learn from clinical experience. Research on the value of clinical experience and clinical training will be reviewed along with research on cognitive processes. Comments will be made about the nature of feedback that clinicians receive in clinical settings. Finally, recommendations will be made for improving clinical practice.

THE VALUE OF CLINICAL EXPERIENCE AND TRAINING

Clinical lore suggests that psychologists and mental health professionals "learn by doing," or learn from experience. Experienced clinicians are presumed to make more accurate and valid assessments of personality and psychopathology than novice clinicians, and presumed experts are assumed to be more competent providers of psychological interventions than other clinicians. Psychology training programs adhere to these assumptions, and common supervisory practices emphasize the value of experience in the development of competent clinicians. The inherent message to mental health trainees is that clinical acumen develops over time and with increased exposure to various patients and presenting problems.

Despite common lore, a large body of research contradicts the popular belief that experience and clinical competence are positively related. In fact, research suggests that it is very difficult for mental health workers to learn from experience. Numerous studies investigating clinical judgment have demonstrated that when clinicians are given identical sets of information, experienced clinicians are no more accurate than less experienced clinicians (Dawes, 1994; Garb, 1989, 1998; Garb & Schramke, 1996; Goldberg, 1968; Wiggins, 1973; see also Meehl, 1997). Moreover, judgmental validity appears to be unrelated to experience *regardless of the type of information presented to clinicians*. Studies demonstrating the lack of a relation between experience and accuracy in the assessment of personality and psychopathology are alarming, particularly because assessment is a primary task for psychologists as well as other mental health professionals. Given the importance of these findings, individual studies will be described.

The validity of judgments will be described for (1) experienced versus less experienced clinicians, (2) clinicians versus graduate students, (3) graduate students followed over time, (4) clinicians and graduate students versus lay judges, and (5) clinicians differing in experience and specialized training. The results describe the relation between (1) training and validity and (2) experience and validity.

Experienced versus Less Experienced Clinicians

For the task of interpreting personality assessment test results, alleged experts have not been more accurate than other clinicians, and experienced clinicians have not been more accurate than less experienced clinicians (Graham, 1967; Levenberg, 1975; Silverman, 1959; Turner, 1966; Walters,

White, & Greene, 1988; Wanderer, 1969; Watson, 1967). For example, Graham (1967) presented Minnesota Multiphasic Personality Inventory (MMPI) protocols to two groups of psychologists with differing levels of experience with the MMPI. The first group consisted of PhD-level psychologists who had used the MMPI routinely in clinical practice for approximately 5 years. The second group consisted of PhD-level psychologists who had used the MMPI much more frequently in clinical practice for over 5 years and who also demonstrated a broad knowledge of the research literature on the MMPI. Clinicians were asked to perform Q-sorts to describe patients' personality features, and clinician ratings were compared with criterion Q-sorts that were generated on the basis of patient and family member interviews. Although results indicated that overall judgmental validity was moderate, with correlations ranging from .29 to .37, judgmental validity was *unrelated* to experience with the MMPI. That is, clinicians with more MMPI experience and knowledge were no more accurate in their interpretations of MMPI data than were clinicians with significantly less MMPI experience and knowledge.

The relation between experience and validity has also been investigated among psychiatrists. In one study, Kendell (1973) studied the relation between experience and diagnostic accuracy among practicing psychiatrists with varying degrees of experience in the field (each had a minimum of 4 years of practice). Psychiatrists observed segments of initial clinical interviews with psychiatric inpatients and were asked to provide diagnoses on the basis of the interview data. Their diagnoses were compared to diagnoses that were based on more complete information including full interviews with the patients and the patients' relatives, information from the case notes of earlier admissions, and additional information collected during patients' stays in the hospital. Results indicated that experience was unrelated to the validity of diagnoses. Similarly, in another study (Muller & Davids, 1999), experienced psychiatrists were no more adept than less experienced clinicians when the task was to assess positive and negative symptoms of schizophrenia.

In a final study using psychiatrists as participants (Hermann, Ettner, Dorwart, Langman-Dorwart, & Kleinman, 1999), number of years of clinical experience was *negatively* related to validity. Hermann et al. reported that "psychiatrists trained in earlier eras were more likely to use ECT [electroconvulsive therapy] for diagnoses outside evidence-based indications" (p. 1059). In this study, older psychiatrists may have made less valid judgments than younger psychiatrists because education regarding the proper and improper uses of ECT has improved in recent years. If this is true, then having years of clinical experience did not compensate for not having up-to-date training.

Similar results have been obtained in the area of neuropsychology: Neuropsychologists with the American Board of Professional Psychology

(ABPP) diploma are generally no more accurate than less experienced doctoral-level neuropsychologists (Faust et al., 1988; Gaudette, 1992; Heaton, Smith, Lehmann, & Vogt, 1978; Wedding, 1983). One of the best-known studies was conducted by Faust and colleagues (1988). They examined the validity of judgments made by 155 neuropsychologists. The neuropsychologists evaluated results from several commonly used neuropsychological tools (including the Halstead–Reitan Battery) and made ratings regarding the presence/absence of neurological impairment, as well as ratings of the likely location, process, and etiology of the neurological injury. In addition, the clinicians' levels of training and experience were assessed. Measures of training included cumulative practicum experience in neuropsychology, cumulative supervised neuropsychology hours, relevant coursework, specialized neuropsychology internship training, and the completion of postdoctoral training in neuropsychology. Measures of experience included years of practice in neuropsychology and total career hours spent on issues related to neuropsychology. ABPP status was used as a measure of alleged expertise. Training, experience, and alleged expertise were *not* related to the validity of judgments.

In only one study has experience been related to validity. Brammer (2002) reported that when psychologists were required to request information in a simulated interview, more experienced practitioners made more accurate diagnoses, even when level of training was controlled for. Thus, more experienced clinicians may be better at knowing what information to collect.

In conclusion, when clinicians are given identical sets of information, experienced clinicians are no more accurate than less experienced clinicians. When practitioners are required to search for information or decide what judgments should be made, experience may be related to validity for some judgment tasks.

Clinicians versus Graduate Students

One would assume that clinical and counseling psychologists are more accurate than psychology graduate students. However, with few exceptions, this difference has not been found. In empirical studies, clinicians have rarely been more accurate than graduate students, regardless of the type of information provided to clinicians. Studies have revealed no differences in accuracy between experienced clinicians and graduate students when judgments are made on the basis of interview data (Anthony, 1968; Grigg, 1958; Schinka & Sines, 1974), biographical and history information (Oskamp, 1965; Soskin, 1954), behavioral observation data (Garner & Smith, 1976; Walker & Lewine, 1990), data from therapy sessions (Brenner & Howard, 1976), MMPI protocols (Chandler, 1970; Danet, 1965; Goldberg, 1965, 1968; Graham, 1967, 1971; Oskamp, 1962;

Walters et al., 1988; Whitehead, 1985), projective-drawing protocols (Levenberg, 1975; Schaeffer, 1964; Stricker, 1967), Rorschach protocols (Gadol, 1969; Turner, 1966; Whitehead, 1985; see also Chapter 3), screening instruments for detecting neurological impairment (Goldberg, 1959; Leli & Filskov, 1981, 1984; Robiner, 1978), and all of the data that clinical and counseling psychologists usually have available in clinical practice (Johnston & McNeal, 1967).

Clinicians did outperform graduate students in two studies. In both studies, the graduate students were just beginning their training. In the first study (Grebstein, 1963; reanalyzed by Hammond, Hursch, & Todd, 1964), the task was to predict IQ scores on the basis of projective (Rorschach) test data (see also Chapter 3). Psychologists were more accurate than graduate students. However, when the data were reanalyzed after graduate students were separated into two groups, those with and without practicum experience, the clinical psychologists were no more accurate than the graduate students with practicum training. In a second study (Falvey & Hebert, 1992), the task was to read case histories and write treatment plans. Criterion scores were obtained by having clinicians with special expertise in the treatment of anxiety and mood disorders read the case histories and formulate treatment plans. Ratings were averaged across the criterion judges: Having a group of judges make ratings and averaging their ratings is one way to improve the reliability and validity of ratings (e.g., Horowitz, Inouye, & Siegelman, 1979). Treatment plans written by certified clinical mental health counselors were more valid than those written by graduate students in master's degree programs. About half of the graduate students had not yet completed a single class related to diagnosis and treatment planning.

Though clinicians were sometimes more accurate than beginning graduate students, this was not always the case. In one study (Whitehead, 1985), psychologists, advanced clinical psychology graduate students, and beginning clinical psychology graduate students were instructed to make differential diagnoses on the basis of Rorschach (see Chapter 3) or MMPI results (e.g., they were instructed to differentiate back pain patients from psychiatric patients). The beginning graduate students had received training in the use of the MMPI, but they had not yet received training in the use of the Rorschach. Thus, the only Rorschach data given to beginning graduate students were transcripts of the Rorschach sessions. In contrast, the Rorschach data given to psychologists and advanced graduate students included transcripts of the Rorschach sessions, response location sheets, and Rorschach scores (using the Comprehensive System Structural Summary; Exner, 1974). The psychologists (and the advanced graduate students) were not more accurate than the beginning graduate students, both when they were given Rorschach data and when they were given MMPI data.

Graduate Students Followed over Time

To study the relations between (1) training and validity and (2) experience and validity, it is helpful to conduct longitudinal studies. In one study (Aronson & Akamatsu, 1981), 12 graduate students' judgments were evaluated three times: (1) after the first year of graduate education in psychology, (2) following the completion of a course on MMPI interpretation, and (3) following the completion of a year-long assessment and therapy practicum. Graduate students' personality ratings were then compared with criterion ratings made on the basis of patient and family interviews. Results revealed a validity coefficient of .20 at time 1, .42 at time 2, and .44 at time 3. Thus, graduate students were able to make more accurate judgments of client profiles following specialized didactic training, but additional practicum experience did not improve accuracy (for related results, see Whitehead, 1985).

Clinicians and Graduate Students versus Lay Judges

When given nonpsychometric data, clinicians and graduate students tend to be more accurate than lay judges, depending on characteristics of the lay judges and characteristics of the subjects (e.g., patients). For example, when instructed to describe psychopathology using interview data, clinicians and graduate students outperformed undergraduate students and individuals with bachelor's degrees (Brammer, 2002; Grigg, 1958; Waxer, 1976). However, clinicians and graduate students did not outperform physical scientists (Luft, 1950). The differential rates of accuracy for this task may be related to differences among groups in intellectual functioning and maturity (presumably physical scientists are more intelligent and mature than undergraduate students). When asked to make similar judgments on the basis of biographical and history data, clinicians outperformed lay judges with respect to the assessment of psychiatric patients (Horowitz, 1962; Lambert & Wertheimer, 1988; Stelmachers & McHugh, 1964; see also Holmes & Howard, 1980), but not with respect to the assessment of normal subjects (Griswold & Dana, 1970; Oskamp, 1965; Weiss, 1963). Of course, clinicians rarely provide assessments for individuals who are not seeking, or are not currently involved, in treatment. As a consequence, clinicians may overpathologize normals because they are not used to working with them.

When given psychometric data, clinicians and graduate students were more accurate than lay judges (e.g., undergraduates, secretaries) depending on the type of data they were given and the specific judgment task. Psychologists were not more accurate than lay judges when they were given results from projective tests, including results from the Rorschach Inkblot Method and Human Figure Drawings (Cressen, 1975; Gadol, 1969; Hiler

& Nesvig, 1965; Levenberg, 1975; Schaeffer, 1964; Schmidt & McGowan, 1959; Todd, 1954, cited in Hammond, 1955; Walker & Linden, 1967). Nor were clinical psychologists more accurate than lay judges when the task was to use screening instruments (e.g., the Bender–Gestalt test) to detect neurological impairment (Goldberg, 1959; Leli & Filskov, 1981, 1984; Nadler, Fink, Shontz, & Brink, 1959; Robiner, 1978). For example, in one of these studies (Goldberg, 1959), clinical psychologists were not more accurate than their own secretaries! Finally, when given MMPI protocols, psychologists and graduate students were more accurate than lay judges (Aronson & Akamatsu, 1981; Goldberg & Rorer, 1965, and Rorer & Slovic, 1966, cited in Goldberg, 1968; Karson & Freud, 1956; Oskamp, 1962). For example, Aronson and Akamatsu (1981) compared the ability of graduate and undergraduate students to perform Q-sorts to describe the personality characteristics of patients with psychiatric conditions on the basis of MMPI protocols. Students' level of training differed in that graduate students had taken coursework in the MMPI and had some experience administering and/or interpreting the instrument, whereas undergraduates had only attended two lectures on the MMPI. Criterion ratings were based on family and patient interviews. Correlations between judges' ratings and criterion ratings were .44 and .24 for graduate and undergraduate students' ratings, respectively. Graduate student ratings were significantly more accurate than undergraduate ratings.

Clinicians Differing in Experience and Specialized Training

Not only are mental health professionals more accurate than lay judges for some tasks, they are also more accurate than other mental health professionals for some tasks when they have received special training. For example, neuropsychologists are more accurate than clinical psychologists when the task is to detect neurological impairment (e.g., Goldstein, Deysach, & Kleinknecht, 1973), psychologists with a background in forensic psychology are more accurate than other psychologists at detecting lying (Ekman, O'Sullivan, & Frank, 1999), and psychiatrists do a better job than other physicians at prescribing antidepressant medicine (e.g., making sure a patient is on a therapeutic dose; Fairman, Drevets, Kreisman, & Teitelbaum, 1998).

Summary and Discussion

Clinicians who use pseudoscientific methods often do not discover that these methods are invalid because it is difficult to learn from clinical experience. Systematic research supports the value of training in psychology and other mental health fields, but it calls into question the value of clinical experience. Judgments and decisions made by experienced clinicians are generally no more accurate than those made by less experienced clinicians when all of the judges are given identical sets of information. Similarly, experienced clinicians are generally no more accurate than advanced graduate students. On the other hand, clinicians and graduate students frequently outperform lay judges, and in some instances mental health professionals with specialized training and interests outperform other mental health professionals. Obviously, longitudinal results that show that graduate students become more accurate after didactic training but not after training at a practicum site also suggest that training is of value but that it can be difficult to learn from clinical experience. To obtain a deeper understanding of why clinicians continue to use pseudoscientific methods, it is important to understand why it is difficult to learn from clinical experience.

IMPEDIMENTS TO LEARNING FROM EXPERIENCE

There are many reasons why it can be difficult for mental health professionals to learn from experience. Psychologists and other mental health workers are routinely confronted with ambiguous and complex decision-making tasks in which they must interpret and manipulate large amounts of data to formulate diagnostic impressions. Research has shown that in such situations professionals are susceptible to numerous cognitive and environmental influences that can result in poor judgments and a failure to learn from experience (Arkes, 1981; Brehmer, 1980; Dawes, 1994; Dawes, Faust, & Meehl, 1989; Einhorn, 1988; Garb, 1998).

These cognitive factors include biases, heuristics, and memory processes, and environmental influences include the unavailability of adequate and appropriate feedback. These cognitive and environmental influences can exert a major negative impact on clinical care. Erroneous cognitive processes and poor feedback systems often result in the use of suboptimal hypothesis testing and decision-making strategies. When poor decision-making strategies are used, the likelihood that mental health workers will make accurate judgments and effectively learn from experience is diminished.

Cognitive Processes and Errors in Judgment

Biases, heuristics, and memory processes can compromise the ability of clinicians to use optimal decision-making strategies. Biases are beliefs or preconceptions that adversely influence clinicians' interpretations of available data. Heuristics are simple rules or shortcuts that describe how clinicians make judgments, treatment decisions, or both. Reliance on heuristics can be efficient, but they are fallible and can lead clinicians to fail to learn from their experiences.

Biases include (but are not limited to) confirmatory bias, overconfidence, hindsight bias, race bias, gender bias, and bias to perceive psychopathology. Confirmatory bias occurs when clinicians knowingly or unknowingly review patient information in such a way that they seek and attend to information that can support but not counter their initial hypotheses. For example, in one study (Haverkamp, 1993), when psychology graduate students watched a videotape of an initial counseling session and listed the questions they would like to ask the client, their style of hypothesis testing was confirmatory 64% of the time (their questions could confirm but not refute their impressions of the client), neutral 21% of the time, and disconfirmatory only 15% of the time.

As revealed in another study, confirmatory information seeking strategies occur early in the diagnostic decision-making process and can minimize the likelihood that clinicians will make accurate judgments. Gauron and Dickinson (1969) asked psychiatrists to describe their diagnostic impressions of patients on the basis of videotaped interviews. Many diagnoses were made within 30–60 seconds of viewing the interview and most never changed, even when the psychiatrists received disconfirming evidence. Presumably, because the clinicians did not actively seek out and attend to disconfirming evidence, they were less apt to change their initial opinions. When the psychiatrists received disconfirming evidence, they may have ignored it or, even more likely, they may have reinterpreted the contradictory evidence so that it became consistent with their initial beliefs.

Confirmatory bias can lead to overconfidence, and overconfidence can in turn lead to a greater reliance on confirmatory bias. Oskamp (1965) conducted a study in which the combined influence of overconfidence and confirmatory strategies was highlighted. Oskamp investigated the relation between incremental data gathering, validity of personality judgments, and confidence in the accuracy of judgments. Interestingly, clinicians' confidence in their personality judgments increased with the presentation of additional case history information. However, as confidence increased, accuracy remained at roughly the same level. Oskamp's data suggest that overconfidence led practitioners to emphasize information that confirmed their initial hypotheses and to ignore or reinterpret information that did not support these hypotheses. The combination of confirmatory hypothesis testing strategies and overconfidence may have prevented clinicians from attending to relevant patient data and contributed to diagnostic inaccuracy.

Though confirmatory bias can lead to overconfidence, it is important to note that little research has been done on the appropriateness of confidence ratings in clinical judgment (Garb, 1986). For example, overconfidence has been investigated in only a few studies. Clinicians have been overconfident in some studies (e.g., Oskamp, 1965) but underconfident in others (Wedding, 1983). In general, the greater the validity of assessment information, the stronger the relation between confidence and validity. For example, confidence has not been positively related to validity when clinicians have been given Rorschach or Thematic Apperception Test (TAT) protocols (Albert, Fox, & Kahn, 1980; Gadol, 1969; Holsopple & Phelan, 1954; see also Chapter 3).

Confirmatory bias and overconfidence can help to explain what goes wrong once a clinician has formed a hypothesis, but they do not help us understand how hypotheses are initially formulated. Consider the task of diagnosis. Clinicians may form hypotheses when they learn that a client meets at least some of the criteria for a diagnosis, but insidious influences are also sometimes at work. Clinicians can be influenced by a number of biases, such as race bias, social class bias, gender bias, age bias, labeling bias, and a tendency to overpsychopathologize clients (Garb, 1998). Thus, when interviewing an African American client, they may consider a diagnosis of schizophrenia before they consider a diagnosis of bipolar (manic–depressive) disorder. When clinicians engage in confirmatory hypothesis testing and become overconfident, they are unlikely to overcome the biases that led to their formulating a hypothesis.

Research on illusory correlations can also help us understand how hypotheses are initially formulated. This area of research also demonstrates that it can be difficult for clinicians to learn from clinical experience and that once clinicians formulate a hypothesis they tend to hold onto it despite disconfirming evidence (Garb, 1998, pp. 23–25). An illusory correlation occurs when a clinician believes there is a correlation between events that are not truly correlated, are only weakly correlated, or are correlated in the opposite manner from that assumed by the clinician.

In a pioneering study, Chapman and Chapman (1967) attempted to determine why clinicians continue to use the Draw-A-Person test in spite of a large body of research documenting no relation between picture characteristics (e.g., peculiar or emphasized eyes) and personality characteristics (e.g., suspiciousness) (see also Chapter 3). Chapman and Chapman conducted a two-part study. First, they asked clinicians to identify which features of drawings are associated with particular symptoms and traits. Second, they presented human figure drawings to undergraduates. Undergraduates were to examine each drawing and then read a statement on the back that described a symptom or trait that was said to be possessed by the client who had drawn the picture. Undergraduates were unaware that the drawings and statements on the back of the drawings were randomly paired. Remarkably, undergraduates reported observing the same relations that had been reported by the clinicians, even though these relations were nonexistent in the stimulus materials. These results demonstrate that clinicians respond to verbal associations (e.g., between "eyes" and "watchfulness or suspiciousness"). Typically, they do not respond to the actual co-occurrence of particular picture features and psychiatric symptomatology (in most cases, picture features are unrelated to psychiatric symptomatology, even though some clinicians think that they are related; Groth-Marnat & Roberts, 1998; Kahill, 1984; Motta, Little, & Tobin, 1993; Swensen, 1957; Thomas & Jolley, 1998).

Hindsight bias describes the mental processes that occur when individuals generate explanations for events that have occurred. For example, when clinicians learn that a client has committed suicide, they are likely to make high ratings if asked to rate the likelihood of the client committing suicide given the information they had about the client before the client committed suicide. Clinicians are generally unaware that the knowledge of an outcome influences the perceived likelihood of that outcome (Fischhoff, 1975). To put it another way, after an event has occurred, people are likely to believe that the event was bound to occur. This finding has been widely replicated across a range of judgment tasks (Hawkins & Hastie, 1990), such as the diagnosis of neurological impairment (Arkes, Faust, Guilmette, & Hart, 1988) and even the occurrence (or nonoccurrence) of events related to Y2K (M. B. Garb, 2000). Hindsight bias is important for understanding why clinicians have difficulty learning from clinical experience because it suggests that clinicians think in deterministic (not probabilistic) terms. In reality, all assessment information is fallible, and we frequently cannot make predictions with a high degree of certainty. To think otherwise is likely to lead clinicians to the erroneous belief that a particular combination of symptoms or behaviors is almost invariably associated with a particular outcome.

Additional errors in judgment can result from the use of heuristics. As already noted, heuristics are simple rules that describe how people make judgments (Kahneman, Slovic, & Tversky, 1982). They allow people to make judgments with a minimum of time and effort, and they frequently lead to accurate judgments. Nevertheless, in certain circumstances, they can also lead to mistakes in judgment.

The heuristic that is most relevant to understanding why clinicians can have a difficult time learning from experience is the availability heuristic. The availability heuristic describes the role of memory in judgmental error. Clinicians may have trouble learning from experience because of the way clinicians remember or misremember information. Given that it is difficult, or even impossible, to retain all details of cases and clients, clinicians often recall only selected information about each case. The recalled information, however, may not adequately describe the case or may be irrelevant to its central features.

According to the availability heuristic, a clinician's judgments are influenced by the ease with which the clinician remembers particular cases.

The ease with which information can be remembered is related to several factors (e.g., the vividness of information and the strength of verbal associative connections between events). For example, clinicians are more likely to remember a case that is striking or unusual in some way. Similarly, the strength of verbal associative connections can make it easier for a clinician to remember whether a test indicator and a symptom or behavior co-occurred. Finally, clinicians are more likely to remember instances when a test indicator and symptom were present than cases when a test indicator was absent and a symptom was either present or absent (Arkes, 1981; Kayne & Alloy, 1988). To accurately determine how two events covary, one has to remember instances when the symptom or behavior did not occur as well as instances when they did occur. Of course, when clinicians cannot accurately determine how two events covary, an illusory correlation is said to be present.

In addition to the inherent fallibility of memory, Arkes and Harkness (1980) suggested that the act of making a diagnosis can influence how one remembers a client's symptoms. That is, a clinician's memory can be altered by the very act of making a diagnosis. A psychologist is likely to "recall" a patient having a symptom that is typical of the diagnosis, even though the client may not have that symptom. Similarly, the psychologist may forget that a client has a particular symptom because the symptom is atypical of the diagnosis rendered. Clinicians are unlikely to learn from experience when the details of cases are remembered incorrectly.

The Nature of Feedback in Clinical Practice

Mental health professionals typically do not receive feedback on the validity of their judgments and decisions. In most cases, to determine the accuracy of a judgment or decision, one would have to collect longitudinal or outcome data. This is accomplished in empirical studies, but most clinicians find it to be too expensive and time-consuming to perform in clinical practice.

This state of affairs can be contrasted with most areas of medicine. Physicians frequently receive accurate feedback from laboratory results, radiology studies, and, in some cases, autopsies. These outcome measures are significantly more objective than those commonly used for mental health interventions (e.g., client reports of improved functioning). The paucity of appropriate outcome measures for psychology and psychiatry reflects both the difficulties of obtaining criterion information for mental health tasks and a lack of training in outcome evaluation techniques.

When mental health clinicians receive feedback, this feedback is sometimes misleading. For example, a clinician may seek feedback from a client to determine if a test report is accurate or if a treatment has caused a reduction in distress. This method of obtaining feedback can be problematic for several reasons. First, clients may be reluctant to dispute their therapists' hypotheses. This may be due to passivity or suggestibility, fear of authority, or social desirability. Second, clients may be unaware of, or unable to describe, some of their own traits. Similarly, their reports of whether they have improved may be powerfully influenced by how they feel when they are asked. Third, psychological test reports often describe traits that are common to people in general, but do not describe traits that are specific to a client (e.g., "You are sensitive to other people's needs," "You have a great deal of unused potential," "You occasionally have difficulty making decisions"). Clients may accept the validity of the test report on face value.

This phenomenon has been labeled the P. T. Barnum effect, after the circus entrepreneur P. T. Barnum (Meehl, 1956), who once said that "I try to give a little something to everyone." Thus, a client may feel that a test report is accurate even though the report yields little individualized information. A client may be even more likely to believe that a test report is accurate if the report includes positive Barnum statements (this is termed the "Pollyanna principle"). For the client to say, "Yes, that describes me!" would be misleading to clinicians who are trying to understand the validity of their case conceptualizations, test reports, or both.

The Barnum effect was illustrated in a study by Logue, Sher, and Frensch (1992). They administered a personality inventory to 224 undergraduates, 112 of whom were adult children of alcoholics. Participants were informed that the purpose of the study was to validate a new personality questionnaire. Following completion of the questionnaire, participants were given a personality profile. They were told the profile was based on their responses to the test items, and they were asked to rate the accuracy of the profile description. Participants were randomly given one of two profiles, regardless of their test responses. The first was a general profile that was descriptive of many individuals (the Barnum profile) and the second was an "Adult Child of an Alcoholic" profile (based on commonly assumed characteristics of adult children of alcoholics). Examples of statements for the Barnum and Adult Child of an Alcoholic profiles are, respectively, "You are able to take criticism occasionally" and "In times of crisis you tend to take care of others."

Both profiles received widespread endorsement by all subjects. Of those who received the Barnum profile, 79% of the adult children of alcoholics and 70% of the remaining participants reported that the profile described them very well or better. Of those who received the Adult Child of an Alcoholic profile, 71% of the adult children of alcoholics and 63% of the remaining population reported that the profile described them very well or better. Clearly, participants were unaware that test profiles had been randomly assigned to them and that the profiles were not really designed to describe their specific personality traits.

Clinicians also receive misleading feedback when they make incorrect interpretations but convince their clients that they are correct. For example, some clinicians tell their clients that they believe they were abused, even when their clients have no memory of having been abused. To help them "remember" having been abused, therapists may tell them that they were abused and repeatedly ask them to remember the events. Similarly, they may interpret their dreams, hypnotize them, or refer them to incest-survivor groups, all in an effort to help them "remember" an episode of abuse that may have never occurred. Too often, clients falsely remember having been abused (Loftus, 1993; Ofshe & Watters, 1994; see also Chapter 8).

SUMMARY AND DISCUSSION

Clinicians who use pseudoscientific assessment and treatment methods continue to use them in part because they have not learned from clinical experience that they do not work. Empirical studies may raise questions about the validity and utility of pseudoscientific methods, but clinical experience is less likely to do so. A great deal of research has been conducted on cognitive processes, the nature of feedback, and the reasons why it is difficult to learn from experience. However, empirical studies have not focused on studying clinicians who use pseudoscientific methods. That is, studies have not focused on understanding why clinicians who use pseudoscientific methods have trouble learning from experience. Put another way, no study has looked at the cognitive processes, personality traits, and belief structures (cognitive schemas) of clinicians who use pseudoscientific methods. Nor has any study looked at social factors that may reinforce clinicians for using pseudoscientific methods.

One can wonder whether individual differences exist among clinicians in their attraction to pseudoscientific methods. For example, if a clinician is attracted to one pseudoscientific method, will the clinician also be attracted to others? Will there be some pseudoscientific methods that the clinician is not attracted to? If individual differences are present, then studies need to be conducted and theories need to be developed to help us understand these differences. Similarly, it would also be interesting to learn if some clinicians who use pseudoscientific methods graduate from training programs that reject pseudoscientific methods.

It is surprisingly difficult for clinicians to learn from clinical experience. This is not to say that clinical experience is never valuable. For example, experience may help clinicians structure judgment tasks (Brammer, 2002). That is, it may help clinicians decide what judgments and decisions need to be made. Similarly, more experienced clinicians may be better at knowing what information to collect in an interview. However, experience does *not* seem to be useful for helping clinicians evaluate the validity of an assessment instrument. Nor does experience seem to help clinicians make more valid judgments when the task is structured for them (e.g., when they are all given the same information).

Because it is difficult to learn from clinical experience, mental health professionals should not use an assessment instrument or treatment method solely because it seems to work in clinical practice. Instead, clinicians should become familiar with the research literature to learn if the assessment instrument or treatment method is supported by empirical research.

Mental health professionals also need to become familiar with the research literature on clinical judgment. Hundred of studies have been conducted on the validity of judgments made by mental health professionals. By becoming familiar with the results of these studies, clinicians can avoid making judgments for tasks that are surprisingly difficult and for which they are unlikely to be accurate. To give just one example, interrater reliability is generally poor for generating psychodynamic formulations (Garb, 1998, pp. 90–92). Even more relevant for the controversies surrounding the use of pseudoscientific assessment instruments, theories, and treatment interventions, clinicians may become more scientifically minded if they understand why and how clinical experience can be inconclusive or misleading.

To bring about positive change, admissions policies may need to be changed for graduate school programs. Snyder (1995) addressed this issue:

> Are there forces attracting students to graduate training who are not predisposed toward scientific approaches to clinical psychology? . . . Unless changes occur in the type of students recruited to our field and in the work environment for graduates who become practicing clinicians, my sense is that all the efforts exerted in training programs, licensure, and continuing education will not accomplish any greater emphasis on the scientific principles underlying the helping process. (p. 423)

Thus, when selecting students for graduate school, one should select for scientific-mindedness as well as for intelligence and personality factors (e.g., warmth and empathy). Students should be selected who are likely to use an assessment instrument or a treatment intervention because it has been repeatedly supported by research, not because a charismatic figure has praised it or because in their experience they have found it to be helpful.

Additional changes will need to be made if empirically supported assessment instruments and treatment interventions are to be used more widely. For example, in addition to making changes to training programs, licensure exams should be critically appraised. Specifically, licensing exams should evaluate applicants' knowledge of empirically supported assessment instruments and treatment interventions. Only when such changes are made will clinicians become less likely to use pseudoscientific methods.

In conclusion, clinical lore suggests that psychologists "learn from doing" or learn from experience. However, empirical research indicates that it is difficult to learn from experience. To become more accurate, psychologists need to understand why it can be difficult to learn from experience, and they need to place greater emphasis on scientific findings.

GLOSSARY

Availability heuristic: The tendency for an individual's judgments to be influenced by the ease with which the individual remembers particular cases. This heuristic can lead to incorrect judgments. The ease with which information can be remembered is related to several factors (e.g., the strength of verbal associative connections between events may influence how well one "remembers" the co-occurrence of those events).

Biases: Beliefs or preconceptions that adversely influence clinicians' interpretations of available data. Also, cognitive processes that relate to the occurrence of cognitive biases (e.g., overconfidence, confirmatory bias).

Confirmatory bias: The tendency to seek, attend to, or remember information that can support but not counter a belief or preconception.

Gender bias: This bias occurs when, for a particular task, judgments are more valid for one gender than another.

Heuristics: Simple rules or shortcuts by which individuals, including clinicians, make judgments, decisions, or both.

Hindsight bias: The tendency for knowledge of a particular outcome event to influence the perceived likelihood of that event, leading to incorrect explanations for the occurrence of the event.

Illusory correlation: The belief that events are correlated when in reality the events are not correlated, are only weakly correlated, or are correlated in the opposite direction from that assumed by the clinician.

Q-sort: A judgment task in which clinicians are instructed to describe a client by sorting items into categories ranging from least characteristic to most characteristic of the client. Items typically describe personality traits, psychiatric symptoms, or both.

Race bias: This bias occurs when, for a particular task, judgments are more valid for one racial group than another.

REFERENCES

Albert, S., Fox, H. M., & Kahn, M. W. (1980). Faking psychosis on the Rorschach: Can expert judges detect malingering? *Journal of Personality Assessment, 44,* 115–119.

Anthony, N. (1968). The use of facts and cues in clinical judgments from interviews. *Journal of Clinical Psychology, 24,* 37–39.

Arkes, H. R. (1981). Impediments to accurate clinical judgment and possible ways to minimize their impact. *Journal of Consulting and Clinical Psychology, 49,* 323–330.

Arkes, H. R., Faust, D., Guilmette, T. J., & Hart, K. (1988). Eliminating the hindsight bias. *Journal of Applied Psychology, 73,* 305–307.

Arkes, H. R., & Harkness, A. R. (1980). Effect of making a diagnosis on subsequent recognition of symptoms. *Journal of Experimental Psychology: Human Learning and Memory, 6,* 568–575.

Aronson, D. E., & Akamatsu, T. J. (1981). Validation of a Q-sort task to assess MMPI skills. *Journal of Clinical Psychology, 37,* 831–836.

Brammer, R. (2002). Effects of experience and training on diagnostic accuracy. *Psychological Assessment, 14,* 110–113.

Brehmer, B. (1980). In one word: Not from experience. *Acta Psychologica, 45,* 223–241.

Brenner, D., & Howard, K. I. (1976). Clinical judgment as a function of experience and information. *Journal of Clinical Psychology, 32,* 721–728.

Chandler, M. J. (1970). Self-awareness and its relation to other parameters of the clinical inference process. *Journal of Consulting and Clinical Psychology, 35,* 258–264.

Chapman, L. J., & Chapman, J. P. (1967). Genesis of popular but erroneous psychodiagnostic observations. *Journal of Abnormal Psychology, 72,* 193–204.

Cressen, R. (1975). Artistic quality of drawings and judges' evaluations of the DAP. *Journal of Personality Assessment, 39,* 132–137.

Danet, B. N. (1965). Prediction of mental illness in college students on the basis of "nonpsychiatric" MMPI profiles. *Journal of Consulting Psychology, 29,* 577–580.

Dawes, R. M. (1994). *House of cards: Psychology and psychotherapy built on myth.* New York: Free Press.

Dawes, R. M., Faust, D., & Meehl, P. E. (1989). Clinical versus actuarial judgment. *Science, 243,* 1668–1674.

Einhorn, H. J. (1988). Diagnosis and causality in clinical and statistical prediction. In D. C. Turk & P. Salovey (Eds.), *Reasoning, inference, and judgment in clinical psychology* (pp. 51–70). New York: Free Press.

Ekman, P., O'Sullivan, M., & Frank, M. G. (1999). A few can catch a liar. *Psychological Science, 10,* 263–266.

Exner, J. E., Jr. (1974). *The Rorschach: A comprehensive system* (Vol. 1). New York: Wiley.

Fairman, K. A., Drevets, W. C., Kreisman, J. J., & Teitelbaum, F. (1998). Course of antidepressant treatment, drug type, and prescriber's specialty. *Psychiatric Services, 49,* 1180–1186.

Falvey, J. E., & Hebert, D. J. (1992). Psychometric study of the Clinical Treatment Planning Simulations (CTPS) for assessing clinical judgment. *Journal of Mental Health Counseling, 14*, 490–507.

Faust, D., Guilmette, T. J., Hart, K., Arkes, H. R., Fishburne, F. J., & Davey, L. (1988). Neuropsychologists' training, experience, and judgment accuracy. *Archives of Clinical Neuropsychology, 3*, 145–163.

Fischhoff, B. (1975). Hindsight–foresight: The effect of outcome knowledge on judgment under uncertainty. *Journal of Experimental Psychology: Human Perception and Performance, 1*, 288–299.

Gadol, I. (1969). The incremental and predictive validity of the Rorschach test in personality assessments of normal, neurotic, and psychotic subjects. *Dissertation Abstracts, 29*, 3482–B. (University Microfilms No. 69–4469)

Garb, H. N. (1986). The appropriateness of confidence ratings in clinical judgment. *Journal of Clinical Psychology, 42*, 190–197.

Garb, H. N. (1989). Clinical judgment, clinical training, and professional experience. *Psychological Bulletin, 105*, 387–396.

Garb, H. N. (1998). *Studying the clinician: Judgment research and psychological assessment.* Washington, DC: American Psychological Association.

Garb, H. N., & Schramke, C. J. (1996). Judgment research and neuropsychological assessment: A narrative review and meta-analyses. *Psychological Bulletin, 120*, 140–153.

Garb, M. B. (2000). *Y2K and the hindsight bias.* Unpublished manuscript, Solomon Schecter Community Day School, Pittsburgh, PA.

Garner, A. M., & Smith, G. M. (1976). An experimental videotape technique for evaluating trainee approaches to clinical judging. *Journal of Consulting and Clinical Psychology, 44*, 945–950.

Gaudette, M. D. (1992). Clinical decision making in neuropsychology: Bootstrapping the neuropsychologist utilizing Brunswik's lens model (Doctoral dissertation, Indiana University of Pennsylvania, 1992). *Dissertation Abstracts International, 53*, 2059B.

Gauron, E. F., & Dickinson, J. K. (1969). The influence of seeing the patient first on diagnostic decision making in psychiatry. *American Journal of Psychiatry, 126*, 199–205.

Goldberg, L. R. (1959). The effectiveness of clinicians' judgments: The diagnosis of organic brain damage from the Bender–Gestalt test. *Journal of Consulting Psychology, 23*, 25–33.

Goldberg, L. R. (1965). Diagnosticians versus diagnostic signs: The diagnosis of psychosis versus neurosis from the MMPI. *Psychological Monographs, 79*(9, Whole No. 602).

Goldberg, L. R. (1968). Simple models or simple processes? Some research on clinical judgments. *American Psychologist, 23*, 483–496.

Goldstein, S. G., Deysach, R. E., & Kleinknecht, R. A. (1973). Effect of experience and amount of information on identification of cerebral impairment. *Journal of Consulting and Clinical Psychology, 41*, 30–34.

Graham, J. R. (1967). A Q-sort study of the accuracy of clinical descriptions based on the MMPI. *Journal of Psychiatric Research, 5*, 297–305.

Graham, J. R. (1971). Feedback and accuracy of clinical judgments from the MMPI. *Journal of Consulting and Clinical Psychology, 36*, 286–291.

Grebstein, L. (1963). Relative accuracy of actuarial prediction, experienced clinicians, and graduate students in a clinical judgment task. *Journal of Consulting Psychology, 37*, 127–132.

Grigg, A. E. (1958). Experience of clinicians, and speech characteristics and statements of clients as variables in clinical judgment. *Journal of Consulting Psychology, 22*, 315–319.

Griswold, P. M., & Dana, R. H. (1970). Feedback and experience effects on psychological reports and predictions of behavior. *Journal of Clinical Psychology, 26*, 439–442.

Groth-Marnat, G., & Roberts, L. (1998). Human Figure Drawings and House-Tree-Person drawings as indicators of self-esteem: A quantitative approach. *Journal of Clinical Psychology, 54*, 219–222.

Hammond, K. R. (1955). Probabilistic functioning and the clinical method. *Psychological Review, 62*, 255–262.

Hammond, K. R., Hursch, C. J., & Todd, F. J. (1964). Analyzing the components of clinical inference. *Psychological Review, 71*, 438–456.

Haverkamp, B. E. (1993). Confirmatory bias in hypothesis testing for client-identified and counselor self-generated hypotheses. *Journal of Counseling Psychology, 40*, 303–315.

Hawkins, S. A., & Hastie, R. (1990). Hindsight: Biased judgments of past events after the outcomes are known. *Psychological Bulletin, 107*, 311–327.

Heaton, R. K., Smith, H. H., Jr., Lehman, R. A. W., & Vogt, A. T. (1978). Prospects for faking believable deficits on neuropsychological testing. *Journal of Consulting and Clinical Psychology, 46*, 892–900.

Hermann, R. C., Ettner, S. L., Dorwart, R. A., Langman-Dorwart, N., & Kleinman, S. (1999). Diagnoses of patients treated with ECT: A comparison of evidence-based standards with reported use. *Psychiatric Services, 50*, 1059–1065.

Hiler, E. W., & Nesvig, D. (1965). An evaluation of criteria used by clinicians to infer pathology from figure drawings. *Journal of Consulting Psychology, 29*, 520–529.

Holmes, C. B., & Howard, M. E. (1980). Recognition of suicide lethality factors by physicians, mental health professionals, ministers, and college students. *Journal of Consulting and Clinical Psychology, 48*, 383–387.

Holsopple, J. Q., & Phelan, J. G. (1954). The skills of clinicians in analysis of projective tests. *Journal of Clinical Psychology, 10*, 307–320.

Horowitz, L. M., Inouye, D., & Siegelman, E. Y. (1979). On averaging judges' ratings to increase their correlation with an external criterion. *Journal of Consulting and Clinical Psychology, 47*, 453–458.

Horowitz, M. J. (1962). A study of clinicians' judgments from projective test protocols. *Journal of Consulting Psychology, 26*, 251–256.

Johnston, R., & McNeal, B. F. (1967). Statistical versus clinical prediction: Length of neuropsychiatric hospital stay. *Journal of Abnormal Psychology, 72*, 335–340.

Kahill, S. (1984). Human figure drawing in adults: An update of the empirical evidence, 1967–1982. *Canadian Psychology, 25*, 269–292.

Kahneman, D., Slovic, P., & Tversky, A. (Eds.). (1982). *Judgment under uncertainty: Heuristics and biases.* New York: Cambridge University Press.

Karson, S., & Freud, S. L. (1956). Predicting diagnoses with the MMPI. *Journal of Clinical Psychology, 12*, 376–379.

Kayne, N. T., & Alloy, L. B. (1988). Clinician and patient as aberrant actuaries: Expectation-based distortions in assessment of covariation. In L. Y. Abramson (Ed.), *Social cognition and clinical psychology: A synthesis* (pp. 295–365). New York: Guilford Press.

Kendell, R. E. (1973). Psychiatric diagnoses: A study of how they are made. *British Journal of Psychiatry, 122*, 437–445.

Lambert, L. E., & Wertheimer, M. (1988). Is diagnostic ability related to relevant training and experience? *Professional Psychology: Research and Practice, 19*, 50–52.

Leli, D. A., & Filskov, S. B. (1981). Clinical-actuarial detection and description of brain impairment with the W-B Form I. *Journal of Clinical Psychology, 37*, 623–629.

Leli, D. A., & Filskov, S. B. (1984). Clinical detection of intellectual deterioration associated with brain damage. *Journal of Clinical Psychology, 40*, 1435–1441.

Levenberg, S. B. (1975). Professional training, psychodiagnostic skill, and Kinetic Family Drawings. *Journal of Personality Assessment, 39*, 389–393.

Loftus, E. F. (1993). The reality of repressed memories. *American Psychologist, 48*, 518–537.

Logue, M. B., Sher, K. J., & Frensch, P. A. (1992). Purported characteristics of adult children of alcoholics: A possible "Barnum Effect." *Professional Psychology: Research and Practice, 23*, 226–232.

Luft, J. (1950). Implicit hypotheses and clinical predictions. *Journal of Abnormal and Social Psychology, 45*, 756–760.

Meehl, P. E. (1956). Wanted—a good cookbook. *American Psychologist, 11*, 263–272.

Meehl, P. E. (1997). Credentialed persons, credentialed knowledge. *Clinical Psychology: Science and Practice, 4*, 91–98.

Motta, R. W., Little, S. G., & Tobin, M. I. (1993). The use and abuse of human figure drawings. *School Psychology Quarterly, 8*, 162–169.

Muller, M. J., & Davids, E. (1999). Relationship of psychiatric experience and interrater reliability in assessment of negative symptoms. *Journal of Nervous and Mental Diseases, 187*, 316–318.

Nadler, E. B., Fink, S. L., Shontz, F. C., & Brink, R. W. (1959). Objective scoring vs. clinical evaluation of the Bender-Gestalt. *Journal of Clinical Psychology, 15*, 39–41.

Ofshe, R., & Watters, E. (1994). *Making monsters: False memories, psychotherapy, and sexual hysteria.* New York: Scribner's.

Oskamp, S. (1962). The relationship of clinical experience and training methods to several criteria of clinical prediction. *Psychological Monographs, 76* (28, Whole No. 547).

Oskamp, S. (1965). Overconfidence in case-study judgments. *Journal of Consulting Psychology, 29*, 261–265.

Robiner, W. N. (1978). *An analysis of some of the variables influencing clinical use of the Bender-Gestalt.* Unpublished manuscript.

Schaeffer, R. W. (1964). Clinical psychologists' ability to use the Draw-A-Person Test as an indicator of personality adjustment. *Journal of Consulting Psychology, 28*, 383.

Schinka, J. A., & Sines, J. O. (1974). Correlates of accuracy in personality assessment. *Journal of Clinical Psychology, 30,* 374–377.

Schmidt, L. D., & McGowan, J. F. (1959). The differentiation of human figure drawings. *Journal of Consulting Psychology, 23,* 129–133.

Silverman, L. H. (1959). A Q-sort study of the validity of evaluations made from projective techniques. *Psychological Monographs, 73*(7, Whole No. 477).

Snyder, C. R. (1995). Clinical psychology building inspection: Slipping off its science-based foundation [Review of the book *House of cards: Psychology and psychotherapy built on myth*]. *Contemporary Psychology, 40,* 422–424.

Soskin, W. F. (1954). Bias in postdiction from projective tests. *Journal of Abnormal and Social Psychology, 49,* 69–74.

Stelmachers, Z. T., & McHugh, R. B. (1964). Contribution of stereotyped and individualized information to predictive accuracy. *Journal of Consulting Psychology, 28,* 234–242.

Stricker, G. (1967). Actuarial, naive clinical, and sophisticated clinical prediction of pathology from figure drawings. *Journal of Consulting Psychology, 31,* 492–494.

Swensen, C. H. (1957). Empirical evaluations of human figure drawings. *Psychological Bulletin, 54,* 431–466.

Thomas, G. V., & Jolley, R. P. (1998). Drawing conclusions: A re-examination of empirical and conceptual bases for psychological evaluation of children from their drawings. *British Journal of Clinical Psychology, 37,* 127–139.

Todd, F. J. (1954). *A methodological analysis of clinical judgment.* Unpublished doctoral dissertation, University of Colorado, Boulder.

Turner, D. R. (1966). Predictive efficiency as a function of amount of information and level of professional experience. *Journal of Projective Techniques and Personality Assessment, 30,* 4–11.

Walker, C. D., & Linden, J. D. (1967). Varying degrees of psychological sophistication in the interpretation of sentence completion data. *Journal of Clinical Psychology, 23,* 229–231.

Walker, E., & Lewine, R. J. (1990). Prediction of adult-onset schizophrenia from childhood home movies of the patients. *American Journal of Psychiatry, 147,* 1052–1056.

Walters, G. D., White, T. W., & Greene, R. L. (1988). Use of the MMPI to identify malingering and exaggeration of psychiatric symptomatology in male prison inmates. *Journal of Consulting and Clinical Psychology, 56,* 111–117.

Wanderer, Z. W. (1969). Validity of clinical judgments based on human figure drawings. *Journal of Consulting and Clinical Psychology, 33,* 143–150.

Watson, C. G. (1967). Relationship of distortion to DAP diagnostic accuracy among psychologists at three levels of sophistication. *Journal of Consulting Psychology, 31,* 142–146.

Waxer, P. (1976). Nonverbal cues for depth of depression: Set versus no set. *Journal of Consulting and Clinical Psychology, 44,* 493.

Wedding, D. (1983). Clinical and statistical prediction in neuropsychology. *Clinical Neuropsychology, 5,* 49–55.

Weiss, J. H. (1963). The effect of professional training and amount and accuracy of information on behavioral prediction. *Journal of Consulting Psychology, 27,* 257–262.

Whitehead, W. C. (1985). Clinical decision making on the basis of Rorschach, MMPI, and automated MMPI report data (Doctoral dissertation, University of Texas at Southwestern Medical Center at Dallas, 1985). *Dissertation Abstracts International, 46–08B,* 2828.

Wiggins, J. S. (1973). *Personality and prediction: Principles of personality assessment.* Reading, MA: Addison-Wesley.

3

Controversial and Questionable Assessment Techniques

JOHN HUNSLEY
CATHERINE M. LEE
JAMES M. WOOD

At the heart of the scientific enterprise, including a scientific approach to psychological assessment, lie the principles of falsifiability and methodological skepticism (e.g., Alcock, 1991; Bunge, 1991; Popper, 1959). At a minimum, these principles require that claims about the scientific merits or validity of a hypothesis, measure, or theory be framed in a such a way that they can be (1) subjected to empirical investigation (i.e., by data-based investigation, rather than by reliance on appeals to anecdotal evidence or to special knowledge or authority), (2) refuted or disconfirmed by empirical investigation, and (3) independently investigated (and ideally replicated) by both proponents and critics of the claims. Moreover, there is a presumption in the scientific enterprise that the burden of proof to evaluate or demonstrate the validity of such claims rests with those who are making them (Lett, 1990). It is therefore incumbent on proponents of an assessment strategy to demonstrate empirical evidence of its reliability and validity and to supply norms for relevant populations.

In this chapter, we focus on a particular class of assessment approaches and techniques that are widely used, but considered questionable by most psychologists who adhere to scientific principles. The assessment techniques that we discuss may have some limited merit as indicators of psychological phenomena, but they are commonly used in clinical practice in a manner that goes well beyond what is appropriate or justifiable based on scientific evidence.

PSYCHOLOGICAL TESTS

Psychological assessment is not synonymous with psychological testing (cf. Matarazzo, 1986), but psychological tests commonly comprise a major part of the assessment process. We therefore focus on specific problematic psychological tests. There are thousands of psychological tests, which vary enormously in their complexity and scientific merit. By definition, a psychological test is the measurement of a sample of behavior obtained under standardized conditions and that has established rules for scoring or interpreting this sample (Anastasi, 1988).

Standards for psychological tests and for their appropriate professional use are well-developed and widely known (*Standards for Educational and Psychological Testing*, 1985, 1999). These standards set out the criteria against which psychological tests are evaluated. They also serve to ensure that test developers and test users meet consensually defined expectations, held by the profession and the public, with regard to the scientifically appropriate use of tests. Proponents of questionable and controversial tests frequently claim the legitimacy that is associated with scientifically sound measures. However, they also sometimes deny that their test should be subjected to the high standards expected of a psychological test because it is not "really" a test, but merely a method for collecting information.

TEST CONSTRUCTION AND PSYCHOMETRIC PRINCIPLES

We next focus on elements that are required for a test to be both psychometrically sound and clinically useful. These elements, which hold for all types of psychological tests, are standardization (of stimuli, administration, and scoring), reliability, validity, and norms.

Standardization is essential for a psychological test, as it is the first step in ensuring that obtained results can be replicated by another assessor. Unless there is standardization, any results are likely to be highly specific to the unique aspects of the testing situation. Standardization is necessary to ensure that the influence of unique aspects of the testing situation and the assessor are minimized. To this end, test developers typically provide detailed instructions regarding the nature of the stimuli, administrative procedures, time limits (if relevant), and the types of verbal probes and responses to the examinee's questions that are permitted. Instructions must also be provided for the scoring of the test. In some cases, only simple addition of responses is required to obtain a test result; however, even in these cases, there is clear evidence that computational errors that compromise the validity of the results often arise (e.g., Allard, Butler, Faust, & Shea, 1995). For many tests, complex scoring rules may require that assessors receive extensive training to achieve proficiency in accurate scoring.

Reliability is the next criterion that must be addressed in the development of a scientifically sound test. The basic issue addressed by reliability is one of consistency—whether (1) all aspects of the test contribute in a meaningful way to the data obtained (internal consistency), (2) similar results would be obtained if the test was conducted and/or scored by another evaluator (interrater reliability), and (3) similar results would be obtained if the person was retested after the initial test (retest reliability or test stability). That is, standardization of stimuli, administration, and scoring are necessary, but not sufficient, to establish reliability. Reliable results are crucial for generalizing the results and their psychological implications beyond the immediate context of the assessment. Even thorough and complete test standardization cannot guarantee reliability. For example, the test may consist of too many components that are influenced by ephemeral characteristics of the examinee or by contextual characteristics of the testing, including demand characteristics associated with the purpose of the testing or the behavior of the examiner. Alternatively, the scoring criteria for the test may be too complicated or insufficiently detailed to ensure reliable scoring across different assessors.

Validity addresses the issue of whether the test measures what it purports to measure. A standardized and reliable test does not necessarily yield valid data. Validity is a matter of ensuring that the test samples the type of behavior that is relevant to the purpose of the test (content validity), provides data consistent with theoretical postulates associated with the phenomena being assessed (concurrent and predictive validity), and provides a measure of the phenomenon that is minimally contaminated by other psychological phenomena (discriminant validity). In applied contexts, an additional form of validity should be considered, namely incremental validity—the extent to which data from a test add to our knowledge over and above the information gleaned from other data (Sechrest, 1963). Although it is common to talk about a test as either valid or invalid, actual validity is far more complex. Many psychological tests consist of subscales designed to measure discrete aspects of a more global construct. In such situations, it is erroneous to talk about the validity of the test, because the validity of each subscale must be established. Moreover, global validity of a test or subscale does not exist because validity is always established within certain parameters, such that a test may be valid for specific purposes within specific groups of people (e.g., specific ages or genders). Finally, a test may be used for multiple purposes, but its validity for each purpose must be empirically established. For example, knowing that a self-report test of psychological distress is a valid indicator of diagnostic status does not automatically support its use for such forensic purposes as determining competency or child custody arrangements.

For a test to be clinically useful, it must meet the criteria of standardization, reliability, and validity. However, to meaningfully interpret the results obtained from a single individual, it is essential to have norms, specific criterion-related cutoff scores, or both (*Standards for Educational and Psychological Testing*, 1999). Without such reference points, it is impossible to determine the meaning of the test results. The results must be compared with some type of standard to have meaning: Knowing that a person scored low or high on a test (i.e., relative to the range of possible scores) provides no meaningful information. Comparisons must be made with either criteria that have been set for a test (e.g., a certain degree of accuracy as demonstrated in the test is necessary for the satisfactory performance of a job) or with population norms. Selecting the target population(s) for the establishment of norms and then actually developing the norms are challenging tasks. For example, are the norms to be used for comparing a specific score with those that might be obtained within the general population or within specific subgroups of this population (e.g., gender-specific norms), or are the norms to be used for establishing the likelihood of membership in specific categories (e.g., nondistressed versus psychologically disordered groups)? As with validity considerations, it may be necessary to develop multiple norms for a test, based on the group being assessed and the intent of the assessment.

DISTINGUISHING BETWEEN VALID AND INVALID USE OF ASSESSMENT TECHNIQUES: OR, WHEN IS A TEST NOT A TEST?

Building on these considerations, the appropriate use of psychometrically sound tests requires that guidelines for administration and scoring are followed and that relevant validity data and group norms are used to interpret the obtained data. Care must be taken to ensure that the test is valid for the assessment purpose at hand and for the person being assessed.

Widely accepted definitions of psychological tests should enable psychologists to determine whether an assessment technique should be considered as a test. Specifically, there are two necessary conditions for defining an information-gathering activity as a psychological test. First, a sample of behavior is collected in order to generate statements about a person, a person's experiences, or a person's psychological functioning. Second, a claim is made or implied that the accuracy or validity of these statements stem from the way in which the sample was collected (i.e., the nature of the stimuli, technique, or process that gave rise to the sample of behavior), not just from the expertise, authority, or special qualifications of the assessor. When both conditions are present, we consider that the process used to collect and interpret the behavioral sample is a psychological test. This is consistent with the recently revised standards for psychological tests, which emphasize that an assessment method that relies on or uses the concepts and techniques of psychological testing is a test (*Standards for Educational and Psychological Testing*, 1999). Despite the apparent clarity of this definition, proponents of questionable techniques sometimes employ the term "psychological test" loosely, arguing simultaneously that scientific and professional standards, expectations, and responsibilities are inapplicable to their techniques, while also claiming a valid approach that is supported by scientific evidence. Thus, the issue of whether a specific form of data collection constitutes a test is far from an ivory tower concern for semantic hair-splitting.

For example, the Rorschach Inkblot Test has been used by clinical psychologists for many decades. Some Rorschach proponents have argued that the Rorschach is not a psychological test at all, but that it is instead a method of interviewing that generates data relevant to the practice of clinical assessment (e.g., Aronow, Reznikoff, & Moreland, 1995; Weiner, 1994). A slight variation on this approach is to treat the Rorschach as a test (by using a recognized scoring system), but then "enriching" the test results with personalized, interpretive speculations stemming from selected aspects of the examinee's test responses (e.g., Acklin, 1995; Fischer, 1994). Such positions allow the Rorschach assessor to claim that there is scientific evidence supporting the use of the Rorschach, while simultaneously freeing the assessor to use the data in a manner unconstrained by issues of administration, norms, reliability, or validity. An example of the problem associated with failing to recognize a test *as* a test is contained in a recent guide to conducting child custody evaluations (Ackerman, 1995). The author recommended that a Rorschach protocol be scored with Exner's (1993) Comprehensive System (a scoring system which, as we will demonstrate in a subsequent section, has some limited scientific merits) to comply with professional standards. However, he then contradicted this position by suggesting that it was not always necessary to score a Rorschach protocol, for an experienced clinician can allegedly assess anxiety, depression, and thought disorder on the Rorschach without going through the rigor of formal scoring (p. 116). This type of contradictory reasoning is common among some users of controversial tests.

CONTROVERSIAL AND QUESTIONABLE ASSESSMENT TECHNIQUES: SOME EXAMPLES

At this point, we consider a number of problematic assessment techniques that, according to surveys of assessment practices, are used by large numbers of clinical psychologists. Of course, there are many other examples of unscientific psychological assessment techniques that one could consider (e.g., for a thorough critique of graphology, see Beyerstein & Beyerstein, 1992). However, we have chosen to focus on five questionable assessment

techniques that continue to be routinely used by psychologists: the Rorschach Inkblot Test, the Thematic Apperception Test (TAT), projective
drawings, anatomically detailed dolls (ADDs), and the Myers–Briggs Type
Indicator (MBTI).

Psychologists in the domain of personality assessment have long distinguished between projective tests and self-report inventories (Anastasi,
1988). Projective tests such as the Rorschach or TAT generally present the
person being tested with an ambiguous stimulus (such as an inkblot or a
picture without a caption) and ask for an open-ended response to the stimulus (e.g., "What might this be?" or "What do you think is happening in
this picture?"). In contrast, self-report inventories generally present the
examinee with a statement (e.g., "I often feel like crying") and ask the person to choose among two or more responses to indicate the extent to
which the statement accurately reflects the person's experience.

Among problematic techniques discussed in this chapter, the majority
fit the definition of projective techniques. As we will demonstrate, problems of standardization are rife among projective techniques. Questionable
techniques are not, however, limited to projectives. To illustrate this point,
we review a self-report personality measure, the MBTI. Although standardization is not an issue with this test, concerns about its reliability and
validity highlight the need for clinicians to select tests that have firm scientific support.

THE RORSCHACH INKBLOT TEST

The Rorschach Inkblot Test consist of 10 cards, each containing symmetri-
cal inkblots, some in color and some in black and white. Examinees are
asked to report what they see in these ambiguous stimuli. According to
Rorschach proponents, important evidence regarding psychological functioning can be obtained from the Rorschach when one considers the nature
of what is seen, what aspects of the card are used in the responses, the sequence of responses given during testing, and even the examinee's nonverbal reactions to the inkblots. For much of the 20th century, several distinct
approaches to the administration and scoring of the Rorschach existed,
and many clinicians tended to use elements of different systems and to
"personalize" the scoring and interpretation of the Rorschach based on
their own experiences (Exner & Exner, 1972). However, Exner's Comprehensive System (CS; Exner, 1974, 1993) has become the prevailing approach to teaching and researching the Rorschach (Hilsenroth & Handler,
1995; Shontz & Green, 1992). Indeed, it has been suggested that the CS
should now be considered the primary scoring system in evaluating the scientific status of the Rorschach (Weiner, 2001). Exner's approach focuses
on structural elements of Rorschach responses (i.e., the specific features of

the inkblot that are involved in the response) and emphasizes the need to use appropriate scientific data in interpreting the test. In contrast to many Rorschach proponents (e.g., Weiner, 1994), Exner has always insisted that the Rorschach is a psychological test and, as such, must meet the standards expected of a test (e.g., Exner, 1997).

As the most commonly researched and used projective measure (Butcher & Rouse, 1996; Watkins, Campbell, Nieberding, & Hallmark, 1995), the Rorschach has been the focus of a great deal of scientific attention over the past 50 years. Even Rorschach proponents have accepted the fact that most early research (i.e., before 1970) was so poor that it should not be regarded as offering evidence for the validity of the test (Exner, 1986). As a result of the ascendancy of the CS, this Rorschach scoring method has been the subject of increased scientific scrutiny from both proponents and critics of the Rorschach. It is to this evidence that we now turn.

Standardization

The Rorschach is a complex measure to administer, score, and interpret, requiring a modal time of 3 hours of clinician time (Ball, Archer, & Imhof, 1994). The CS offers very clear information on administration and scoring, with extensive tables and computer software to aid in the interpretation of the test results. Assessors are provided directions on the seating arrangement to be used, the sequence of card administration, the instructions to be given to examinees, and the permissible type of assessor probes and responses to questions. The CS also requires that responses to all cards be obtained before the assessor queries the examinee, response by response, on the elements of the card that influenced the responses of the examinee (known as "determinants").

As the evidence from surveys on the clinical use of the Rorschach suggest that the majority of clinical psychologists use the test, at least occasionally, it is surprising that there are no data on the extent of assessors' fidelity in following CS administration and scoring requirements. Because many graduate courses on the Rorschach include information on multiple scoring systems, and about one third of these courses do not even teach the CS (Hilsenroth & Handler, 1995), there is no reason to believe that the traditional tendency of Rorschach users to "borrow" scores from different scoring systems and to personalize the scoring has diminished. This is a key issue in evaluating the scientific basis of the Rorschach in clinical use, for without evidence that Rorschach data were obtained in a fashion consistent with CS requirements, research stemming from the CS cannot be used to support the assessor's interpretation of the examinee's responses. Even if CS administrative requirements are scrupulously followed, there is extensive evidence that relatively innocuous contextual factors in Rorschach administration, such as the layout of the testing room and the appearance of the assessor, affect examinees' responses (Masling, 1992). Thus, the bottom line with regard to the routine clinical use of the Rorschach is that there is no certainty that a Rorschach has been administered according to CS standards, nor is there any certainty that test data have not been contaminated by extraneous influences.

Norms

Since developing the CS, Exner has published numerous norms for different age groups (e.g., Exner, 1993) that have become a cornerstone of the scientific basis of the CS for years. For the 1993 norms, 700 nonpatient adults were selected from a larger pool of participants in an attempt to approximate a stratified, representative sample. Although members of some minority groups were included in this selected sample, there are neither separate norms nor interpretive guidelines for any minority groups, which poses a significant problem for the clinical use of the Rorschach with members of these groups (cf. Garb, Wood, Nezworski, Grove, & Stejskal, 2001; Gray-Little & Kaplan, 1998). As research frequently finds that minority groups score differently on the Rorschach, and as there has been little systematic examination of differential validity among ethnic groups, it is unclear whether the CS norms are appropriate for use in testing members of minority groups (see, however, Meyer, 2002).

Two major questions have been raised about the clinical value and accuracy of the CS norms. Vincent and Harman (1991) compared the 1989 norms with data reported by Exner (1985, 1989) for comparison samples of patients with schizophrenia, depression, or personality disorders. After examining group differences on over 20 key CS variables, the researchers found that over four fifths of the variables did not differentiate between the nonpatient and the patient groups. These findings led Vincent and Harman to suggest that most of the variables were meaningless for routine clinical use of the Rorschach. The other vexing problem for the CS norms is the likelihood that nonpatient norms tend to overpathologize normal individuals, a phenomenon found for both child and adult samples (e.g., Meyer, 1991; Wideman, 1998). The extent of this problem was made vividly apparent in a recent study by Shaffer, Erdberg, and Haroian (1999), who administered the CS Rorschach, the Minnesota Multiphasic Personality Inventory, Second Edition (MMPI-2), and the Wechsler Adult Intelligence Scale—Revised (WAIS-R) to a sample of 123 nonpatient adults selected to be representative of the American population. Data from their sample closely matched the normative data for both the MMPI-2 and the WAIS-R. However, for the CS, sample means for numerous variables deviated substantially from the CS norms, with most discrepancies leading to the appearance of maladjustment in their sample compared with the norms.

Wood, Nezworski, Garb, and Lilienfeld (2001) reviewed 14 CS variables in 32 studies of nonpatient adults. The findings from these 32 studies were very similar to those of Shaffer et al. Nonpatient adults showed statistically and clinically significant discrepancies from the CS norms for all 14 variables. Overall, the nonpatient adults appeared strikingly pathological when compared with CS norms. In light of these findings, Wood and colleagues recommended that psychologists not use the CS norms in clinical or forensic settings.

Reliability

As there is a long-standing debate among Rorschach scholars regarding the relevance of internal consistency in assessing the reliability of the Rorschach (Reznikoff, Aronow, & Rauchway, 1982), evaluations of reliability have usually focused on interrater and test–retest reliability. One of the challenges involved in evaluating the interrater reliability of the CS Rorschach is the lack of consensus regarding what data unit should be evaluated for reliability (individual responses or summary scores gathered across responses) and what method of assessing reliability should be used (percentage agreement, Cohen's kappa, or intraclass correlation coefficients; see Meyer, 1997a, 1997b; Wood, Nezworski, & Stejskal, 1996a, 1996b, 1997). Leaving aside these considerations, how reliable is the CS across assessors when the best evidence is used? Acklin, McDowell, and Verschell (2000) recently reported intraclass coefficient values for most CS scores, for both normal and clinical samples. The median reliability was slightly above .80 (with a range of approximately .20 to 1.0), suggesting that many CS scores fall below the level commonly regarded as indicative of good interrater reliability. In contrast, the intraclass correlations for the WAIS-III subtests are consistently above .90 (Psychological Corporation, 1997). Moreover, given the complexity of CS scoring, data on the field reliability (i.e., interrater reliability among practicing clinicians) are urgently needed. Simply because highly trained and supervised scorers can attain good reliability for some scores does not imply that the typical Rorschach assessor can match these accomplishments.

As we next turn to consider the test–retest reliability of the CS Rorschach, it is important to note that even Rorschach proponents have stated that such values are likely to overestimate the Rorschach's reliability, as such values are especially prone to inflation due to memory effects (Aronow et al., 1995). Garb and colleagues (2001; see also Wood & Lilienfeld, 1999) recently reviewed the test–retest reliability values for the CS. They were able to locate test–retest values for approximately 40% of the 125 CS variables. Thus, over the course of several revisions of the CS manuals, Exner has not published stability data on approximately 60% of the CS variables. Test–retest coefficients have apparently never been reported for key variables of the CS, such as the Schizophrenia Index, Depression Index, and Hypervigilance Index.

Validity

The literature on the validity of the Rorschach is so large that it is impossible to adequately review it within the constraints of this chapter. Interested readers should consult recent reviews, both supportive and critical, of this literature (Garb, 1999; Garb et al., 2001; Hunsley & Bailey, 1999, 2001; Viglione, 1999; Weiner, 1996, 1997; Wood & Lilienfeld, 1999; Wood, Lilienfeld, Garb, & Nezworski, 2000; Wood, Nezworski, Stejskal, Garven, & West, 1999).

A number of meta-analyses have been conducted on the Rorschach over the past 20 years. The earliest (Atkinson, 1986; Parker, 1983) used meta-analytic techniques that are now considered inappropriate. Later meta-analyses (Hiller, Rosenthal, Bornstein, Berry, & Brunell-Neulieb, 1999; Parker, Hanson, & Hunsley, 1988), although providing some limited evidence for the validity of the Rorschach, have also been criticized on a number of methodological and statistical grounds (Garb, Florio, & Grove, 1998; Garb et al., 2001; Hunsley & Bailey, 1999). Taken together, these studies provide at least some evidence for the validity of a small number of CS variables. But as both critics and proponents of the Rorschach now agree, the validity of the Rorschach must be established for every scale (Hunsley & Bailey, 1999, 2001; Weiner, 2001; Wood et al., 1996a).

As the Rorschach is regarded as a test of personality and psychological functioning, it should correlate significantly with other measures of these qualities. Interestingly, this is not the case. Meta-analytic data indicate virtually no relation with other projective measures (a weighted mean r of .03; Hiller et al., 1999). If one considers the vast array of self-report measures of psychological functioning, the results are somewhat better (a weighted mean r of .28). However, in the face of hundreds of studies indicating weak associations between Rorschach scores and self-report indices purportedly assessing the same constructs, some Rorschach proponents have denied that one should expect such relations (e.g., Ganellen, 1996; Viglione, 1996, 1999).

In addition, many investigators have examined the links between Rorschach responses and diagnostic measures. Wood, Lilienfeld, Garb, and Nezworski (2000) examined over 150 Rorschach studies that examined such diagnoses such as schizophrenia, depression, posttraumatic stress disorder, dissociative identity disorder, dependent personality disorder, narcissistic personality disorder, borderline personality disorder, antisocial personality disorder, and psychopathy. Given the prominence accorded the Rorschach by many clinicians, Wood and colleagues' conclusions are sobering. They found that deviant verbalizations and bad form (i.e., providing responses that did not fit the nature of the inkblot) are associated with schizophrenia and perhaps bipolar disorder and schizotypal personality disorder. Similarly, they found that patients with borderline personality disorder tended to produce more deviant verbalizations than did individuals without this disorder. As disorganized, odd, or pressured speech are diagnostic criteria for most of these disorders, it is hardly surprising that these abnormalities are evident in Rorschach responses. Wood and colleagues found no strong evidence that the Rorschach could consistently detect depression, posttraumatic stress disorder, antisocial personality disorder, or any other psychiatric diagnoses. This conclusion is consistent with the results of the Hiller and colleagues (1999) meta-analysis, which found a weighted mean r of .18 when psychiatric diagnoses were used as the criterion in Rorschach validity studies. As the Rorschach has been touted for decades as a key measure of psychiatric disorders (e.g., Exner, 1993; Rapaport, Gill, & Shafer, 1946; Weiner, 1966), attempts by some Rorschach proponents to dismiss this negative research evidence by arguing that the Rorschach was never intended to be a diagnostic test (e.g., Weiner, 1999) appear to be little more than post hoc rationalizations for consistently negative results.

Rorschach proponents have often suggested that the best way to evaluate the validity of the Rorschach is to examine its incremental validity (e.g., Widiger & Schilling, 1980). However, Garb (1984) concluded that the addition of Rorschach data to demographic or self-report personality data never led to an increase in accuracy of personality assessments. It should be noted, though, that none of the studies included in the review used the CS. Given the limited evidence of convergent validity between the Rorschach and self-report measures, some Rorschach proponents have argued that this provides an opportunity for the Rorschach to add important clinical data beyond that available from such measures as the MMPI (e.g., Weiner, 1993). To date, evidence does not appear to support this contention. Archer and Gordon (1988) found that CS indices of depression and schizophrenia, when added to MMPI data, did not improve upon diagnostic efficiency. Similarly, Archer and Krishnamurthy (1997) reported that Rorschach indices did not improve upon the accuracy of MMPI-A indices in diagnosing depression and conduct disorder.

Conclusions

Of the tests we review in this chapter, the Rorschach has the longest history of empirical investigation. The CS has brought some order to the field and inspired a more scientific approach to the Rorschach. Unfortunately, there are no data on the extent to which the CS is used appropriately by assessors. Although many Rorschach proponents continue to insist upon the scientific merits of the Rorschach, there are serious problems with the norms, reliability, and validity of the CS. There is little evidence that the Rorschach possesses adequate convergent validity when examined vis-à-vis data from other projective tests, self-report measures of personality or psychological functioning, and diagnostic categories. Despite decades of research, there has been no convincing accumulation of data supporting the use of the Rorschach in routine clinical practice. As a result, contemporary critics of the Rorschach have suggested that there is insufficient scientific evidence to justify the continued use of the test in clinical settings (Garb, 1999; Hunsley & Bailey, 1999, 2001).

THEMATIC APPERCEPTION TEST

The Thematic Apperception Test (TAT; Murray, 1943) is a projective test in which examinees are asked to tell stories about pictures printed on cards. According to its developer, in creating these stories examinees reveal dominant drives, emotions, and conflicts of their personality, some of which may not be consciously accessible to the examinee. The TAT consists of 31 cards, with some cards intended for administration to male examinees and others intended for female examinees. Research does not support the clinical utility of the gender-specific card sets, as examinee gender and sex role are unrelated to the stories given to gender-matched and unmatched cards (Katz, Russ, & Overholser, 1993). Although the TAT was the first major "storytelling" test developed, there are a number of other such tests, including some designed for use with children, the elderly, and minority groups (Bellak & Abrams, 1997; Constantino, Malgady, Rogler, & Tsui, 1988; Kroon, Goudena, & Rispens, 1998). The TAT and similar tests are commonly used by clinical psychologists, and the proportion of users has remained relatively constant over the past decades (Watkins et al., 1995). Based on a survey of practitioners, the modal time for administration, scoring, and interpretation of the TAT appears to be about 1.5 hours (Ball et al., 1994).

Standardization and Norms

There is little information on the extent to which practitioners follow or modify the original instructions developed by Murray (1943) for the TAT. It is clear that there is little consistency in how many cards are selected, which cards are administered, and in which order they are presented (Groth-Marnat, 1997). For this reason, Vane (1981) concluded such that variability in administration renders comparisons across the research literature virtually impossible, and discussions of reliability and validity point-less. Almost a decade later, Keiser and Prather (1990) found that, across TAT studies, there was little consistency in card selection and even whether cards described as comprising the TAT stimuli were in the original set developed by Murray.

With regard to scoring and interpretation, a number of differing systems, other than that proposed by Murray (1943), have been developed for the TAT in the past 50 years. However, unlike the Rorschach, no single scoring system has been consistently recognized as offering the promise of valid results. The earliest efforts to establish the TAT as a scientifically sound test were made by Eron (1950, 1953) and Murstein (1965, 1972), who developed normative data and a listing of themes typically obtained for each card. Using some of the TAT cards and adding other picture stimuli, McClelland and colleagues conducted a programmatic series of studies on achievement, power, and affiliative needs (for reviews, see McClelland, Koestner, & Weinberger, 1989; Spangler, 1992). These stimuli and the associated scoring systems have not been routinely incorporated into clinical practice. Perhaps the most consistently used scoring and interpretational system in recent decades is that developed by Bellak (e.g., Bellak & Abrams, 1997). A set series of cards is prescribed in this system, and summary scores are obtained for a number of coding categories (e.g., unconscious structure and drives of the examinee, relationship to others, main defenses used). Specific, theoretically developed criteria are used to assist in the rating of the examinee's ego functions. After completing the scoring, the data are interpreted at the descriptive, interpretive, and diagnostic levels.

Even ardent proponents of the TAT admit that most clinicians do not use these scoring and interpretative systems and have thus abandoned a psychometric approach to the test (Dana, 1985; Rossini & Moretti, 1997). For example, in a survey of 100 psychologists practicing in juvenile and family courts, Pinkerman, Haynes, and Keiser (1993) found that only 3% formally scored the TAT. The TAT is therefore currently best characterized as a test that (1) is taught and used in a manner that ignores scientific and professional standards and (2) emphasizes the clinician's intuitive interpretative skills (Rossini & Moretti, 1997; Telgasi, 1993). The problems with such a stance are clear, and they have been raised repeatedly by TAT proponents and critics alike (e.g., Garb, 1998; Holt, 1999).

Reliability and Validity

Given the current state of the TAT clinical literature, there is little point in attempting to review the reliability and validity of the test as it is typically used by clinical psychologists. We instead focus on McClelland's need-based scoring and recent efforts to revitalize the TAT through the use of coding systems that have demonstrated encouraging reliability and validity.

Spangler (1992) conducted a meta-analytic review of research on TAT-based measures of achievement needs. He found little association between TAT and self-report measures of achievement needs (a mean correlation of .09). The two types of measures were comparable in their ability to predict respondent behavior such as academic performance (the mean correlations were .19 for TAT measures and .15 for the self-report measures). However, TAT measures were superior to the self-report measures in predicting long-term operant outcomes such as income or career success (mean correlations of .22 and .13, respectively). These patterns of results are generally consistent with McClelland's theoretical formulations about (1) the importance of differentiating between implicit motives (i.e., needs) and explicit self-knowledge and (2) the relative values of these characteristics in predicting future behavior.

Over the past decade, Cramer has developed a scoring system for assessing defense mechanisms from TAT stories. As with other standardized systems, clear instructions are available for card selection, administration, and scoring. As reported in numerous studies by Cramer and collaborators, the interrater reliabilities for the measures of denial, projection, and identification are usually in the acceptable range. However, values for internal consistency, alternate forms reliability, and retest reliability are unacceptably low (Cramer, 1991). Cramer (1999) recently reviewed over a dozen studies suggesting that the scoring system had demonstrated validity in a range of populations, including children, adolescents, nonpatient adults, and adults with psychiatric conditions. However, closer examination of these results reveals that there is little consistency across studies in terms of precisely how the defense mechanism scores are related to measures of adjustment and distress.

Westen has developed a psychodynamically oriented scoring system for TAT responses. His system focuses on the assessment of object relations (specifically, complexity of representations of people, affect tone of relationship schemas, capacity for emotional investment in relationships, and understanding of social causality). Using a detailed scoring manual and data from five to seven TAT cards, high interrater reliability has been obtained in several studies for the Social Cognition and Object Relations Scale (e.g., Westen, Lohr, Silk, Gold, & Kerber, 1990). Data from nonpatient and patient samples indicate convergent validity with a range of self-report, interview, and projective measures (see Westen, 1991). Recent studies have found that the system can differentiate between clinical and nonclinical samples, including children with and without a history of physical abuse (Freedenfeld, Ornduff, & Kelsey, 1995), and among individuals with personality disorders (Ackerman, Clemence, Weatherill, & Hilsenroth, 1999).

TAT scoring systems have also been developed from nonpsychodynamic theoretical orientations. Peterson and Ulrey (1994), for example, developed a coding scheme to evaluate attributional style. Using written responses to four TAT cards chosen for negative content, they found that attributional dimensions of stability and globality could be reliably rated, and that the globality index correlated significantly with a self-report measure of attributional style. Ronan and colleagues (Ronan, Colavito, & Hammontree, 1993; Ronan, Date, & Weisbrod, 1995) have developed a scoring system to tap personal problem-solving strategy. In their system, three TAT cards are used. Their research has demonstrated both reliability and validity (convergent relations with self-report measures of problem solving) for this system. In randomized control studies, participants who received training in decision-making and problem-solving skills scored higher on the TAT index than did participants who received only minimal exposure to these skills.

Conclusions

Several lines of research have demonstrated that responses to TAT and similar stimuli can yield valid information about focused aspects of psychological functioning. However, these encouraging findings are almost totally irrelevant to the clinical use of the TAT, as most clinicians use the test as a global measure and fail to use the available standardized scoring systems that have some empirical support. It is now becoming almost routine for TAT proponents to inappropriately overgeneralize from the results of this research, such as that conducted by McClelland (McClelland et al., 1989; Spangler, 1992). As a result, there are an increasing number of statements in the literature that the TAT and other projective tests are valid and that they outperform self-report measures in predicting long-term behavioral patterns (e.g., Masling, 1997). Such claims are unfounded and largely misleading. A careful examination of the literature reveals that, as typically used in clinical practice, the TAT is a potentially useful measure that falls woefully short of professional and scientific test standards.

PROJECTIVE DRAWINGS

Various projective drawing techniques require the examinee to draw a person (Draw-A-Person [DAP]; Harris, 1963; Human Figure Drawing [HFD]; Koppitz, 1968), a house, a tree and a person (House–Tree–Person [HTP]; Buck, 1948), or a family engaged in some joint activity (Kinetic Family Drawing [KFD]; Burns & Kaufman, 1970). Advocates of each variant of projective drawing propose that their strategy allows a richer assessment of the psychological functioning of the examinee than is the case with other projective drawing techniques. For example, Handler and Habenicht (1994) emphasized that the introduction of movement into drawings dramatically changes the experience of the examinee.

Despite their alleged distinctions, surveys of psychologists' use of different assessment tools group these techniques together. Projective drawings have been ranked among the ten most commonly used assessment strategies by clinical psychologists (Watkins et al., 1995). Watkins and colleagues (1995) concluded that psychological assessment currently relies on similar tools to those that were central to practice 30 years ago.

Drawings are used to assess intellectual or emotional functioning in adults and children. In a recent survey, Ackerman and Ackerman (1997) found that projective drawings were among the top ten assessment strategies used in evaluating both adults and children in custody disputes. Projective drawings are employed by mental health practitioners of various disciplines that traditionally have varied in their degree of respect for or adherence to scientific principles, including art therapists, school counselors, psychiatrists, and psychologists. Proponents view drawings as providing access to unconscious material that the person would otherwise be unable or unwilling to communicate (Handler, 1985). They consider projective drawings as especially useful in the assessment of persons who are guarded or lack verbal skills. Proponents suggest that drawings can be used as a springboard for discussion, as well as for assessing progress in psychotherapy.

An abundant literature describes the importance of different characteristics of the drawings, including their size, the inclusion or absence of various features, the heaviness of the lines, the relative distance of figures from one another, and the complexity of the drawing. Machover (1949) proposed links between features of the drawings and various psychological features. For example, large eyes were assumed to reflect paranoia, heavy shading aggressive impulses, and repeated erasures anxiety. Efforts to integrate clinical lore surrounding the meaningfulness of diverse indicators have resulted in the publication of numerous scoring systems. Koppitz (1968) was the first to promote interpretation based on the whole drawing, rather than on interpretation of single indicators of pathology. Applying Koppitz's integrative principles, Naglieri and Pfeiffer (1992) developed the Draw-A-Person Screening Procedure for Emotional Disturbance (DAP-SPED), which shows promise in distinguishing clinical from nonclinical samples.

We know of no data on the numbers of practitioners who apply various scoring systems. Thus we are again faced with the dilemma of determining the pertinence of validity studies for actual clinical practice. Of great concern are articles in journals advocating the use of drawings to assess indications of sexual abuse in children's artwork (e.g., Riordan & Verdel, 1991). Proponents of projective drawings clearly attach great weight to their interpretations and attribute special powers to certain clinicians judged to possess particular acumen in interpreting drawings.

Standardization and Norms

There is variability in the instructions given to examinees completing projective drawings. Typically, examinees are provided with a supply of blank sheets of paper, pencils, and erasers. Instructions specify the size of the paper provided, but these instructions vary across protocols. In the DAP respondents are instructed to draw a picture of a person (Handler, 1985). The HTP requires the person to draw as good a house, tree, and person as possible (Hammer, 1985). The KFD requires the child to draw his or her family doing something. Directions are kept to a minimum, although some instructions explicitly state that the drawing should be of a person rather than a stick figure or cartoon character. In some approaches, examinees are asked to create a story about the drawing or are asked about their associations to the drawing, such as whether the person depicted is happy or sad.

Although a number of scoring systems have been developed, there is considerable use of idiosyncratic scoring based on each practitioner's experience and beliefs. There is an emerging consensus that data do not support the use of single indicators or signs of pathology, but that the drawings must be interpreted in a holistic fashion within the context of other assessment data (Handler & Habenicht, 1994).

Given the large number of different projective drawing techniques and the myriad scoring systems, it is not surprising that there are inadequate norms (Handler & Habenicht, 1994). One important issue that has not been sufficiently addressed is the examinee's level of competence in drawing or willingness to draw (Feldman & Hunt,1958; Nichols & Strumpfer, 1962). Before projective techniques could be used as part of a scientifically based assessment, it would be necessary to develop knowledge of the characteristics of drawings produced by examinees of different ages, of both genders, and different levels of aptitude and interest in drawing.

Reliability and Validity

There is some evidence of reliability in the qualities of drawings produced over a short interval, although reliability between raters tends to be poor (Palmer et al., 2000; Vass, 1998). One factor that mitigates against reliable interpretation is that a given feature can lead to different hypotheses (Thomas & Jolley, 1998). For example, in West's (1998) meta-analysis of the efficacy of projective techniques in discriminating abused and non-abused children, variations in head size were seen as indicative of sexual abuse in one study and physical abuse in another.

An evaluation of the validity of projective drawings is rendered more difficult by the existence of diverse techniques and scoring systems. There is intense and acrimonious discussion regarding the validity of projective drawings (e.g., Holtzman, 1993; Joiner, Schmidt, & Barnett, 1996; Motta, Little, & Tobin, 1993; Riethmiller & Handler, 1997). Critics note the lack of evidence for their validity (Joiner et al.,1996; Motta et al., 1993), whereas proponents castigate critics for their failure to recognize the rich clinical material that is accessible to nonskeptics (Reithmiller & Handler, 1997). Notably, there is little evidence that projective drawing "experts" are accurate in their capacity to identify different types of psychopathology (Wanderer, 1997; see also Chapter 3).

Recent research indicates one must distinguish quantitative approaches that rely on single indicators of pathology from qualitative approaches that use a more integrative approach (Tharinger & Stark, 1990). Tharinger and Stark (1990) found that holistic approaches to the DAP were useful in distinguishing children with mood and mood/anxiety disorders from children without such disorders. However, the qualitative approach to the DAP was not useful in distinguishing between children with and without anxiety disorders. Qualitative approaches to the KFD distinguished children with mood disorders (but not mood/anxiety disorders) from children without mood disorders.

A fundamental assumption of projective techniques is that they provide access to the unconscious and that by communicating with the client through a more "primitive" channel, the clinician may discover the client's true feelings and experiences. Thus, drawings are assumed to circumvent the client's defenses and provide invaluable material about psychological functioning that the client might otherwise be unable or unwilling to acknowledge. This assumption does not meet the scientific criterion of falsifiability, because the criterion against which the technique should be assessed is not measurable through other means.

Conclusions

Projective drawings maintain their place in the armamentarium of many psychologists despite the paucity of scientific evidence for their usefulness. Currently, diverse techniques with various scoring systems are used to discover aspects of functioning that the examinee is assumed to be unable or unwilling to express directly. Until hypotheses based on projective drawings are formulated in a manner that can be subjected to scientific scrutiny and are supported in rigorous studies, there can be no basis to the claims for the validity of these approaches. Given advances in other methods of assessing intelligence and psychological functioning, it is questionable whether resources should be devoted to the use of projective techniques that are vulnerable to a host of weaknesses and errors in administration, scoring, and interpretation. Indeed, a recent review concluded that projective drawings do not meet current standards for admissibility of evidence in a court of law (Lally, 2001).

ANATOMICALLY DETAILED DOLLS

The use of dolls in pediatric mental health services has a long history (Sattler, 1998). Dolls have been employed by clinicians working with very young children who possess limited cognitive and verbal skills on the assumption that through the dolls the children can express material that they are unable or unwilling to express verbally, such as experiences of sexual abuse. Mental health professionals may assist the courts in determining the accuracy of an allegation of child sexual abuse. This task is rendered more difficult by the fact that there is no syndrome of problem behaviors that is consistently or uniquely associated with sexual abuse (Kendall-Tackett, Williams, & Finkelhor, 1993).

In the search for strategies to evaluate children suspected of having been sexually abused, health professionals and law enforcement personnel developed dolls equipped with such anatomical features as anal and vaginal orifices, penises, pubic hair, and breasts (Koocher et al., 1995). These dolls are referred to as anatomically correct dolls, anatomically explicit dolls, or anatomically detailed dolls (ADDs). As these dolls do not always faithfully represent the human body, having sexual characteristics but sometimes lacking such facial details as ears (Koocher et al., 1995), we use the term ADDs here. Surveys have established widespread use of ADDs among professionals working with children who may have been abused (Conte, Sorenson, Fogarty, & Rosa, 1991; Kendall-Tackett & Watson, 1992). However, recent evidence suggests that only a minority (36%) of professionals who interview children to investigate alleged sexual abuse use ADDs (Davey & Hill, 1999). It is unclear whether the lower figure obtained by Davey and Hill reflects sampling differences or a decrease in the dolls' popularity.

Standardization and Norms

Standardized ADDs do not exist. Dolls are produced by many manufacturers and are available with different facial expressions and facial features. Dolls of different racial physiques are used, but there is no evidence to guide the choice of dolls, especially in the case of allegations of abuse in which the victim and perpetrator are of different racial backgrounds.

Everson and Boat (1994) identified 16 sets of published guidelines and 4 other unpublished, but widely disseminated, protocols describing the ways that dolls may be used in interviews. From these protocols, they established six major uses of the dolls, including comforter, icebreaker, anatomical model, demonstration aid, memory stimulus/diagnostic screen, and diagnostic test. Everson and Boat's analysis indicated that of the 20 protocols they evaluated, the most common functions of the dolls were as anatomical models ($n = 16$), demonstration aids ($n = 18$), and memory stimulus/diagnostic screen ($n = 11$). We know of no data indicating either the frequency with which each protocol is used, or the frequency with which clinicians use the dolls for a particular function.

Users vary in the number of evaluation sessions with ADDs and little is known about the effects on children of multiple exposure to ADDs (Ceci & Bruck, 1995). Moreover, some advocate that dolls are an integral part of the interview, whereas others recommend that they be produced only after a child has made a statement about having been abused. Dolls may be clothed, semiclothed, or naked. In the former cases, the examiner may undress the doll or ask the child to do so. Some protocols include questioning the child about names of various parts of the body. In some cases the child is simply left to play with the doll, either in the presence of the examiner, or alone (but unobtrusively observed).

Several researchers have attempted to determine the range of behaviors with ADDs typical of children who have and who have not been abused. However, differences in recruitment strategies, screening methods for abuse, stimulus materials, procedures, and scoring render comparisons almost impossible.

There is no universally accepted scoring system for the observational data gathered with ADDs. Proponents debate whether it is reasonable to make inferences based solely on the child's behavior with the dolls or whether verbal corroboration of abuse is required. Following scholarly reviews, some proponents argue that decisions about whether a child has been abused should not be made solely on the basis of their behavior with dolls (Everson & Boat, 1994; Koocher et al., 1995). However, in a relatively recent psychiatry textbook, the use of ADDs is promoted unequivocally as a means of determining the child's sexual experiences (Yates, 1997). This is particularly troublesome in light of evidence from proponents of ADDs that in one sample of children who had not been abused the majority of children engaged in touching, rubbing, poking and pinching body parts. Furthermore, 25% of 5-year-old boys responded to the direction "show me what the dolls can do together" by placing the dolls in a position suggestive of sexual intercourse (Boat & Everson, 1994; Everson & Boat, 1990). Thus, there is evidence that a significant minority of children who have not been abused engage in sexual exploration with ADDs.

Reliability and Validity

Given the lack of standardization across ADDs, it is not surprising that little research has addressed the reliability of assessments using ADDs. In one study the researchers reported that it was even difficult to assess objectively some parts of the interview (Levy, Markovic, Kalinowski, Ahart, & Torres, 1995). This lack of reliability in the rating of the objective aspects of the interview was dismissed by Levy and colleagues, who concluded that although there may be disagreement over individual statements and gestures there may be full agreement that the child's behavior over the entire interview was indicative of abuse.

There has been little examination of the stability of children's behavior with ADDs. One pilot study conducted by advocates of ADDs reevaluated 10 children who placed dolls in intercourse positions and 10 who did not. Sixteen months after the initial evaluation, changes in the frequency of sexualized and avoidant behavior with the dolls occurred in both groups (Boat, Everson, & Amaya-Jackson, 1996). This study sheds little light on the stability of doll play due to the long interval between sessions as well as the extremely small sample.

The use of ADDs is predicated on the assumption that children's behavior with the dolls is indicative of the child's sexual experiences. Reviews (Aldridge, 1998; Ceci & Bruck, 1995; Koocher et al., 1995; Wolfner, Faust, & Dawes, 1993) show remarkable consistency in their selection of pertinent studies and in the reporting of findings. Nevertheless, proponents and critics differ in their interpretation of the research findings and their willingness to tolerate Type I and Type II errors. Advocates focus on possible increases in the reporting of sensitive material with ADDs, whereas critics focus on possible errors and inaccuracies in reporting that are associated with the use of ADDs.

Having identified various uses of ADDs, Everson and Boat (1994) argued that questions of validity are pertinent only to the use of ADDs as a diagnostic test. They reject the use of ADDs for this purpose and thereby dismiss concerns about the lack of validity data. They instead promote the use of ADDs as "memory stimuli" in which the dolls are presumed to trigger memories of sexual experiences and as "diagnostic screens" in which dolls provide an opportunity for children to spontaneously reveal sexual knowledge. According to the *Standards for Educational and Psychological Testing* (1999), a screening test is used to make broad categorizations as a first step in selection or diagnostic decisions. Thus, if ADDs are used to screen for sexual abuse, even if they are used simply to generate initial hypotheses, they must meet the same standards as other psychological tests. That is, test developers must demonstrate that children's behavior in response to the stimuli is indicative of their experiences. To date, no studies have clearly established this link. On the contrary, even proponents of ADDs have found that children's sexualized behavior with the dolls may vary according to socioeconomic status and race, and that some play may reflect cultural differences in openness about sexuality rather than evidence that the child has been abused (Everson & Boat, 1990, 1994).

Everson and Boat (1994) illustrated the memory stimulus function of ADDs: "A clear example . . . is the case of a young child who, after noticing the pattern on the male doll's underwear stated, 'Granddaddy's underpants had hearts on them.' " (p. 117). This is an excellent example of how clinicians who are sensitized to child sexual abuse could misconstrue an ambiguous response. It is possible that the child has seen grandfather in his underwear, without there being any sexual abuse, or that the child has seen grandfather's underwear without him wearing it.

The American Psychological Association (APA) has commissioned two task forces to examine the validity of ADDs. The first concluded that although the dolls are not standardized and although there are no normative data and no uniform standards for conducting interviews, doll-centered assessment "used as part of a psychological evaluation and interpreted by experienced and competent examiners may be the best available practical solution for a pressing and frequent clinical problem (i.e., the investigation of the possible presence of sexual abuse of a child)" (American Psychological Association, 1991, p. 722). Furthermore, the task force exhorted psychologists who undertake doll-centered assessment to be competent (although this was not defined), to document their procedures, and to provide clinical and empirical rationales for their procedures and interpretations. These recommendations reflect a puzzling mixture of reliance on unspecified clinical wisdom coupled with reference to a research literature that the task force concluded was nonexistent.

The Anatomical Doll Working Group, funded by the APA (Koocher et al., 1995), reiterated the conclusion of the first task force, noting that ADDs do not meet any of the criteria for a valid psychological test or a projective technique. Koocher and colleagues (1995) advised that conclusions about child sexual abuse cannot be made on the basis of doll play alone and that reports of children under 4 years of age are particularly prone to be affected by misleading questions. These cautions notwithstanding, Koocher and colleagues reasserted the original APA task force position. Both APA resolutions reflect the tensions in psychological practice and the lip service paid to science by some psychologists who are willing to examine research literature, but equally willing to dismiss it if it does not correspond to views founded on their clinical experience.

Various reviewers have concluded that it is not clear what children's sexualized play with ADDs indicates (Babiker & Herbert, 1998). Critics charge that the incremental validity of ADDs must be demonstrated (e.g., Ceci & Bruck, 1995; Wolfner et al., 1993). That is, they argue that ADDs must be shown to consistently *add* to our ability to determine whether a child has been abused above and beyond already available information, such as interviews, observations, and rating scales. Advocates argue that ADDs are no worse than other assessment strategies (Aldridge, 1998; Koocher et al., 1995). This latter view stands in sharp contrast to the prototypical scientific position we noted earlier, namely that the onus of demonstration of the utility of a particular assessment strategy rests with its proponents.

Conclusion

Many proponents of ADDs adopt scientific language by referring to "evidence," "studies," "research," and "empirical support." However, they seek to absolve the procedures from the scrutiny of scientific standards by denying that ADDs constitute a psychological test. Paradoxically, some proponents promote their approaches as scientifically supported while rejecting arguments that these measures be held to scientific standards. We reiterate previous findings that neither the stimuli nor the procedures used in ADD assessments are standardized. Given this lack of standardization, it is impossible to collect normative data on the behavior of abused and nonabused children. We reject claims that ADDs can be used as screening instruments without meeting the standards for psychological tests and therefore strongly advise against their use for this purpose in investigations of child sexual abuse.

MYERS–BRIGGS TYPE INDICATOR

The Myers–Briggs Type Indicator (MBTI; Myers & McCaulley, 1985) is a self-report test based on Jung's personality theory. Jung's theory of personality types, designed to be a comprehensive account of personality functioning, posits four basic personality preferences that are operationalized in the MBTI as bipolar, continuous constructs: extraversion–intraversion (oriented outwardly or inwardly), sensing–intuition (reliance on sensorial information versus intuition), thinking–feeling (tendency to make judgments based on logical analysis or personal values), and judgment–perception (preference for using either thinking–feeling or sensing–intuition processes for interacting with the world). Based on scores obtained for these four dimensions, established cutoff scores are used to assign examinees to one of 16 different personality type categories (e.g., extraverted, sensing, thinking, judgment). The use of these 16 categories has been controversial, as they are consistent with neither Jungian theory nor data gathered from the MBTI (Barbuto, 1997; Garden, 1991; Girelli & Stake, 1993; Pittenger, 1993).

The MBTI is available in several versions, although the standard version is a forced-choice 126-item test. During the past two decades, the MBTI has been translated and normed in many languages, and it is among the most commonly used measures of normal personality (McCaulley, 1990). Although it was developed to be useful in education, counseling/therapy, career guidance, and workplace team-building, it is within the assessment practices of career guidance and personnel selection that the MBTI has gained dominance, so much so that it is routinely used by psychologists for gathering information on possible career paths and job placement (Coe, 1992; Jackson, Parker, & Dipboye, 1996; McCaulley & Martin, 1995; Turcotte, 1994). The research on the MBTI is impressive in scope, with hundreds of studies published in the past two decades on a range of personality, educational, and vocational constructs.

Standardization

Given that the MBTI is a published self-report test, standardization of test instructions and test items should be assured when used appropriately. Several short form versions of the test are available. However, because of concerns about limited comparability vis-à-vis the full test (Harvey, Murry, & Markham, 1994), use of these short forms is not recommended.

The MBTI manual (Myers & McCaulley, 1985) provides detailed instructions on scoring the MBTI and converting the scores to 1 of the 16 personality types. Information is also provided on how the results of the test should be interpreted, both in general terms and with reference to counseling, educational, and career counseling contexts. One of the problems with the use of the 16 types that has consistently emerged in the research literature is the appropriateness of the cutoffs used to assign examinees to a type. Researchers have found that scale scores close to the cutoffs frequently lead to classification errors. To address this issue, there have been calls for changes in response format and scale scoring (Girelli & Stake, 1993; Harvey & Murry, 1994; Harvey & Thomas, 1996; Tzeng, Ware, & Chen, 1989).

Norms

The normative information reported in the manual is based on data from tens of thousands of research participants. Normative data for men and women are available across a wide range of ages (15–60+ years) and occupations. Research has tended to support the appropriateness of these norms and to find them applicable across minority groups and cultures (e.g., Kaufman, Kaufman, & McLean, 1993). However, as the data for minority groups are limited and there is some question about the interpretation of age-related factors influencing these data (Cummings, 1995), users of the MBTI would be well advised also to consider data from a recent study designed to obtain normative data from a representative sample of American adults (Hammer & Mitchell, 1996).

Reliability and Validity

The MBTI has typically been found to exhibit acceptable levels of internal consistency and test–retest reliability (Carlson, 1985). However, these data typically focus on the reliability of the four preference scores (e.g., extraversion–intraversion), and far less evidence is available on the reliability of the 16 types.

Dozens of validity studies of the MBTI are available in the scientific literature. They tend to focus on relating MBTI preference scores and types to a myriad of personality constructs, ability measures, and occupations. Nevertheless, there has been no real attempt to integrate the data from these studies to guide the valid interpretation of the test results. Moreover, there is relatively limited information on the predictive validity (i.e., whether accurate predictions of educational and career choices can be made on the basis of the MBTI) or the incremental validity and utility (i.e., whether the MBTI meaningfully adds to the prediction of these decisions; whether there are optimal educational, career, or employment decisions made on the basis of MBTI data) of the MBTI.

One aspect of the MBTI that has received extensive attention in the literature is the validity of the 16 personality types. Using a range of analytical procedures, including exploratory factor analysis, confirmatory factor analysis, and cluster analysis, researchers have generally found that (1) the observed factor structure of the MBTI is consistent with the hypothesized four personality preferences (Thompson & Borrello, 1986; Tischler, 1994), although often at a less than optimal level (Harvey, Murry, & Stamoulis, 1995; Jackson et al., 1996; Sipps, Alexander, & Friedt, 1985), and (2) the fit between the hypothesized 16 types and actual test data is poor (Lorr, 1991; Pittenger, 1993; but see also Pearman & Fleenor, 1996).

As a measure of global personality, the MBTI has been criticized for its failure to relate to other well-established vocational and personality measures. Although the efforts of the test developers to include concurrent validity data with a range of such measures in the test manual is laudable, there is little consistent evidence that the four personality preferences relate to comparable constructs assessed by other measures. Published research suggests that the MBTI bears little correspondence to measures of vocational preferences and job performance (e.g., Apostal & Marks, 1990; Furnham & Stringfield, 1993). Additionally, as a measure of global personality, the MBTI has been found to have limited correspondence with either of the two prevailing scientific models of personality structure, namely Eysenck's three-factor model and the five-factor model (Furnham, 1996; McCrae & Costa, 1989; Saggino & Kline, 1996; Zumbo & Taylor, 1993; but see MacDonald, Anderson, Tsagarakis, & Holland, 1994). One can only conclude that the MBTI is insufficient as a contemporary measure of personality.

Conclusions

The MBTI is based on a explicit theory of personality, was developed and normed in a manner consistent with current standards, and has typically been found to be reliable at the level of the four personality preferences. However, questions about the reliability and validity of the 16 personality types and evidence of limited correspondence between the MBTI and other global measures of personality and vocational interests render the test suspect as an assessment tool. In the absence of a major revision of the test that addresses these shortcomings, psychologists are advised to rely on personality and vocational interest tests that have a sounder empirical basis (cf. Boyle, 1995).

CONCLUSIONS AND RECOMMENDATIONS

Psychologists face a daunting task in making sense of the vast literature on psychological assessment. In considering ways to address pressing clinical questions, they have access to a panoply of potential tools. Unfortunately, there are no simple ways to determine whether a test is scientifically valid. The fact that it is marketed in a prestigious professional newsletter or described in a scholarly journal provides no guarantee that it meets adequate test standards. For example, a recent meta-analysis (West, 1998) provided data that appeared to support the use of projective techniques in detecting sexual abuse in children. However, reexamination of the data revealed that the author had included in her calculations of effect sizes only significant findings, thereby inflating the apparent power of projectives to identify abused children (Garb, Wood, & Nezworski, 2000). Reference to research citations may therefore be inadequate in determining whether a test is appropriate. Many of the articles we reviewed contained abstracts claiming support for an assessment approach, although the article itself offered at best mixed support.

We urge psychologists to use as a reference the most recent edition of the *Standards for Educational and Psychological Testing* (1999), which restate and expand on the principles that have guided a scientifically based approach to assessment. Psychologists are required to engage in reasoned decision making as they select assessment tools. Knowledge of an assessment procedure may become obsolete as it is replaced by a more sophisticated understanding of its limitations. Psychologists using assessment procedures that lack a published manual are required to conduct their own scholarly review of the pertinent literature to determine whether the test meets basic standards of reliability and validity, and whether suitable norms exist. Those using published materials are also required to familiarize themselves with the data relevant to the use of the test. The fact that a published manual exists does not guarantee that the test meets standards of reliability and validity or that appropriate norms are available. Professional and ethical standards indicate that each psychologist is responsible for determining (1) the question that the psychological assessment is designed to answer, (2) whether there is a test that is adequately standardized and that yields reliable and valid information, and (3) whether pertinent norms allow interpretation of the responses on the test in a given circumstance. We caution psychologists against uncritically accepting the argument that a given assessment procedure is absolved from the obligation to meet accepted standards.

Among the tests we reviewed we found scant support for the Rorschach, some promising avenues for the TAT (although no support for this measure as it is currently used in clinical practice), only very limited promise for holistic scoring of some projective drawings, no support for ADDs as a screening instrument for evidence of sexual abuse, and evidence that the MBTI is a potentially reliable measure that lacks convincing validity data. A lack of standardization in the use of many of these techniques and an overreliance on unsubstantiated beliefs that certain people possess special interpretive powers (see also Chapter 2) has thwarted the possibility of advancing these techniques into the realm of scientifically supported assessment strategies.

Responsibility for demonstrating the adequacy of an assessment procedure rests first with those developing the procedure, and second with psychologists electing to use it. Proponents of specific assessment procedures are responsible for elucidating a standardized protocol that fully explains administration procedure. In the case of the Rorschach, TAT, projective drawings, and ADDs, it is necessary that proponents of each approach reach consensus on standardized administration and scoring. The maintenance of idiosyncratic versions of these tests mitigates against their establishment as scientifically sound assessment strategies.

Having established a standard protocol, research must address issues of reliability. Decision rules must be established that permit independent raters to reach the same judgments concerning a response. Once it has been established that a technique can be administered in a standardized fashion and the examinee's responses judged consistently, the issue of validity can be addressed. Tests that purport to measure a construct that cannot be independently measured by other tests or other assessment techniques are inherently unfalsifiable and therefore unscientific (see also Chapter 1). Finally, norms must be developed so that scores for an individual can be meaningfully interpreted. If clinical psychology is ever to be a scientific discipline, it is essential that established criteria for psychological tests be applied consistently and demanded by researchers and practitioners alike.

GLOSSARY

Clinical utility: The extent to which the assessment makes a meaningful, desirable difference in clinical decision making, treatment planning, and/or treatment outcome.

Falsifiability: The extent to which a hypothesis, measure, or theory be framed so that it can be subjected to empirical investigation and potentially refuted by such an investigation.

Norms: Normative data obtained from a comparison group of similar individuals that, ideally, is representative of the population to which the comparison group belongs. Interpretation of the obtained test results requires a comparison between the examinee's test data and relevant norms.

Projective tests: Either ambiguous test stimuli and/or relatively unstructured tasks that, putatively, require examinees to structure their test responses in a manner that reveals basic, unconscious personality characteristics.

Psychological tests: The measurement of a sample of behavior obtained under standardized conditions and the use of established rules for scoring or interpreting the behavioral sample. Additionally, whenever a claim is made or implied that the accuracy or validity of assessment-based inferences stem from the way in which the sample was collected (i.e., the nature of the stimuli, technique, or process that gave rise to the sample of behavior), not just from the expertise, authority, or special qualifications of the assessor, then the process used to collect and interpret the behavioral sample should be considered a psychological test.

Reliability: Refers to a test's consistency, including whether (1) all aspects of the test contribute in a meaningful way to the data obtained (internal consistency), (2) similar results would be obtained if the test was conducted and/or scored by another evaluator (interrater reliability), and (3) similar results would be obtained if the person was retested at some point after the initial test (retest reliability or test stability).

Standardization: Necessary to ensure that the influence of unique aspects of the testing situation and the assessor are minimized and involves the provision of (1) comparable test stimuli across assessors, (2) detailed instructions regarding the administrative procedures, and (3) detailed descriptions of scoring procedures for obtained test data.

Type I and Type II errors: A Type I error involves accepting a hypothesis when the data do not support the hypothesis; a Type II error involves rejecting a hypothesis when the data are supportive of the hypothesis.

Validity: Refers to whether the test measures what it purports to measure, including whether (1) the test samples the type of behavior that is relevant to the purpose of the test (content validity), (2) it provides data consistent with theoretical postulates associated with the phenomenon being assessed (concurrent and predictive validity), (3) it provides a relatively pure measure of the phenomenon that is minimally contaminated by other psychological characteristics (discriminant validity), and (4) it adds to our assessment-based knowledge above and beyond other information gathered in an assessment (incremental validity).

REFERENCES

Ackerman, M. J. (1995). *Clinician's guide to child custody evaluations*. New York: Wiley.

Ackerman, M. J., & Ackerman, M. C. (1997). Custody evaluation practices: A survey of experienced professionals. *Professional Psychology: Research and Practice, 28,* 137–145.

Ackerman, S. J., Clemence, A. J., Weatherill, R., & Hilsenroth, M. J. (1999). Use of the TAT in the assessment of DSM-IV Cluster B Personality Disorders. *Journal of Personality Assessment, 73,* 422–448.

Acklin, M. W. (1995). Integrative Rorschach interpretation. *Journal of Personality Assessment, 64,* 235–238.

Acklin, M. W., McDowell, C. J., & Verschell, M. S. (2000). Interobserver agreement, intraobserver reliability, and the Rorschach Comprehensive System. *Journal of Personality Assessment, 74,* 15–47.

Alcock, J. E. (1991). On the importance of methodological skepticism. *New Ideas in Psychology, 9,* 151155.

Aldridge, N. C. (1998). Strengths and limitations of forensic child sexual abuse interviews with anatomical dolls: An empirical review. *Journal of Psychopathology and Behavioral Assessment, 20,* 1–41.

Allard, G., Butler, J., Faust, D., & Shea, M. T. (1995). Errors in hand scoring objective personality tests: The case of the Personality Diagnostic Questionnaire-Revised (PDQ-R). *Professional Psychology: Research and Practice, 26,* 304–308.

American Psychological Association. (1991). Minutes of the Council of Representatives. *American Psychologist, 46,* 722.

Anastasi, A. (1988). *Psychological testing* (6th ed.). New York: Macmillan.

Apostal, R., & Marks, C. (1990). Correlations between the Strong–Campbell and Myers–Briggs scales of introversion–extraversion and career interests. *Psychological Reports, 66,* 811–816.

Archer, R. P., & Gordon, R. A. (1988). MMPI and Rorschach indices of schizophrenic and depressive diagnoses among adolescent inpatients. *Journal of Personality Assessment, 52,* 276–287.

Archer, R. P., & Krishnamurthy, R. (1997). MMPI-A and Rorschach indices related to depression and conduct disorder: An evaluation of the incremental validity hypothesis. *Journal of Personality Assessment, 69,* 517–533.

Aronow, E., Reznikoff, M., & Moreland, K. L. (1995). The Rorschach: Projective technique or psychometric test? *Journal of Personality Assessment, 64,* 213–228.

Atkinson, L. (1986). The comparative validities of the Rorschach and MMPI: A meta-analysis. *Canadian Psychology, 27,* 238–247.

Babiker, G., & Herbert, M. (1998). Critical issues in the assessment of child sexual abuse. *Clinical Child and Family Psychology Review, 1,* 231–252.

Ball, J. D., Archer, R. P., & Imhof, E. A. (1994). Time requirements of psychological testing: A survey of practitioners. *Journal of Personality Assessment, 63,* 239–249.

Barbuto, J. E. (1997). A critique of the Myers–Briggs Type Indicator and its operationalization of Carl Jung's psychological types. *Psychological Reports, 80,* 611–625.

Bellak, L., & Abrams, D. M. (1997). *The Thematic Apperception Test, the Children's Apperception Test, and the Senior Apperception Technique in clinical use* (6th ed.). Boston: Allyn & Bacon.

Beyerstein, B. L., & Beyerstein, D. F. (Eds.). (1992). *The write stuff: Evaluations of graphology—the study of handwriting analysis.* Buffalo, NY: Prometheus Books.

Boat, B. W., & Everson, M. D. (1994). Exploration of anatomical dolls by non-referred preschool-aged children: Comparisons by age, gender, race, and socio-economic status. *Child Abuse and Neglect, 18,* 139–153.

Boat, B. W., Everson, M. D., & Amaya-Jackson, L. (1996). Consistency of children's sexualized or avoidant reactions to anatomical dolls: A pilot study. *Journal of Child Abuse, 5,* 89–104.

Boyle, G. J. (1995). Myers–Briggs Type Indicator (MBTI): Some psychometric limitations. *Australian Psychologist, 30,* 71–74.

Buck, J. N. (1948). The HTP test. *Journal of Clinical Psychology, 4,* 151–159.

Bunge, M. (1991). A skeptic's beliefs and disbeliefs. *New Ideas in Psychology, 9,* 131149.

Burns, R. C., & Kaufman, S. H. (1970). *Kinetic Family Drawings (K-F-D): An introduction to understanding children through kinetic drawings.* New York: Brunner/Mazel.

Butcher, J., & Rouse, S. (1996). Personality: Individual differences and clinical assessment. *Annual Review of Psychology, 47,* 87–111.

Carlson, J. G. (1985). Recent assessments of the Myers–Briggs Type Indicator. *Journal of Personality Assessment, 49,* 356–365.

Ceci, S. J., & Bruck, M. (1995). *Jeopardy in the courtroom: A scientific analysis of children's testimony.* Washington, DC: American Psychological Association.

Coe, C. K. (1992). The MBTI: Potential uses and misuses in personnel administration. *Public Personnel Management, 21,* 511–522.

Conte, J. R., Sorenson, E., Fogarty, L., & Rosa, J. D. (1991). Evaluating children's reports of sexual abuse: Results from a survey of professionals. *American Journal of Orthopsychiatry, 61,* 428–437.

Costantino, G., Malgady, R. G., Rogler, L. H., & Tsui, E. C. (1988). Discriminant analysis of clinical outpatients and public school children by TEMAS: A thematic apperception test for Hispanics and blacks. *Journal of Personality Assessment, 52,* 670–678.

Cramer, P. (1991). *The development of defense mechanisms: Theory, research, and assessment.* New York: Springer-Verlag.

Cramer, P. (1999). Future directions for the Thematic Apperception Test. *Journal of Personality Assessment, 72,* 74–92.

Cummings, W. H. (1995). Age group differences and estimated frequencies of the Myers–Briggs Type Indicator preferences. *Measurement and Evaluation in Counseling and Development, 28,* 69–77.

Dana, R. H. (1985). Thematic Apperception Test (TAT). In C. S. Newmark (Ed.), *Major psychological assessment instruments* (pp. 89–134). Boston: Allyn & Bacon.

Davey, R. I., & Hill, J. (1999). The variability of practice in interviews used by professionals to investigate child sexual abuse. *Child Abuse and Neglect, 23,* 571–578.

Eron, L. D. (1950). A normative study of the Thematic Apperception Test. *Psychological Monographs, 64* (No. 315).

Eron, L. D. (1953). Response of women to the Thematic Apperception Test. *Journal of Consulting Psychology, 17,* 269–282.

Everson, M. D., & Boat, B. W. (1990). Sexualized doll play among young children: Implications for the use of anatomical dolls in sexual abuse evaluations. *Journal of the American Academy of Child and Adolescent Psychiatry, 29,* 736–742.

Everson, M. D., & Boat, B. W. (1994). Putting the anatomical doll controversy in perspective: An examination of the major uses and criticisms of the dolls in child sexual abuse evaluations. *Child Abuse and Neglect, 18,* 113–129.

Exner, J. E. (1974). *The Rorschach: A comprehensive system* (Vol. 1). New York: Wiley.

Exner, J. E. (1985). *A Rorschach workbook for the Comprehensive System* (2nd ed.). Bayville, NY: Exner Workshops.

Exner, J. E. (1986). *The Rorschach: A comprehensive system: Vol. 1. Basic foundations* (2nd ed.). New York: Wiley.

Exner, J. E. (1989). *A Rorschach workbook for the Comprehensive System* (3rd ed.). Ashville, NC: Exner Workshops.

Exner, J. E. (1993). *The Rorschach: A comprehensive system. Vol. 1. Basic foundations* (3rd ed.). New York: Wiley.

Exner, J. E. (1997). The future of the Rorschach in personality assessment. *Journal of Personality Assessment, 68,* 37–46.

Exner, J. E., & Exner, D. E. (1972). How clinicians use the Rorschach. *Journal of Personality Assessment, 36,* 403–408.

Feldman, M., & Hunt, R. G. (1958). A relation of difficulty in drawing and ratings of adjustment based on human figure drawings. *Journal of Consulting Psychology, 22,* 217220.

Fischer, C. T. (1994). Rorschach scoring questions as access to dynamics. *Journal of Personality Assessment, 62,* 515–524.

Freedenfeld, R. N., Ornduff, S. R., & Kelsey, R. M. (1995). Object relations and physical abuse: A TAT analysis. *Journal of Personality Assessment, 64,* 552–568.

Furnham, A. (1996). The Big Five versus the Big Four: The relationship between the Myers–Briggs Type Indicator (MBTI) and the NEO-PI five factor model of personality. *Personality and Individual Differences, 21,* 303–307.

Furnham, A., & Stringfield, P. (1993). Personality and work performance: Myers–Briggs Type Indicator correlates of managerial performance in two cultures. *Personality and Individual Differences, 14,* 145–153.

Ganellen, R. J. (1996). Exploring MMPI–Rorschach relationships. *Journal of Personality Assessment, 67,* 529–542.

Garb, H. N. (1984). The incremental validity of information used in personality assessment. *Clinical Psychology Review, 4,* 641–655.

Garb, H. N. (1998). Recommendations for training in the use of the Thematic Apperception Test (TAT). *Professional Psychology: Research and Practice, 29,* 621–622.

Garb, H. N. (1999). Call for a moratorium on the use of the Rorschach inkblot test in clinical and forensic settings. *Assessment, 6,* 313–317.

Garb, H. N., Florio, C. M., & Grove, W. M. (1998). The validity of the Rorschach and the Minnesota Multiphasic Personality Inventory: Results from meta-analyses. *Psychological Science, 9,* 402–404.

Garb, H. N., Wood, J. M., & Nezworski, M. T. (2000). Projective techniques and the detection of child sexual abuse. *Child Maltreatment, 5,* 161–168.

Garb, H. N., Wood, J. M., Nezworski, M. T., Grove, W. M., & Stejskal, W. J. (2001). Towards a resolution of the Rorschach controversy. *Psychological Assessment, 13,* 433–448.

Garden, A.-M. (1991). Unresolved issues with the Myers–Briggs Type Indicator. *Journal of Psychological Type, 22,* 3–14.

Girelli, S. A., & Stake, J. E. (1993). Bipolarity in Jungian type theory and the Myers–Briggs Type Indicator. *Journal of Personality Assessment, 60,* 290–301.

Gray-Little, B., & Kaplan, D. A. (1998). Interpretation of psychological tests in clinical and forensic evaluations. In J. Sandoval, C. L. Frisby, K. F. Geisinger, J. D. Scheuneman, & J. R. Grenier (Eds.), *Test interpretation and diversity: Achieving equity in assessment* (pp. 141–178). Washington, DC: American Psychological Association.

Groth-Marnat, G. (1997). *Handbook of psychological assessment* (3rd ed.). New York: Wiley.

Hammer, A. L., & Mitchell, W. D. (1996). The distribution of MBTI types in the US by gender and ethnic group. *Journal of Psychological Type, 37,* 2–15.

Hammer, E. F. (1985). The House–Tree–Person test. In C. S. Newmark (Ed.), *Major psychological assessment instruments* (pp. 135–164). Boston: Allyn & Bacon.

Handler, L. (1985). The clinical use of the Draw-A-Person test (DAP). In C. S. Newmark (Ed.), *Major psychological assessment instruments* (pp. 165–216). Boston: Allyn & Bacon.

Handler, L., & Habenicht, D. (1994). The Kinetic Family Drawing: A review of the literature. *Journal of Personality Assessment, 62,* 440–464.

Harris, D. B. (1963). *Children's drawings as a measure of intellectual maturity.* New York: Harcourt, Brace & Wood.

Harvey, R. J., & Murry, W. D. (1994). Scoring of the Myers–Briggs Type Indicator: Empirical comparison of perference score versus latent-trait methods. *Journal of Personality Assessment, 62,* 116–129.

Harvey, R. J., Murry, W. D., & Markham, S. E. (1994). Evaluation of three short-form versions of the Myers–Briggs Type Indicator. *Journal of Personality Assessment, 63,* 181–184.

Harvey, R. J., Murry, W. D., & Stamoulis, D. T. (1995). Unresolved issues in the dimensionality of the Myers–Briggs Type Indicator. *Educational and Psychological Measurement, 55*, 535–544.

Harvey, R. J., & Thomas, L. A. (1996). Using item response theory to score the Myers–Briggs Type Indicator: Rationale and research findings. *Journal of Psychological Type, 37*, 16–60.

Hiller, J. B., Rosenthal, R., Bornstein, R. F., Berry, D. T. R., & Brunell-Neuleib, S. (1999). A comparative meta-analysis of Rorschach and MMPI validity. *Psychological Assessment, 11*, 278–296.

Hilsenroth, M. J., & Handler, L. (1995). A survey of graduate students' experiences, interests, and attitudes about learning the Rorschach. *Journal of Personality Assessment, 64*, 243–257.

Holt, R. R. (1999). Empiricism and the Thematic Apperception Test: Validity is the payoff. In L. Gieser & M. I. Stein (Eds.), *Evocative images: The Thematic Apperception Test and the art of projection* (pp, 99–105). Washington, DC: American Psychological Association.

Holtzman, W. H. (1993). An unjustified, sweeping indictment by Motta et al. of human figure drawings for assessing psychological functioning. *School Psychology Quarterly, 8*, 189–190.

Hunsley, J., & Bailey, J. M. (1999). The clinical utility of the Rorschach: Unfulfilled promises and an uncertain future. *Psychological Assessment, 11*, 266–277.

Hunsley, J., & Bailey, J. M. (2001). Whither the Rorschach? An analysis of the evidence. *Psychological Assessment, 13*, 472–485.

Jackson, S. L., Parker, C. P., & Dipboye, R. L. (1996). A comparison of competing models underlying responses to the Myers–Briggs Type Indicator. *Journal of Career Assessment, 4*, 99–115.

Joiner, T. E., Schmidt, K. L., & Barnett, J. (1996). Size, detail, and line heaviness in children's drawings as correlates of emotional distress: (More) negative evidence. *Journal of Personality Assessment, 67*, 127–141.

Katz, H. E., Russ, S. W., & Overholser, J. C. (1993). Sex differences, sex roles, and projection on the TAT: Matching stimulus to examinee gender. *Journal of Personality Assessment, 60*, 186–191.

Kaufman, A. S., Kaufman, N. L., & McLean, J. E. (1993). Profiles of Hispanic adolescents and adults on the Myers–Briggs Type Indicator. *Perceptual and Motor Skills, 76*, 628–630.

Keiser, R. E., & Prather, E. N. (1990). What is the TAT? A review of ten years of research. *Journal of Personality Assessment, 55*, 800–803.

Kendall-Tackett, K. A., & Watson, M. W. (1992). Use of anatomical dolls by Boston-area professionals. *Child Abuse and Neglect, 16*, 423–428.

Kendall-Tackett, K. A., Williams, L. M., & Finkelhor, D. (1993). Impact of sexual abuse on children: A review and synthesis of recent empirical studies. *Psychological Bulletin, 113*, 164–180.

Koocher, G. P., Goodman, G. S., White, C. S., Friedrich, W. N., Sivan, A. B., & Reynolds, C. R. (1995). Psychological science and the use of anatomically detailed dolls in child sexual abuse assessments. *Psychological Bulletin, 118*, 199–122.

Koppitz, E. M. (1968). *Psychological evaluation of children's human figure drawings*. New York: Grune & Stratton.

Kroon, N., Goudena, P. P., & Rispens, J. (1998). Thematic apperception tests for a child and adolescent assessment: A practitioner's consumer guide. *Journal of Psychoeducational Assessment, 16,* 99–117.

Lally, S. J. (2001). Should human figure drawings be admitted into court? *Journal of Personality Assessment, 76,* 135–149.

Lett, J. (1990). A field guide to critical thinking. *Skeptical Inquirer, 14*(2), 153–160.

Levy, H. B., Markovic, J., Kalinowski, M. N., Ahart, S., & Torres, H. (1995). Child sexual abuse interviews: The use of anatomic dolls and the reliability of information. *Journal of Interpersonal Violence, 10,* 334–353.

Lorr, M. (1991). An empirical evaluation of the MBTI typology. *Personality and Individual Differences, 12,* 1141–1145.

MacDonald, D. A., Anderson, P. E., Tsagarakis, C. I., & Holland, C. J. (1994). Examination of the relationship between the Myers–Briggs Type Indicator and the NEO Personality Inventory. *Psychological Reports, 74,* 339–344.

Machover, K. (1949). *Personality projection in the drawing of the human figure.* Springfield IL: Charles C Thomas.

Masling, J. M. (1992). The influence of situation and interpersonal variables in projective testing. *Journal of Personality Assessment, 59,* 616–640.

Masling, J. M. (1997). On the nature and utility of projective tests and objective tests. *Journal of Personality Assessment, 69,* 257–270.

Matarazzo, J. D. (1986). Computerized clinical psychological test interpretations: Unvalidated plus all mean and no sigma. *American Psychologist, 41,* 14–24.

McCaulley, M. H. (1990). The Myers–Briggs Type Indicator: A measure for individuals and groups. *Measurement and Evaluation in Counseling and Development, 22,* 181–195.

McCaulley, M. H., & Martin, C. R. (1995). Career assessment and the Myers–Briggs Type Indicator. *Journal of Career Assessment, 3,* 219–239.

McClelland, D. C., Koestner, R., & Weinberger, J. (1989). How do self-attributed and implicit motives differ? *Psychological Bulletin, 96,* 690–702.

McCrae, R. R., & Costa, P. T. (1989). Reinterpreting the Myers–Briggs Type Indicator from the perspective of the five-factor model of personality. *Journal of Personality, 57,* 17–40.

Meyer, G. J. (1991). An empirical search for fundamental personality and mood dimensions within the Rorschach test (Doctoral dissertation, Loyola University of Chicago, 1991). *Dissertation Abstracts International, 52,* 1071B-1072B.

Meyer, G. J. (1997a). Assessing reliability: Critical corrections for a critical examination of the Rorschach Comprehensive System. *Psychological Assessment, 9,* 480–489.

Meyer, G. J. (1997b). Thinking clearly about reliability: More critical corrections regarding the Rorschach Comprehensive System. *Psychological Assessment, 9,* 495–498.

Meyer, G. J. (2002). Exploring possible ethnic differences and bias in the Rorschach Comprehensive System. *Journal of Personality Assessment, 78,* 104–129.

Motta, R. W., Little, S. G., & Tobin, M. I. (1993). The use and abuse of human figure drawings. *School Psychology Quarterly, 8,* 162–169.

Murray, H. A. (1943). *Thematic Apperception Test manual.* Cambridge, MA: Harvard University Press.

Murstein, B. L. (1965). *Handbook of projective techniques.* New York: Basic Books.

Murstein, B. L. (1972). Normative written TAT responses for a college sample. *Journal of Personality Assessment, 36,* 104–107.

Myers, I. B., & McCaulley, M. H. (1985). *Manual: A guide to the development and use of the Myers–Briggs Type Indicator.* Palo Alto, CA: Consulting Psychologists Press.

Naglieri, J. A., & Pfeiffer, S. I. (1992). Performance of disruptive behavior-disordered and normal samples on the Draw A Person: Screening Procedure for Emotional Disturbance. *Psychological Assessment, 4,* 156–159.

Nichols, R. C. & Strumpfer, D. J. (1962). A factor analysis of Draw-A-Person test scores. *Journal of Consulting Psychology, 26,* 156–161.

Palmer, L., Farrar, A. R., Valle, M., Ghahary, N., Panella, M., & DeGraw, D. (2000). An investigation of the clinical use of the House–Tree–Person projective drawings in the psychological evaluation of child sexual abuse. *Child Maltreatment, 5,* 169–175.

Parker, K. C. H. (1983). A meta-analysis of the reliability and validity of the Rorschach. *Journal of Personality Assessment, 47,* 227–231.

Parker, K. C. H., Hanson, R. K., & Hunsley, J. (1988). MMPI, Rorschach, and WAIS: A meta-analytic comparison of reliability, stability, and validity. *Psychological Bulletin, 103,* 367–373.

Pearman, R. R., & Fleenor, J. (1996). Differences in observed and self-reported qualities of psychological types. *Journal of Psychological Type, 39,* 3–17.

Peterson, C., & Ulrey, L. M. (1994). Can explanatory style be scored from TAT protocols? *Personality and Individual Differences, 20,* 102–106.

Pinkerman, J. E., Haynes, J. P, & Keiser, T. (1993). Characteristics of psychological practice in juvenile court clinics. *American Journal of Forensic Psychology, 11*(2), 3–12.

Pittenger, D. J. (1993). The utility of the Myers–Briggs Type Indicator. *Review of Educational Research, 63,* 467–488.

Popper, K. R. (1959). *The logic of scientific discovery.* New York: Basic Books.

Psychological Corporation. (1997). *Wechsler Adult Intelligence Scale, Third Edition: Technical manual.* San Antonio, TX: Author.

Rapaport, D., Gill, M., & Shafer, R. (1946). *Diagnostic psychological testing.* Chicago: Year Book.

Reznikoff, M., Aronow, E., & Rauchway, A. (1982). The reliability of inkblot content scales. In C. D. Spielberger & J. D. Butcher (Eds.), *Advances in personality assessment: Vol. 1* (pp. 83–113). Hillsdale, NJ: Erlbaum.

Riethmiller, R. J., & Handler, L. (1997). Problematic methods and unwarranted conclusions in DAP research: Suggestions for improved research procedures. *Journal of Personality Assessment, 69,* 459–475.

Riordan, R., & Verdel, A. C. (1991). Evidence of sexual abuse in children's art products. *School Counselor, 39,* 116–121.

Ronan, G. F., Colavito, V. A., & Hammontree, S. R. (1993). Personal problem-solving system for scoring TAT responses: Preliminary validity and reliability data. *Journal of Personality Assessment, 61,* 28–40.

Ronan, G. F., Date, A. L., & Weisbrod, M. (1995). Personal problem-solving scoring of the TAT: Sensitivity to training. *Journal of Personality Assessment, 64,* 119–131.

Rossini, E. D., & Moretti, R. J. (1997). Thematic Apperception Test (TAT) interpretation: Practice recommendations from a survey of clinical psychology doctoral programs accredited by the American Psychological Association. *Professional Psychology: Research and Practice, 28,* 393–398.

Saggino, A., & Kline, P. (1996). The location of the Myers–Briggs Type Indicator in personality factor space. *Personality and Individual Differences, 21,* 591–597.

Sattler, J. M. (1998). *Clinical and forensic interviewing of children and families: Guidelines for the mental health, education, pediatric, and child maltreatment fields.* San Diego, CA: Author.

Sechrest, L. (1963). Incremental validity: A recommendation. *Educational and Psychological Measurement, 23,* 153–158.

Shaffer, T. W., Erdberg, P., & Haroian, J. (1999). Current nonpatient data for the Rorschach, WAIS-R, and MMPI-2. *Journal of Personality Assessment, 73,* 305–316.

Shontz, F. C., & Green, P. (1992). Trends in research on the Rorschach: Review and conclusions. *Applied and Preventive Psychology, 1,* 149–156.

Sipps, G. J., Alexander, R. A., & Friedt, L. (1985). Item analysis of the Myers–Briggs Type Indicator. *Educational and Psychological Measurement, 45,* 789–796.

Spangler, W. D. (1992). Validity of questionnaire and TAT measures of need for achievement: Two meta-analyses. *Psychological Bulletin, 112,* 140–154.

Standards for Educational and Psychological Testing. (1985). Washington, DC: American Psychological Association.

Standards for Educational and Psychological Testing. (1999). Washington, DC: American Psychological Association.

Telgasi, H. (1993). *Clinical use of story telling: Emphasizing the TAT with children and adolescents.* Boston: Allyn & Bacon.

Tharinger, D. J., & Stark, K. (1990). A qualitative versus quantitative approach to evaluating the Draw-A-Person and Kinetic Family Drawing: A study of mood and anxiety-disorder children. *Psychological Assessment, 2,* 365–375.

Thomas, G. V., & Jolley, R. P. (1998). Drawing conclusions: A re-examination of empirical and conceptual bases for psychological evaluations of children from their drawings. *British Journal of Clinical Psychology, 37,* 127–139.

Thompson, B., & Borrello, G. M. (1986). Second-order factor structure of the MBTI: A construct validity assessment. *Measurement and Evaluation in Counseling and Development, 18,* 148–153.

Tischler, L. (1994). The MBTI factor structure. *Journal of Psychological Type, 31,* 24–31.

Turcotte, M. (1994). Use of tests in the Canadian employment services. *Journal of Employment Counseling, 31,* 188–199.

Tzeng, O. C., Ware, R., & Chen, J.-M. (1989). Measurement and utility of continuous unipolar ratings for the Myers–Briggs Type Indicator. *Journal of Personality Assessment, 53,* 727–738.

Vane, J. R. (1981). The Thematic Apperception Test: A review. *Clinical Psychology Review, 1,* 319–336.

Vass, Z. (1998). The inner formal structure of the H-T-P Drawings: An exploratory study. *Journal of Clinical Psychology, 54,* 611–619.

Viglione, D. J. (1996). Data and issues to consider in reconciling self-report and the Rorschach. *Journal of Personality Assessment, 67,* 579–587.

Viglione, D. J. (1999). A review of recent research addressing the utility of the Rorschach. *Psychological Assessment, 11,* 251–263.

Vincent, K. R., & Harman, M. J. (1991). The Exner Rorschach: An analysis of its clinical utility. *Journal of Clinical Psychology, 47,* 596–599.

Wanderer, Z. W. (1997). Validity of clinical judgments based on human figure drawings. In E. F. Hammer (Ed.), *Advances in projective drawing interpretation* (pp. 301–315). Springfield, IL: Charles C Thomas.

Watkins, C. E., Jr., Campbell, V. L., Nieberding, R., & Hallmark, R. (1995). Contemporary practice of psychological assessment by clinical psychologists. *Professional Psychology: Research and Practice, 26,* 54–60.

Weiner, I. B. (1966). *Psychodiagnosis in schizophrenia.* New York: Wiley.

Weiner, I. B. (1993). Clinical considerations in the conjoint use of the Rorschach and the MMPI. *Journal of Personality Assessment, 60,* 148–152.

Weiner, I. B. (1994). The Rorschach Inkblot Method (RIM) is not a test: Implications for theory and practice. *Journal of Personality Assessment, 62,* 498–504.

Weiner, I. B. (1996). Some observations on the validity of the Rorschach Inkblot Method. *Psychological Assessment, 8,* 206–213.

Weiner, I. B. (1997). Current status of the Rorschach Inkblot Method. *Journal of Personality Assessment, 68,* 5–19.

Weiner, I. B. (1999). What the Rorschach can do for you: Incremental validity in clinical applications. *Assessment, 6,* 327–339.

Weiner, I. B. (2001). Advancing the science of psychological assessment: The Rorschach inkblot method as exemplar. *Psychological Assessment, 13,* 423–432.

West, M. M. (1998). Meta-analysis of studies assessing the efficacy of projective techniques in discriminating child sexual abuse. *Child Abuse and Neglect, 11,* 1151–1166.

Westen, D. (1991). Clinical assessment of object relations using the TAT. *Journal of Personality Assessment, 56,* 56–74.

Westen, D., Lohr, N. E., Silk, K., Gold, L., & Kerber, K. (1990). Object relations and social cognition in borderlines, major depressives, and normals: A Thematic Apperception Test analysis. *Psychological Assessment: A Journal of Consulting and Clinical Psychology, 2,* 355–364.

Wideman, B. G. (1998). Rorschach responses in gifted and nongifted children: A comparison study (Doctoral dissertation, Georgia State University, 1998). *Dissertation Abstracts International, 59,* 905B.

Widiger, T. A., & Schilling, K. M. (1980). Toward a construct validation of the Rorschach. *Journal of Personality Assessment, 44,* 450–459.

Wolfner, G., Faust, D., & Dawes, R. M. (1993). The use of anatomically detailed dolls in sexual abuse evaluations: The state of the science. *Applied and Preventive Psychology, 2,* 1–11.

Wood, J. M., & Lilienfeld, S. O. (1999). The Rorschach inkblot test: A case of overstatement? *Assessment, 6,* 341–349.

Wood, J. M., Lilienfeld, S. O., Garb, H. N., & Nezworski, M. T. (2000). The Rorschach test in clinical diagnosis: A critical review, with a backward look at Garfield (1947). *Journal of Clinical Psychology, 56,* 395–430.

Wood, J. M., Nezworski, M. T., Garb, H. N., & Lilienfeld, S. O. (2001). The misperception of psychopatholgy: Problems with the norms of the Comprehensive System for the Rorschach. *Clinical Psychology: Science and Practice, 8,* 350–373.

Wood, J. M., Nezworski, M. T., & Stejskal, W. J. (1996a). The Comprehensive System for the Rorschach: A critical examination. *Psychological Science, 7,* 3–10.

Wood, J. M., Nezworski, M. T., & Stejskal, W. J. (1996b). Thinking critically about the Comprehensive System for the Rorschach: A reply. *Psychological Science, 7,* 14–17.

Wood, J. M., Nezworski, M. T., & Stejskal, W. J. (1997). The reliability of the Comprehensive System for the Rorschach: A comment on Meyer (1997). *Psychological Assessment, 9,* 490–494.

Wood, J. M., Nezworski, M. T., Stejskal, W. J., Garven, S., & West, S. G. (1999). Methodological issues in evaluating Rorschach validity: A comment on Burns and Viglione (1996), Weiner (1996), and Ganellen (1996). *Assessment, 6,* 115–120.

Yates, A. (1997). Sexual abuse of children. In J. M. Wiener (Ed.), *Textbook of child and adolescent psychiatry* (2nd ed., pp. 699–709). Washington, DC: American Psychiatric Press.

Zumbo, B. D., & Taylor, S. V. (1993). The construct validity of the Extraversion subscale of the Myers–Briggs Type Indicator. *Canadian Journal of Behavioural Science, 25,* 590–604.

4

The Science and Pseudoscience of Expert Testimony

JOSEPH T. McCANN
KELLEY L. SHINDLER
TAMMY R. HAMMOND

In recent years significant attention has been accorded to the role of mental health professionals as expert witnesses in legal proceedings. Several factors account for this trend, including more mental health professionals turning to forensic work as a way of coping with managed care and greater attention being given by the courts to serious social problems, such as child abuse, sexual harassment, and domestic violence. According to Ciccone (1992), the use of expert witnesses dates back many centuries in that early Egyptian and Greek societies used forensic medicine to resolve legal issues. Over the centuries, litigants and their attorneys have gained greater control over the selection, preparation, and presentation of expert witnesses in courts (Landsman, 1995).

The use of expert testimony pertaining to issues involving psychological or mental health issues also has a fairly lengthy history. Cases involving questions of a criminal defendant's sanity, for example, have been at the forefront of most debates about the appropriate role of mental health professionals in legal proceedings. In 1843, Daniel McNaughton shot and killed the secretary of the British Prime Minister and was found not guilty by reason of insanity (Steadman et al., 1993). Although there was considerable public outcry over the verdict, the legal test for insanity arising from this case has endured.

The use of behavioral science and mental health expert testimony has expanded considerably over the last few decades to include such issues as competency to stand trial, diminished capacity, mitigation and aggravating factors at sentencing, and the accuracy of eyewitness testimony. In civil and family court cases, expert testimony is frequently offered on such issues as claims of psychological injury or neuropsychological impairment, the veracity of child sexual abuse allegations, and domestic violence. Along with the expanding use of experts in court has come considerable debate about the validity, reliability, and appropriateness of permitting experts from the behavioral sciences to testify in court proceedings, as well as the scientific basis of theories, constructs, and diagnostic syndromes that form the basis of their testimony (Faust & Ziskin, 1988; Ziskin & Faust, 1988).

In this chapter we review legal and professional standards pertaining to the admissibility of expert testimony by mental health professionals and behavioral scientists, and attempt to distinguish scientifically appropriate and scientifically inappropriate uses of such testimony. We review the extant standards for admissibility in state and federal courts, as well as professional guidelines that govern the ethics and standards of such testimony. We then review several major areas addressed by expert testimony, including the accuracy of eyewitnesses, psychiatric diagnoses and syndromes, psychometric testing, and the prediction of violent behavior. In addition, we review several controversial syndromes and constructs that have either been proposed or proffered in legal settings. Throughout this discussion, we attempt to provide some guidance for distinguishing between those areas that have an adequate scientific basis from those that are pseudoscientific or that possess questionable validity.

ADMISSIBILITY OF SCIENTIFIC EVIDENCE IN THE COURTROOM

Legal Standards

The determination of whether certain evidence is admitted in any legal proceeding is governed by rules of evidence. Because the legal system in the United States is federalist in nature, in that there are separate state and federal courts, evidentiary rules can vary across jurisdictions. Federal courts rely on the *Federal Rules of Evidence* (FRE; Green & Nesson, 1992), whereas state courts typically rely on either codified rules of evidence, which in some instances may be modeled after the FRE, or an extensive body of case law. Regardless of whether the specific jurisdiction is state or federal, one of two major legal standards typically governs the admissibility of expert testimony. One standard is the *Frye* test, which was outlined in *United States v. Frye* (1923). The other is the FRE, which was further expanded on in the landmark case *Daubert v. Merrell Dow Pharmaceuticals, Inc.* (1993), also known as the *Daubert* standard. Because of its importance, as well as some inconsistencies in the manner in which principles outlined in *Daubert* were applied by various courts, some important post-*Daubert* decisions set forth by the United States Supreme Court have clarified the standards for admissibility of expert testimony in federal courts.

The Frye Test

Although the *Frye* decision was a federal opinion issued in the early part of the 20th century by the Court of Appeals of the District of Columbia, the *Frye* test was widely adopted by other federal jurisdictions and many state courts. Interestingly, the *Frye* test, also referred to as the "general acceptance" standard, arose from a case addressing the admissibility of a systolic blood pressure deception test, which was an early precursor of the polygraph (i.e., "lie detector") examination. In ruling that such a test was not admissible because it did not have adequate scientific recognition, the court in *Frye* stated that:

> Just when a scientific principle or discovery crosses the line between the experimental and demonstrable states is difficult to define. Somewhere in this twilight zone the evidential force of the principle must be recognized, and while courts will go a long way in admitting expert testimony deduced from a well-recognized scientific principle or discovery, the thing from which the deduction is made must be sufficiently established to have gained *general acceptance in the particular field in which it belongs*. (*United States v. Frye*, 1923, p. 1014, emphasis added)

When adopting the *Frye* standard, courts typically examine whether a particular theory or technique is generally accepted within the field from which the expert's testimony is derived. Some examples of how general acceptance can be established include examining peer-reviewed literature, looking at surveys of common techniques or practices used by professionals, and referring to scholarly treatises or books.

Federal Rules of Evidence

In 1961, the Chief Justice of the United States Supreme Court, Earl Warren, appointed a special committee to determine whether a formal set of federal evidentiary laws was both possible and desirable (Green & Nesson, 1992). The FRE were subsequently signed into law in 1975 and have become the formal legal standard for determining admissibility of evidence in federal courts. Many states have enacted codes of evidence that are based largely on the FRE, making them "the most significant single source of evidence law in America" (Green & Nesson, 1992, p. xii).

The admissibility of expert testimony is governed by Article VII of the FRE, which includes Rule 702: "If scientific, technical, or other specialized knowledge will assist the trier of fact to understand the evidence or to determine a fact in issue, a witness qualified as an expert by knowledge, skill, experience, training, or education, may testify thereto in the form of an opinion or otherwise." The FRE can be conceptualized as a "helpfulness" standard in that testimony that is of assistance to the trier of fact (i.e., judge or jury) in understanding evidence or factual circumstances in a case is admissible.

Rule 703 of the FRE pertains to the basis of an expert witness' opinion: "The facts or data in the particular case on which an expert bases an opinion or inference may be those perceived by or made known to the expert at or before the hearing. If of a type reasonably relied upon by experts in the particular field in forming opinions or inferences upon the participant, the facts or data need not be admissible in evidence." Therefore, when judging the admissibility of an expert's opinion, the court can examine the reasonableness of the expert's reliance on a particular technique, theory, body of research, and the like by examining the practices of other experts in the field.

Two additional provisions in the FRE pertaining to expert testimony are worth noting. Rule 704 governs the controversial issue of whether experts may offer opinions on the "ultimate issue," such as whether a specific accident caused the plaintiff's injuries, if a criminal defendant is competent to stand trial, and so forth. Rule 704 of the FRE states that expert testimony that embraces the ultimate issue is not objectionable, except that no expert may testify in a federal court "as to whether the defendant did or did not have the mental state or condition constituting an element of the crime charged or of a defense thereto" (Green & Nesson, 1992, p. 131). This rule essentially overrules previous case law that limited the extent to which experts could testify on ultimate issues (Goodman-Delahunty, 1997). According to Green and Nesson (1992), however, Rule 704 was drafted to facilitate the admissibility of ultimate issue testimony because restricting such testimony "generally served to deprive the trier of fact of useful information" (p. 132). The sole restriction of ultimate opinion testimony under Rule 704 pertains to the issue of a federal criminal defendant's mental state during commission of an offense and was implemented as part of the Insanity Defense Reform Act that followed the controversial acquittal of John Hinkley, Jr., for the assassination attempt on President Ronald Reagan (McPherson, 1999; Steadman et al., 1993). In addition, Rule 705 of the FRE pertains to the disclosure of facts upon which the expert relied in forming his or her opinion. In this context, facts would refer to research studies, data from clinical examinations, and other information that the expert utilized when forming an opinion. According to Rule 705, experts do not have to disclose such facts before offering their opinions unless the court requires them to do so, although they may be required to disclose them on cross-examination.

The Daubert Standard

The *Daubert* opinion arose from a civil case in which a pharmaceutical company was sued for damages related to birth defects that were allegedly caused by an antinausea drug manufactured by the company and that was ingested by pregnant women. The major focus of the *Daubert* opinion was the appropriate standard for admissibility of expert testimony offered by the plaintiffs; the testimony was based on scientific principles determined by the trial court to not meet the applicable "general acceptance" test outlined in *United States v. Frye* (1923).

Both the FRE and *Frye* test are federal standards governing admissibility, one a statutory code (i.e., FRE) and the other a published legal opinion (i.e., *Frye*). The issue in *Daubert* was a determination of the appropriate standard for admissibility in federal courts, given that federal jurisdictions had been essentially divided on whether the FRE or *Frye* test was the appropriate standard. The United States Supreme Court held that "the Federal Rules of Evidence, not *Frye*, provide the standard for admitting expert scientific testimony in a federal trial" (*Daubert v. Merrell Dow Pharmaceuticals, Inc.*, 1993, p. 2790). Moreover, the *Daubert* opinion held that the FRE "assign to the trial judge the task of ensuring that an expert's testimony both rests on a reliable foundation and is relevant to the task at hand" (p. 2799).

The most interesting aspect of the *Daubert* decision, and the one of greatest relevance to expert witnesses, is the delineation of four factors that trial judges may consider when making a determination as to whether expert testimony is admissible. These four major factors include the following:

1. The theory or technique constitutes scientific knowledge that is testable.
2. The theory or technique has been subjected to peer review.
3. There is a known or potential rate of error.
4. There is general acceptance of the theory or technique in the field.

With respect to the first of these factors, the Supreme Court stated that the critical question is whether hypotheses can be developed and tested to determine their validity. The second factor recommends that judges determine the extent to which a theory or technique has been subjected to peer review. Although not entirely controlling of admissibility, peer review helps to "increase the likelihood that substantive flaws in methodology will be detected" (p. 2797). The third factor applies to "particular" scientific techniques and refers also to the "existence and maintenance of standards controlling the technique's operation" (p. 2797). Fourth and finally, the general acceptance of a theory or technique, as outlined earlier in *Frye*, remains an important consideration in determining the admissibility of expert testimony. However, under *Daubert* general acceptance is no longer the sole determining factor for admissibility.

There has been considerable academic discussion concerning the implications of the *Daubert* decision (e.g., Goodman-Delahunty, 1997; Lubit, 1998). The FRE standard of helpfulness has typically been construed as a more liberal standard that permits greater leniency when deciding what evidence is admissible, whereas the *Frye* general acceptance test has been construed as more stringent (Blau, 1998). Given that the *Daubert* standard offers specific factors that judges may consider when deciding on the admissibility of expert testimony, the *Daubert* decision raised some questions that required further elaboration. One such issue was whether *Daubert* would make it more difficult for certain types of expert testimony to be ruled admissible, thereby making the *Daubert* standard more stringent than the liberal FRE standard dictates. With respect to the scope of the *Daubert* standard, another issue was raised concerning whether the social sciences, including psychology, would be characterized as "scientific, technical, or other knowledge" as outlined in Rule 702 of the FRE (Faigman, 1995). In addition, the *Daubert* decision placed judges, who are often untrained in science, in the role of determining the scientific adequacy of certain forms of expert testimony.

Post-Daubert Rulings

In *General Electric Co. v. Joiner* (1997), the "gatekeeper" role of the trial judge outlined in *Daubert* was affirmed. More importantly, the *Joiner* decision held that an "abuse of discretion" standard is to be applied to appellate review of rulings of the trial judge on the admissibility of expert testimony. The abuse of discretion standard is applied in all federal courts for appellate review of evidentiary matters and the *Joiner* decision held that *Daubert* did not create a more stringent or higher standard for review. Also, the trial judge in *Joiner* reached different conclusions than did some of the experts when reviewing the scientific research on which the experts based their opinions. The Supreme Court did not find this practice an abuse of discretion on the part of the trial judge, and *Joiner* appears to hold that "trial courts have broad discretion to reject proffered expert opinions if they are inadequately supported by the data" (Grudzinskas & Appelbaum, 1998, p. 502).

A second major United States Supreme Court case on the application of the *Daubert* standard was outlined in *Kumho Tire Co., Ltd. v. Carmichael* (1999). The case involved civil litigation over personal injuries resulting from a traffic accident in which the plaintiffs offered expert testimony on alleged defects in a tire on one of the vehicles. The significant holding in *Kumho* was that the admissibility of the expert's testimony, even though characterized as "technical" and not necessarily scientific, was to be analyzed according to the *Daubert* criteria. As a result of this ruling, the *Daubert* standard applied to all expert testimony, not just that which is scientific (Cavanagh, 1999). That is, the *Daubert* criteria are not to be applied in a strict and inflexible manner, but according to the specific nature of the testimony offered. Therefore, expert testimony that is based on a procedure or methodology that has not been subjected to extensive peer review may still be admissible if other factors, such as reliability and general acceptance by others in the field, support the testimony.

As a result of the rulings in *Joiner* and *Kuhmo*, trial judges in federal courts are empowered to exercise their discretion when attempting to exclude junk science from the courtroom, while permitting expert testimony that is not only relevant, but reliable and based on acceptable methodologies (Cavanagh, 1999; Littleton, 1999). Given the broad discretion accorded trial judges under *Daubert* and the post-*Daubert* rulings, expert testimony must withstand an independent analysis by the trial judge of its relevance and reliability, as well as the methodologies upon which it is based. Grudzinskas (1999) noted that the implications of these recent Supreme Court cases include the following:

1. Opinions should be based on data that are collected and observed.
2. Inferences should be differentiated from data.
3. Consideration should be given to the selection of methodologies used to collect data.
4. The expert should be prepared to support the efficacy of methodology selected. These factors would extend to such issues as the selection of certain methodologies (e.g., interview, psychological testing, collateral interviews), diagnostic concepts or terminology, and explanatory theories.

Standards for Admissibility across Various Jurisdictions

The two major standards that remain for judging admissibility of expert testimony are the "general acceptance" test outlined in *Frye* and the relevant, helpful, and reliable standard outlined in the FRE and expanded upon in *Daubert*. Although the FRE and *Frye* are both federal standards, most state courts have adopted one of these standards for determining the admissibility of expert testimony. Because state courts are not bound to follow the rulings of federal courts, unless there is a state law that violates individual rights or privileges guaranteed by the United States Constitution, there may be considerable variability in legal standards not only across states but also between federal and state jurisdictions within the same state.

Hamilton (1998) conducted a study on trends in state courts following the *Daubert* ruling and found that the "trend toward adopting *Daubert*, although initially significant, may be slowing" (pp. 201–202). According to Hamilton, by the end of 1997, 17 states that had utilized the *Frye* test prior to the *Daubert* ruling continued to apply the *Frye* test as the standard for admissibility of expert testimony in state courts even after *Daubert*. Likewise, 21 states or jurisdictions had a *Daubert* or *Daubert*-type standard based on the FRE both prior to and after the *Daubert* ruling. On the other hand, 12 states changed from the *Frye* test to the *Daubert* or a *Daubert*-type standard after the United States Supreme Court ruling in 1993. One state (i.e., North Dakota) had no clear evidentiary standard prior to the *Daubert* ruling but later adopted the *Daubert* standard.

Therefore, two major legal standards continue to govern the admissibility of expert testimony in U.S. courts. The *Frye* "general acceptance" test is applied in those states that have chosen to retain this standard in spite of the *Daubert* ruling. The FRE standard, as expanded upon in *Daubert*, is the appropriate standard in all federal courts in the United States, as well as in those states that have explicitly adopted this standard in state appellate decisions. In jurisdictions where the *Daubert* standard is applied, general acceptance is a factor to be considered, but this does not form the sole basis for the admissibility of expert testimony. In some states (e.g., New York, Florida) there may be two different standards, with the *Frye* test applicable in state courts and the *Daubert* standard applicable in federal courts within the state. The application of either the *Frye* or *Daubert* standard requires that expert witnesses be familiar with the governing standard in the particular court in which they seek to testify.

Professional Standards for Expert Testimony

Although legal standards provide the ultimate test for determining whether an expert's testimony is admitted in court, professional standards in the behavioral sciences provide guidance as well. The most recent version of the Ethical Principles of Psychologists and Code of Conduct published by the American Psychological Association (1992) provides a section on forensic activities. These standards state that psychologists who perform psychological services in forensic settings, including assessment, consultation, and treatment, must comply with all other provisions of the ethical code (Section 7.01). Additionally, psychologists are directed to base their assessments, recommendations, and conclusions on information and techniques that can adequately substantiate findings and that, unless it is not feasible, psychologists should provide opinions about an individual only after having conducted an examination of that individual. Otherwise, clarification should be provided on the effects of limited information on the reliability and validity of reports and testimony (Section 7.02). The ethical principles also direct psychologists to clarify their role and to avoid adopting multiple, conflicting roles (Section 7.03). For example, therapists who are in the helping role should avoid shifting to the role of a neutral forensic examiner (Greenberg & Shuman, 1997). Finally, the ethical principles direct psychologists to be truthful and candid in their testimony and reports (Section 7.04), to clarify the distinction between expert and fact witness (Section 7.05), and to comply with legal rules (Section 7.06).

Although the ethical principles are instructive in many respects, they are silent on a number of issues that often arise when providing expert testimony. Therefore, the Committee on Ethical Guidelines for Forensic Psychologists (1991) in Division 41 of the American Psychological Association developed *Specialty Guidelines for Forensic Psychologists* to provide further guidance. The *Specialty Guidelines* recommend that forensic psychologists take steps to assure that their work, including communications in the form of reports or testimony, is not misrepresented or misused in legal proceedings. Therefore, forensic psychologists have "a special responsibility for fairness and accuracy in their public statements" (Committee on Ethical Guidelines for Forensic Psychologists, 1991, p. 664), although this principle does not prevent psychologists from being persuasive and forceful in presenting their data and conclusions.

Because expert testimony by mental health professionals most often involves the assessment of an individual and the rendering of a psychiatric diagnosis, additional concerns arise when formal diagnostic classification systems are used. Bloom and Rogers (1987) argued that although legal standards and principles provide the framework for developing issues that are the focus of forensic mental health evaluations, psychiatric knowledge and ethical concerns should dictate how the professional functions in his or her role. Consequently, one important source of guidance on the use of expert testimony derives from the *Diagnostic and Statistical Manual of Mental Disorders*, fourth edition (DSM-IV; American Psychiatric Association, 1994), which can be viewed as a significant learned treatise for mental health professionals with respect to the diagnostic conclusions that are drawn (McCann & Dyer, 1996). Learned treatises are published research, texts, or summaries that are often used to reflect consensus agreement within a particular field against which a particular expert's statements, opinions, and methods can be compared. Despite criticisms that have been made with respect to the reliability and validity of DSM-IV, it "reflects a consensus about the classification and diagnosis of mental disorders derived at the time of its initial publication" (American Psychiatric Association, 1994, p. xxiii). It is important to recognize that DSM-IV explicitly states that dangers "arise because of the imperfect fit between the questions of ultimate concern to the law and the information contained in clinical diagnosis." Consequently, the rendering of a DSM-IV diagnosis does not equate with a specific legal standard (American Psychiatric Association, 1994, p. xxiii).

For instance, the presence of a major mental disorder, such as schizophrenia, in a criminal defendant does not equate with a legal finding that the defendant is incompetent to stand trial or was insane at the time of a criminal act. It must be shown that the defendant's mental disorder caused him or her to lack an appreciation of the charges, to be incapable of assisting defense counsel, or to lack an appreciation of the nature, consequences or wrongfulness of the criminal act. Although the diagnosis may be relevant to the case, issues of legal blameworthiness or causality are established by the trier of fact after all evidence presented at trial is weighed.

Despite the imperfect fit that sometimes exists between psychiatric diagnoses and legal standards, as well as concerns that may be raised about the reliability and validity of its diagnostic criteria, DSM-IV reflects a consensus within the mental health community regarding the classification and diagnosis of mental disorders. However, the relationship between specific diagnoses and legal standards remains an area in which reliance on research, accepted psychological theory, and reliable and valid assessment techniques are needed to form a scientific basis for the expert's reasoning about connections between a diagnosis (e.g., schizophrenia) and specific legal standard (e.g., insanity).

COMMON AREAS OF EXPERT TESTIMONY

Several topics have been repeatedly introduced into legal settings where their application seems appropriate or relevant. Issues surrounding the admissibility of expert testimony on these topics have received considerable attention, including psychological assessment methods, prediction of violent behavior, the accuracy of eyewitness accounts, battered woman syndrome, and rape trauma syndrome. Many of these topics are controversial, and several legal cases have addressed the admissibility of these concepts and principles.

Psychological Testing and Assessment

The use of psychological assessment methods, including psychometric tests, has been the focus of increasing attention in legal settings (McCann, 1998; McCann & Dyer, 1996; Pope, Butcher, & Seelen, 1993). Although legal rules of evidence provide the standards under which the admissibility of psychological assessment methods is determined, guidelines have been set forth in the psychological literature that offer direction for the selection of psychometric tests in forensic settings. These professional standards and guidelines provide useful frameworks for selecting instruments that are likely to be viewed as relevant, reliable, and valid (see also Chapter 3).

Heilbrun (1992) noted that the selection of psychological assessment instruments in forensic evaluations should be guided by the relevance of the instrument to the legal standard that gives rise to the issues being evaluated. That is, whether the legal issue is dangerousness, insanity, presence or absence of emotional injury, competence, or some other matter, the psychological tests used for evaluating a criminal defendant or civil plaintiff should be related in some way to the legal issue at hand. In addition, Heilbrun noted that there are two types of relevance guiding the selection of psychometric instruments and that it is misleading to argue or assume that just because an instrument is indirectly related to the ultimate legal issue that it is inappropriate for forensic applications. The first type of relevance involves the use of instruments that are direct measures of a specific legal issue. Examples of such instruments would include the Gudjonsson Suggestibility Scales as measures of interrogative suggestibility (Gudjonsson, 1997), the Rogers Criminal Responsibility Assessment Scales (Rogers, 1984), and the Instruments for Assessing Understanding and Appreciation of Miranda Rights (Grisso, 1998). The second form of relevance noted by Heilbrun (1992) is when a psychometric instrument measures a specific construct that is one component of a broader legal issue. Examples of this more remote form of relevance include measurement of personality disorders (e.g., Millon Clinical Multiaxial Inventory-III [MCMI-III]), impulsivity (e.g., Minnesota Multiphasic Personality Inventory, second edition [MMPI-2]; Rorschach), and other constructs in violence risk assessments (Quinsey, Harris, Rice, & Cormier, 1998), intellectual and neuropsychological assessment in personal injury cases (Reynolds, 1998), and the assessment of formal thought disorder in insanity evaluations (Rogers, 1984; Shapiro, 1999).

In addition, Heilburn (1992) outlined seven general guidelines that professionals can follow when selecting appropriate instruments for use in forensic setting:

1. The test should be commercially available, have an adequately documented manual, and have been peer reviewed.
2. The reliability of the instrument should be established, with a coefficient of .80 advisable, or explicit justification for lower coefficients. In this regard, Heilbrun stated that test–retest reliability is most important; although McCann and Dyer (1996) argued that internal consistency is more appropriate because it pertains to the precision of measurement, rather than the stability of the construct as measured by test–retest reliability.
3. The test should be relevant to the legal issue, or measure a construct that underlies the legal issue, with available validation research.

4. The test should have a standard method of administration.
5. The test should be applicable to the population and purpose for which it is used.
6. Objective (i.e., structured) tests and actuarial data applications are preferred.
7. There should be some method for interpreting test results within the context of the individual's response style (e.g., defensiveness, positive impression management, malingering).

Psychometric instruments vary in the extent to which they attain these individual standards (McCann, 1998; see also Chapter 3). Although most well-established tests are commercially available, have documented technical manuals, and have been subjected to peer review, some instruments may have excellent reliability but scant actuarial data for making decisions (e.g., Millon Adolescent Clinical Inventory; McCann, 1999), whereas other instruments may have weaker reliability yet extensive actuarial data supporting interpretive decisions (e.g., MMPI-2; McCann & Dyer, 1996).

Another model for assessing the admissibility of psychometric evidence is Marlowe's (1995) hybrid model, which blends scientific and legal principles. According to this model, the analysis of admissibility for psychometric evidence follows a logical course from initial questions about the expert witness' qualifications, the falsifiability and level of acceptance of the data collection procedures and psychological tests utilized, and the availability of proper procedures for collecting and analyzing data (e.g., norms, standardized administration). In the latter stages of Marlowe's hybrid model, questions are directed at issues related to how the expert utilizes test data. For instance, issues about the relevance, social policies (e.g., discrimination, racial bias), and validity of the expert's reasoning when drawing conclusions from the data are additional considerations that must be addressed.

The admissibility of assessment data in forensic psychological evaluations, including the use of psychometric tests, is guided by a number of factors, including the level of acceptance, standardization, reliability, and validity of the test. If one selects psychological tests or other assessment techniques (e.g., structured interviews) in light of the guidelines outlined by Heilbrun (1992) and Marlowe (1995), then the scientific basis of the expert's opinions will be stronger. Nevertheless, the expert bears the burden of providing clear reasoning concerning why a specific instrument was selected and how psychometric data relate to the psycholegal issue at hand.

Prediction of Violent Behavior

A key issue in many civil and criminal cases is the potential for violence posed by a specific individual. This is a key consideration in civil cases involving involuntary commitment, as well as in criminal cases in which future dangerousness is often an issue to be considered during sentencing. For example, the presence of a mental illness or a mental abnormality, coupled with a risk of danger to self or others, is legally permissible for civilly committing an individual (*Allen v. Illinois*, 1986). Furthermore, the United States Supreme Court case of *Kansas v. Hendricks* (1997) established that it is permissible for states to civilly commit felons who have completed their sentences if evidence exists of a mental abnormality or personality disorder that makes it likely the individual will engage in predatory acts of sexual violence. Therefore, courts are likely to seek out expert testimony on a particular individual's propensity for violence with greater frequency.

It has often been asserted that mental health professionals are no better predictors of future violence than are informed nonprofessionals. To support this claim, attention is often directed to Monahan's (1981/1995) conclusion that mental health professionals are correct only 1 out of 3 times in their predictions of violence. However, much has changed in the last two decades, including a second generation of research on violence prediction (Monahan, 1992; Otto, 1992) that shows (1) mental health professionals' predictions are better than chance (Mossman, 1994), (2) accuracy of predicting future sexual violence is improved (Rice, 1997), and (3) more is known about the demographic and clinical correlates of violent behavior (Monahan & Steadman, 1994). In addition, the practice of evaluating a person's potential for violence has been reconceptualized as risk assessment, rather than prediction, of violent behavior (Borum, 1996; Monahan & Steadman, 1996), wherein specific clinical, demographic, and situational variables are identified that raise or lower the likelihood of violence. Definitive statements that a person will or will not become violent are avoided in risk assessment, as such predictions are prone to error and often in the direction of overprediction of violent behavior.

Research on risk assessment for violent behavior has resulted in considerable advances in our understanding of the correlates of violence and our ability to identify factors that raise or lower a person's propensity for harm to others (e.g., Klassen & O'Connor, 1988, 1990; Monahan & Steadman, 1994; Quinsey et al., 1998). However, the question remains regarding how mental health professionals can best communicate opinions about risk for violence in a manner that is based in science.

Three general types of testimony are theoretically possible with respect to an individual's risk for violence. One involves offering opinions about a person's psychological functioning, history, and psychiatric diagnosis without any opinions offered about dangerousness. Testimony of this type is likely to be of limited use to the courts. A second offers an assessment of the person's psychological functioning, history, and diagnosis along with an assessment of variables that raise or lower the person's risk for violence and a general estimate (i.e., low, moderate, high) of the person's risk at various times (e.g., imminent risk, short-term risk, long-term risk). Third, expert testimony could be offered in the form of a definitive statement that the person will or will not become violent. Based on a review of the existing literature, testimony of the latter type has a very limited scientific basis and could be appropriately viewed as pseudoscientific. Expert testimony of the second type, in which general estimates are offered based on research findings from the risk assessment literature, is likely to be of greatest use to courts, under the helpfulness standard of both *Daubert* and the FRE, while also remaining firmly grounded in research. Heilbrun, Philipson, Berman, and Warren (1999) found that the most commonly cited preferences among a sample of psychiatrists and psychologists for communicating violence risk are statements about how specific risk factors raise or lower risk and the use of general estimates (e.g., low, moderate, high) of risk.

Eyewitness Testimony

The testimony of eyewitnesses is highly probative, meaning that jurors rely heavily on the accounts of individuals who have witnessed an event or crime. Although jurors are often instructed to examine such testimony and form their own opinions about the reliability of specific witnesses, research demonstrates that jurors often make errors regarding the veracity of eyewitness accounts. Penrod and Cutler (1995) cited research showing that jurors have difficulty differentiating eyewitness testimony that is accurate from that which is inaccurate. Moreover, witness confidence in memory is a poor indicator of accuracy, yet jurors often view witness confidence as strongly indicative of accuracy. In addition, witness confidence in memory is often malleable and influenced by such postidentification factors as suggestions and leading questioning (see also Chapter 8 for a discussion of the fallibility of memory). For example, witnesses who are repeatedly questioned about an event grow more confident in the accuracy of what they report (Hastie, Landsman, & Loftus, 1978), as do those who are given information about the behavior and reports of other witnesses (Penrod & Cutler, 1995).

A related issue in the accuracy of eyewitnesses is the use of police lineups to identify criminal suspects. Research has shown that several factors influence the accuracy of eyewitness identification, including how police question eyewitnesses during police lineups, how similar the suspect is to other participants in the lineup, and the types of instructions that are given to eyewitnesses during the identification process. Wells and Seelau (1995) concluded that the potential for false identification can be reduced by instituting four rules

1. Inform eyewitnesses that the guilty party may not be in the lineup.
2. Make sure the suspect does not stand out in the lineup.

3. Have the lineup administered by someone who does not know who the culprit is.
4. Obtain an assessment of eyewitness confidence before any additional information is given.

These procedures, according to Wells and Seelau (1995), may reduce the risk of false eyewitness identifications. In fact, many wrongful convictions are attributable to false identification by eyewitnesses (Wells, 1995).

One way to increase juror scrutiny of eyewitness accounts is to present expert testimony on variables that influence the accuracy and reliability of eyewitness accounts. Jurors tend to make fewer errors, such as placing excessive trust in witnesses, when such testimony is presented (Penrod & Cutler, 1995). Despite research suggesting improved accuracy in jury decision making when expert testimony is provided, many courts have not deemed such testimony admissible. In *United States v. Amador-Galvan* (1997), for example, the exclusion of expert testimony on eyewitness identification was upheld on appeal as permissible because such testimony could confuse the jury and waste time. In addition, the court viewed the testimony as relying on scientific data that was suspect, abstract, and incomplete in that it did not take into account many known variables that influence juror decision making. However, the court failed to note which juror-influencing variables were excluded in the testimony and claimed that such testimony is unnecessary because of effective voir dire, cross examination, argument, and juror instructions. In other cases, expert testimony on eyewitness identification has been ruled as inadmissible. For instance, in *United States v. Hall* (1999), the court ruled that such testimony would not assist the jury because it addressed issues of which the jury was already aware and would not contribute to jurors' understanding of the case. Likewise, *United States v. Kime* (1996) questioned the scientific basis of eyewitness expert testimony, stating that it failed to qualify as "scientific knowledge" under *Daubert*. Other courts (e.g., *Bachman v. Leapley*, 1992) have excluded such testimony when it was introduced for the sole purpose of casting doubt on the credibility of a witness.

In some cases, however, expert testimony on the validity of eyewitness reports has been deemed admissible. The case of *People v. McDonald* (1984) is one in which the exclusion of such testimony at trial was ruled as reversible error because it deprived the jury of important information about the inaccuracy of eyewitnesses that would have assisted them in reaching a decision. Moreover, some researchers argue that courts should make it mandatory to include an expert witness on eyewitness accounts in all criminal trials with juries (Gross, 1999), as standard instructions about conflicting eyewitness accounts do little to improve the ability of jurors to evaluate the reliability of eyewitnesses (Penrod & Cutler, 1995).

Contrary to the opinion of some appellate courts, research on the accuracy of eyewitness identification and juror decision making is extensive and provides a sound basis for communicating information to courts. Nevertheless, the admissibility of expert testimony in this area is not uniformly accepted and whether such testimony may be deemed admissible depends on the judge's ruling.

Battered Woman Syndrome

Battered woman syndrome is a term coined by Walker (1984) to describe the cyclical nature of violence in domestic relationships. This concept incorporates widely accepted psychological constructs, such as learned helplessness, to explain why some women who are battered remain in violent relationships. Although battered woman syndrome is not a formal diagnosis, it is commonly associated with the DSM-IV diagnosis of posttraumatic stress disorder (PTSD; American Psychiatric Association, 1994) because many women who are victims of battering exhibit either symptoms of, or a formal diagnosis of PTSD (Walker, 1994). Battered woman syndrome has recently been the subject of expert testimony in a variety of cases, including the prosecution of accused batterers and trials of battered women who have killed their abusive partners and claimed self-defense (Blowers & Bjerregaard, 1994; Magnum, 1999).

Battered woman syndrome has traditionally been applied in self-defense arguments in which a woman who has been battered, claiming to reasonably believe that she was in imminent physical danger at the time of the killing, killed an abusive partner. Often, the invocation of this syndrome is necessary in these trials to attempt to prove that the woman who has been battered did not provoke the attack, did not use excessive force during the killing of an abusive partner, and that no other recourse was available other than murdering this partner. Thus, battered woman syndrome may be offered as a conceptual framework for understanding the reasonableness of a victim's actions as self-defense, despite the fact that such actions may not conform to the usual standards for reasonableness (Blowers & Bjerregaard, 1994).

There is considerable variability across jurisdictions as to whether battered woman syndrome is admissible. Many states admit expert testimony that incorporates the battered woman syndrome when offered by the defense, although some courts do so with limitations or under specific conditions (Magnum, 1999). In most jurisdictions in which battered woman syndrome testimony has been allowed, the testimony is confined to a general discussion of existing research on the syndrome, including characteristics of battered women and common beliefs or misconceptions that lay persons may have about battered women (Blowers & Bjerregaard, 1994; Schuller & Vidmar, 1992). In some cases, experts may offer opinions regarding whether a defendant exhibits behaviors that are consistent with battered woman syndrome, although testimony about a criminal defendant's mental state at the time of the offense is generally disallowed.

Blowers and Bjerregaard (1994) examined 72 appellate court decisions pertaining to the admissibility of testimony on battered woman syndrome over a 15-year period (1979–1994). Their analysis reveals a trend toward increasing acceptance of testimony on battered woman syndrome. In general, courts have ruled that such testimony is relevant for providing a context within which to understand the defendant's actions, unless the defense in criminal cases has not raised issues related to the defendant's sanity or if self-defense is not raised. Although acceptance of the scientific basis of battered woman syndrome has been a subject of debate, courts have generally been more accepting of such testimony as the body of scientific research on the topic has expanded (Schuller & Vidmar, 1992). By 1993 battered woman syndrome gained legal acceptance as a scientifically acceptable construct in all state courts (Blowers & Bjerregaard, 1994). In general, battered woman syndrome may be used to assist the jury in evaluating the reasonableness of a defendant's belief of being in mortal or imminent danger (e.g., *People v. Humphrey*, 1996). Nevertheless, the construct is typically not permitted as a means of allowing experts to testify about a defendant's state of mind at the time of the killing (e.g., *People v. Erikson*, 1997).

One criticism of battered woman syndrome is that its clinical characteristics do not appear consistently among women who have experienced long-term abuse. Because learned helplessness does not appear universally, as evidenced by the wide range of coping efforts among different battered women and the cyclical nature of violence in domestic relationships, questions have been raised about the reliability with which the syndrome can be identified across various cases. Because battered woman syndrome has not been adopted as a formal diagnosis, many courts permit experts to testify about research findings but often restrict them from offering opinions regarding whether a defendant exhibits this syndrome (Schuller & Vidmar, 1992).

Rape Trauma Syndrome

Rape trauma syndrome is most often viewed as a subtype of PTSD. However, the specific reference to rape trauma syndrome as a unique form of trauma response is based on the assumption that victims of rape may exhibit behavioral responses that are seemingly inconsistent with having been traumatized. These contradictory behaviors may include returning to the scene of the rape as a gesture of defiance or refusal to surrender to fear (Stefan, 1994), continuing to have contact with the assailant following the assault (Ritchie, 1998), and delaying reporting of an assault once it has occurred.

Expert testimony on the responses of rape victims, and rape trauma syndrome in particular, has been admitted inconsistently across various jurisdictions. For instance, the defendant in *United States v. Smith* (1998) argued that the victim was unreliable because she failed to report the rape immediately. A prosecution expert was permitted to testify that victims of rape often do not report their assaults immediately for various reasons, including fear, guilt, or shame. This evidence was permitted only for the purpose of rebutting a defense claim that the victim's delay in reporting was evidence of unreliability. In a more liberal use of testimony on rape trauma syndrome, the court in *State v. Allewalt* (1986) permitted an expert to testify that a victim's PTSD was caused by rape. Such testimony could be criticized, however, in that it went beyond the bounds of scientific knowledge and addressed questions that are reserved solely for the jury (Boeschen, Sales, & Koss, 1998). In *Henson v. State* (1989), the defense was permitted to present expert testimony on rape trauma syndrome to support its argument that a rape had not occurred. The testimony suggested that the alleged rape victim's behavior was inconsistent with rape trauma syndrome.

Although a close connection between rape trauma syndrome and the generally accepted diagnosis of PTSD might argue in favor of the admissibility of expert testimony on this syndrome, there is a risk of such testimony being misapplied or used improperly. Because the characteristics of rape trauma syndrome are not universal in all rape victims, the syndrome is not validated as a definitive sign that a rape did or did not occur. Moreover, some critics of the syndrome argue that although expert testimony may bolster a claim of nonconsensual sexual contact for the victim, it has the effect of putting the victim on trial by placing emphasis on the diagnosis as a sign that the rape occurred (Ritchie, 1998; Stefan, 1994). Stefan (1994) proposed that a more accurate description of the symptoms of rape trauma would be silence, survival, and a desire for being perceived as normal.

CONTROVERSIAL SYNDROMES AND DIAGNOSES

Some proposed syndromes and diagnoses have limited empirical support or have received only provisional acceptance in formal classification systems (see also Chapter 5). Many of these syndromes and diagnoses can be considered controversial when introduced into legal settings. In considering the validity of these conditions, it is useful to have a basic framework for evaluating theoretical and empirical support for a particular construct. The criteria outlined by Robins and Guze (1970) represent a fairly straightforward set of guidelines for determining whether a syndrome possesses adequate validity. These guidelines call for a diagnosis to (1) be sufficiently described, (2) have specific laboratory or psychometric findings that are reliable and reproducible, (3) differentiate individuals with the diagnosis from individuals with other disorders, (4) provide a means for predicting clinical course and outcome, and (5) have a specific familial pattern.

Sexual Addiction

Some researchers and clinicians have compared compulsive sexual behavior with substance dependence or addiction, the latter of which is included in DSM-IV as a mental disorder (American Psychiatric Association, 1994). However, sexual addiction can be conceptualized as a tolerance or compulsive need to engage in sexual behavior or to become sexually aroused, with the occurrence of withdrawal symptoms in the absence of such behavior. Moreover, sexual addiction is often viewed as encompassing excessive sexual behavior, failed efforts to reduce such behavior, and interference with important activities (e.g., work, relationships) despite knowledge of detrimental effects of the behavior. Nevertheless, Gold and Hefner (1998) noted that the literature on sexual addiction consists largely of theories that are based on clinical observation and that there is little research to support its validity.

The lack of such research suggests that expert testimony on sexual addiction would fail under most legal standards for admissibility. With respect to the criteria for evaluating diagnostic validity outlined by Robins and Guze (1970), there appear to have been attempts to provide a clinical description of sexual addiction. However, no studies are available at this time to show that it can be reliably distinguished from other disorders, that individuals with sexual addiction produce reliable and reproducible patterns of responses on psychological testing, and that the course, family patterns, and outcomes of sexual addiction can be predicted.

Despite the lack of research support for the concept of sexual addiction, some courts are willing to entertain the notion, and even to misuse the term by deviating from its proposed definition. In *United States v. Romualdi* (1996), the defendant was charged with possession of child pornography and admitted to fantasizing about sex with young girls, despite the fact that he had no previous criminal record and his behavior was seemingly out of character. Expert testimony was presented suggesting the defendant might have a sexual addiction. However, the facts of the case indicate that the defendant had fantasies only and had not engaged in any sexual activities with children or nonconsenting partners, pointing to a diagnosis of paraphilia and not a sexual addiction. Expert testimony surrounding compulsive sexual behavior or disturbed patterns of sexual arousal should be based on recognized diagnoses in DSM-IV, such as the paraphilias, personality disorders, and mood disorders.

Homosexual Panic

The term homosexual panic has been loosely defined as a state of rage, mixed with anxiety and tension, experienced by an individual with latent homosexual tendencies and that are aroused by a homosexual advance (Chuang & Addington, 1988). Although homosexual panic does not appear as a diagnosis in DSM-IV (American Psychiatric Association, 1994), Chuang and Addington (1988) argued that the characteristics of this state could fit under the rubric of either adjustment disorder or brief reactive psychosis. Nevertheless, these researchers observed that homosexual panic is essentially a term that attempts to remove behaviors from their social context. Furthermore, Chuang and Addington noted that legal defenses in criminal cases based on the notion of homosexual panic should more appropriately be construed as hate crimes based on phobic beliefs about homosexuality. They concluded that homosexual panic does not have wide acceptance in the scientific community. Nevertheless, homosexual panic has been invoked as a defense in murder cases (*People v. Milner*, 1988; *State v. Escamilla*, 1994). In the case of *State v. Escamilla* (1994), the court did not allow expert testimony on homosexual panic, whereas in a previous case such testimony was allowed (*Parisie v. Greer*, 1983). Recent trends suggest that homosexual panic is not likely to be deemed admissible, which is consistent with the weak scientific foundation that exists for this concept.

Black Rage

A black rage defense in criminal cases relies on the assertion that an African American defendant's conduct resulted from an uncontrollable rage induced by the experience of racism in a predominantly white society or by specific individuals who provoked the defendant (Goldklang, 1997). The defense asserts further that the rage so impaired the defendant's mental state that his or her criminal responsibility should be negated. In most cases, a defense based on black rage is used in conjunction with such defenses as insanity or diminished capacity, rather than self-defense.

Although introduced in 1846 as a legal defense in conjunction with an insanity defense (*People v. Freeman*, 1847), black rage defenses have not been particularly successful. Although courts may be willing to consider a defense of insanity based on a related mental disorder (*People v. Ferguson*, 1998; *United States v. Robertson*, 1974), courts generally will not permit a defense of black rage when an insanity defense is explicitly rejected by the defendant. Overall, there is little scientific support for a distinct diagnosis of black rage. It is more likely to be accepted if the principal focus is on a more widely accepted mental disorder (e.g., delusional disorder; personality disorder) that forms the basis of an insanity or diminished capacity defense.

Road Rage

Road rage is another popular term that has received considerable attention in the media as a syndrome, or pattern of aggressive behavior, for which scientific and legal recognition is being sought. Typically, road rage involves impulsive acts of violence committed against people whose driving incurs the wrath of the perpetrator. The victim may be a pedestrian, bicyclist, or other driver, and the offender's behavior may include rude conduct, obscene gestures, aggressive retaliatory maneuvers, physical confrontation, and property damage. Although road rage has appeared tangentially in some legal cases, as in *People v. Ilieveski* (1998)—in which a driver was ticketed for driving at the speed limit in the passing lane out of concern that such behavior might inspire road rage in others—the construct has not been the subject of expert testimony. In one study, police reports in Western Australia were examined over a 4-year period for instances of road rage, which was defined as impulsive driving-related violence between strangers (Harding, Morgan, Indermaur, Ferrante, & Blagg, 1998). This study found that a majority of road rage cases occurred in urban settings, involved male perpetrators and victims, and involved victims who were threatened or assaulted by the perpetrator. Moreover, the risk of involvement in incidents of road rage was greatest among drivers who were younger, on the road more frequently, and driving during afternoon rush hour. Despite this initial attempt to examine the characteristics of road rage, the concept remains a behavioral descriptor, rather than a formal diagnosis. As such, expert testimony in cases involving instances of road rage should rely on generally accepted diagnostic categories such as personality disorders, substance abuse, and other relevant conditions.

Premenstrual Dysphoric Disorder

Unlike many other controversial syndromes and diagnoses, premenstrual dysphoric disorder (PDD) has achieved conditional acceptance by being adopted in the appendix of DSM-IV as a diagnostic criterion meriting further study (American Psychiatric Association, 1994). Considered more severe and less prevalent than premenstrual syndrome (Steiner, 1997), PDD is defined as a distinct mood-related disturbance that includes at least one of four emotional symptoms: feelings of sadness, hopelessness, or worthlessness; tension; emotional lability; or persistent irritability. Women who are diagnosed with PDD experience severe depressive-type symptoms during most menstrual cycles that interfere with occupational or social functioning.

Despite its inclusion in the appendix of DSM-IV, PDD is not extensively validated. The criteria are not firmly established and causes of this condition are not well understood, although biological models focus on hormonal changes or deficits in specific neurotransmitters (e.g., serotonin; Steiner, 1997). Consequently, there remains considerable debate regarding whether PDD is a distinct mental disorder. Moreover, although the broader construct of premenstrual syndrome has been considered a form of insanity in France and a mitigating factor in English courts, PDD is not recognized as a criminal defense in the United States (Grose, 1998). Although premenstrual syndrome has been raised in some isolated cases, including forgery and bankruptcy cases, courts have not accepted testimony based on this syndrome. There appears to be insufficient psychiatric consensus on the diagnostic criteria, etiology, and treatment of this condition to permit acceptance under most legal evidentiary standards (Grose, 1998).

Paraphilic Coercive Disorder

The preliminary drafts of DSM-III-R (American Psychiatric Association, 1987) included a diagnosis of paraphilic coercive disorder, which was defined as a preoccupation with recurrent and intense sexual urges and sexually arousing fantasies involving the act of forcible sexual contact on a nonconsenting partner. Although this proposed diagnosis was withdrawn because of problems with differentiating it from other disorders as well as concerns that it could be misused as an exculpatory defense by rapists, Fuller (1990) found that clinicians could agree on its features and that it might constitute an accurate and useful diagnosis. Aside from the validity of an insanity defense based on paraphilic coercive disorder, it might be argued that concerns regarding a diagnosis's misuse are irrelevant to its validity.

Perhaps because it does not appear in formal diagnostic classification systems, paraphilic coercive disorder has not been cited in legal cases. Although research is needed to establish the reliability and validity of paraphilic coercive disorder, it is likely to raise controversy if it is again proposed as a formal diagnosis. In light of recent sexually violent predator laws, whereby criminal defendants who have committed an act of sexual violence are civilly committed for treatment of a personality disorder or another mental disturbance that renders them a threat to others (e.g., *Kansas v. Hendricks*, 1997), this diagnosis may again become a focus of attention.

Codependency

Originally developed to describe a pattern of behavior in spouses of chemically dependent individuals, the term codependency has gained popular use in the context of expert testimony. In general, codependency refers to the tendency of an individual, typically a spouse or intimate partner, to rely excessively on another person, typically the chemically dependent spouse or partner, for identity. Granello and Beamish (1998) noted that there is no scientific research to support a disease-based concept of codependency. Most research on codependency has based the construct within the personality disorders. Specifically, certain forms of character pathology may lead some individuals to seek relationships with addicted individuals (Loughead, Spurlock, & Ting, 1998; Wells, Glickauf-Hughes, & Bruss, 1998). A search of legal databases in several large state appellate courts revealed no cases in which expert testimony cited the concept of codependency. Therefore, although codependency may have some utility in formulating or conceptualizing cases for treatment purposes, it does not hold wide acceptance in legal settings, where formal diagnoses (e.g., personality disorders) are more likely to be accepted.

Factitious Disorder by Proxy

The diagnosis of factitious disorder by proxy, sometimes called Munchausen's by proxy, has been included in the appendix of DSM-IV as a condition requiring further study (American Psychiatric Association, 1994). Factitious disorder by proxy is defined as a caregiver, typically the mother, who intentionally induces or causes repeated physical illness or symptoms in a child. The caregiver must be acting with deliberate intent to gain medical attention and not for financial or other secondary gain. Despite its provisional recognition in DSM-IV, factitious disorder by proxy presents many problems from a scientific and evidentiary perspective. Mart (1999) noted that the empirical basis for factitious disorder by proxy is questionable, given that only a small number of preliminary controlled studies exist. Furthermore, Mart argued that most of the literature on this condition is based on clinical observations, rather than systematic studies (see also Mart, 2002, for a critical examination of the literature).

Although Vollaro (1993) suggested that factitious disorder by proxy is underdiagnosed and may be more prevalent than originally believed, Mart (1999) argued that the condition may be overdiagnosed. The major problems noted with making a diagnosis of factitious disorder by proxy include its likely low base rate and the frequent absence of direct evidence of a parent's creation of physical symptoms.

Expert testimony on factitious disorder by proxy is typically sought to aid the prosecution in cases of child abuse. In *People v. Phillips* (1981), a prosecution expert who had not examined the defendant responded to a question pertaining to hypothetical findings that the defendant's actions were consistent with those of a person with factitious disorder by proxy. Despite defense arguments at trial and later on appeal, this evidence was deemed admissible because such expert testimony was considered beyond the common experiences of jurors and would assist the trier of fact.

At this time, it is not clear if individuals with factitious disorder by proxy produce reliable and reproducible patterns of behavior in research studies, and there is equivocal evidence as to whether the course, outcome, and familial pattern of the disorder can be predicted. There is a pressing need for more controlled research on this condition due to the importance of protecting children where there is bona fide evidence of intentional harm to the child by a parent.

Neonaticide/Infanticide Syndrome

Neonaticide is defined as the killing of a newborn baby within hours of delivery, whereas infanticide is the killing of a child who is over 1 day old. Research has demonstrated meaningful differences between individuals, typically mothers, who kill a newborn infant and those who kill an older child (Bookwalter, 1998; Haapasalo & Petaja, 1999). In DSM-IV, postpartum is an onset specifier for the major mood disorders and brief psychotic disorder (American Psychiatric Association, 1994). Therefore, postpartum mental disorders have attained some formal recognition. In legal settings, neonaticide/infanticide syndrome is commonly linked to postpartum depression or postpartum psychosis in which the defendant attempts to prove that she was insane at the time of the killing of the child (Nonacs & Cohen, 1998).

There has been inconsistency in how neonaticide/infanticide syndrome has been applied in legal cases. Bookwalter (1998) observed that in three cases with similar facts, different outcomes occurred, with one woman convicted of murder, another convicted of second-degree murder, and another convicted of criminally negligent homicide. In some cases, particularly those arising in jurisdictions outside the United States, a criminal defendant may be found not guilty by reason of insanity due to a postpartum mental disorder (Haapasalo & Petaja, 1999). In *People v. Wernick* (1995) the New York State Court of Appeals upheld the exclusion of expert testimony on neonaticide syndrome in a case involving a woman who delivered her baby in a college dormitory bathroom and then asphyxiated the infant and disposed of the body. Although the defendant sought to raise an insanity defense without evoking the term neonaticide syndrome, the appellate court still ruled that because a *Frye* hearing was not held to determine whether such a syndrome was generally accepted in psychology, the expert testimony was properly excluded by the trial judge.

Although the decision in *Wernick* could be criticized because expert testimony pertaining to the defendant's sanity was based solely on a recognized mental disorder, namely brief reactive psychosis, the use of neonaticide syndrome as a formal term in legal settings may be met with resistance. However, DSM-IV explicitly recognizes the postpartum onset of certain mental disorders, including depression and mania. Therefore, in cases involving questions about the mental state of a woman charged with the death of an infant or neonate, it is recommended that experts adhere to standards outlined in formal diagnostic classification systems.

Child Sexual Abuse Accommodation Syndrome

Another controversial syndrome that is often the subject of expert testimony is child sexual abuse accommodation syndrome (CSAAS). Like battered woman syndrome, CSAAS was formulated to explain a pattern of contradictory and misunderstood responses frequently observed in child victims of sexual abuse (Summit, 1983). The characteristics of CSAAS are descriptive, not diagnostic, and include five general clusters of behaviors that seek to explain why some victims of sexual abuse delay reporting or retract their claims. The first is secrecy, whereby the perpetrator swears the child victim to secrecy, often with threats of physical harm or the dissolution of the family. A second is helplessness, as the perpetrator is often someone close to, or trusted by the child, thereby widening the power differential between perpetrator and child and leading to passive acceptance of the perpetrator's abusive behavior. The remaining three features of CSAAS constitute a complex series of events in which the child victim assumes feelings of responsibility for the abuse, followed by conflict that may precipitate a delayed or unconvincing disclosure.

In legal settings, CSAAS has been invoked to explain seemingly inconsistent or illogical behavior on the part of child victims of sexual abuse, including delayed reporting, the lack of witnesses or physical evidence, and retraction by the victim. Summit (1983) asserted that the testimony of social science experts may be critical in clarifying the victim's seemingly illogical behavior and to overcome jurors' misconceptions about the claims of child victims. However, application of CSAAS in the prosecution of child sexual abuse cases is extremely controversial because the syndrome is often used not only to explain the reactions of child victims, but also to prove that sexual abuse occurred. Among the major difficulties with the scientific adequacy of CSAAS is that behaviors characterizing the syndrome have been noted in children who have not been sexually abused (Levy, 1989) and the syndrome is essentially unfalsifiable because the defining features are contradictory. That is, if a child claims victimization at any time, CSAAS provides an explanation; if that same person recants, CSAAS explains the behavior and thus claims of child sexual abuse cannot be falsified.

Steele (1999) suggested that such testimony be considered technical or specialized knowledge, rather than scientific. Moreover, Summit (1992) responded to criticisms of CSAAS by attempting to clarify its proper role in research and forensic settings. He asserted that CSAAS was never designed for the purpose of proving sexual abuse in any given case, despite the fact that the syndrome has been so applied in several cases. Levy (1989) stated that CSAAS has not been empirically tested as clinical opinion. Therefore, application of CSAAS in legal settings may be misleading and confusing to fact finders. The case of *United States v. Bighead* (1997) illustrates one application of CSAAS testimony that was admitted as specialized knowledge to explain the general characteristics of victims of child sexual abuse. The expert who testified had not examined the alleged victim, who had not reported the abuse at the time it allegedly occurred, and the testimony was offered to explain why delayed reporting can be common among those who have experienced sexual abuse. The testimony offered no speculation concerning whether the victim actually exhibited signs of CSAAS and merely provided a context within which the victim's behavior might be understood. Although this testimony may serve to inform the trier of fact, the question remains whether such testimony may be misleading or lead to improper use of the CSAAS construct as providing proof that sexual abuse occurred in a specific case when the construct has not been properly validated for such a purpose.

IDENTIFYING SUITABLE AND UNSUITABLE EXPERT TESTIMONY UNDER EXTANT STANDARDS

We would like to conclude with some general principles that can be used to distinguish suitable and scientifically based expert testimony from testimony that could be considered unsuitable or pseudoscientific. These principles are offered with a major caveat, in that it must be remembered that judges remain the ultimate gatekeepers for determining whether expert testimony is deemed admissible or inadmissible. Nevertheless, sound forensic practice necessitates that experts appraise the scientific basis and support for their testimony.

With respect to the admissibility of psychiatric diagnoses, expert testimony that has been deemed suitable is based on reliable, valid, and generally accepted principles of psychiatric diagnosis. DSM-IV offers experts a set of standardized diagnostic criteria that represent a consensus in the field that has been subjected to empirical testing for reliability and validity. Those syndromes that are novel, tentative, or speculative may at times overlap with established diagnoses. However, their general acceptance, reliability, and validity remain unclear. Therefore, it is recommended that mental health professionals frame their diagnostic formulations around DSM-IV diagnostic criteria, and avoid controversial syndromes, such as sexual addiction, road rage, homosexual panic, black rage, and codependency. A few proposed diagnoses, such as premenstrual dysphoric disorder, factitious disorder by proxy, and paraphilic coercive disorder, require further study but have not been formally accepted in DSM-IV.

Some areas of expert testimony appear to have adequate research support. These areas include risk assessment of violent behavior, the accuracy of eyewitness testimony, and certain psychological assessment methods. Testimony that is based on research and assessment methods that have been subjected to peer review, that are widely available (e.g., psychological tests that are commercially available and have a technical manual), and that have been evaluated with respect to their reliability and validity provide experts with a scientific basis for their testimony. Although courts appear unwilling to admit some forms of expert testimony (e.g., eyewitness testimony) in certain cases, this appears to be a function of the extent to which this testimony addresses ultimate legal opinions that remain within the province of the trier of fact. In most instances, it is incumbent on the expert to be able to defend the data that were relied upon when drawing conclusions and to cite adequate research in support of the use of specific techniques, the making of certain assumptions, and the drawing of specific conclusions.

GLOSSARY

Codependency: Typically refers to the tendency of an individual, typically the spouse or intimate partner, to excessively rely on another person, who is often chemically dependent or abusive, for a sense of personal identity.

Daubert **standard:** A legal standard based on the U.S. Supreme Court ruling in *Daubert v. Merrell Dow Pharmaceuticals*, 509 U.S. 579 (1993), which holds that the Federal Rules of Evidence govern admissibility in federal courts; specific criteria that a court may examine when ruling on admissibility of expert testimony include (1) whether a theory or technique can be tested, (2) peer review, (3) rate of error, and (4) general acceptance.

Expert testimony: Scientific, technical, or other specialized knowledge that will assist judges or juries to understand legal evidence or determine facts in a case. To be considered expert testimony, the subject matter must be outside the lay person's general knowledge.

Expert witness: A person whose knowledge, skill, experience, training, or education qualifies that person to provide opinions and other forms of expert testimony.

Federal Rules of Evidence (FRE): A set of legal rules that govern the admissibility of evidence in federal courts.

Frye **test:** Also known as the "general acceptance" test; a legal standard for determining the admissibility of expert testimony which examines whether or not the scientific principle, theory, or procedures relied upon by the expert have been generally accepted in the particular field in which it belongs.

Homosexual panic: A state of rage, mixed with anxiety and tension, that is purportedly experienced by a person with latent homosexual tendencies that are aroused by homosexual advances. It has been proffered, but usually rejected by courts, as a legal defense in criminal cases.

Learned treatise: A legal term referring to written material such as a book, chapter, or published article that represents an expert compilation of scientific theories and principles that are used as a standard against which expert testimony is compared.

Road rage: Impulsive acts of violence committed by a driver against other people whose behavior evokes rage or anger in the driver.

Trier of fact: Either a judge or a jury. The trier of fact evaluates legal evidence, establishes facts, and renders verdicts in civil and criminal trials.

REFERENCES

Allen v. Illinois, 478 U.S. 364 (1986).

American Psychiatric Association. (1987). *Diagnostic and statistical manual of mental disorders* (3rd ed. rev.). Washington, DC: Author.

American Psychiatric Association. (1994). *Diagnostic and statistical manual of mental disorders* (4th ed.). Washington, DC: Author.

American Psychological Association. (1992). Ethical principles of psychologists and code of conduct. *American Psychologist, 47,* 1597–1611.

Bachman v. Leapley, 953 F.2d 440 (9th Cir. 1992).

Blau, T. H. (1998). *The psychologist as expert witness.* New York: Wiley.

Bloom, J. D., & Rogers, J. L. (1987). The legal basis of forensic psychiatry: Statutorily mandated psychiatric diagnoses. *American Journal of Psychiatry, 144,* 847–853.

Blowers, A. N., & Bjerregaard, B. (1994, Winter). The admissibility of expert testimony on the battered woman syndrome in homicide cases. *Journal of Psychiatry and Law, 22,* 527–560.

Boeschen, L. E., Sales, B. D., & Koss, M. P. (1998). Rape trauma experts in the courtroom. *Psychology, Public Policy, and Law, 4,* 414–432.

Bookwalter, B. E. (1998). Throwing the bath water out with the baby: Wrongful exclusion of expert testimony on neonaticide syndrome. *Boston University Law Review, 78,* 1185–1210.

Borum, R. (1996). Improving the clinical practice of violence risk assessment. *American Psychologist, 51,* 945–956.

Cavanagh, E. D. (1999). Decision extends *Daubert* approach to all expert testimony. *New York State Bar Journal, 71*(6), 9, 19–20.

Chuang, H. T., & Addington, D. (1988). Homosexual panic: A review of its concept. *Canadian Journal of Psychiatry, 33,* 613–617.

Ciccone, J. R. (1992). Murder, insanity, and medical expert witnesses. *Archives of Neurology, 49,* 608–611.

Committee on Ethical Guidelines for Forensic Psychologists. (1991). Specialty guidelines for forensic psychologists. *Law and Human Behavior, 15,* 655–665.

Daubert v. Merrell Dow Pharmaceuticals, Inc., 509 U.S. 579, 113 S.Ct. 2786 (1993).

Faigman, D. L. (1995). The evidentiary status of social science under *Daubert*: Is it "scientific," "technical," or "other" knowledge? *Psychology, Public Policy, and Law, 1,* 960–979.

Faust, D., & Ziskin, J. (1988). The expert witness in psychology and psychiatry. *Science, 241,* 31–35.

Fuller, K. A. (1990). Paraphilic coercive disorder. *Journal of Sex Education and Therapy, 16,* 164–171.

General Electric Co. v. Joiner, 118 S.Ct. 512 (1997).

Gold, S. N., & Heffner, C. L. (1998). Sexual addiction: Many conceptions, minimal data. *Clinical Psychology Review, 18,* 367–381.

Goldklang, D. L. (1997). Post-traumatic stress disorder and black rage: Clinical validity, criminal responsibility. *Virginia Journal of Social Policy and the Law, 5,* 213–235.

Goodman-Delahunty, J. (1997). Forensic psychological expertise in the wake of *Daubert*. *Law and Human Behavior, 21,* 121–140.

Granello, D. H., & Beamish, P. M. (1998). Reconceptualizing codependency in women: A sense of connectedness, not pathology. *Journal of Mental Health Counseling, 20,* 344–358.

Green, E. D., & Nesson, C. R. (1992). *Federal rules of evidence: With selected legislative history and new cases and problems.* Boston: Little, Brown.

Greenberg, S. A., & Shuman, D. W. (1997). Irreconcilable conflict between therapeutic and forensic roles. *Professional Psychology: Research and Practice, 28,* 50–57.

Grisso, T. (1998). *Instruments for assessing understanding and appreciation of Miranda rights.* Sarasota, FL: Professional Resource Press.

Grose, N. R. (1998). Premenstrual dysphoric disorder as a mitigating factor in sentencing: Following the lead of English criminal courts. *Valparaiso University Law Review, 33,* 201–230.

Gross, W. D. (1999). The unfortunate faith: A solution to the unwarranted reliance upon eyewitness testimony. *Texas Wesleyan Law Review, 5,* 307–331.

Grudzinskas, A. J. (1999). Kuhmo Tire Col, Ltd. v. Carmichael. *Journal of the American Academy of Psychiatry and the Law, 27,* 482–488.

Grudzinskas, A. J., & Appelbaum, K. L. (1998). General Electric Co. v. Joiner: Lighting up the post-Daubert landscape? *Journal of the American Academy of Psychiatry and the Law, 26,* 497–503.

Gudjonsson, G. (1997). *The Gudjonsson suggestibility scales manual.* East Sussex, England: Psychology Press.

Haapasalo, J., & Petaja, S. (1999). Mothers who killed or attempted to kill their child: Life circumstances, childhood abuse, and types of killing. *Violence and Victims, 14,* 219–239.

Hamilton, H. G. (1998). The movement from *Frye* to *Daubert*: Where do the states stand? *Jurimetrics, 38,* 201–213.

Harding, R. W., Morgan, F. H., Indermaur, D., Ferrante, A. M., & Blagg, H. (1998). Road rage and the epidemiology of violence: Something old, something new. *Studies on Crime and Prevention, 7,* 221–238.

Hastie, R., Landsman, R., & Loftus, E. F. (1978). Eyewitness testimony: The dangers of guessing. *Jurimetrics, 19,* 1–8.

Heilbrun, K. (1992). The role of psychological testing in forensic assessment. *Law and Human Behavior, 16,* 257–272.

Heilbrun, K., Philipson, J., Berman, L., & Warren, J. (1999). Risk communication: Clinicians' reported approaches and perceived values. *Journal of the American Academy of Psychiatry and the Law, 27,* 397–406.

Henson v. State, 535 N.E.2d 1189 (Ind. 1989).

Kansas v. Hendricks, 117 S.Ct. 2072 (1997).

Klassen, D., & O'Connor, W. (1988). A prospective study of predictors of violence in adult male mental patients. *Law and Human Behavior, 12,* 143–158.

Klassen, D., & O'Connor, W. (1990). Assessing the risk of violence in released mental patients: A cross-validation study. *Psychological Assessment, 1,* 75–81.

Kumho Tire Co., Ltd. v. Carmichael 119 S.Ct. 1167 (1999).

Landsman, S. (1995). Of witches, madmen, and products liability: An historical survey of the use of expert testimony. *Behavioral Sciences and the Law, 13,* 131–157.

Levy, R. J. (1989). Using "scientific" testimony to prove child sexual abuse. *Family Law Quarterly, 23,* 383–409.

Littleton, R. W. (1999). Supreme court dramatically changes the rules on experts. *New York State Bar Journal, 71*(6), 8, 10–18.

Loughead, T. A., Spurlock, V. L., & Ting, Y. (1998). Diagnostic indicators of codependence: An investigation using the MCMI-II. *Journal of Mental Health Counseling, 20,* 64–76.

Lubit, B. W. (1998). The time has come for doing science: A call for rigorous application of *Daubert* standards for the admissibility of expert evidence in the impending silicone breast implant litigation. *New York Law School Law Review, 42,* 147–178.

Magnum, P. F. (1999). Reconceptualizing battered woman syndrome evidence: Prosecution use of expert testimony on battering. *Boston College Third World Law Journal, 19,* 593–624.

Marlowe, D. B. (1995). A hybrid decision framework for evaluating psychometric evidence. *Behavioral Sciences and the Law, 13,* 207–228.

Mart, E. G. (1999). Problems with the diagnosis of factitious disorder by proxy in forensic settings. *American Journal of Forensic Psychology, 17,* 69–82.

Mart, E.G. (2002). Munchausen's syndrome (factitious disorder) by proxy: A brief review of its scientific and legal status. *Scientific Review of Mental Health Practice, 1,* 55–61.

McCann, J. T. (1998). *Malingering and deception in adolescents: Assessing credibility in clinical and forensic settings.* Washington, DC: American Psychological Association.

McCann, J. T. (1999). *Assessing adolescents with the MACI: Using the Millon Adolescent Clinical Inventory.* New York: Wiley.

McCann, J. T., & Dyer, F. J. (1996). *Forensic assessment with the Millon inventories.* New York: Guilford Press.

McPherson, S. B. (1999). Insanity and mitigation to murder. In H. V. Hall (Ed.), *Lethal violence: A sourcebook on fatal domestic, acquaintance and stranger violence* (pp. 442–467). Boca Raton, FL: CRC Press.

Monahan, J. (1992). Mental disorder and violent behavior: Perceptions and evidence. *American Psychologist, 47,* 511–521.

Monahan, J. (1995). *The clinical prediction of violent behavior.* Northvale, NJ: Aronson. (Original work published 1981)

Monahan, J., & Steadman, H. J. (Eds.). (1994). *Violence and mental disorder: Developments in risk assessment.* Chicago: University of Chicago Press.

Monahan, J., & Steadman, H. J. (1996). Violent storms and violent people: How meteorology can inform risk communication in mental health law. *American Psychologist, 51,* 931–938.

Mossman, D. (1994). Assessing prediction of violence: Being accurate about accuracy. *Journal of Consulting and Clinical Psychology, 62,* 783–792.

Nonacs, R., & Cohen, L. S. (1998). Postpartum mood disorders: Diagnosis and treatment guidelines. *Journal of Clinical Psychiatry, 59*(2), 34–40.

Otto, R. K. (1992). Prediction of dangerous behavior: A review and analysis of "second-generation" research. *Forensic Reports, 5,* 103–133.

Parisie v. Greer 705 F.2d 882 (7th Cir. 1983).

Penrod, S., & Cutler, B. (1995). Witness confidence and witness accuracy: Assessing their forensic relation. *Psychology, Public Policy, and Law, 1,* 817–845.

People v. Erikson, 67 Cal.Rptr. 740 (Cal. 1997).

People v. Ferguson, 248 A.D. 2d 725, 670 N.Y.S. 2d 327 (N.Y. App. Div. 1998).

People v. Freeman, 4 Denio 9 (N.Y. Sup. Ct. 1847).

People v. Humphrey, 56 Cal.Rptr. 142, 921 P.2d 1 (Cal. 1996).

People v. Ilieveski, 670 N.Y.S.2d 1004 (Monroe Co. 1998).

People v. McDonald, 37 Cal.3d 351, 690 P.2d 709 (Cal. 1984).

People v. Milner, 45 Cal.3d 227, 753 P.2d 669 (Sup. Ct. of Cal. 1988).

People v. Phillips, 122 Cal. Rptr. 703 (Cal. Ct. App. 1981).

People v. Wernick, 37 Cal. 3d 351, 690 P.2d 709 (N.Y. App. Div. 1995).

Pope, K. S., Butcher, J. N., & Seelen, J. (1993). *The MMPI, MMPI-2, and MMPI-A in court.* Washington, DC: American Psychological Association.

Quinsey, V. L., Harris, G. T., Rice, M. E., & Cormier, C. A. (1998). *Violent offenders: Appraising and managing risk.* Washington, DC: American Psychological Association.

Reynolds, C. R. (Ed.). (1998). *Detection of malingering during head injury litigation.* New York: Plenum Press.

Rice, M. E. (1997). Violent offender research and implications for the criminal justice system. *American Psychologist, 52,* 414–423.

Ritchie, E. C. (1998). Reactions to rape: A military forensic psychiatrist's perspective. *Military Medicine, 163,* 505–509.

Robins, E., & Guze, S. B. (1970). Establishment of diagnostic validity in psychiatric illness: Its application to schizophrenia. *American Journal of Psychiatry, 126,* 107–111.

Rogers, R. (1984). *Rogers Criminal Responsibility Assessment scales.* Odessa, FL: Psychological Assessment Resources.

Schuller, R. A., & Vidmar, N. (1992). Battered woman syndrome evidence in the courtroom: A review of the literature. *Law and Human Behavior, 16,* 273–291.

Shapiro, D. L. (1999). *Criminal responsibility evaluations: A manual for practice.* Sarasota, FL: Professional Resource Press.

State v. Allewalt, 308 Md. 89, 517 A.2d 741 (Md. 1986).

State v. Escamilla, 245 Neb. 13, 511 N.W.2d 58 (Neb. 1994).

Steadman, H. J., McGreevy, M. A., Morrissey, J. P., Callahan, L. A., Robbins, P. C., & Cirincione, C. (1993). *Before and after Hinckley: Evaluating insanity defense reform.* New York: Guilford Press.

Steele, D. L. (1999). Expert testimony: Seeking an appropriate admissibility standard for behavioral science in child sexual abuse prosecutions. *Duke Law Journal, 48,* 933–973.

Stefan, S. (1994). The protection racket: Rape trauma syndrome, psychiatric labeling, and law. *Northwestern University Law Review, 88,* 1271–1345.

Steiner, M. (1997). Premenstrual syndromes. *Annual Review of Medicine, 48,* 447–455.

Summit, R. C. (1983). The child sexual abuse accommodation syndrome. *Child Abuse and Neglect, 7,* 177–193.

Summit, R. C. (1992). Abuse of the child sexual abuse accommodation syndrome. *Journal of Child Sexual Abuse, 1,* 153–163.

United States v. Amador-Galvan, 9 F.3d 1414 (9th Cir. 1997).

United States v. Bighead, 128 F.3d 1329 (9th Cir. 1997).

United States v. Frye, 293 F. 1013 (D.C. Cir. 1923).

United States v. Hall, 165 F.3d 1095 (7th Cir. 1999).

United States v. Kime, 99 F.3d 870 (8th Cir. 1996).

United States v. Robertson, 507 F.2d 1148 (D.C. Cir. 1974).

United States v. Romualdi, 101 F.3d 971 (3rd Cir. 1996).

United States v. Smith, 1998 LEXIS 5772 (6th Cir. 1998).

Vollaro, T. (1993). Muchausen syndrome by proxy and its evidentiary problems. *Hofstra Law Review, 22,* 495–520.

Walker, L. E. (1984). *The battered woman syndrome.* New York: Springer.

Walker, L. E. (1994). *Abused women and survivor therapy: A practical guide for the psychotherapist.* Washington, DC: American Psychological Association.

Wells, G. L. (1995). Scientific study of witness memory: Implications for public and legal policy. *Psychology, Public Policy, and Law, 1,* 726–731.

Wells, G. L., & Seelau, E. P. (1995). Eyewitness identification: Psychological research and legal policy on lineups. *Psychology, Public Policy, and Law, 1,* 765–791.

Wells, M., Glickauf-Hughes, C., & Bruss, K. (1998). The relationship of co-dependency to enduring personality characteristics. *Journal of College Student Psychotherapy, 12,* 25–38.

Ziskin, J., & Faust, D. (1988). *Coping with psychiatric and psychological testimony* (4th ed.). Marina del Rey, CA: Law and Psychology Press.

5

Dissociative Identity Disorder

Multiple Personalities, Multiple Controversies

SCOTT O. LILIENFELD
STEVEN JAY LYNN

Dissociative identity disorder (DID), known formerly as multiple personality disorder (MPD), is among the most controversial of all psychiatric diagnoses (see Chapter 4 for a review of other controversial psychiatric diagnoses and their legal status). The controversies surrounding DID have centered primarily on its descriptive psychopathology, diagnosis, etiology, and treatment (see also Elzinga, van Dyck, & Spinhoven, 1998). Although these controversies have a lengthy history, they have become especially divisive and even acrimonious over the past decade.

Some researchers (e.g., Ross, 1997) contend that DID is one of the most commonly overlooked diagnoses in psychiatry and clinical psychology, and that DID's prevalence has been greatly underestimated (see also Dell, 2001). Yet surveys of clinicians indicate that numerous professionals are deeply skeptical of the DID diagnosis and of many prevailing theories of its etiology (Cormier & Thelen, 1998; Dell, 1988; Pope, Oliva, Hudson, Bodkin, & Gruber, 1999).

In this chapter, we provide an overview of the major controversies regarding the scientific status of DID.[1] In addition, we outline areas of po-

---

[1]One important controversy regarding DID that we touch on only briefly in this chapter is the question of whether this condition is overdiagnosed using structured interviews or other assessment methods (see Elzinga et al., 1998). This issue is extremely difficult to settle at the present time owing to the absence of dependable external validating "criteria" for the presence or absence of DID. See Elzinga et al. (1988), Gleaves (1996), Lilienfeld et al. (1999), and Ross (1991) for discussions of this controversy.

109

tential common ground among individuals who hold markedly differing viewpoints regarding DID, and to delineate fruitful areas for further investigation.

DID: A BRIEF HISTORY

Early Conceptions of DID

Reports of DID in the popular and clinical literature date back at least to the 19th century. Robert Louis Stevenson's classic 1885 novel, *The Strange Case of Dr. Jekyll and Mr. Hyde*, which describes the case of a scientist who ingests a mysterious potion that transforms him into an entirely different person, is among the first tales reminiscent of the modern-day notion of DID.

Around the turn of the century, the French neurologist Pierre Janet introduced the concept of dissociation (which he termed "desagregation"), conceptualized as a means of walling off disturbing experiences from conscious awareness. Freud and his followers, however, were skeptical of the notion of multiple personality disorder, and suggested that most or all cases of this condition were due largely to the suggestive influence of therapists upon patients. Freud jettisoned Janet's concept of dissociation (i.e., horizontal splitting within different parts of the unconscious), and replaced it with the concept of repression (i.e., vertical splitting between the conscious and unconscious).

Although the remarkable signs and symptoms of DID captured the imagination of authors and researchers throughout the 19th and 20th centuries, reports of this condition were extremely rare until the late 20th century. As of 1970, there was a total of 79 well-documented cases of DID in the world literature. Perhaps the best-known early case of DID was that of "Miss Beachamp," which was reported by psychologist Morton Prince around the turn of the century (Prince, 1905). Another relatively early celebrated case of DID was that of a patient, Chris Sizemore, which formed the basis of the book (and later the Hollywood film) *The Three Faces of Eve* (Thigpen & Cleckley, 1957). Chris Sizemore reported three personalities, Eve White, Eve Black, and a third personality named Jane. As in many cases of DID (see "DID: Descriptive Features and Correlates" later in this chapter), two of the personalities exhibited almost diametrically opposed personality characteristics. Eve White was reserved, traditional, and demure, whereas Eve Black was flamboyant, fun loving, and seductive. This case attracted considerable public attention, largely because it was one of the few clear-cut cases of DID known at that time.

The DID Epidemic Begins

Beginning in the mid- to late 1970s, however, cases of DID cases began to be reported in substantial numbers. As of 1986, the number of reported

DID cases had swollen to approximately 6,000. This massive increase followed closely upon the release of the best-selling book (later made into a widely viewed television film), *Sybil* (Schreiber, 1973) in the mid-1970s, which told the story of a young woman with 16 personalities who reported a history of severe and sadistic child abuse at the hands of her mother.

Interestingly, however, a well-known psychiatrist who was intimately involved with the Sybil case recently contended that Sybil's DID was largely the product of therapeutic suggestion. Herbert Spiegel, who served as a backup therapist for Sybil, maintained that Sybil's primary therapist, Cornelia Wilbur, encouraged her to develop and display different personalities in therapy. According to Spiegel, Wilbur referred to Sybil's personalities by different names and communicated with them individually. Spiegel further maintained that Wilbur and Flora Schreiber, who authored the best-selling book about Sybil, insisted that Sybil be described in the book as a "multiple" to make the book more appealing to the publisher (see Acocella, 1998). As we will see shortly, the role of therapeutic suggestion in Sybil's case and in other cases of DID is probably the most contentious issue in the DID literature.

The number of reported DID cases at the turn of the 21st century is difficult to ascertain, although one estimate places the number of DID cases as of 1998 at approximately 40,000 (Marmer, 1998). Moreover, a number of celebrities, including Roseanne Arnold, have announced that they suffer from DID, and television coverage of DID has skyrocketed over the past two decades (Showalter, 1997; Spanos, 1996). The reasons for the recent "epidemic" (Boor, 1982) in the number of reported DID cases remain controversial.

Two other historical changes in the characteristics of patients with DID are worth noting. First, the number of DID personalities has increased dramatically over time. Whereas most cases of DID prior to the 1970s were characterized by only one or two personalities, recent cases of DID are typically characterized by considerably more personalities (North, Ryall, Ricci, & Wetzel, 1993). For example, Ross, Norton, and Wozney (1989) reported that the mean number of DID personalities was 16, precisely the number reported by Sybil (Acocella, 1998). Second, although few individuals with DID prior to Sybil reported a history of child abuse, a substantial proportion of DID cases that followed in the wake of Sybil reported such a history (Spanos, 1996).

DID: DESCRIPTIVE FEATURES AND CORRELATES

Major Diagnostic Features

According to the *Diagnostic and Statistical Manual of Mental Disorders*, fourth edition (DSM-IV; American Psychiatric Association [APA], 1994), DID is one of several "dissociative disorders," all of which are marked by

profound disturbances in memory, identity, consciousness, and/or perception of the external environment. DID is characterized by the presence of
two or more distinct personalities or "personality states" (i.e., temporary
patterns of behavior) that recurrently assume control over the individual's
behavior. These alternate personalities, or "alters," often exhibit personality features that differ markedly from those of the primary or "host" personality. In some cases, these features appear to be the exact opposite of
those exhibited by the host personality. For example, if the host personality
is shy and retiring, one or more of the alters may be outgoing or flamboyant. Some therapists (e.g., Allison, 1974) have even argued that patients
with DID possess an "inner self-helper," a part of the personality that is
aware of everything that is occurring to the alters and that can assist in
their integration.

In addition, according to DSM-IV, individuals with DID report significant episodes of amnesia for important personal information. For example,
they may report periods of "lost time" lasting hours or days in which they
cannot recall where they were or what they were doing. This amnesia is often reported to be asymmetrical, whereby the host personality knows little
about the behaviors of the alters, but not vice versa (American Psychiatric
Association, 1994).

Nevertheless, the scientific standing of amnesia as a feature of DID is
controversial. Allen and Iacono (2001) concluded that controlled laboratory studies examining the transfer of explicit and implicit memories offer
relatively little support for the claim that patients with DID actually experience amnesia across alters (but see Dorahy, 2001, for a somewhat different conclusion). In addition, research by Read and his colleagues (see, e.g.,
Read & Lindsay, 2000) demonstrates that one can readily induce reports
of autobiographical memory gaps in normal subjects by asking them to recall multiple events from early childhood. Specifically, individuals who are
asked to recall multiple events from early childhood (as often occurs in
depth-oriented psychotherapy) typically do so obligingly. As a consequence, when they are asked such questions as "Was there ever a period of
time when you remembered less of your childhood than you do now?"
they will typically respond "Yes," because they are accurately reporting
that they now recall (or at least believe that they recall) more of their childhood history than they once did. In fact, these and similar questions are
used commonly in investigations of DID to verify the presence of amnesia
(see Ross, 1997). Self-reports of autobiographical memory gaps in patients
with DID must therefore be interpreted with caution.

Demographic and Familial Correlates

Relatively little is known about the demographic or familial correlates of
DID. Until recently, it was widely assumed that DID is exceedingly uncom-

mon. DSM-III (American Psychiatric Association, 1980), for example, stated that MPD, as it was then called, "is apparently extremely rare" (p. 258). Nevertheless, DSM-IV is conspicuously silent regarding DID's prevalence, and notes only that reports of its prevalence have been highly variable across studies. Indeed, although some authors (e.g., Piper, 1997) claim that genuine DID is very rare (see also Rifkin, Ghisalbert, Dimatou, Jin, & Sethi, 1998), other authors maintain that DID is at least as common as schizophrenia. For example, Ross (1997) estimated that between 1% and 2% of the North American population meets criteria for DID. These discrepancies among authors are difficult to resolve given the absence of clear-cut external validating variables (Robins & Guze, 1970) for DID (see footnote 1).

Virtually all prevalence studies show a marked female predominance, with most sex ratios ranging from 3 to 1 to 9 to 1 across clinical samples (American Psychiatric Association, 1994). Some authors, however, argue that this imbalanced sex ratio may be an artifact of selection and referral biases, and that a large proportion of males with DID end up in prisons (or other forensic settings) rather than in clinical settings (Putnam & Loewenstein, 2000).

Alters

The nature and features of DID alters are highly variable both across and within individuals. The number of alters has been reported to range from one (the so-called "split" personality) to hundreds or even thousands. One clinician reported a case of a patient with DID who had 4,500 alters (Acocella, 1998). These alters are not uncommonly of different sexes, ages, and even races. There have even been reported alters of Mr. Spock, Teenage Mutant Ninja Turtles, lobsters, chickens, gorillas, tigers, unicorns, God, the bride of Satan, and the rock star Madonna (Acocella, 1998; Ganaway, 1989).

Some of the reported differences among alters have been striking. For example, alters have been reported to differ in their allergies, handwriting, voice patterns, eyeglass prescriptions, handedness, and other psychological and physical characteristics. Frank Putnam, a major DID researcher, even reported a case of DID in which one alter, but not other alters, exhibited cardiac arrhythmias (Lichtenstein Creative Media, 1998).

Nevertheless, virtually all of these reported differences derive from anecdotal and uncontrolled reports. Moreover, most of these reports have not controlled adequately for naturally occurring variability in these characteristics over time. Both handwriting and voice, for example, often show at least some variability over time within individuals, especially in response to situational variables (e.g., fatigue, stress), and some allergies have been demonstrated to be susceptible to classical conditioning. As a consequence, these and other reported differences across alters are difficult to interpret with confidence (see also Merkelbach, Devilly, & Rassin, 2002, and Spanos, 1996, for a critique).

Several researchers have also reported psychophysiological differences across alters. For example, investigators have reported differences among alters in respiration rate (e.g., Bahnson & Smith, 1975), electroencephalographic (brain wave) activity (e.g., Ludwig, Brandsma, Wilbur, Bendefeldt, & Jameson, 1972), and skin conductance responses (e.g., Brende, 1984). Nevertheless, these and other differences (see also Putnam, Zahn, & Post, 1990) do not provide especially compelling evidence for the existence of qualitatively distinct differences among alters. As Allen and Movius (2000) noted, such differences could be attributable to changes in mood or cognition over time or to temporal changes in variables (e.g., levels of muscle tension) that are largely under volitional control (see also Merkelbach et al., 2002). Moreover, at least some of these differences may be attributable to Type I error given the large number of psychophysiological variables examined in many of these investigations (Allen & Movius, 2000).

The "Multiple Personalities" Controversy

One long-standing controversy concerns the question of whether individuals with DID harbor qualitatively distinct "personalities," each with its own unique pattern of life experiences, personality traits, and attitudes. Some authors, like Braun (1986), maintain that patients with DID possess separate personalities in addition to "fragments," that is, aspects of personalities. Indeed, the older term "multiple personality disorder" in DSM-III and DSM-III-R (American Psychiatric Association, 1987) clearly implies the existence of largely independent cohabiting personalities.

Nevertheless, many advocates of the DID diagnosis now argue that DID is not characterized by the presence of independent and fully developed personalities (Ross, 1990, 1997). Coons (1984), for example, contended that "it is a mistake to consider each personality totally separate, whole, or autonomous. The other personalities might best be described as personality states, other selves, or personality fragments" (p. 53). Ross (1989) similarly asserted that "much of the skepticism about MPD is based on the erroneous assumption that such patients have more than one personality, which is, in fact, impossible" (p. 81; see also Spiegel, 1993). This caveat notwithstanding, the first major criterion for DID in DSM-IV is "the presence of two or more distinct identities or personality states (each with its own relatively enduring pattern of perceiving, relating to, and thinking about the environment and self)" (p. 487). This wording implies the presence of more than one discrete and fully developed personality.

The question of whether patients with DID possess distinct coexisting personalities is of more than semantic significance. For example, in legal cases questions have arisen concerning whether individuals with DID should be held criminally responsible if one of their alter personalities committed a crime or whether each alter personality is entitled to separate legal representation. Some trial judges have even required all DID personalities to be sworn in before providing testimony (Slovenko, 1999). In addition, if patients with DID truly possess independent and fully developed personalities, this poses significant challenges to models of DID's etiology. For example, how do these ostensibly complete personalities, each presumably with its own set of personality traits and attitudes, form? For patients who possess hundreds of alters, is each personality genuinely independent of the others, or are certain personalities merely variants or slightly different manifestations of the others?

ETIOLOGY: TWO COMPETING MODELS

DID's "Existence": A Pseudocontroversy

The principal controversy regarding DID's scientific status has often been framed in terms of whether this condition "exists" (e.g., Arrigo & Pezdek, 1998; Dunn, Paolo, Ryan, & van Fleet, 1994; Mai, 1995; see also Hacking, 1995). Nevertheless, as we have argued elsewhere (Lilienfeld et al., 1999), the question of DID's "existence" is a pseudocontroversy. There is little dispute that DID "exists," in that individuals with this condition exhibit multiple identity enactments (i.e., apparent alters). This point was aptly put by McHugh (1993): "Students often ask me whether multiple personality disorder (MPD) really exists. I usually reply that the symptoms attributed to it are as genuine as hysterical paralysis and seizures" (p. 4). Somatoform conditions, like DID, are clearly genuine, although their origins remain largely obscure. The central question at stake is not DID's existence but rather its etiology. As we will learn shortly, some researchers contend that DID is a spontaneously occurring response to childhood trauma, whereas others contend that it emerges in response to suggestive therapist cueing, media influences, and broader sociocultural expectations.

There is general agreement, however, that at least some individuals have successfully malingered DID. For example, Kenneth Bianchi, one of the Hillside Strangler murderers, is widely believed to have faked DID to escape criminal responsibility (Orne, Dinges, & Orne, 1984). Nevertheless, outside of criminal settings, cases of malingered DID are believed to be quite rare, and there is agreement among both proponents and skeptics of the DID diagnosis that the substantial majority of individuals with this condition are not intentionally producing their symptoms (see Draijer & Boon, 1999, for a discussion of the problem of intentionally produced DID).

The Central Controversy: Two Competing Etiological Models

In general, two major competing views regarding the etiology of DID have emerged (see Gleaves, 1996): the posttraumatic model (PTM) and the sociocognitive model (SCM). To oversimplify these views slightly, the former model posits that core DID features, particularly alters, are discovered by therapists, whereas the latter model posits that these features are largely created by therapists. Because we believe that the bulk of the research evidence supports the SCM, we devote much of the remainder of the chapter to a discussion of this model. Nevertheless, we also believe that certain aspects of the PTM have yet to be convincingly falsified and therefore require additional investigation. Moreover, we believe that a meaningful rapprochement between at least certain aspects of these two models may ultimately prove possible.

The Posttraumatic Model

Proponents of the PTM (e.g., Gleaves, 1996; Gleaves, May, & Cardena, 2001; Ross, 1997) posit that DID is a posttraumatic condition that arises primarily from a history of severe physical and/or sexual abuse in childhood. They typically argue that individuals who undergo horrific trauma in early life often dissociate or compartmentalize their personalities into alters as a means of coping with the intense emotional pain of this trauma. According to Ross (1997), "MPD is a little girl imagining that the abuse is happening to someone else" (p. 59). In support of this assertion, proponents of the PTM cite data suggesting that a large proportion—perhaps 90% or more—of individuals with DID report a history of child abuse (Gleaves, 1996).

The essence of the PTM has been articulated by philosopher Daniel Dennett (1991):

> . . . the evidence is now voluminous that there are not a handful or a hundred but thousands of cases of MPD diagnosed today, and it almost invariably owes its existence to prolonged early childhood abuse, usually sexual, and of sickening severity. . . . These children have often been kept in such extraordinarily terrifying and confusing circumstances that I am more amazed that they survive psychologically at all than I am that they manage to preserve themselves by a desperate redrawing of their boundaries. (p. 150)

Proponents of the PTM attribute the dramatic recent increase in the reported prevalence of DID to the heightened awareness and recognition of this condition by psychotherapists. Specifically, they maintain that clinicians have only recently become attuned to the presence of possible DID in their clients and as a consequence now inquire more actively about symptoms of this condition (Gleaves, 1996). They also point out that a number of conditions, such as posttraumatic stress disorder (PTSD) and obsessive–compulsive disorder, were apparently underdiagnosed until recently (e.g., Zohar, 1998), and that a relatively abrupt massive increase in the reported prevalence of a condition does not necessarily call into question its validity. In many cases, proponents of the PTM advocate the use of hypnosis, sodium amytal (so-called "truth serum"; see Piper, 1993, for a critique of the claim that sodium amytal is a "truth serum"), guided imagery, and other suggestive therapeutic techniques to call forth alters that are otherwise inaccessible and to recover apparently repressed memories of child abuse.

The Sociocognitive Model

In contrast, proponents of the SCM (Spanos, 1994, 1996; see also Aldridge-Morris, 1989; Lilienfeld et al., 1999; Lynn & Pintar, 1997; McHugh, 1993; Merskey, 1992; Sarbin, 1995) contend that DID is a socially constructed condition that results from inadvertent therapist cueing (e.g., suggestive questioning regarding the existence of possible alters), media influences (e.g., film and television portrayals of DID), and broader sociocultural expectations regarding the presumed clinical features of DID. For example, proponents of the SCM believe that the release of the book and film *Sybil* in the 1970s played a substantial role in shaping conceptions of DID in the minds of the general public and psychotherapists (see Spanos, 1996). Interestingly, as noted earlier, reported cases of child abuse in DID patients became widespread only following the release of Sybil.

Spanos (1994) and other proponents of the SCM contend that individuals with DID are engaged in a form of "role playing" that is similar in some ways to the intense sense of imaginative involvement that some actors report when playing a part. Because individuals who engage in role playing essentially "lose themselves" in the enacted part, this phenomenon should be not be confused with simulation or conscious deception. Some authors have erroneously assumed that the SCM posits that individuals with DID are intentionally producing these features. But the SCM is careful to distinguish role playing from simulation (Lilienfeld et al., 1999; in contrast, see Gleaves, 1996).

According to the SCM, the dramatic "epidemic" in DID cases over the past several decades stems largely from iatrogenic (therapist-induced) influences and the increased media attention accorded to DID. Specifically, as DID has become more familiar to psychotherapists and the general public, an autocatalytic feedback loop (see Shermer, 1997, for examples) has been set in motion. In this feedback loop, therapeutic and societal expectations regarding the features of DID have given rise to greater numbers of cases of DID, in turn influencing therapeutic and societal expectations regarding the features of DID, in turn giving rise to greater number of cases of DID, and so on. It is critical to emphasize that the SCM does not contend that DID is entirely iatrogenic, because media influences and broader sociocultural expectations often play an important role in the genesis of DID. The notion that the SCM posits that DID is entirely iatrogenic represents another frequent misconception concerning this model. For example, Gleaves and colleagues (2001) referred to the SCM as the "iatrogenic" theory of DID (see Brown, Frischholz, & Scheflin, 1999; and Gleaves, 1996, for other examples).

Nevertheless, proponents of the SCM maintain that suggestive therapeutic practices—such as hypnosis, guided imagery, and repeated prompting of alters (see Chapter 8 for a discussion of these and other suggestive practices)—often play a substantial role in the genesis of DID. For example, they point to evidence demonstrating that detailed, complex, and nontrivial pseudomemories of life experiences can be elicited by suggestive memory recovery procedures. These experiences include being lost in a shopping mall (Loftus & Pickrell, 1995; Pezdek, Finger, & Hodge, 1997), knocking over a punchbowl at a wedding (Hyman, Husband, & Billings, 1995; Hyman & Pentland, 1996), being discouraged from using one's left hand (see Lindsay, 1996), choking and witnessing an occurrence of demonic possession as a child (Mazzoni, Loftus, & Kirsch, 2001), and being abused as a child in a past life (Spanos, Menary, Gabora, DuBreuil, & Dewhirst, 1991). Lindsay (1998) contended that such laboratory studies come nowhere near to "approximating the power of the suggestive influences that are brought to bear in some forms of memory-recovery work, in which individuals may be exposed to suggestions several hours per week for months or even years" (p. 490). Proponents of the SCM therefore maintain that suggestive therapeutic procedures can quite plausibly induce the production of alters and the autobiographical memories (e.g., child abuse) associated with them.

Another important brick in the edifice of the SCM is the assumption that DID is merely one variant of a broader constellation of conditions characterized by multiple identity enactments, including cases of purported demonic possession, channeling, mass hysteria, transvestism, and glossolalia (speaking in tongues), that traverse cultural and historical boundaries (Spanos, 1996). From this perspective, DID is not a unique condition but rather a superficially different manifestation of the same diathesis that gives rise to other conditions marked by dramatically different behaviors over time. Although the protean manifestations of these role enactments are shaped by cultural and historical expectations, their underlying commonalities are suggestive of a shared etiology (Lilienfeld et al., 1999; see also Hacking, 1995).

Some proponents of the SCM (e.g., Spanos, 1994, 1996) have placed more emphasis on social role expectations and iatrogenic influences than on individual difference variables. Nevertheless, the SCM is compatible with the possibility that individual differences in certain personality traits, such as fantasy proneness (Lynn, Rhue, & Green, 1988) or absorption (Tellegen & Atkinson, 1974), render certain individuals especially susceptible to suggestive therapeutic, media, and cultural influences. In addition, this model is compatible with findings indicating that a substantial proportion of patients with DID meet criteria for borderline personality disorder (BPD) and other psychiatric conditions marked by unstable and unpredictable behavior, such as bipolar disorder (Ganaway, 1995; Lilienfeld et al., 1999). For example, clients with BPD—who typically exhibit severe disturbances of identity, dramatic mood swings, sudden changes in feelings toward other people, and impulsive and seemingly inexplicable behaviors (e.g., self-mutilation)—may often be seeking an explanation for these puzzling symptoms, as may their therapists. Therapists who repeatedly ask such questions as "Is it possible that there is another part of you with whom I haven't yet spoken?" may gradually begin to elicit previously "latent alters" that ostensibly account for their clients' otherwise enigmatic behaviors.

Many of the key features of the SCM were summed up by Frances and First (1998), who ironically were two of the principal architects of DSM-IV:

> Dissociative Identity Disorder . . . is a fascinating condition. Perhaps too much so. The idea that people can have distinct, autonomous, and rapidly alternating personalities has captured the attention of the general public, of some therapists, and of hordes of patients. As a result, especially in the United States, there has been a marked increase in the diagnosis of Dissociative Identity Disorder. Much of the excitement followed the appearance of books and movies (like *Sybil* and *The Three Faces of Eve*) and the exploitation of the diagnosis by enthusiastic TV talk show guests. . . . Many therapists feel that the popularity of Dissociative Identity Disorder represents a kind of social contagion. It is not so much that there are lots of personalities as that there are lots of people and lots of therapists who are very suggestible and willing to climb onto the bandwagon of this new fad diagnosis. As the idea of multiple personality pervades our popular culture, suggestible people coping with a chaotic current life and a severely traumatic past express discomfort and avoid responsibility by uncovering "hidden personalities" and giving each of them a voice. This is especially likely when there is a zealous therapist who finds multiple personality a fascinating topic of discussion and exploration. (pp. 286–287)

Advocates of the SCM have invoked a variety of pieces of evidence in support of this position (Lilienfeld et al., 1999; Spanos, 1994, 1996). We next present the major sources of evidence consistent with the SCM and examine common criticisms of this model.

EVIDENCE FOR THE SOCIOCOGNITIVE MODEL OF DID

Typical Treatment Practices

One important source of evidence in favor of the SCM are the typical treatment practices employed by many proponents of the PTM. Claims by some proponents of the PTM to the contrary (Brown et al., 1999; Gleaves, 1996), many standard therapeutic practices for DID are geared toward encouraging the appearance of alters and treating them as though they were distinct identities.

Inspection of the mainstream DID treatment literature reveals that therapists are often encouraged to reify the existence of multiple identities by mapping the system of alters and to establish contact with alters if they are not otherwise forthcoming (Piper, 1997). These reifying techniques are especially common in the early stages of psychotherapy (Ross, 1997).

For example, Kluft (1993) argued that "when information suggestive of MPD is available, but an alter has not emerged spontaneously, asking to meet an alter directly is an increasingly accepted intervention" (p. 29). Kluft has further acknowledged that his most frequent hypnotic instruction to patients with DID is "Everybody listen" (see Ganaway, 1995). Braun (1980) wrote that "after inducing hypnosis, the therapist asks the patient 'if there is another thought process, part of the mind, part, person or force that exists in the body' " (p. 213). Bliss (1980) noted in the treatment of DID that "alter egos are summoned, and usually asked to speak freely. . . . When they appear, the subject is asked to listen. [The subject] is then introduced to some of the personalities" (p. 1393). Putnam (1989) suggested using a technique known as the "bulletin board," which allows patients with DID to have a "place where personalities can 'post' messages to each other. . . . I suggest that the patient buy a small notebook in which personalities may write messages to each other" (p. 154). Ross (1997) and other therapists (e.g., Putnam, 1989) have recommended giving names to each alter in order to " 'crystallize' it and make it more distinct" (p. 311). Ross also advocated the use of "inner board meetings" as "a good way to map the system, resolve issues, and recover memories" (p. 350). He described this technique as follows:

> The patient relaxes with a brief hypnotic induction, and the host personality walks into the boardroom. The patient is instructed that there will be one chair for every personality in the system. . . . Often there are empty chairs because some alters are not ready to enter therapy. The empty chairs provide useful information, and those present can be asked what they know about the missing people. (p. 351)

These and other treatment recommendations derived from the mainstream DID literature (see Piper, 1997, pp. 61–68, for additional examples) strongly suggest that many therapists are explicitly encouraged to reify the existence of alters by acknowledging and validating their independent existence. From a behavioral or social learning perspective, the process of attending to and reifying alters may adventitiously reinforce patients' displays of multiplicity.

Another treatment practice that may inadvertently facilitate the emergence of alters is hypnosis. Clinicians who treat patients with DID frequently use hypnosis in an effort to discover or call forth presumed latent alters (Spanos, 1994, 1996). The evidence regarding the use of hypnosis with patients with DID provides mixed support for the SCM. On the one hand, the results of several studies reveal few or no differences in the diagnostic features (e.g., alters, number of DID criteria) of patients with DID who have and have not been hypnotized (e.g., Putnam, Guroff, Silberman, Barban, & Post, 1986; Ross & Norton, 1989; see also Gleaves, 1996, for a review). In addition, several studies indicate that many or most patients with DID have never been hypnotized (Gleaves, 1996), strongly suggesting that hypnosis is not necessary for the emergence of DID.

On the other hand, the finding that hypnotized and nonhypnotized patients with DID do not differ significantly in many characteristics (e.g., number of DID criteria) is difficult to interpret in light of ceiling effects (Lilienfeld et al., 1999; Powell & Gee, 1999). Specifically, given that almost all of the patients in these studies met criteria for DID according to various diagnostic criterion sets (e.g., DSM-III), the differences in the number of DID criteria between hypnotized and nonhypnotized patients is not surprising.

In addition, in a reanalysis of the data set of Ross and Norton (1989), Powell and Gee (1999) found that hypnotized patients exhibited greater variance in the number of alters at the time of diagnosis and in later treatment. Although the meaning of this finding is not entirely clear, it may reflect bimodal attitudes toward iatrogenesis among practitioners who use hypnosis, with some (who believe that hypnosis is potentially iatrogenic) using hypnosis never or rarely and others (who believe that hypnosis is not iatrogenic) using hypnosis frequently. Powell and Gee also found that clinicians who used hypnosis reported a significantly higher number of patients with DID in their caseloads than did practitioners who did not use hypnosis. Although this finding is open to several interpretations (e.g., DID specialists may be more likely to use hypnosis than are other clinicians), it is consistent with iatrogenesis.

Moreover, the SCM does not posit that hypnosis is necessary for the creation of DID alters. Hypnotic procedures do not possess any inherent or unique features that are necessary to facilitate responsivity to suggestion (Spanos & Chaves, 1989). Other methods, such as suggestive and leading questions, may be equally likely to induce clients' adoption of multiple identities (Spanos, 1996).

Clinical Features of Patients with DID before and after Psychotherapy

There is compelling evidence that a large proportion—perhaps even a substantial majority—of patients with DID exhibit very few or no unambiguous signs of this condition (e.g., alters) prior to psychotherapy. For example, Kluft (1991) estimated that only 20% of patients with DID exhibit unambiguous signs of this condition and that the remaining 80% exhibit only transient "windows of diagnosability," that is, short-lived periods during which the core features of DID are observable. Moreover, individuals with DID typically are in treatment for an average of 6–7 years before being diagnosed with this condition (Gleaves, 1996). Such evidence raises the possibility that these patients often develop unambiguous features of DID only after receiving psychotherapy.

Moreover, although systematic data are lacking, there is general agreement in the DID literature that many or most patients with DID are unaware of the existence of their alters prior to psychotherapy. For example, Putnam (1989) estimated that 80% of patients with DID possess no knowledge of their alters before entering treatment, and Dell and Eisenhower (1990) reported that all 11 of their adolescent patients with DID had no awareness of their alters at the time of diagnosis. Similarly, Lewis, Yeager, Swica, Pincus, and Lewis (1997) reported that none of the 12 murderers with DID in their sample reported any awareness of their alters.

Some authors have also reported that the number of DID alters tends to increase over the course of treatment (Kluft, 1988; Ross et al., 1989). In addition, although the number of alters per DID case at the time of initial diagnosis has remained roughly constant over time (Ross et al., 1989), the number of alters per DID case in treatment has increased over time (North et al., 1993).

These findings are consistent with the SCM, as they suggest that many therapeutic practices for DID may inadvertently encourage the emergence of new alters. Moreover, as we noted elsewhere (Lilienfeld et al., 1999), one would be hard-pressed to find another DSM-IV disorder whose principal feature (i.e., alters) is often unobservable prior to standard treatment and becomes substantially more florid following this treatment.

Nevertheless, some proponents of the PTM argue that these findings are potentially consistent with this model. Specifically, they maintain that the alters were "latent" at the time of diagnosis and became observable only after elicitation by therapists (Gleaves, 1996). Nevertheless, without independent evidence of these alters this position raises concerns regarding the falsifiability of the PTM. That is, if the number of alters either decreased or remained constant over the course of therapy, proponents of the PTM could maintain that treatment for DID either ameliorated the symptoms of DID or held potential deterioration at bay. In contrast, the finding that the number of alters increases over the course of therapy has been interpreted by proponents of the PTM as indicating that psychotherapy successfully uncovered alters that were latent (Gleaves, 1996). Because a model that is consistent with any potential set of observations is impossible to falsify and is therefore of questionable scientific utility (Popper, 1959), proponents of the PTM will need to make explicit what types of evidence could falsify this model.

Some critics of the SCM (e.g., Brown et al., 1999; Gleaves, 1996) have attempted to argue that suggestive therapeutic practices can produce additional alters in patients who already meet criteria for DID, but that these practices cannot create DID itself. This assertion hinges on the assumption that iatrogenic influences can lead patients with one alter to develop additional alters, but cannot lead patients with no alters to develop one or more alters. The theoretical basis underlying this assumption has not been clearly articulated by critics of the SCM (Lilienfeld et al., 1999). Moreover, this assertion appears extremely difficult, if not impossible, to falsify given that many critics of the SCM maintain that DID alters can be "latent" (e.g., Kluft, 1991). That is, if a patient with no alters developed alters following suggestive therapeutic practices, critics of the SCM could readily maintain that this patient merely had latent alters and in fact suffered from DID all along (Piper, 1997). In addition, even some of the most ardent proponents of the PTM acknowledge that DID can be iatrogenically created in certain cases. Ross (1997), for example, estimated that approximately 17% of DID cases are predominantly iatrogenic (see also Coons, 1989). Thus, the more important question appears to be not whether DID can be largely created by iatrogenic factors, but rather the relative importance of iatrogenesis compared with other potential causal variables, including media influences, sociocultural factors, and individual differences in personality.

Distribution of Cases across Clinicians

The distribution of DID cases across therapists is strikingly nonrandom, demonstrating that a relatively small number of clinicians account for a large number of cases of DID. For example, a 1992 survey study in Switzerland revealed that 66% of DID diagnoses were made by .09% (!) of all clinicians. Moreover, 90% of respondents reported that they had never seen a single patient with DID, whereas three psychiatrists reported that they had seen over 20 patients with DID (Modestin, 1992). Ross and colleagues (1989) reported that members of the International Society for the Study of Multiple Personality and Dissociation were between 10 and 11 times more likely than members of the Canadian Psychiatric Association to report having seen a case of DID. In addition, Mai (1995) found evidence for substantial variability in the number of DID diagnoses across Canadian psychiatrists and reported that the lion's share of DID diagnoses derived from a relatively small number of psychotherapists. These findings dovetail with those of Qin, Goodman, Bottoms, and Shaver (1998), who reported that reports of satanic ritual abuse derive from a small number of psychotherapists. Reports of satanic ritual abuse are closely associated with diagnoses of DID (Mulhern, 1991).

Findings on the nonrandom distribution of DID cases are compatible with several explanations. For example, such findings could be explained by positing that patients with actual or possible DID are selectively referred to DID experts. Alternatively, perhaps certain therapists are especially adept at either detecting or eliciting the features of DID. Nevertheless, these findings are consistent with the SCM and with Spanos's (1994, 1996) contention that only a handful of clinicians are diagnosing DID, producing DID symptoms in their patients, or both.

At this point the data do not permit one to select among these possibilities, which are not mutually exclusive. Nevertheless, these findings provide one useful test of the SCM, because if DID diagnoses were not made disproportionately by a subset of clinicians—namely those who are ardent proponents of the DID diagnosis—the SCM would be called into question. Longitudinal investigations examining whether patients tend to exhibit the core features of DID prior to or following referrals to DID specialists would help to determine whether these findings are attributable primarily to iatrogenesis or to either differential referral patterns or the use of more sensitive diagnostic practices.

Role-Playing Studies

Another source of evidence in support of the SCM derives from laboratory studies of role playing. These investigations are designed to test the hypothesis, derived from the SCM, that cues, prompts, and suggestions from a psychotherapist can trigger participants without DID to display the overt features of this condition.

In one of these studies, Spanos, Weekes, and Bertrand (1985) provided participants with suggestions for DID (e.g., "I think perhaps there might be another part of [you] that I haven't talked to") in the context of a simulated psychiatric interview. They found that many role-playing participants, but not control participants (who were not provided with these suggestions), spontaneously adopted a different name, referred to their host personality in the third person (e.g., "He"), and exhibited striking differences between the host and alter "personalities" on psychological measures (e.g., sentence completion tests, semantic differential questionnaires). In addition, most role-playing participants, but not control participants, spontaneously reported amnesia for their alters following hypnosis. It is crucial to note that participants were not explicitly told or asked to display any of these features, which are similar to those exhibited by patients with DID. These findings were essentially replicated with a similar methodology by Spanos, Weekes, Menary, and Bertrand (1986; but see Frischholz & Sachs, 1991, cited in Brown et al., 1999). Stafford and Lynn (1998) similarly found that given adequate situational inducements, normal participants can readily role play a variety of life history experiences often reported among patients with DID, including reports of physical, sexual, and satanic ritual abuse.

Role-playing studies have been commonly misinterpreted by critics of the SCM. For example, Gleaves (1996) argued that "to conclude that these studies prove that DID is simply a form of role-playing is unwarranted" (p. 47). Similarly, Brown and colleagues (1999) contended that role playing studies do not demonstrate that DID "can be created in the laboratory" (p. 580) and that "these role enactments are not identical with alter behavior in MPD patients, nor are they proof that a major psychiatric condition, MPD, has been created" (p. 581). But role-playing studies were not designed to reproduce the full range or subjective experience of DID symptoms, nor to create DID itself, but rather to demonstrate the ease with which subtle cues and prompts can trigger normal participants to display some of the key features of this condition. The findings of these studies provide support for the SCM, because they demonstrate that (1) the behaviors and reported experiences of DID are familiar to many members of the population, and (2) individuals without DID can be readily induced to exhibit some of the key features of DID following prompts and cues, even though these features were not explicitly suggested to them. Were this not the case, the SCM could not account for many of the core features of DID. Role-playing studies therefore provide corroboration for one important and falsifiable precondition of the SCM, although they do not provide dispositive evidence for this model (Lilienfeld et al., 1999).

Cross-Cultural Studies

As noted earlier, the SCM posits that the overt expression of multiple identity enactments is shaped by cultural and historical factors. Consistent with this claim is the fact that until fairly recently DID was largely unknown outside of North America (see also Hochman & Pope, 1997, for data suggesting considerably greater acceptance of DID in North American countries compared with non–North American English-speaking countries). For example, a 1990 survey in Japan (Takahashi, 1990) revealed no known cases of DID in that country. In addition, until recently DID was rare in England, Russia, and India (Spanos, 1996). Interestingly, the cross-cultural expression of DID appears to be different in India than in North America. In the relatively rare cases of DID reported in India, the transition between alters is almost always preceded by sleep, a phenomenon not observed in

North American cases of DID. Media portrayals of DID in India similarly include periods of sleep prior to the transitions between alters (North et al., 1993).

Gleaves (1996) noted that DID has recently been diagnosed in Holland (see also Sno & Schalken, 1999) and several other European countries, and used this finding to argue against the SCM. Nevertheless, this finding is difficult to interpret. In Holland, for example, the writings of several well-known researchers, (e.g., van der Hart, 1993; van der Kolk, van der Hart, & Marmar, 1996) have resulted in substantially increased media and professional attention to DID.

Moreover, "culturally influenced" is not equivalent to "culture-bound." In other words, the fact that a condition initially limited to only a few countries subsequently spreads to other countries does not necessarily indicate that this condition is independent of cultural influence. To the contrary, the fact that the features of DID are becoming better known in certain countries would lead one to expect DID to be diagnosed with increasing frequency in these countries. Indeed, the spread of DID to countries in which the characteristics of this condition are becoming more familiar constitutes one important and potentially falsifiable prediction of the SCM.

Summary

A variety of pieces of evidence, including the typical treatment practices of DID proponents, the clinical features of patients with DID before and after psychotherapy, the distribution of DID cases across psychotherapists, data from role-playing studies, and cross-cultural epidemiological data, provide support for several predictions of the SCM. In addition, these data call into question a "strong" form of the PTM (e.g., Gleaves, 1996), namely, a version of the PTM that essentially excludes sociocultural influence as an explanation of DID's etiology. These data may, however, be consistent with a "weak" form of the PTM that accords a predisposing role to early trauma but also grants a substantial causal role to sociocultural influences, including iatrogenesis. Nevertheless, to provide more compelling support for the PTM, the proponents of this model will need to make more explicit predictions that could in principle permit this model to be falsified.

ETIOLOGY: THE CHILD ABUSE CONTROVERSY

As noted earlier, a linchpin of the PTM is the assumption that DID is caused by early trauma, particularly severe abuse, in childhood. Indeed, some authors regard DID as a form or variant of PTSD (see Gleaves,

1996). Many authors have accepted rather uncritically the claim that severe abuse is an important precursor, if not cause, of DID. For example, Carson and Butcher (1992) asserted that "while it is somewhat amazing that this connection [between DID and child abuse] was not generally recognized until 1984, there is now no reasonable doubt about the reality of this association" (p. 208). Gleaves and colleagues (2001) concluded that "there is a clear body of evidence linking DID or dissociative experiences in general with a history of childhood trauma" (p. 586). In contrast, our reading of the research literature suggests a considerably more complex and ambiguous picture, and raises important questions regarding the hypothesized association between early abuse and DID.

Corroboration of Abuse Reports

Some investigators have reported high prevalences of child abuse among patients with DID (see Gleaves, 1996, p. 53). Nevertheless, in virtually none of these studies was the abuse independently corroborated (e.g., Boon & Draijer, 1993; Coons, Bowman, & Milstein, 1988; Ellason, Ross, & Fuchs, 1996; Putnam et al., 1986; Ross et al., 1989, 1990; Schultz, Braun, & Kluft, 1989; Scroppo, Drob, Weinberger, & Eagle, 1998). The absence of corroboration in these studies is problematic in light of findings that memory is considerably more malleable and vulnerable to suggestion than previously believed (Loftus, 1993, 1997; Malinowski & Lynn, 1995; see also Chapter 8). Recent evidence demonstrates that memories of traumatic experiences (e.g., wartime combat) are not immune to this problem (Southwick, Morgan, Nicolaou, & Charney, 1997).

In addition, the phenomenon of "effort after meaning," whereby individuals interpret potentially ambiguous events (e.g., hitting, fondling) in accord with their implicit theories regarding the causes of their conditions, renders some reports of relatively mild or moderate child abuse difficult to interpret without independent corroboration (see Rind, Tromovitch, & Bauserman, 1998). Furthermore, it is difficult to exclude the possibility that the same inadvertent cues emitted by therapists that promote the creation of alters may also promote the creation of false abuse memories (Spanos, 1994), although little is known about the prevalence of suggestive therapeutic practices among DID therapists. As a consequence, it is difficult to rule out the possibility that the reported association between DID and child abuse is at least partly spurious and contaminated by therapists' methods of eliciting information.

Another reason for emphasizing the importance of corroboration in child abuse research with patients with DID is research indicating that high scorers on the Dissociative Experiences Scale (Bernstein & Putnam, 1986), who are prone to DID, (1) exhibit a response bias toward endorsing a large number of autobiographical events on life events questionnaires, including memories of both negative and neutral life events (Merckelbach, Muris, Horselenberg, & Stougie, 2000), and (2) are especially likely to accept as veridical misleading statements, including those concerning autobiographical events (Ost, Fellows, & Bull, 1997). It has yet to be established whether these findings are directly pertinent to reports of child abuse among patients with DID. Nevertheless, these findings raise the possibility that individuals prone to DID are especially likely to report life events that did not occur (Merckelbach & Muris, 2001).

Several investigators have attempted to corroborate the retrospective abuse reports of patients with DID. For example, Coons and Milstein (1986) and Coons (1994) claimed to provide objective documentation for the abuse reports of some DID patients. Close inspection of these studies, however, reveals various methodological shortcomings. In neither study were diagnoses of DID made blindly of previous abuse reports. This methodological shortcoming is problematic because certain therapists may be especially likely to attempt to elicit features of DID among patients with a history of severe abuse. In the Coons study, DID diagnoses were made only after medical histories and psychiatric records (many of which may have contained information regarding abuse histories) were reviewed. Moreover, because standardized interviews were not administered in Coons and Milstein and were administered only to an unknown number of participants in Coons, the possibility of diagnostic bias is heightened. Finally, the patients in Coons "were diagnosed personally by the first author over an 11 year period" (p. 106). Because there is no evidence concerning whether these patients met criteria for DID prior to treatment, the possibility of iatrogenic influence is difficult to exclude.

More recently, Lewis and colleagues (1997) reported findings from a study of 12 murderers with DID that in their words, "establishes, once and for all, the linkage between early severe child abuse and dissociative identity disorder" (p. 1703). Some authors have cited Lewis and colleagues' findings as providing strong evidence for the corroboration of abuse reports among patients with DID (e.g., Gleaves et al., 2001). Nevertheless, the objective documentation of abuse provided by Lewis and colleagues was often quite vague (see also Klein, 1999). For example, in several cases, there are indications only that the "mother [was] charged as unfit" or that "emergency room records report[ed] severe headaches." In addition, their findings are difficult to interpret for several other reasons. First, the objective documentation of childhood DID symptoms was similarly vague in many cases and was often based on the presence of imaginary playmates and other features (e.g., marked mood changes) that are extremely common in childhood. Second, because violent individuals tend to have high rates of abuse in childhood (Widom, 1988), Lewis and colleagues' findings are potentially attributable to the confounding of DID with violence. Third, diagnoses of DID were not performed blindly with respect to knowledge of reported abuse history. Fourth, the murderers' handwriting samples, which differed over time and were used by Lewis and colleagues to buttress the claim that these individuals had DID, were not evaluated by graphoanalysts or compared with the handwriting samples of normals over time. Fifth, the possibility of malingering (which is often a particular problem among criminals) was not evaluated with psychometric indices. These methodological limitations raise serious questions regarding Lewis and colleagues' claim that their study convincingly demonstrates an association between child abuse and later DID.

A more indirect approach to the corroboration of child abuse among patients with DID was adopted by Tsai, Condie, Wu, and Chang (1999), who used magnetic resonance imaging with a 47-year-old female with DID. Reasoning from previous investigations that had reported a reduction in hippocampal volume in individuals with combat trauma (e.g., Bremner, Randall, Scott, & Bronen, 1995) and child abuse (Bremner, Randall, Vermetten, & Staib, 1997; Stein, Koverola, Hanna, & Torchia, 1997), Tsai and colleagues hypothesized that patients with DID (given their presumed history of early abuse) would similarly exhibit decreased hippocampal volume. As predicted, they found significant bilateral reductions in hippocampal volume in their patient with DID, which is broadly consistent with predictions derived from the PTM. Nevertheless, this finding must be interpreted cautiously for two major reasons. First, because it is based on only one patient, its generalizability to other individuals with DID is unclear. Second, decreased hippocampal volume is not specific to PTSD or other conditions secondary to trauma, and has also been reported in schizophrenia (Nelson, Saykin, Flashman, & Riordan, 1998) and depression (Bremner et al., 2000). Consequently, decreased hippocampal volume may be a nonspecific marker of long-term stress (Sapolsky, 2000).

Moreover, several pieces of data raise questions regarding the veracity of some reports of child abuse in studies of DID. In the study by Ross and colleagues (1991), 26% of patients with DID reported being abused prior to age 3, and 10.6% reported being abused prior to age 1. Dell and Eisenhower (1990) noted that 4 of 11 adolescent patients with DID reported that their first alter emerged at age 2 or earlier, and 2 of these patients reported that their first alter emerged between the ages 1 of 2. Memories reported prior to age 3 are of extremely questionable validity, and it is almost universally accepted that adults and adolescents are unable to remember events that occurred prior to age 1 (Fivush & Hudson, 1990). It is possible that the memories reported in these studies were accurate, but that they were dated incorrectly. Nonetheless, the nontrivial percentages of individuals in the studies of Ross and colleagues and Dell and Eisenhower who reported abuse and the emergence of alters at very young ages raise concerns regarding the accuracy of these memories.

Finally, Ross and Norton (1989) found that patients with DID who had been hypnotized reported higher rates of child abuse than patients with DID who had not been hypnotized. Because there is little evidence that hypnosis enhances memory (Lynn, Lock, Myers, & Payne, 1997; see Chapter 8), this finding is consistent with the possibility that hypnosis produces an increased rate of false abuse reports. Nevertheless, this conclusion must remain tentative in view of the absence of corroboration of the abuse reports and the correlational nature of Ross and Norton's data.

Interpretation of the Child Abuse–DID Association

Even if the child abuse reports of most patients with DID were corroborated, several important questions arise concerning the interpretation of these reports. In particular, it remains to be determined whether a history of child abuse is (1) more common among patients with DID than among psychiatric patients in general and (2) causally associated with risk for subsequent DID.

With respect to the first issue, base rates and referral biases pose potential problems for interpreting the child abuse data. Because the prevalence of reported child abuse among psychiatric patients tends to be high (e.g., Pope & Hudson, 1992), these data are difficult to interpret without a psychiatric comparison group. Moreover, the co-occurrence between reported abuse and DID could be a consequence of several selection artifacts that increase the probability that individuals with multiple problems seek treatment. Berksonian bias (Berkson, 1946) is a mathematical artifact that results from the fact that an individual with two problems can seek treatment for either problem. Clinical selection bias (see du Fort, Newman, & Bland, 1993) reflects the increased likelihood that patients with one problem will seek treatment if they subsequently develop another problem. Either or both of these artifacts could lead to the apparent relation between child abuse and DID. Indeed, Ross (1991) found that nonclinical participants with DID reported substantially lower rates of child abuse than did patients with DID recruited from a clinical population. This finding is consistent with the hypothesis that selection biases account at least partly for the high levels of co-occurrence between reported child abuse and DID. Moreover, Ross and colleagues (1989) reported that American psychiatrists reported a substantially higher prevalence of child abuse among patients with DID (81.2%) than did Canadian psychiatrists (45.5%). This finding suggests the possibility of biases in the assessment or elicitation of child abuse reports and raises questions concerning the claim that child abuse is necessary for most cases of DID (Spanos, 1994).

If a clear correlation between early child abuse and DID were demonstrated, it would still be necessary to demonstrate that this abuse plays a causal role in subsequent DID. This task will be difficult given that studies of child abuse in patients with DID are necessarily quasi-experimental. Nevertheless, data from causal modeling studies could help to shed light on this question. In addition, studies of monozygotic (identical) twins discordant for early abuse history could provide more compelling evidence for a causal role of abuse in DID. Specifically, if it could be demonstrated that only the MZ twin with a history of early abuse exhibited significant levels of dissociative features (including features of DID), then this finding would buttress the contention that early abuse, rather than a host of other nuisance variables that distinguish patients with dissociative disorders from other individuals (e.g., genetic differences in the propensity toward suggestibility), plays an etiological role in DID.

Summary

The PTM hinges on the assumption that early trauma, particularly child abuse, is a risk factor for DID. Consistent with this assumption, many authors have found that a large proportion, and probably a majority, of patients with DID report a history of early and sometimes severe child abuse. Nevertheless, careful inspection of this literature raises significant questions concerning the child abuse–DID link. Most of the reported confirmations of this association derive from studies lacking objective corroboration of child abuse (e.g., Ross et al., 1990). Moreover, even those studies that purport to provide such corroboration (e.g., Coons, 1994; Lewis et al., 1997) are plagued by methodological shortcomings. In addition, the reported high levels of child abuse among patients with DID may be attributable to selection and referral biases. Finally, it is unclear whether early abuse plays a causal role in DID. These limitations suggest the need for further controlled research before strong conclusions regarding the child abuse–DID link (e.g., Gleaves, 1996; Gleaves et al., 2001) can be drawn.

CONCLUSIONS

The literature on DID has recently been engulfed in numerous divisive controversies (see also Elzinga et al., 1998). In particular, there has been substantial scientific disagreement over whether DID is (1) a "genuine" condition, (2) truly characterized by the coexistence of multiple in-dwelling and fully developed personalities, (3) a socially constructed product of iatrogenic, media, and cultural influences, and (4) a consequence of childhood trauma. As we have argued, controversy (1) is actually a pseudoissue, as there is no longer much dispute that DID "exists" in the sense that most individuals with this condition exhibit signs and symptoms of psychopathology and experience intense subjective distress.

Furthermore, controversy (2) is difficult to resolve with existing data, although it is clear that most DID researchers, even those who are fervent proponents of the PTM (e.g., Ross, 1997), do not believe that the alters of patients with DID constitute fully developed and independent personalities. Moreover, the proposition that alters constitute fully developed and independent personalities poses significant challenges and problems for models of DID's etiology, particularly for patients with very large numbers of alters. It is therefore troubling that DSM-IV (American Psychiatric Association, 1994) continues to refer to the presence of two or more co-occurring identities in its diagnostic criteria for DID.

Perhaps the primary controversy surrounding DID is the question of whether it is a socially constructed and culturally influenced condition rather than a naturally occurring response to early trauma (Merskey, 1992). As we have argued elsewhere (Lilienfeld et al., 1999), a number of important lines of evidence converge to provide support for the SCM. Specifically, 10 findings are consistent with the major theses of the SCM:

1. The number of patients with DID has increased dramatically over the past few decades (Elzinga et al., 1998).
2. The number of alters per individual with DID has similarly increased over the past few decades (North et al., 1993), although the number of alters at the time of initial diagnosis appears to have remained constant (Ross et al., 1989).
3. Both of these increases coincide with dramatically increased therapist and public awareness of the major features of DID (Fahy, 1988).
4. Mainstream treatment techniques for DID appear to reinforce patients' displays of multiplicity, reify alters as distinct personalities, and encourage patients to establish contact with presumed latent alters (Spanos, 1994, 1996).
5. Many or most patients with DID show few or no clear-cut signs of this condition (e.g., alters) prior to psychotherapy (Kluft, 1991).
6. The number of alters per individual with DID tends to increase substantially over the course of DID-oriented psychotherapy (Piper, 1997).
7. Psychotherapists who use hypnosis tend to have more patients with DID in their caseloads than do psychotherapists who do not use hypnosis (Powell & Gee, 1999).
8. The majority of diagnoses of DID derive from a relatively small number of psychotherapists, many of whom are specialists in DID (Mai, 1995).
9. Laboratory studies suggest that nonclinical participants provided

with appropriate cues and prompts can reproduce many of the overt features of DID (Spanos et al., 1985).

10. Until fairly recently, diagnoses of DID were limited largely to North America, where the condition has received widespread media publicity (Spanos, 1996), although DID is now being diagnosed with considerable frequency in some countries (e.g., Holland) in which it has recently become more widely publicized.

These 10 sources of evidence do not imply, however, that DID can typically be created in vacuo by iatrogenic or sociocultural influences. As noted earlier, a large proportion of patients with DID have histories of co-occurring psychopathology, particularly borderline personality disorder (BPD; Ganaway, 1995). Therefore, it seems plausible that iatrogenic and sociocultural influences often operate on a backdrop of preexisting psychopathology, and exert their impact primarily on individuals who are seeking a causal explanation for their instability, identity problems, and impulsive and seemingly inexplicable behaviors.

We should also note that several of these 10 sources of evidence are fallible and open to multiple causal interpretations (Lilienfeld et al., 1999). For example, the finding that the number of alters per individual tends to increase over the course of psychotherapy is potentially consistent with the assertion (Ross, 1997) that psychotherapy for DID is often accompanied by a progressive uncovering of previously latent alters. In addition, the finding that diagnoses of DID have increased dramatically over the past few decades is potentially attributable to the advent of superior diagnostic and assessment practices among DID practitioners. Moreover, diagnoses of several other disorders, including PTSD and obsessive–compulsive disorder (OCD), have increased dramatically over the past two decades (Zohar, 1998).

Although none of these 10 lines of evidence is by itself dispositive, the convergence of evidence across all of these sources of data provides a potent argument for the validity of the SCM (Lilienfeld et al., 1999; see also Lynn & Pintar, 1997). Our conclusions differ sharply from those of Brown and colleagues (1999), who contended that "the entire data base of 'scientific evidence' [for the SCM] consists of a grand total of three experimental studies—all coming out of the same laboratory" (p. 617). Brown and colleagues were referring here to the laboratory role-playing studies of Spanos and his colleagues (e.g., Spanos et al., 1985).

Nevertheless, Brown and colleagues (1999) drew this conclusion only because they restricted themselves entirely to strictly experimental studies (i.e., those involving random assignment to conditions and manipulation of a discrete independent variable) when evaluating the scientific status of the SCM. This approach is grossly underinclusive, because a variety of lines of quasi-experimental and observational evidence (e.g., the higher rates of psychopathology of patients with DID after versus before psychotherapy, the markedly nonrandom distribution of DID cases across practitioners) are relevant to the validity of the SCM. In many well-developed "hard" sciences, including geology, astronomy, meteorology, and paleontology, nonexperimental evidence is used routinely to test causal hypotheses, and the same evidentiary guidelines should hold in psychology. Indeed, as the 19th century philosopher William Whewell observed, most scientific hypotheses are tested by evaluating the "consilience of evidence" across diverse and maximally independent sources of information (Shermer, 2001). The consilience of evidence for the SCM is striking, and strongly suggests that iatrogenic and sociocultural influences play at least some etiological role in DID.

This conclusion does not imply, however, that the PTM has been falsified. With respect to the fourth major controversy examined in this chapter, namely, the child abuse–DID link, extant studies provide relatively weak support for the contention that child abuse is a causal risk factor for DID (cf. Gleaves et al., 2001). Nevertheless, this possibility cannot be excluded on the basis of existing data. Studies that provide corroborated abuse reports and psychiatric comparison groups, and that control for selection and referral biases, are required to bring clarity to this area (Lilienfeld et al., 1999). In addition, causal modeling studies may help to exclude alternative hypotheses for the high levels of co-occurrence between reported child abuse and later DID. If such abuse can be corroborated and shown to be associated with risk for DID, such studies will be especially informative if they incorporate potential third variables that could account for this correlation (e.g., adverse home environment).

If future studies provide more convincing evidence for the child abuse–DID association, such evidence might necessitate a rapprochement between the SCM and PTM. Indeed, some important aspects of these two models may ultimately prove commensurable. For example, early trauma could predispose individuals to develop high levels of fantasy proneness (Lynn et al., 1988), absorption (Tellegen & Atkinson, 1974), or related traits. In turn, such traits may render individuals susceptible to the kinds of iatrogenic and cultural influences posited by the SCM, thereby increasing the likelihood that they will develop DID and related dissociative disorders following exposure to suggestive influences. This and even more sophisticated etiological models of DID await direct empirical tests.

Given the converging support for the SCM across multiple sources of evidence, however, we believe that the burden of proof now falls squarely on proponents of the PTM to provide more compelling evidence for this position (cf. Brown et al., 1999). If they are successful, the multiple controversies that have swirled around the concept of multiple personality disorder virtually since its inception could move closer to a satisfactory resolution.

GLOSSARY

Alter: One of the presumed "personalities" or "personality states" of individuals with dissociative identity disorder.

Borderline personality disorder: A personality disorder characterized by identity confusion, mood instability, erratic and unpredictable interpersonal relationships, and impulsive and self-damaging behaviors, among other features.

Dissociation: A defense mechanism characterized by the compartmentalization or "walling off" of negative experiences from consciousness.

Dissociative disorders: A set of disorders, including dissociative identity disorder, characterized by disturbances in memory, identity, consciousness, and/or perception of the external environment.

Dissociative identity disorder (DID): A condition, known formerly as multiple personality disorder, characterized by the presence of distinct personalities or personality states that recurrently take control over the individual's behavior. This condition is also characterized by marked memory gaps for autobiographical information.

Host personality: The "original" or primary personality of the individual with DID.

Iatrogenic: Produced by physicians or mental health professionals.

Inner self-helper: As proposed by Allison (1974), a part of the personality of individuals with dissociative identity disorder that is aware of what is occurring to the alters and can assist in their integration.

Posttraumatic model: A model positing that dissociative identity disorder is a naturally occurring response to childhood trauma, particularly child physical and/or sexual abuse.

Sociocognitive model: A model positing that dissociative identity disorder is a socially constructed condition resulting primarily from inadvertent therapist prompting, media influences, and sociocultural expectations regarding the presumed features of this condition.

ACKNOWLEDGMENTS

Selected portions of this chapter are based on Lilienfeld et al. (1999). Copyright 1999 by the American Psychological Association. Adapted by permission.

REFERENCES

Acocella, J. (1998, April 6). The politics of hysteria. *New Yorker*, pp. 64–79.

Aldridge-Morris, R. (1989). *Multiple personality: An exercise in deception*. Hillsdale, NJ: Erlbaum.

Allen, J. J. B., & Iacono, W. G. (2001). Assessing the validity of amnesia in dissociative identity disorder: A dilemma for the DSM and the courts. *Psychology, Public Policy, and Law, 7*, 311–344.

Allen, J. J. B., & Movius, H. L. (2000). The objective assessment of amnesia in dissociative identity disorder using event-related potentials. *International Journal of Psychophysiology, 38*, 21–41.

Allison, R. (1974). A new treatment approach for multiple personality. *American Journal of Clinical Hypnosis, 17*, 15–32.

American Psychiatric Association. (1980). *Diagnostic and statistical manual of mental disorders* (3rd ed.). Washington, DC: Author.

American Psychiatric Association. (1987). *Diagnostic and statistical manual of mental disorders* (3rd ed., rev.). Washington, DC: Author.

American Psychiatric Association. (1994). *Diagnostic and statistical manual of mental disorders* (4th ed.). Washington, DC: Author.

Arrigo, J. M., & Pezdek, K. (1998). Textbook models of multiple personality: Source, bias, and social consequences. In S. J. Lynn & K. M. McConkey (Eds.), *Truth in memory* (pp. 372–393). New York: Guilford Press.

Bahnson, C. B., & Smith, K. (1975). Autonomic changes in a multiple personality. *Psychosomatic Medicine, 37*, 85–86.

Berkson, J. (1946). Limitations of the application of the four-fold table analysis to hospital data. *Biometrics Bulletin, 2*, 47–53.

Bernstein, E. M., & Putnam, F. W. (1986). Development, reliability, and validity of a dissociation scale. *Journal of Nervous and Mental Disease, 174*, 727–735.

Bliss, E. L. (1980). Multiple personalities: A report of 14 cases with implications for schizophrenia and hysteria. *Archives of General Psychiatry, 37*, 1388–1397.

Boon, S., & Draijer, N. (1993). Multiple personality disorder in the Netherlands: A clinical investigation of 71 cases. *American Journal of Psychiatry, 150*, 489–494.

Boor, M. (1982). The multiple personality epidemic: Additional cases and inferences regarding diagnosis, etiology, dynamics, and treatment. *Journal of Nervous and Mental Disease, 170*, 302–304.

Braun, B. G. (1980). Hypnosis for multiple personalities. In H. J. Wain (Ed.), *Clinical hypnosis in medicine* (pp. 209–217). Chicago: Year Book Medical.

Braun, B. G. (1986). Issues in the psychotherapy of multiple personality disorder. In B. G. Braun (Ed.), *Treatment of multiple personality disorder* (pp. 1–28). Washington, DC: American Psychiatric Press.

Bremner, J. D., Narayan, M., Anderson, E. R., Staib, L. H., Miller, H. L., & Charney, D. S. (2000). Hippocampal volume reduction in major depression. *American Journal of Psychiatry, 157*, 115–117.

Bremner, J. D., Randall, P., Scott, T. M., & Bronen, R. (1995). MRI-based measurement of hippocampal volume in patients with combat-related posttraumatic stress disorder. *American Journal of Psychiatry, 152*, 973–981.

Bremner, J. D., Randall, P., Vermetten, E., & Staib, L. (1997). Magnetic resonance imaging-based measurement of hippocampal volume in posttraumatic stress disorder related to childhood physical and sexual abuse: A preliminary report. *Biological Psychiatry, 41*, 23–32.

Brende, J. O. (1984). The psychophysiologic manifestations of dissociation: Electodermal responses in a multiple personality patient. *Psychiatric Clinics of North America, 7*, 41–50.

Brown, D., Frischholtz, E. J., & Scheflin, A. W. (1999). Iatrogenic dissociative identity disorder: An evaluation of the scientific evidence. *Journal of Psychiatry and Law, 27*, 549–637.

Carson, R. C., & Butcher, J. N. (1992). *Abnormal psychology and modern life* (9th ed.). New York: HarperCollins.

Coons, P. M. (1984). The differential diagnosis of multiple personality disorder: A comprehensive review. *Psychiatric Clinics of North America, 7*, 51–67.

Coons, P. M. (1989). Iatrogenic factors in the misdiagnosis of multiple personality disorder. *Dissociation, 2*, 70–76.

Coons, P. M. (1994). Confirmation of childhood abuse in child and adolescent cases of multiple personality disorder and dissociative identity disorder not otherwise specified. *Journal of Nervous and Mental Disease, 182*, 461–464.

Coons, P. M., Bowman, E. S., & Milstein, V. (1988). Multiple personality disorder: A clinical investigation of 50 cases. *Journal of Nervous and Mental Disease, 176*, 519–527.

Coons, P. M., & Milstein, V. (1986). Psychosexual disturbances in multiple personality: Characteristics, etiology, and treatment. *Journal of Clinical Psychiatry, 47*, 106–111.

Cormier, J. F., & Thelen, M. H. (1998). Professional skepticism of multiple personality disorder. *Professional Psychology: Research and Practice, 29*, 163–167.

Dell, P. F. (1988). Professional skepticism about multiple personality. *Journal of Nervous and Mental Disease, 176*, 528–531.

Dell, P. F. (2001). Why the diagnostic criteria for dissociative identity disorder should be changed. *Journal of Trauma and Dissociation, 2*, 7–37.

Dell, P. F., & Eisenhower, J. W. (1990). Adolescent multiple personality disorder: A preliminary study of eleven cases. *Journal of the American Academy of Child and Adolescent Psychiatry, 29*, 359–366.

Dennett, D. C. (1991). *Consciousness explained.* Boston: Little, Brown.

Dorahy, M. J. (2001). Dissociative identity disorder and memory dysfunction: The current state of experimental research and its future directions. *Clinical Psychology Review, 21*, 771–795.

Draijer, N., & Boon, S. (1999). The limitations of dissociative identity disorder: Patients at risk, therapists at risk. *Journal of Psychiatry and Law, 27*, 423–458.

du Fort, G. G., Newman, S. C., & Bland, R. C. (1993). Psychiatric comorbidity and treatment seeking: Sources of selection bias in the study of clinical populations. *Journal of Nervous and Mental Disease, 181*, 467–474.

Dunn, G. E., Paolo, A. M., Ryan, J. J., & van Fleet, J. N. (1994). Belief in the existence of multiple personality disorder among psychologists and psychiatrists. *Journal of Clinical Psychology, 50*, 454–457.

Ellason, J. W., Ross, C. A., & Fuchs, D. L. (1996). Lifetime Axis I and Axis II comorbidity and childhood trauma history in dissociative identity disorder. *Psychiatry: Interpersonal and Biological Processes, 59*, 255–266.

Elzinga, B. M., van Dyck, R., & Spinhoven, P. (1998). Three controversies about dissociative identity disorder. *Clinical Psychology and Psychotherapy, 5*, 13–23.

Fahy, T. A. (1988). The diagnosis of multiple personality disorder: A critical review. *British Journal of Psychiatry, 153*, 597–606.

Fivush, R., & Hudson, J. A. (Eds.). (1990). *Knowing and remembering in young children*. New York: Cambridge University Press.

Frances, A., & First, M. B. (1998). *Your mental health: A layman's guide to the Psychiatrist's Bible*. New York: Scribner.

Ganaway, G. K. (1989). Historical versus narrative truth: Clarifying the role of exogenous trauma in the etiology of MPD and its variants. *Dissociation, 2*, 205–220.

Ganaway, G. K. (1995). Hypnosis, childhood trauma, and dissociative identity disorder: Toward an integrative theory. *International Journal of Clinical and Experimental Hypnosis, 43*, 127–144.

Gleaves, D. H. (1996). The sociocognitive model of dissociative identity disorder: A reexamination of the evidence. *Psychological Bulletin, 120*, 42–59.

Gleaves, D. H., May, M. C., & Cardena, E. (2001). An examination of the diagnostic validity of dissociative identity disorder. *Clinical Psychology Review, 21*, 577–608.

Hacking, I. (1995). *Rewriting the soul: Multiple personality and the science of memory*. Princeton, NJ: Princeton University Press.

Hochman, J., & Pope, H. G. (1997). Debating dissociative diagnoses. *American Journal of Psychiatry, 153*, 887–888.

Hyman, I. E., Jr., Husband, T. H., & Billings, F. J. (1995). False memories of childhood experiences. *Applied Cognitive Psychology, 9*, 181–197.

Hyman, I. E., Jr., & Pentland, J. (1996). The role of mental imagery in the creation of false childhood memories. *Journal of Memory and Language, 35*, 101–117.

Klein, D. F. (1999). Multiples: No amnesia for child abuse. *American Journal of Psychiatry, 156*, 976–977.

Kluft, R. P. (1988). The phenomenology and treatment of extremely complex multiple personality disorder. *Dissociation, 1*, 47–58.

Kluft, R. P. (1991). Multiple personality disorder. In A. Tasman & S. M. Goldfinger (Eds.), *American Psychiatric Press Review of Psychiatry* (Vol. 10, pp. 161–188). Washington, DC: American Psychiatric Association Press.

Kluft, R. P. (1993). Multiple personality disorders. In D. Spiegel (Ed.), *Dissociative disorders: A clinical review* (pp. 17–44). Lutherville, MD: Sidran Press.

Lewis, D. O., Yeager, C. A., Swica, Y., Pincus, J. H., & Lewis, M. (1997). Objective documentation of child abuse and dissociation in 12 murderers with dissociative identity disorder. *American Journal of Psychiatry, 143*, 1703–1710.

Lichtenstein Creative Media. (1998). *The infinite mind* [Radio broadcast]. National Public Radio.

Lilienfeld, S. O., Lynn, S. J., Kirsch, I., Chaves, J. F., Sarbin, T. R., Ganaway, G. K., & Powell, R. A. (1999). Dissociative identity disorder and the sociocognitive model: Recalling the lessons of the past. *Psychological Bulletin, 125*, 507–523.

Lindsay, D. (1996). Commentary on informed clinical practice and the standard of care: Proposed guidelines for the treatment of adults who report delayed memories of childhood trauma. In J. D. Read & D. S. Lindsay (Eds.), *Recollections of trauma: Scientific evidence and clinical practice* (pp. 361–370). New York: Plenum Press.

Lindsay, D. S. (1998). Depolarizing views on recovered memory experiences. In S. J. Lynn & K. M. McConkey (Eds.), *Truth in memory* (pp. 481–494). New York: Guilford Press.

Loftus, E. F. (1993). The reality of repressed memories. *American Psychologist, 48,* 518–537.

Loftus, E. F. (1997, September). Creating false memories. *Scientific American,* pp. 70–75.

Loftus, E. F., & Pickrell, J. E. (1995). The formation of false memories. *Psychiatric Annals, 25,* 720–725.

Ludwig, A. M., Brandsma, J. M., Wilbur, C. B., Bendefeldt, F., & Jameson, D. H. (1972). The objective study of a multiple personality: Or, are four heads better than one? *Archives of General Psychiatry, 26,* 298–310.

Lynn, S. J., Lock, T. G., Myers, B., & Payne, D. (1997). Recalling the unrecallable: Should hypnosis be used to recover memories in psychotherapy? *Current Directions in Psychological Science, 6,* 79–83.

Lynn, S. J., & Pintar, J. (1997). A social narrative model of dissociative identity disorder. *Australian Journal of Clinical and Experimental Hypnosis, 25,* 1–7.

Lynn, S. J., Rhue, J. W., & Green, J. P. (1988). Multiple personality and fantasy proneness: Is there an association or dissociation? *British Journal of Experimental and Clinical Hypnosis, 5,* 138–142.

Mai, F. M. (1995). Psychiatrists' attitudes to multiple personality disorder: A questionnaire study. *Canadian Journal of Psychiatry, 40,* 154–157.

Malinowski, P., & Lynn, S. J. (1995, August). *The pliability of early memory reports.* Paper presented at the Annual Convention of the American Psychological Association, Washington, DC.

Marmer, S. S. (1998, December). Should dissociative identity disorder be considered a bona fide psychiatric diagnosis? *Clinical Psychiatry News.*

Mazzoni, G. A., Loftus, E. F., & Kirsch, I. (2001). Changing beliefs about implausible autobiographical memories. *Journal of Experimental Psychology: Applied, 7,* 51–59.

McHugh, P. R. (1993). Multiple personality disorder. *Harvard Mental Health Newsletter, 10*(3), 4–6.

Merckelbach, H., Devilly, G. J., & Rassin, E. (2002). Alters in dissociative identity disorder: Metaphors or genuine entities? *Clinical Psychology Review, 22,* 481–497.

Merckelbach, H., & Muris, P. (2001). The causal link between self-reported trauma and dissociation: A critical review. *Behaviour Research and Therapy, 39,* 245–254.

Merckelbach, H., Muris, P., Horselenberg, R., & Stougie, S. (2000). Dissociative experiences, response bias, and fantasy proneness in college students. *Personality and Individual Differences, 28,* 49–58.

Merskey, H. (1992). The manufacture of personalities: The production of multiple personality disorder. *British Journal of Psychiatry, 160,* 327–340.

Modestin, J. (1992). Multiple personality disorder in Switzerland. *American Journal of Psychiatry, 149,* 88–92.

Mulhern, S. (1991). Satanism and psychotherapy: A rumor in search of an inquisition. In J. T. Richardson, J. Best, & D. G. Bromley (Eds.), *The Satanism scare* (pp. 145–172). New York: Aldine de Gruyter.

Nelson, M. D., Saykin, A. J., Flashman, L. A., & Riordan, H. J. (1998). Hippocampal volume reduction in schizophrenia as assessed by magnetic resonance imaging: A meta-analytic study. *Archives of General Psychiatry, 55*, 433–440.

North, C. S., Ryall, J-E. M., Ricci, D. A., & Wetzel, R. D. (1993). *Multiple personalities, multiple disorders*. New York: Oxford University Press.

Orne, M. T., Dinges, D. F., & Orne, E. C. (1984). On the differential diagnosis of multiple personality in the forensic context. *International Journal of Clinical and Experimental Hypnosis, 32*, 118–169.

Ost, J., Fellows, B., & Bull, R. (1997). Individual differences and the suggestibility of human memory. *Contemporary Hypnosis, 14*, 132–137.

Pezdek, K., Finger, K., & Hodge, D. (1997). Planting false childhood memories: The role of event plausibility. *Psychological Science, 8*, 437–441.

Piper, A. (1993). "Truth serum" and "recovered memories" of sexual abuse: A review of the evidence. *Journal of Psychiatry and Law, 21*, 447–471.

Piper, A. (1997). *Hoax and reality: The bizarre world of multiple personality disorder*. Northvale, NJ: Aronson.

Pope, H. G., & Hudson, J. I. (1992). Is childhood sexual abuse a risk factor for bulimia nervosa? *American Journal of Psychiatry, 149*, 455–463.

Pope, H. G., Oliva, P. S., Hudson, J. I., Bodkin, J. A., & Gruber, A. J. (1999). Attitudes toward DSM-IV dissociative disorders diagnoses among board-certified American psychiatrists. *American Journal of Psychiatry, 156*, 321–323.

Popper, K. R. (1959). *The logic of scientific discovery*. London: Hutchinson.

Powell, R. A., & Gee, T. L. (1999). The effects of hypnosis on dissociative identity disorder: A reexamination of the evidence. *Canadian Journal of Psychiatry, 44*, 914–916.

Prince, M. (1905). *The dissociation of a personality: A biographical study in abnormal psychology*. New York: Longmans, Green.

Putnam, F. W. (1989). *Diagnosis and treatment of multiple personality disorder*. New York: Guilford Press.

Putnam, F. W., Guroff, J. J., Silberman, E. K., Barban, L., & Post, R. M. (1986). The clinical phenomenology of multiple personality disorder: Review of 100 recent cases. *Journal of Clinical Psychiatry, 47*, 285–293.

Putnam, F. W., & Lowenstein, R. J. (2000). Dissociative identity disorder. In B. J. Sadock & V. A. Sadock (Eds.), *Kaplan and Sadock's comprehensive textbook of psychiatry* (7th ed., Vol. 1, pp. 1552–1564). Philadelphia: Lippincott Williams & Wilkins.

Putnam, F. W., Zahn, T. P., & Post, R. M. (1990). Differential autonomic nervous system activity in multiple personality disorder. *Psychiatry Research, 31*, 251–260.

Qin, J. J., Goodman, G. S., Bottoms, B. L., & Shaver, P. R. (1998). Repressed memories of ritualistic and religion-related child abuse. In S. J. Lynn & K. M. McConkey (Eds.), *Truth in memory* (pp. 284–303). New York: Guilford Press.

Read, J. D., & Lindsay, D. S. (2000). "Amnesia" for summer camps and high school graduation: Memory work increases reports of prior periods of remembering less. *Journal of Traumatic Stress, 13*, 129–147.

Rifkin, A., Ghisalbert, D., Dimatou, S., Jin, C., & Sethi, M. (1998). Dissociative identity disorder in psychiatric inpatients. *American Journal of Psychiatry, 155*, 844–845.

Rind, B., Tromovitch, P., & Bauserman, R. (1998). A meta-analytic examination of assumed properties of child sexual abuse using college samples. *Psychological Bulletin, 124,* 22–53.

Robins, E., & Guze, S. B. (1970). Establishment of diagnostic validity in psychiatric illness: Its application to schizophrenia. *American Journal of Psychiatry, 126,* 107–111.

Ross, C. A. (1989). *Multiple personality disorder: Diagnosis, clinical features, and treatment.* New York: Wiley.

Ross, C. A. (1990). Twelve cognitive errors about multiple personality disorder. *American Journal of Psychotherapy, 44,* 348–356.

Ross, C. A. (1991). Epidemiology of multiple personality disorder and dissociation. *Psychiatric Clinics of North America, 14,* 503–517.

Ross, C. A. (1997). *Dissociative identity disorder: Diagnosis, clinical features, and treatment of multiple personality.* New York: Wiley.

Ross, C. A., Anderson, G., Fleisher, W. P., & Norton, G. R. (1991). The frequency of multiple personality disorder among psychiatric inpatients. *American Journal of Psychiatry, 148,* 1717–1720.

Ross, C. A., Miller, S. D., Reagor, P. Bjornson, L., Fraser, G. A., & Anderson, G. (1990). Structured interview data on 102 cases of multiple personality disorder from four centers. *American Journal of Psychiatry, 147,* 596–601.

Ross, C. A., & Norton, G. R. (1989). Effects of hypnosis on the features of multiple personality disorder. *Dissociation, 3,* 99–106.

Ross, C. A. ., Norton, G. R., & Wozney, K. (1989). Multiple personality disorder: An analysis of 236 cases. *Canadian Journal of Psychiatry, 34,* 413–418.

Sapolsky, R. M. (2000). Glucocorticoids and hippocampal atrophy in neuropsychiatric disorders. *Archives of General Psychiatry, 57,* 925–935.

Sarbin, T. R. (1995). On the belief that one body may be host to two or more personalities. *International Journal of Clinical and Experimental Hypnosis, 43,* 163–183.

Schreiber, F. R. (1973). *Sybil.* New York: Warner.

Schultz, R., Braun, B. G., & Kluft, R. P. (1989). Multiple personality disorder: Phenomenology of selected variables in comparison to major depression. *Dissociation, 2,* 45–51.

Scroppo, J. C., Drob, S. L., Weinberger, J. L., & Eagle, P. (1998). Identifying dissociative identity disorder: A self-report and projective study. *Journal of Abnormal Psychology, 107,* 272–284.

Shermer, M. (1997). *Why people believe weird things: Pseudoscience, superstition, and other confusions of our time.* New York: Freeman.

Shermer, M. (2001). *The borderlands of science: Where sense meets nonsense.* New York: Oxford University Press.

Showalter, E. (1997). *Hystories: Hysterical epidemics and modern culture.* New York: Columbia University Press.

Slovenko, F. (1999). The production of multiple personalities. *Journal of Psychiatry and Law, 27,* 215–253.

Sno, H. N., & Schalken, H. F. (1999). Dissociative identity disorder: Diagnosis and treatment in the Netherlands. *European Psychiatry, 5,* 270–277.

Southwick, S., Morgan, A. C., Nicolaou, A. L., & Charney, D. S. (1997). Consistency of memory for combat-related traumatic events in veterans of Operation Desert Storm. *American Journal of Psychiatry, 154,* 173–177.

Spanos, N. P. (1994). Multiple identity enactments and multiple personality disorder: A sociocognitive perspective. *Psychological Bulletin, 116*, 143–165.

Spanos, N. P. (1996). *Multiple identities and false memories: A sociocognitive perspective.* Washington, DC: American Psychological Association.

Spanos, N. P., & Chaves, J. F. (1989). *Hypnosis: The cognitive-behavioral perspective.* Buffalo, NY: Prometheus.

Spanos, N. P., Menary, E., Gabora, M. J., DuBreuil, S. C., & Dewhirst, B. (1991). Secondary identity enactments during hypnotic past-life regression: A sociocognitive perspective. *Journal of Personality and Social Psychology, 61*, 308–320.

Spanos, N. P., Weekes, J. R., & Bertrand, L. D. (1985). Multiple personality: A social psychological perspective. *Journal of Abnormal Psychology, 94*, 362–376.

Spanos, N. P., Weekes, J. R., Menary, E., & Bertrand, L. D. (1986). Hypnotic interview and age regression procedures in the elicitation of multiple personality symptoms. *Psychiatry, 49*, 298–311.

Spiegel, D. (1993, May 20). Letter to the Executive Council, International Study for the Study of Multiple Personality and Dissociation. *News, International Society of the Study of Multiple Personality and Dissociation, 11*, 15.

Stafford, J., & Lynn, S. J. (1998). *Cultural scripts, childhood abuse, and multiple identities: A study of role-played enactments.* Manuscript submitted for publication.

Stein, M. B., Koverola, C., Hanna, C., & Torchia, M. G. (1997). Hippocampal volume in women victimized by childhood sexual abuse. *Psychological Medicine, 27*, 951–959.

Takahashi, Y. (1990). Is multiple personality really rare in Japan? *Dissociation, 3*, 57–59.

Tellegen, A., & Atkinson, G. (1974). Openness to absorbing and self-altering experiences ("absorption"), a trait related to hypnotic susceptibility. *Journal of Abnormal Psychology, 83*, 268–277.

Thigpen, C. H., & Cleckley, H. M. (1957). *The three faces of Eve.* New York: McGraw Hill.

Tsai, G. E., Condie, D., Wu, M-T., & Chang, I.-W. (1999). Functional magnetic resonance imaging of personality switches in a woman with dissociative identity disorder. *Harvard Review of Psychiatry, 72*, 119–122.

van der Hart, O. (1993). Multiple personality disorder in Europe: Impressions. *Dissociation, 6*, 102–118.

van der Kolk, B. A., van der Hart, O., & Marmar, C. R. (1996). Dissociation and information processing in posttraumatic stress disorder. In B. A. van der Kolk, A. C. McFarlane, & L. Weisaeth (Eds.), *Traumatic stress: The effects of overwhelming experience on mind, body, and society* (pp. 303–327). New York: Guilford Press.

Widom, C. S. (1988). Does violence beget violence? A critical examination of the literature. *Psychological Bulletin, 106*, 3–28.

Zohar, J. (1998). Post-traumatic stress disorder: The hidden epidemic of modern times. *CNS Spectrums, 3*(7, Suppl. 2), 4–51.

PART II

GENERAL CONTROVERSIES IN PSYCHOTHERAPY

Toward a Science of Psychotherapy Research

Present Status and Evaluation

JOHN P. GARSKE
TIMOTHY ANDERSON

Psychotherapy is the stock-in-trade of many professions. Practiced in many forms and hybrids by psychologists, physicians, clergymen, social workers, counselors, and the like, psychotherapy has been applied as a curative for a panorama of human ills and miseries. The number of psychotherapies, their domain of application, and their utilization by the public have increased dramatically over the past few decades. It has been estimated recently that there are now 250 distinct psychotherapy approaches, which are described and discussed in more than 10,000 books (Wampold, 2001). The psychotherapy professions comprise a loosely knit guild that predictably functions to provide both service to a suffering public and self-perpetuation.

The proliferation of psychotherapies has fueled clashes among paradigms, systems, and schools. With theoretical status and professional existence at stake, certain psychotherapies continue to claim superiority over their rivals in the absence of definitive empirical support (Smith, Glass, & Miller, 1980). The private and public sectors are closely scrutinizing the role of psychotherapy in the provision of health care. Social critics, health care managers, and policymakers are clamoring to make psychotherapeutic practice accountable.

This climate of crisis has produced a vigorous debate (cf. Wampold,

2001). There appears to be an emerging recognition that the thorny issues facing the profession are best analyzed and resolved by reliance on scientific data rather than armchair philosophy, poorly grounded theory, and unsystematic observations and opinions. With psychologists as the prime movers and mainstays, the knowledge base regarding psychotherapy and the processes of behavior change has burgeoned in recent years (Bergin & Garfield, 1994). Although much remains to be answered, the field of psychotherapy has matured considerably and progressed well beyond its origins as a healing art toward a technical psychosocial intervention.

Does psychotherapy work? This question of effectiveness has long been the bedfellow of the field. Few, if any, professional activities other than psychotherapy have been scrutinized with comparable zeal and vigor. Critics have raised substantive questions regarding the effects of psychotherapy; clinicians and researchers have provided counterpoints. The outcome polemic, although troublesome for the profession, has spawned many related questions and some scientifically based answers. The overarching question—Does psychotherapy work?—has been reconfigured as an array of component questions, such as the following: Do some psychotherapies work and not others? Which psychotherapies work the best? Why? What are the characteristics of an effective therapist? Does professional training and experience make a difference? How about gender? What are the essential ingredients of psychotherapies that work? Do we know how they work? Are there negative or detrimental effects? This chapter will address these and other questions regarding the effects of psychotherapy, and tender some answers. Our intent is to provide a sampling of the discussion and debate, and an evaluation of the present status of the field from a scientific perspective.

DEFINITIONS AND TERMINOLOGY

Let us begin by considering some key terminology. The term "psychotherapy" is commonly used by professionals and nonprofessionals alike, yet it remains remarkably difficult to define. In the acknowledged "holy book" of psychotherapy research, the *Handbook of Psychotherapy and Behavior Change*, the editors, Bergin and Garfield (1994), did not even offer a definition of psychotherapy. One of the present authors, in the introduction to a book on contemporary psychotheories, conceded that a precise definition was elusive (Lynn & Garske, 1985). This apparent problem in definition reflects the divergent perspectives that those in the field have regarding behavior change and how psychotherapy may bring it about.

Yet there appears to be some common ground when using the term psychotherapy. In general, it refers to "a variety of psychological interventions designed to help people resolve emotional, behavioral and interpersonal problems of various kinds and improve the quality of their lives" (Engler & Goleman, 1992, p. 15). Although there are considerable differences of opinion regarding which psychological interventions, if any, work the best and how they operate, there appear to be two points of agreement. The first is that psychotherapy involves a significant interpersonal relationship between a client and therapist. This relationship is special, if not unique, and facilitates the use of therapists' techniques and procedures and may be therapeutic in itself. Second, the general objective of psychotherapy is to promote behavior change—to help people act, think, and feel differently to lessen the problems for which they sought help. The processes by which change is brought about are "psychological," although there is considerable disagreement about the specific psychological mechanisms that may be involved. What is agreed on is that the psychotherapist facilitates change verbally; there are no pills, surgeries, or other material interventions. Even such well-defined procedures as relaxation training and guided homework and practice are verbally mediated.

Frank (Frank & Frank, 1991) attempted to provide a rapprochement among the many disparate views of psychotherapy by suggesting that all psychotherapies share four common features. First, the psychotherapist's office is a setting designated by our culture as a place to receive help for emotional distress. It is a contemporary sanctuary of a sort that is safe, private, and confidential. The office has the accoutrements of expertise and status (e.g., diplomas, licenses, certificates, thick books) and exudes what is humorously referred to as the "edifice complex" (Torrey, 1972). According to Frank, the office strengthens the client's expectations of help.

The second shared feature of psychotherapies is the therapeutic relationship within which the client and therapist possess well-defined roles. According to Frank, the client is demoralized and highly motivated to be helped, regardless of the specific problem, symptoms, or diagnosis with which he or she might present. The client expects the therapist to be an empathic expert, and the therapist responds in kind with support, warmth, skillfulness, and hope.

The setting and the relationship provide the therapist with significant leverage to bring about psychological change. This basis of therapeutic influence is enhanced by the third component common to all psychotherapies—a conceptual scheme or theoretical system to explain the client's suffering. Although psychotherapies are often dramatically different in terms of their underlying concepts and principles, they all address the causes of abnormal symptoms, the pathways and goals of changes, and procedures and techniques for the realization of symptom reduction and positive behavior change. Although the therapist's theory is certainly not unique and is not necessarily scientifically validated (indeed, Frank even used the term "myth"), it nonetheless provides the client with an understanding of his or his symptoms. Knowledge and meaning facilitate mastery and personal control.

The fourth therapeutic feature derives from the therapist's conceptual scheme and constitutes the treatment procedure in which both the therapist and client actively participate. Such procedures are a complex series of operations implemented by the therapist, consistent with his or her theoretical viewpoints and aimed at changing the client's problem. The therapist's technique is composed of a variety of activities such as interpretations, empathic reflections, dream analysis, hypnotic suggestions, role playing, cognitive reframing, homework assignments, and exercises. These theory-based activities strengthen the therapist–client relationship and augment the influence and persuasive power of the therapist. Frank referred to these collective activities and operations on the part of the therapist as *therapeutic rituals*, emphasizing that their effectiveness does not derive from specific theoretical explanations, but rather how well they match the client's perspective on his or her problem and what is necessary for change.

EFFICACY AND EFFECTIVENESS

Let us now return to the fundamental question for psychotherapists and their clients—Does psychotherapy work? This question is asked in at least two ways and answered with data from two methods of investigation (Howard, Moras, Brill, Martinorich, & Lutz, 1996). The first is the efficacy question: Does psychotherapy work under specific, well-controlled, experimental conditions? Efficacy research is the most scientifically rigorous. It involves a methodology that is commonly referred to as a randomized clinical trial, in which a treatment is clearly specified, therapists are highly trained to carry it out, and clients are rigorously selected and their problems carefully measured and matched. The clients are then randomly assigned to a treatment group or a control group for comparison. The ideal design (1) randomly assigns patients to treatment and control conditions, (2) carefully selects patients, (3) consists of both researchers and research participants who are blind to the nature of the treatment being administered (i.e., "double blind"), and (4) carefully controls the conditions of the intervention. Considerable attention is given to "purifying" the treatment conditions so that unique aspects of the treatment are only active within the treatment condition(s) and control conditions do not contain any of the "active ingredients." If a given treatment works better than no treatment, the efficacy method permits us to say that it works, but only under the conditions in which it was studied. The efficacy method permits a scientific conclusion, but only for the particular therapists, procedures, and clients that have been studied. It is said to possess strong internal validity.

External validity is more difficult to establish because it requires generalizability to psychotherapy as it is typically practiced. Moreover, the highly specific therapy protocols used in efficacy designs may not represent those used by most practicing clinicians. The latter point is referred to as ecological representativeness (see Kerlinger & Lee, 2000, pp. 476–477).

A second derived question is referred to as the effectiveness question. It can be stated as such: Does psychotherapy work in actual clinical settings? The effectiveness method is said to be quasi-experimental in that is usually does not possess the scientific rigor of the efficacy method. It involves the naturalistic study of psychotherapy as it is typically practiced. The hallmark of the efficacy methodology—random assignment to experimental versus control groups—is sacrificed to increase generalizability to practicing therapists and clients, and to procedures used in the field. The effectiveness method is thus posited to possess strong external validity but weak internal validity. Because effectiveness studies are less rigorous than efficacy studies, the results are subject to multiple interpretations. For example, if a sample of clients report that being in psychoanalysis has produced personality change, there could be several interpretations. It could be true; it could be that the therapist thought psychoanalysis was essential; it could be that the client changed over time independent of psychoanalysis; or it could be that the client did not change at all from the vantage point of another person, such as a friend, relative, or coworker.

To evaluate the outcomes of psychotherapy, data from both methodologies must be examined. Efficacy studies are necessary but probably not sufficient. Efficacy research will tell us if a therapy works under experimental conditions and that it *might* work in practice. Effectiveness research will tell us if a therapy *does* work in actual clinical settings.

PSYCHOTHERAPY OUTCOMES AND THE EMERGENCE OF EFFICACY RESEARCH

Eysenck (1952) published the first critical review of psychotherapeutic outcomes. His premise was that for psychotherapy to be judged efficacious it must relieve psychological distress demonstrably better than no psychotherapy at all. Hence, it was necessary to compare improvement in psychotherapy patients with improvement in untreated controls. Eysenck restricted his comparisons to so-called neurotic patients, a clinical population assumed to be representative of clientele who seek and who have optimum potential for benefiting from psychotherapy.

The data for psychotherapy outcomes were derived from 24 uncontrolled studies. From these studies Eysenck tabulated rates of improvement specified in percentages. Two rates were presented: Of the patients treated in psychoanalysis, 44% improved; of the patients treated in eclectic psychotherapies, 64% improved. For comparison, Eysenck reported rates of improvement for neurotic patients who had received no formal psycho-therapy. Two uncontrolled studies were used. The improvements came to 72% and were attributed to *spontaneous remission*, a term designating re-covery in the absence of formal psychotherapy.

Eysenck's (1952) conclusions were pointed and have echoed ever since. The data "fail to prove that psychotherapy . . . facilitates the recov-ery of neurotic patients. They show that roughly two-thirds of a group of neurotic patients will recover or improve to a marked extent within about two years of the onset of their illness, whether they are treated by means of psychotherapy or not" (p. 322).

For Eysenck (1952), the implications of these findings were stark and far-reaching. He questioned the continued training of clinical psychologists in psychotherapy in view of the lack of scientifically acceptable evidence regarding its efficacy. Moreover, he challenged clinical researchers to dem-onstrate the positive effects of psychotherapy by means of rigorous, well-controlled investigations. He was thus the first to advocate the use of effi-cacy methodology to evaluate psychotherapy outcomes.

The professional and research communities were staggered by Eys-enck's assertions and responded with an outpouring of critique and rebut-tal (e.g., Bergin, 1963, 1971; Kiesler, 1966; Luborsky, 1954). The diversity of the criticism converged on several conclusions regarding the Eysenck (1952) survey. Most of the criticism focused, somewhat ironically, on the poor methodology used by Eysenck, which arguably weakened his conclu-sions. It is noteworthy, however, that none of the critics contended that the research reviewed by Eysenck clearly demonstrated the efficacy of psycho-therapy.

In the wake of criticism and invective, Eysenck (1961, 1966) redou-bled his polemic regarding the efficacy of psychotherapy. After a review and critical analysis of 12 controlled studies that had been published since his 1952 survey, Eysenck concluded that the positive effects of psychother-apy still had not been demonstrated. Moreover, he contended that the breadth of the apparent inefficacy of psychotherapy extended beyond the treatment of common adult disorders to other clinical disorders, such as those characteristic of childhood. The most significant conclusion, how-ever, pertained to Eysenck's interpretation of comparative therapeutic out-comes. According to Eysenck, learning-theory–based therapies apparently worked, although verbal, insight-oriented therapies apparently did not.

Eysenck's (1961, 1966) remarks rubbed salt in old wounds and opened new ones. The issue of dubious psychotherapeutic efficacy lin-gered, and a new issue regarding the relative superiority of one psychother-apeutic paradigm over another arose. The global question of overall psy-chotherapeutic efficacy had thus evolved into a more specific question of relative psychotherapeutic efficacy. The emergent question to be answered by psychotherapy researchers became "*what* treatment, by *whom*, is most effective for *this* individual with *that* specific problem, and under *which* set of circumstances" (Paul, 1966, p. 111). The increased specificity of research questions generated a growing body of research. The research methodologies improved commensurately.

Since Eysenck's challenge regarding the effects of psychotherapy and his suggestions that some therapies may be better than others, specific questions of psychotherapeutic efficacy have been addressed largely by means of a common research strategy—the controlled, comparative study. As this research paradigm has been refined by clinical scientists over the years it has evolved into the gold standard for efficacy research, the means by which psychotherapy outcomes are evaluated under the best approximation of scientific conditions.

Exemplary of the controlled, comparative investigation is a large-scale psychotherapy project known as the Temple study (Sloane, Staples, Cristal, Yorkston, & Whipple, 1975). The Temple study is noteworthy both for its methodological rigor and close resemblance to clinical practice. The research sample was composed of 94 outpatients typical of those seen by psychotherapists in clinical settings. The majority received neurotic diagnoses; the remainder received diagnoses of personality disorders. The patients were matched for sex and symptom severity and randomly assigned to one of two treatment groups or a control. The therapy in one treatment group was conducted by three psychoanalytically oriented therapists. The treatment in the other therapy group was conducted by three behavior therapists. All therapists were highly experienced, considered good therapists by their peers, and had excellent reputations. Guidelines for the contrasting therapeutic modalities were developed and adhered to by the six therapists. The control patients were asked to wait 4 months before seeing a therapist. They were told that if they were in a crisis they could call the psychiatrist who had conducted the initial interview. A research assistant contacted them by phone occasionally to check on their status and reassure them that they would eventually be assigned a therapist.

To assess the efficacy of the psychotherapeutic treatments, the initial measures and assessments were repeated after 4 months of psychoanalytically oriented psychotherapy, behavior therapy, or minimal contact while waiting for psychotherapy. The average number of therapy sessions during this time was about 14. Follow-up evaluations occurred at 1-year and 2-year intervals after the initial assessment.

The results provided clear support for the efficacy of both the behavioral and psychoanalytic psychotherapies. Although all three groups showed significant improvement with regard to the severity of their specific symptoms, the treated groups improved significantly more than the controls. Moreover, there were no significant differences among the therapies, suggesting that they were equally effective. Ratings by an independent assessor also revealed that more of the treated patients improved overall than the controls. The follow-up data suggested that group improvements were maintained over 1-year and 2-year intervals; thus, the positive outcomes did not appear transitory.

The Temple study, like most controlled comparative studies since, has provided evidence that psychotherapy works and that mainstream approaches like psychoanalytic psychotherapy and behavior therapy are comparably effective. However, the methodological merits of the study also restrict the generalizability of the results. The results pertain only to brief versions of the respective therapies with so-called neurotic patients.

Even state-of-science studies of this ilk are neither definitive nor without controversy. A case in point is the NIMH Treatment of Depression Collaborative Research Program (see Elkin, 1994). This highly funded, elaborate project, unquestionably the most extensive and methodologically sound clinical trial of psychotherapy efficacy yet to be completed, compares the relative effectiveness for treating depression of the two psychotherapy approaches, cognitive therapy and interpersonal therapy, with an antidepressant medication, imipramine (Tofranil). Upon termination, the two psychotherapies and the antidepressant achieved significant and equivalent outcomes relative to a placebo control. Moreover, after an 18-month follow-up the treatment conditions did not differ significantly, and of the patients who had initially improved, 30% or less were without depression symptoms. The controversy revolves around the apparent efficacy of drugs versus psychotherapies. Researchers who have examined the same raw data have reached very different conclusions. Klein (1996), for example, concluded that imipramine was superior for severe depression, whereas Jacobson and Hollon (1996) contended that patients on imipramine dropped out of treatment and relapsed significantly more. Moreover, Jacobson and Hollon noted that all other published studies had shown a superiority for cognitive therapy versus drugs in the treatment of depression. Clearly, good science in psychotherapy research does not necessarily lead to a consensus of opinion.

NEGATIVE EFFECTS

The surgeon's knife is a frequently used analogy for psychotherapy's effectiveness. If psychotherapy is a powerful and effective intervention for ameliorating psychopathology and human suffering then, like the surgeon's knife, it may also exacerbate suffering when misdirected or misapplied. Although the possibility of negative effects in psychotherapy is a serious concern for most psychotherapy researchers, precious little has actually been written that sheds light on this problem (Stricker, 1995).

The oft-cited distillation of Hippocrates' caution for physicians—"Primum Non Nocere" (First do no harm)—pertains to psychotherapists as well. There is little consensus on the definition of a "negative effect" within the psychotherapy research community. We see a number of distinctions that might be made along a continuum, starting with (1) failure to change, but with nonsignificant improvements, (2) absolute negative change in outcome, but with nonsignificant deterioration, and (3) clinically significant deterioration. Most authors who have written about "negative effects" either combine the latter two definitions or focus on some form of "significant deterioration." However, it is also reasonable to assume that lack of any significant change is also a negative effect or at least a negative outcome. After all, if the patient does not respond to surgery, then the illness prevails—clearly a negative outcome. Negative effects can occasionally be even more revealing of the nature of a study than an exclusive focus on improvement. Tarrier and colleagues (2000) compared a variety of mixes of cognitive-behavioral interventions, supportive care, and/or standard care for patients with schizophrenia. Most revealing were follow-up results, on which patients in the standard care condition were shown to have deteriorated on all of the measures.

Initial estimates of the rate of negative effects/deterioration in psychotherapy often included a mix of the aforementioned definitional criteria, which tended to be between 1/10 and 1/3 of all cases (Stricker, 1995). More recent estimates of deterioration using a more operationally formal criterion of clinically significant change indicate that "deterioration" is likely to be a much rarer occurrence. For example, Jacobson and Truax's (1991) statistical definition of clinically significant deterioration was used in a sample of 30 patients who underwent behavioral marital therapy. Only 1 of the 30 patients exhibited scores that would be considered deterioration in clinical significance terms. Of 61 patients with complete data in the Vanderbilt II psychotherapy research project, there was not a single patient with clinically significant deterioration (Bein et al., 2000). Analysis of the NIMH Collaborative Study for Depression found that only 1 of 250 patients exhibited clinically significant deterioration (Ogles, Lambert, & Sawyer, 1995). Using this more clear definition of clinically significant deterioration, the rate of deterioration appears to be infrequent, well below 5%, at least in these large, carefully controlled studies.

It is both fortunate—though paradoxically somewhat unfortunate— that studies demonstrate little actual deterioration within psychotherapy research. Clearly, the lack of significant deterioration, unquestionably a negative effect, reflects the fact that psychotherapy is a highly effective treatment for a wide range of psychosocial ills. Yet careful study of cases with deterioration has the potential to greatly inform the field about areas for improving psychotherapeutic practice.

The majority of psychotherapy cases are more equivocal than the clear-cut success stories that tend to be illustrated in case reports and texts.

This ambiguity may leave some feeling uncomfortable, but many psychotherapy researchers have responded to this challenge by attempting to expand the context of their evaluations. For example, in their study of negative effects, Strupp, Hadley, and Gomez-Schwarz (1977) developed the tripartite model of psychotherapy outcome. They recognized that psychotherapy was infused within a malleable constellation of human values, and suggested that outcomes be characterized by the unique configurations of patient, mental health professional (i.e., "structural"), and societal outcomes that could be achieved within any one case. Hence, negative effects could be dependent on the values advocated by these three agents.

MAKING SENSE OF THE RESEARCH: META-ANALYSIS

Controlled, comparative investigations of psychotherapy efficacy, such as the Temple and NIMH projects, are now myriad. The task at hand is to make sense out of many, at times seemingly disparate, scientific findings.

Historically, scientific literature, including psychotherapy findings, has been evaluated by means of narrative reviews in which research literature is compiled, reviewed, and analyzed by a scholar. The pitfalls are obvious; the values, biases, and preconceptions of the reviewer can significantly affect both the selection and appraisal of the studies and the conclusions. The firestorm created by Eysenck's polemic and its rebuttals is exemplary.

Smith and Glass (1977) and Smith and colleagues (1980) developed a quantitative procedure for integrating the results of psychotherapy outcome studies that largely eliminates the pitfalls of the narrative review. Their procedure used data that are typically available in published articles such as means, variances, t tests, F ratios, and so forth. It involves an analysis of analyses, or meta-analysis. The primary advantage of a meta-analysis over a narrative review is that it relies on statistical rather than human judgment to draw conclusions about the strength of the findings. The pivotal statistic in meta-analysis is effect size. It is calculated by dividing the mean difference between a treated group and a control group by the standard deviation of the control group. Effect size is thus a standardized mean difference that reflects the magnitude of an effect and hence permits comparison across many studies using divergent procedures and measures.

Smith and colleagues (1980) completed an exhaustive meta-analysis in which they reviewed 475 psychotherapy outcome studies, calculating 1,766 effect sizes and performing thousands of tabulations and data summaries. Unlike other surveys, theirs included *all* published studies for which effect sizes could be calculated or derived. Various classification schemes and statistical analyses of the effect-sizes provided data bearing on many specific questions of psychotherapeutic efficacy.

Several major conclusions emerged:

1. In general, various forms of psychotherapy produced positive outcomes. The average effect size was .85. Statistically, this means that the average recipient of psychotherapy is more improved than 80% of those who go untreated. Effect size increases to .93 if placebo treatments and undifferentiated counseling techniques are eliminated. Such effects for psychotherapy are comparable with those of expensive and lengthy interventions in medicine and education.

2. Different theoretical orientations (e.g., psychoanalytic, learning-based, cognitive, and client-centered) and different modalities (verbal, behavioral, or expressive) did not produce different degrees or types of improvement. Simple, uncontrolled comparisons of effect sizes suggested that hypnotherapy, systematic desensitization, cognitive, and cognitive-behavioral therapies were most efficacious, but this apparent superiority vanished when controlled comparisons took into account client type and type of outcome measure. Therapies tended to be most effective, regardless of orientation or modality, when clients with depression, simple phobias, and analogues of these disorders were solicited for treatment.

3. Brief versus long-term interventions, individual versus group therapies, and experienced versus novice therapists yielded similar effect sizes.

4. Two findings temper the positive thrust of the conclusions. The generally good outcomes for psychotherapy diminish somewhat 2 years following treatment; the average effect sizes shrink to .50, and a small percentage of therapeutic outcomes (about 9%) are actually negative.

The major criticism of the Smith and colleagues (1980) meta-analytic study is that it is too inclusive; using all studies necessarily requires that good and bad pieces of research are taken into account (e.g., Howard, Krause, Sanders, & Kopta, 1997). Nevertheless, Smith et al. compared effect sizes on the basis of research quality. The rigor of the research had little or no impact on effect size (Smith & Glass, 1977; Smith et al., 1980). The results, thus, were not artifacts of including methodologically weak investigations in the meta-analysis.

As efficacy research has burgeoned, so have the number of meta-analyses. The primary findings of Smith and colleagues (1980) have been repeatedly affirmed (Wampold, 2001). Not only does psychotherapy appear to be effective, but there is little evidence that one therapy is significantly better than another. The most comprehensive meta-analysis (Wampold et al., 1997) and a meta-analysis of 32 meta-analyses (Grissom, 1996) have corroborated the conclusion reached 65 years ago by Rosenzweig (1936). He characterized the apparent uniform efficacy of psychotherapies at the time as the Dodo bird verdict, after the Dodo's observation at the end of a race in *Alice in Wonderland* that "Everybody has won and all must have prizes" (p. 412). This conclusion bears profound implications for the field of psychotherapy, which for the past five decades has been preoccupied with unearthing the essential, specific findings of behavior change in the form of the best therapy. The verdict so far is that psychotherapies appear to share common, not specific, therapeutic features.

PLACEBO CONTROLS AND COMMON FACTORS

The Dodo bird verdict led psychotherapy researchers to redouble their efforts to identify the specific and active ingredients of psychotherapy. Psychotherapy research borrowed the placebo-control design from medical research in the hopes of partitioning specific from nonspecific factors. Increasingly, attention turned to finding ways of understanding these placebo groups and the factors they were assumed to represent.

Medical placebos involve psychological processes and became of interest to psychotherapy research because of the need to find a control group for comparison with psychological treatments (see also Chapter 11, for a discussion of placebo effects). Beginning in the 1950s, evidence from medical trials demonstrated that on average about 30–40% of patients who were assigned to placebo conditions, and for which there should have been no measurable improvements, often showed significant reductions in symptoms (Harrington, 1997).

Understanding medical placebos may assist in the development of good psychological placebos as well as enhance understanding of the nonspecific components of psychological treatments. These hypotheses could be tested in psychotherapy research. First, there may be greater improvement for patients in psychological placebo conditions who have more extreme psychological pain. Hence, patients who are self-referred and who may even be desperate for relief of suffering may be much more immediately responsive to almost any treatment so long as there is some minimal rationale for improvement. Yet such immediate responsiveness may not lead to long-term treatment success (just as is true with medical placebos). Similarly, psychological placebos may achieve similar outcomes to psychological treatments in the short term (this issue is discussed later in the chapter), but the nature of longer-term improvement and the correction of basic personality patterns has yet to be addressed in studies with a long-term placebo comparison. Second, psychological placebos may be more effective when patient's anxieties and expectancies are heightened. Finally, psychological placebo providers with warm and affective qualities, such as case managers, paraprofessionals, and other supportive helpers, may be expected to achieve better placebo outcomes than those who lack these qualities.

The study of placebos in psychotherapy is best understood within the context of the larger research goal of partitioning the active ingredients of psychotherapy into two components: those that are specifically linked to the application of psychological treatments and those that are related to other, more general, aspects of the treatment environment and that possess some therapeutic value. These latter factors have been referred to as *common factors* because they were generally believed to be shared by all forms of therapy. The difficulty of linking these factors to specific techniques makes them *nonspecific*, meaning that these factors are not simply common but *may* be harnessed and studied in their own right. Nonspecific factors are attributable to both patient and treatment providers and include such phenomena as therapist and patient responsiveness; patient expectancy, enthusiasm, and motivation for change; and interpersonal relationship factors (Kirsch, 1997). The study of the therapeutic alliance is one example of a nonspecific factor that has been demonstrated to exert more specific and positive influences on outcome (Horvath & Symonds, 1991; Martin, Garske, & Davis, 2000).

The main requirement of the psychological placebo group is the inclusion of *some* of the nonspecific factors (it is now generally recognized that it is not possible for a placebo group to control for all nonspecific factors). This can be accomplished through activities that mimic the treatment studied, including reading about psychological processes, distraction tasks, various levels of clinical case management, or receiving sessions from "therapists" who have little or no training in providing psychological treatments. Generally, the more a placebo group mimics the general structure of psychotherapy (without including any specific techniques), the more similar the effect size of the placebo to bona fide psychotherapy (Lambert & Bergin, 1994; Wampold, 2001). Furthermore, findings indicate that patients in placebo groups achieve equivalent outcomes when compared with those in genuine psychotherapy (e.g., Strupp & Hadley, 1979).

PARAPROFESSIONALS AND EMPIRICALLY SUPPORTED THERAPIES

There have been two responses to the puzzling findings that all therapies, irrespective of therapist sophistication and professional lineage, appear equivalent. First, there are those who view equivalent results as evidence that therapy, although effective, can be practiced with minimal training (see, e.g., Dawes, 1996); they see little need for doctoral training and licensure. Such advocates endorse minimal training and the increase of paraprofessional practitioners in therapeutic settings. An implication of this viewpoint is that psychotherapy as it is practiced is likely to become even more diverse and difficult to study properly. Although the field is constantly changing, more rapid alterations in the basic structure of psychotherapy practice result in something of a moving target for researchers. It will be nearly impossible to design studies that will identify these components. Although this may be less of a problem for efficacy research, it is an especially sensitive problem for practitioners of effectiveness research, who are interested in understanding psychotherapy as it is practiced.

A second response, motivated in large part by managed care and other health care reformers that are aimed at cost reduction, has been an attempt on the part of professional organizations to identify treatments that have received some form of support. The American Psychiatric Association and the American Psychological Association have spearheaded this movement. A Task Force from Division 12 of the American Psychological Association has established stringent criteria used to designate what are referred to as *empirically supported therapies* (once referred to as "empirically validated" therapies) for psychological practice (American Psychological Association Task Force, 1995). These criteria are reproduced in Tables 6.1 and 6.2. The Task Force modeled their criteria of acceptable treatment on those used by the Federal Drug Administration in the attempt to select a smaller list of *efficacious* treatments from the much larger list known psychotherapies. Although the Task Force itself did not make any claims that their list of therapies was conclusive, it was clearly implied that by omission a treatment was deemed as empirically unsupported. Some have argued that the short list of psychotherapies has passed some "standards of proof" and by implication should be preferred, if not mandated, for use in clinical practice (cf. Nathan & Gorman, 1998). However, the list of empirically supported therapies was intended to be preliminary and updated on an annual

TABLE 6.1. Criteria for Empirically Supported Treatments: Well-Established Treatments

I.   At least two good group design studies, conducted by different investigators, demonstrating efficacy in one or more of the following ways:
   A. Superior to pill or psychological placebo or to another treatment.
   B. Equivalent to an already established treatment in studies with adequate statistical power.

OR

II. A large series of single-case design studies demonstrating efficacy. These studies must have:
   A. Used good experimental designs.
   B. Compared the intervention to another treatment as in IA.

Further criteria for both I and II.

III. Studies must be conducted with treatment manuals.

IV. Characteristics of the client samples must be clearly specified.

Note. From American Psychological Association Division 12 Task Force (1995, p. 21). Copyright 1995 by the American Psychological Association. Reprinted by permission.

TABLE 6.2. Criteria for Empirically Supported Treatments: Probably Efficacious Treatments

I. Two studies showing the treatment is more effective than a waiting-list control group.

OR

II. Two studies otherwise meeting the well-established treatment criteria I, III, and IV, but both are conducted by the same investigator. Or one good study demonstrating effectiveness by these same criteria.

OR

III. At least two good studies demonstrating effectiveness but flawed by heterogeneity of the client samples.

OR

IV. A small series of single-case design studies otherwise meeting the well-established treatment criteria II, III, and IV.

Note. From American Psychological Association Division 12 Task Force (1995, p. 22). Copyright 1995 by the American Psychological Association. Reprinted by permission.

basis. The Task Force hoped to inspire new research on existing therapies as well as to respond to the real world marketplace dangers that surround the practice of psychotherapy. As such, the list would continue to evolve while establishing minimal standards of care regarding the need to provide more research evidence for the practice of psychotherapy.

The movement to identify empirically supported therapies appears to run counter to our discussion thus far. The creation of a list of empirically supported therapies appears to be scientifically premature for the primary reason that certain psychotherapies, as long as they are bona fide forms of treatment, are likely to be equivalent to other psychotherapies (see Chapter 1 for a somewhat different perspective). The cumulative record of efficacy research and meta-analytic evaluations suggests as much (cf. Wampold, 2001).

Although we believe that the null hypothesis of psychotherapy equivalence cannot be rejected, we acknowledge that others do not agree with this conclusion. On the basis of research evidence, some scholars (e.g., Chambless & Ollendick, 2001; Hunsley & Di Guilio, in press) argue that certain protocols, especially those based on cognitive-behavioral approaches, are more efficacious than others. Two counterpoints to the equivalence view are worth noting. First, there appears to be stronger evidence for the relative effects of behavioral and cognitive-behavioral interventions with children and adolescents than with adults. Second, certain effect size differences in major meta-analyses (e.g., Smith et al., 1980) suggest that cognitive-behavioral interventions appear superior, although these differences are small. Chambless and Ollendick (2001) acknowledged, however, that for many disorders, such as depression in adults, many treatment approaches appear to be comparably effective.

There are two noteworthy implications of the empirically supported therapies debate. The first involves the implications for clinical practice and the ethics of policymaking. Practice guidelines may serve to create limitations on clinicians that are unjustified, including problems in financial reimbursement for service, and to increase liabilities for practice that are legal under the provisions of psychology licensure and yet called into question by exclusion from a preferred list of empirically supported treatments. The second is the specification of empirically supported therapies in terms of psychiatric disorders. Therapies are judged to be valid for specific problems, which are classified under categories from the *Diagnostic and Statistical Manual of Mental Disorders*, fourth edition (DSM-IV), the system for grouping mental disorders developed by the American Psychiatric Association (1994). The reliance on DSM categories further muddies the waters scientifically as its psychometric problems with reliability and validity are legion (cf. Garfield, 1996), and alternative (e.g., dimensional) approaches have been advocated by some psychopathology researchers (Turner & Hersen, 1997).

EFFECTIVE AND INEFFECTIVE THERAPISTS

Research on therapist effects has been largely neglected. Most of the findings have come from meta-analyses and reanalyses of previous studies. The study of therapist effects in an individual research project is difficult, and only larger scale psychotherapy studies have been able to ascertain the potential effects of this variable. Most studies do not include more than a handful of carefully selected therapists, and attempts to control this variable have focused on minimizing individual therapist differences by a forced adherence to treatment protocols.

Therapy manuals have been used as a means of controlling therapist effects through standardizing therapist techniques. For example, Crits-Christoph and Mintz (1991) concluded that individual therapist effects tend to be reduced when a therapy manual is used. One interpretation of these results is that the use of manuals minimizes the unwanted "noise" of therapist effects. However, an alternative interpretation is that many of the potential advantages of therapist effects are lost when therapist behaviors are standardized.

Luborsky and colleagues (1986) reanalyzed four studies for both therapist and treatment effects. Results indicated that the magnitude of the therapist effects in the study were much greater than the effects of the treatments or techniques being used. In a meta-analysis of therapist effects,

Crits-Christoph and colleagues (1991) found that the therapist effect was large and surpassed the typical effects of individual treatment comparisons. Blatt, Sanislow, Zuroff, and Pilkonis (2000) reanalyzed data from the NIMH collaborative study of depression and found that even with careful controls and the use of strictly regimented treatment manuals, significant therapist effects remained. In addition, differences in efficacy were not related to therapists' levels of clinical experience. Differences were related to the therapist's clinical orientation, with more effective therapists having a more psychological (not biological) clinical orientation. More effective therapists were also more cautious in estimating the time needed for effects to emerge, in that they estimated that more, rather than less, therapy would be needed before treatment differences in their patients would be manifested.

There can be little argument that these studies demonstrate the existence of therapist effects. Hence one must wonder why more research has not been conducted on such effects. Interestingly, the aforementioned studies have been cited to argue both for treating therapist effects as a significant variable for further study as well for treating therapist effects as a nuisance variable. Some have argued that the Luborsky and colleagues (1986) study provides evidence for the need for greater experimental control through the use of therapy manuals, as it was conducted prior to the advent of modern treatment manuals (which for some "explains" why the therapist effects were so large). Yet the magnitude of these effects have led others to argue for greater exploration of the therapist qualities that contribute to these effects (e.g., Strupp & Anderson, 1997).

Further exploration of the nature of therapist effects has often led researchers to examine such variables as the therapist's level of experience or the "competence" at which therapists apply techniques (e.g., see Beutler, Machado, & Neufeldt, 1994). However, these research avenues generally have led to dead ends. Beutler (1997), in an interesting argument, suggested that therapist "experience" may have been prematurely shelved as a research variable. The reason for this is that previous studies have defined therapist experience as the number of years since training. Such a definition does not include the variety of experiences with different patient populations and is likely confounded by skill, personality traits, and other variables. Mallinckrodt and Nelson (1991) also reported that therapist experience may be related to the ability to form a therapeutic alliance, although again, this was not a clear, unidirectional relationship.

Psychotherapy process research has provided the best clues about what separates "effective" from "ineffective" therapists. Process research focuses on what happens during therapy sessions and may relate these events to (1) the changes that patients make at the end of therapy, (2) independent assessments about the quality of these events (e.g., What makes for a "good" interpretation?), or (3) both. The following findings have repeatedly emerged with respect to the qualities of effective and ineffective therapists:

1. There is little evidence that professional training distinguishes effective from ineffective therapists. Although there are many important reasons for advanced professional training (e.g., responsibility for difficult cases, maintaining the privacy of client disclosures), there are few demonstrable differences in therapist effectiveness that are related to training (Christensen & Jacobson, 1994). One caveat to this conclusion is that professionally trained therapists may be slightly more effective at brief treatments than are paraprofessionals (Berman & Norton, 1985).

2. Similarly, the number of years of clinical experience does not distinguish effective from ineffective therapists. As noted earlier, a less superficial definition of clinical "experience" has not yet been studied. The same could be said for research on training (see #1) in that the nature of training experiences that therapists receive has been narrowly operationalized.

3. Effective therapists do not differ in their theoretical orientation.

4. Effective therapists tend to develop more positive therapeutic alliances with their patients than do ineffective therapists. Moreover, this tendency is independent of patient variables (e.g., Luborsky, McLellan, Diguer, Woody, & Seligman, 1997).

Unpacking the alliance variable has proven to be more difficult and has led to more inclusive findings. However, some interesting leads have developed, which we note with the caveat that these findings have not been replicated or are complicated by some conflicting findings:

Effective therapists demonstrate a number of positive communication behaviors during treatment sessions. Therapists with positive outcomes tend to have surprisingly few pejorative or disaffiliative communications with their patients compared with ineffective therapists (Henry, Schacht, Strupp, Butler, & Binder, 1993). It also appears that effective therapists tend not to contradict their patients (Friedlander, 1984) and may have a more "coordinated" pattern of communications (Westerman, Foote, & Winston, 1995), which are more warm, straightforward, and nearly devoid of complex communications (Henry et al., 1993).

5. Attempts to identify effective therapists through peer nominations have suggested a variety of potential differences between effective and ineffective therapists. For example, Jennings and Skovholt's (1999) study of peer-nominated "master therapists" led to the identification of numerous variables related to effective therapists. Specifically, they are voracious learners, emotionally receptive, psychologically healthy individuals who possess strong relationship skills. Although interesting, these findings may be more of a reflection of what makes for a "popular" therapist among peers and have less to do with actual effectiveness (Orlinsky, 1999).

6. Effective therapists may differ from ineffective therapists in their understanding of clinical material and identification of significant segments of their sessions with patients (Goldfried, Raue, & Castonguay, 1998). These differences are numerous and may reflect a greater degree of cognitive complexity in the understanding of clinical material (Jennings & Skovholt, 1999). Some limited evidence suggests that effective therapists may spend more time with difficult cases, which could reflect an curiosity or interest in the challenges that such cases provide (Ricks, Thomas, & Roff, 1974).

EFFECTIVENESS RESEARCH

Much of our review has focused on efficacy (as opposed to effectiveness) research, and the vast majority of psychotherapy research has been based upon this research strategy. Efficacy studies have been criticized for their small sample sizes and lack of power. Most studies in psychotherapy are so small that there is often insufficient power to characterize the sample beyond basic group differences, and often even these have insufficient power. As noted by Hsu (1989), the basic assumption within the randomized clinical trial (viz., that randomization creates equivalence) is frequently violated because randomization only guarantees equivalent samples with relatively large sample sizes. These criticisms and others have been used to argue for effectiveness research, in which the solution to small samples has been to slacken numerous methodological controls and to investigate large sample sizes of psychotherapy as it is typically practiced.

Effectiveness research is performed in "real" community settings in which psychotherapy is studied as it is actually practiced. This is in contrast to efficacy research, which includes randomized clinical trials and other forms of controlled, laboratory research on psychotherapy. The potential advantages of effectiveness research are the relative ease of collecting samples, larger sample sizes, and (assuming adequate internal validity) producing findings that are more generalizable. Perhaps the best-known example of effectiveness research was carried out by *Consumer Reports*, a publication that monitors and evaluates a variety of services and products that people buy. In an extensive survey of psychotherapy outcomes, the 180,000 subscribers to the magazine were asked a series of questions about their experiences with mental health professionals, self-help groups, and medications. In general, the results demonstrated the positive effects of psychotherapy and surprised even the project consultant, Martin Seligman (1995, 1998). The respondents who had sought professional help for emotional problems reported being much better; approximately 90% indicated that they had improved. Moreover, the strongest reported effects were for those who saw highly trained and licensed professionals—psychologists, social workers, or psychiatrists—for at least 6 months. No specific thera-peutic modality seemed to fare better than any other and medications did not appear to enhance the reported effects of psychotherapy alone. Thus, highly trained professionals were perceived as effective by those who re-ceived help.

Seligman (1995) acknowledged that effectiveness research, such as that exemplified in the *Consumer Reports* study, lacks the methodological rigor of efficacy research. Chief among the shortcomings is the absence of an untreated control group. Without it, the improvements reported could be attributable to spontaneous remission, that is, improvement over time that is not causally related to treatment. Seligman (1998), however, empha-sized that this and other criticisms aside, effectiveness methodology is in-valuable. It provides the link to clinical practice and to the experience of help-seekers in real-world settings. By contrast, the efficacy research design "omits so many crucial elements of real therapy, and introduces others as alien to real therapy, that it masks, minimizes, and distorts the beneficial results that actual therapy provides" (Seligman, 1998, p. 570).

Seligman (1998) discussed several properties that characterize psycho-therapy as it is practiced that may be essential to client improvement. All are overlooked or underestimated by efficacy studies conducted under con-trolled conditions. These properties are presented in Table 6.3. The col-umns contrast "psychotherapy as practiced" as it is represented in effec-tiveness research and "psychotherapy as operationally defined" as it is represented in efficacy research.

As one can see from examining the table, the definitions of "psycho-therapy" vary greatly as a function of the research perspective. Clearly, effectiveness researchers and efficacy researchers are not studying the same phenomena. Consequently, knowledge garnered from the body of efficacy research does not necessarily apply to the realities of clinical practice.

The efficacy and effectiveness distinction is useful and can be thought of as roughly analogous to the distinction between internal and external validity (see previous discussion). More often than not, the term "effective-ness research" has become a shorthand way of describing the reduction of internal validity (viz., methodological rigor) in the hopes of expanded ex-ternal validity (viz., generalizability). In contrast, "efficacy research" places emphasis on internal validity to gain a more tightly controlled, inter-nally valid understanding of psychotherapy. There is the potential that the distinction will cloud the fact that within any research design the psycho-therapy investigator inevitably makes choices regarding trade-offs on a continuum of internal and external validity. Modern-day psychotherapy research may indeed be classifiable in terms of efficacy versus effectiveness terminology. Yet the categories may also serve to mask the possibility that some unknown variable(s) could account for the magnitude of findings

TABLE 6.3. Psychotherapy as Viewed by Effectiveness versus Efficacy Research Approaches

Effectiveness research: "Psychotherapy as practiced"	Efficacy research: "Psychotherapy as operationally defined"
Duration is not fixed; client continues until he or she improves or quits.	Duration is limited, usually to 8–12 sessions; client need does not determine time spent.
Therapy is self-correcting; if one technique does not work, another is chosen.	Techniques are limited or fixed, and often delivered using a manual.
Clients often actively shop and select a therapist of their choice.	Clients are passively assigned to a treatment condition, independent of preference.
Clients usually have multiple problems and even comorbid diagnoses; therapies are flexible and accommodating.	Clients are highly selected with multiple inclusion and exclusion criteria, and usually a single diagnosis.
Outcomes involve general functioning and symptom reduction of clients.	Outcomes are specific, usually defined by standardized measures and inventories.

Note. Data from Seligman (1995).

that are detected in research that is carefully controlled compared with research that is based on psychotherapy as practiced.

RECOMMENDATIONS FOR SCIENTIFIC PSYCHOTHERAPY RESEARCH

We recommend that psychotherapy would be best served by a more coordinated program of research that includes both efficacy and effectiveness research. Given that the *Consumer Reports* study runs counter to some findings from efficacy research, such as the equivalence of professionals and paraprofessionals, it would be useful to perform additional effectiveness studies (using, for example, professionals and pastoral counselors). Unfortunately, the findings from effectiveness research are not well coordinated with the relatively structured research agendas that have been pursued with efficacy research. It is sometimes easy to forget about the necessary interdependence of efficacy and effectiveness, and especially the principle that science typically advances by mastering problems concerning internal validity prior to developing an explanation that is sound enough to be generalized. This oversight is frequently made. For example, Seligman and Levant (1998) advocated for effectiveness research because "the virtue of the effectiveness method is its realism—it has no threats to external validity because it tests therapy as it is actually conducted in the field. One can generalize from effectiveness studies to therapy as it is actually practiced with impunity" (p. 211).

But this is true if and only if current therapeutic practice has achieved some sort of pristine golden standard, along with theoretical explanations for why these treatments work, and if therapies operate exactly in the manner that proponents say they do.

Perhaps the best scientific strategy is to design "hybrid" studies that will incorporate aspects of both efficacy and effectiveness strategies within a single study. For example, Clarke (1995) suggested collecting a large, clinic-based sample for the purpose of performing effectiveness research and then using a subsample for a more carefully controlled efficacy study. Clarke also recommended other "hybrid" methodological strategies. First, he suggested that in such hybrid studies, therapists be trained with manuals but not required to read or use them. Second, Clarke suggested that effectiveness strategies would allow for comparison of the targeted treatment with a standard care condition that represents a typical mode of treatment in practice, and that this is often a much more rigorous test of a treatment's usefulness than a placebo comparison. Third, such a strategy could allow for the combination of heterogeneous (the larger effectiveness sample) and homogeneous (the efficacy, subset sample) sampling. The advantage is that more specific questions, for example, about a treatment for severe major depression could simultaneously be asked with questions regarding depression in general. A hybrid study such as that recommended by Clarke is presently underway under the auspices of the Pennsylvania Practice Research Network (see Borkovec, Echemendia, Ragusea, & Ruiz, 2001). The effectiveness trial is completed and the efficacy component is planned.

The effectiveness strategy opens up powerful tools to the psychotherapy researcher, but as with any tool, it is necessary to understand how it is used. Effectiveness research tools are most useful in developing the "technology" of therapy in a pragmatic, relatively easy, and cost-effective manner. Researchers can develop these technologies and engage in empirically based model building with relatively large samples.

Effectiveness research has the advantage of studying psychotherapy in actual practice settings. Yet it is ironic that the primary criticism of this approach is that it is not linked to clinical applications and that the data collected are too "detached" from actual clinical processes. How can this be? The main reason is that much of the effectiveness data are derived from questionnaires regarding therapies that are not fully understood. The lack of specificity in research design can sometimes make it more difficult for individual clinicians to apply research findings to the treatment of individual patients. Hybrid research models can also assist in overcoming this problem. For example, much of the late Kenneth Howard's research career focused on developing a dose–response model of psychotherapy. One aspect of his scheme is that improvement in psychotherapy tends to occur quite rapidly, often in the first few sessions of therapy. Howard ultimately used growth curve modeling to identify three different types of dose–response patterns, which correspond to different treatment needs with concomitant increases in the number of required sessions (Howard et al., 1996): (1) remoralization, in which a few sessions will lead to sudden changes, (2) remediation, in which treatment focuses on coping skills for symptomatic relief, and (3) rehabilitation, in which patients engage in unlearning chronic maladaptive patterns over a long period of time. Howard et al. suggested that individual clinicians could track patient change as a means of identifying the type of treatment that their patient requires.

In a variant of Howard's approach, Michael Lambert has used dose–response modeling (e.g., Anderson & Lambert, 2001) to identify types of patient changes, ranging from success to deterioration. Clients complete a symptom checklist at the beginning of each session and after each session, and clinicians receive feedback by means of a "flag" in their patient's chart that represents their individual patient's growth response pattern. Clinicians then make decisions, for example, to change the treatment approach when the patient is deteriorating or to discontinue the case when success has been attained.

These approaches are the best contemporary examples of effectiveness research because of the link created between data collection and individual clinician use of that data, which in turn is studied further by researchers. Such a pattern creates an "empirical dialogue" between researchers and clinicians that allows for an acceleration of hypothesis testing of these more pragmatic models. Effectiveness research might thrive through the development of numerous "empirical dialogues," which would represent the perspectives of the different participants in psychotherapy. For example, empirical dialogues could include the three different perspectives of Strupp and colleagues' (1977) tripartite model of psychotherapy outcomes (clinician, patient, and patient's significant others) or expanded to include the six outcome perspectives suggested by Howard and his colleagues (Howard et al., 1996)—patient, client, clinicians, managers, sponsors, and researchers.

CONCLUSIONS: IS A SCIENCE OF PSYCHOTHERAPY POSSIBLE?

It can be asked whether the attempts to study psychotherapy can rightly be referred to as a science at all. What sort of truth claims can be made? According to one perspective, psychotherapy may fall into a class of questions that arc not possible to answer through science. Koch (1985) quite eloquently described the need to overextend the application of science as deriving from

> the endemic human need for crawling into cozy conceptual boxes—any box, so long as it gives promise of relieving the pains of cognitive uncertainty or easing problematic tension. This poignant human need, at any cost, for a frame, an abacus, a system, map, or set of rules that can seem to offer a wisp of hope for resolving uncertainty makes all of us vulnerable—in one degree or another—to the claims of simplistic, reductive, hypergeneral, or in other ways ontology-distorting frames, so long as they have the appearance of "systematicity." (p. 87)

From this perspective, psychotherapy could be approached with an entirely different set of tools and for an entirely different purpose.

Although it is important to recognize the limitations of what can be known, psychotherapy is a phenomenon like many others that have clearly defined goals and procedures (e.g., the application of techniques). As argued by Erwin (2000), even subjective interpretations of client meaning-making are difficult to observe, but it may be possible to develop scientific methods to better understand these phenomena. In contrast to this position is the constructivist view that human meanings defy objective classification. We believe that science can lead to a better understanding of many, but not all, aspects of psychotherapy. However, it is also important to recognize that psychotherapy research, like so much of clinical psychology, is presently at a basic, *descriptive* phase of development.

Causal, scientific explanation is unlikely to develop without further development of a basic taxonomy for human change processes. A human change taxonomy must occur at two levels in order for the scientific study of psychotherapy to thrive. One level is a more abstract description of treatments, including combinations of psychotherapeutic techniques and relational processes that lead to change. This taxonomy focuses on understanding treatment approaches, individually or in combination, and their relationship to "outcomes." This level of description could examine such questions as "Does systematic desensitization lead to a significant reduction of symptoms in persons with generalized anxiety disorder?" A second level of description would link psychotherapeutic phenomena to basic psychological processes. For example, one might ask "What *psychological, cognitive, and emotional processes* must be activated that lead persons to better create psychological distance from a threatening situation?" Coordinating these two types of questions will assist in establishing a science of psychotherapy research.

The overarching issue in this chapter pertains to research methodology. Is the science of psychotherapy best served by the efficacy paradigm, the effectiveness paradigm, or the integration of the two? In closing, we would like to emphasize an approach that is critically important for both traditions and that could be used to foster the development of psychotherapy research. Qualitative research methods emphasize the detailed, intensive observations of clinical processes. Qualitative research is especially useful because it can be used to generate valuable hypotheses that can later be tested with traditional methods (e.g., Soldz, 1990). Naturalistic observation arguably has been absent throughout traditional psychological research and qualitative research offers the potential to infuse research programs with new databases, models, and perspectives. Goldfried (2000) described a process whereby researchers test theory with empirical studies, which often leads to creating numerous modifications to maintain the integrity of the theory. Interestingly, most researchers are prone either to dismiss the negative findings of their own research on methodological grounds or to attempt to salvage the theory through modification. Additional studies are then conducted, which then lead to further methodological regrets, and so on.

Qualitative researchers differ from traditional researchers in that they generally are not in search of definitive answers. It is often assumed that psychotherapy research will advance in answering some of the field's more basic questions through new statistical procedures and better psychometric measurement (see Stiles, Shapiro, & Elliott, 1986). However, it is equally possible that the field cannot advance without developing more basic scientific tools, including naturalistic observation. The argument made by qualitative researchers is that we have plunged into rapid methodological expansion without "some direct contact with these phenomena prior to experimental manipulation" (Giorgi, 1985/1992, p. 50). In the ever-accelerating search for answers to what treatment is superior, what type of therapy manual permits the best adherence, or what components of a treatment are most active when dismantled, it is important to remember that the foundation of science is the process of formulating the right questions.

GLOSSARY

Common factors: Aspects of psychotherapy that are shared by all other psychotherapies. Common factors include many nonspecific factors (e.g., client expectations) but are completely independent of specific factors.

Effect size: The primary statistic used in meta-analysis. It is often calculated by dividing the mean difference between a treated group and a control group by the standard deviation of the control group.

Effectiveness research: Research on psychotherapy that is "applied" within actual clinical settings, in which there is less experimental control. The nature of the clinical setting is not greatly altered. Effectiveness research may be highly generalizable, but is generally less rigorous.

Efficacy research: Research on psychotherapy that is "experimental" in that there are highly specified selection criteria, randomized selection of patients, and clearly delineated independent groups (e.g., through a treatment manual). Efficacy research is rigorous, but its generalizability tends to be untested.

Meta-analysis: A technique for quantitatively reviewing and cumulating data from previous studies. Decision rules are decided upon in advance for such issues as the selection of studies, criteria for weighting of samples, and procedures for aggregating measures.

Nonspecific factors: Aspects of psychotherapy that are derived from the effects of treatment that are more general and difficult to isolate empirically, but that may be a significant aspect of treatment. Nonspecific factors may include nonprescribed interpersonal phenomena, client involvement, and cultural and personal expectations for change.

Outcome research: The attempt to identify the changes made at the end of a treatment or follow-up period.

Process research: The attempt to identify the events that occur during the course of therapy sessions, often relating these events to (1) the changes that patients make at the end of therapy or (2) independent assessments regarding the quality of these events (e.g., What makes for a "good" therapeutic interpretation?).

Psychotherapy: A set of psychological interventions designed to help people resolve emotional, behavioral, and interpersonal problems and improve the quality of their lives.

Specific factors: Aspects of psychotherapy that are derived from formally defined therapeutic techniques and theoretical orientations.

REFERENCES

American Psychiatric Association. (1994). *Diagnostic and statistical manual for mental disorders* (4th ed.). Washington, DC: Author.

American Psychological Association Task Force. (1995). *Template for developing guidelines: Interventions for mental disorders and psychosocial aspects of physical disorders*. Washington, DC: Author.

Anderson, E. M., & Lambert, M. J. (2001). A survival analysis of clinically significant change in outpatient psychotherapy. *Journal of Clinical Psychology, 57,* 875–888.

Bein, E., Anderson, T., Strupp, H. H., Henry, W. P., Schacht, T. E., Binder, J. L., & Butler, S. F. (2000). The effects of training in time-limited dynamic psychotherapy: Changes in therapeutic outcomes. *Psychotherapy Research, 10,* 119–131.

Bergin, A. E. (1963). The effects of psychotherapy: Negative results revisited. *Journal of Counseling Psychology, 10,* 244–250.

Bergin, A. E. (1971). The evaluation of therapeutic outcomes. In A. E. Bergin & S. L. Garfield (Eds.), *Handbook of psychotherapy and behavior change* (pp. 139–189). New York: Wiley.

Bergin, A. E., & Garfield, S. (1994). *Handbook of psychotherapy and behavior change* (4th ed.). New York: Wiley.

Berman, J. S., & Norton, N. C. (1985). Does professional training make a therapist more effective? *Psychological Bulletin, 98,* 401–407.

Beutler, L. E. (1997). The psychotherapist as a neglected variable in psychotherapy: An illustration by reference to the role of therapist experience and training. *Clinical Psychology: Science and Practice, 4,* 44–52.

Beutler, L. E., Machado, P. P., & Neufeldt, S. (1994). Therapist variables. In A. E. Bergin & S. L. Garfield (Eds.), *Handbook of psychotherapy and behavior change* (4th ed., pp. 229–269). New York: Wiley.

Blatt, S. J., Sanislow, C. A., Zuroff, D., & Pilkonis, P. (2000). Characteristics of the effective therapist: Further analysis of data from the National Institute of Mental Health Treatment of Depression Collaborative Research Program. *Journal of Consulting and Clinical Psychology, 64,* 1276–1284.

Borkovec, T. D., Echemendia, R. J., Ragusea, S. A., & Ruiz, M. (2001). The Pennsylvania Practice Research Network and future possibilities for clinically meaningful and scientifically rigorous psychotherapy effectiveness research. *Clinical Psychology: Science and Practice, 8,* 155–185.

Chambless, D. L., & Ollendick, T. H. (2001). Empirically supported psychological interventions: Controversies and evidence. *Annual Review of Psychology, 52,* 685–716.

Christensen, A., & Jacobson, N. S. (1994). Who (or what) can do psychotherapy: The status and challenge of nonprofessional therapies. *Psychological Science, 5,* 9–13.

Clarke, G. N. (1995). Improving the transition from basic efficacy research to effectiveness studies: Methodological issues and procedures. *Journal of Consulting and Clinical Psychology, 63,* 718–725.

Crits-Christoph, P., Barnackie, K., Kurcias, J., Beck, A. T., Carroll, K., Perry, K., Luborsky, L., McLeallan, A. T., Woody, G., Thompson, L., Gallagher, D., & Zitrin, C. (1991). Meta-analysis of therapist effects in psychotherapy outcome studies. *Psychotherapy Research, 1,* 81–91.

Crits-Christoph, P., & Mintz, J. (1991). Implications of therapist effects for the design and analysis of comparative studies of psychotherapies. *Journal of Consulting and Clinical Psychology, 59,* 20–26.

Dawes, R. M. (1996). *House of cards: Psychology and psychotherapy built on myth.* New York: Free Press.

Elkin, I. (1994). The NIMH Treatment of Depression Collaborative Research Program: Where we began and where we are. In A. E. Gerbin & S. L. Garfield (Eds.), *Handbook of psychotherapy and behavior change* (4th ed., pp. 114–139). New York: Wiley.

Engler, J., & Goleman, D. (1992). *A consumer's guide to psychotherapy.* New York: Simon & Shuster.

Erwin, E. (2000). Is a science of psychotherapy possible? *American Psychologist, 55,* 1133–1138.

Eysenck, H. J. (1952). The effects of psychotherapy: An evaluation. *Journal of Consulting Psychology, 16,* 319–324.

Eysenck, H. J. (1961). The effects of psychotherapy. In H. J. Eysenck (Ed.), *Handbook of abnormal psychology* (pp. 697–725). New York: Basic Books.

Eysenck, H. J. (1966). *The effects of psychotherapy.* New York: International Science Press.

Frank, J. D., & Frank. J. B. (1991). *Persuasion and healing: A comparative study of psychotherapy* (3rd ed.). Baltimore: Johns Hopkins University Press.

Friedlander, M. L. (1984). Psychotherapy talk as social control. *Psychotherapy, 21,* 335–341.

Garfield, S. L. (1996). Some problems associated with "validated" forms of psychotherapy. *Clinical Psychology Science and Practice, 3,* 218–229.

Giorgi, A. (1992). Toward the articulation of psychology as a coherent discipline. In S. Koch & D. E. Leary (Eds.), *A century of psychology as science* (pp. 46–59). Washington, DC: American Psychological Association. (Original work published 1985)

Goldfried, M. R. (2000). Consensus in psychotherapy research and practice: Where have all the findings gone? *Psychotherapy Research, 10,* 1–16.

Goldfried, M. R., Raue, P. J., & Castonguay, L. G. (1998). The therapeutic focus in significant sessions of master therapists: A comparison of cognitive-behavioral and psychodynamic-interpersonal interventions. *Journal of Consulting and Clinical Psychology, 66,* 803–810.

Grissom, R. J. (1996). The magical number .7 + –.2: Meta-meta-analysis of the probability of superior outcome in comparisons involving therapy, placebo, and control. *Journal of Consulting and Clinical Psychology, 64,* 973–982.

Harrington, A. (Ed.). (1997). *The placebo effect: An interdisciplinary exploration.* Cambridge, MA: Harvard University Press.

Henry, W. P., Schacht, T. E., Strupp, H. H., Butler, S. F., & Binder, J. L. (1993). Effects of training in time-limited dynamic psychotherapy: Mediators of therapists' responses to training. *Journal of Consulting and Clinical Psychology, 61,* 441–447.

Horvath, A. O., & Symonds, B. D. (1991). Relation between working alliance and outcome in psychotherapy: A meta-analysis. *Journal of Counseling Psychology, 38,* 139–149.

Howard, K. L., Krause, M. S., Saunders, S. M., & Kopta, S. M. (1997). Trial and tribulations in the meta-analysis of treatment differences: Comment on Wampold et al. (1997). *Psychological Bulletin, 122,* 221–225.

Howard, K. I., Moras, K., Brill, L., Martinorich, Z., & Lutz, W. (1996). Evaluation of psychotherapy efficacy, effectiveness, and patient progress. *American Psychologist, 51,* 1059–1064.

Hsu, L. M. (1989). Random sampling, randomization, and equivalence of contrasted groups in psychotherapy outcome research. *Journal of Consulting and Clinical Psychology, 57,* 131–137.

Hunsley, J., & Di Giulio, G. (in press). Dodo bird, Phoenix or urban legend? The question of psychotherapy equivalence. *Scientific Review of Mental Health Practice.*

Jacobson, N. S., & Hollon, S. D. (1996). Cognitive-behavior therapy versus pharmacotherapy : Now that the jury's returned its verdict, it's time to present the rest of the evidence. *Journal of Consulting and Clinical Psychology, 64,* 74–80.

Jacobson, N. S., & Truax, P. (1991). Clinical significance: A statistical approach to defining meaningful change in psychotherapy research. *Journal of Consulting and Clinical Psychology, 59,* 12–19.

Jennings, L., & Skovholt, T. M. (1999). The cognitive, emotional, and relational characteristics of master therapists. *Journal of Counseling Psychology, 46,* 3–11.

Kerlinger, F. N. & Lee, H. B. (2000). *Foundations of behavioral research* (4th ed.). Fort Worth, TX: Harcourt College.

Kiesler, D. J. (1966). Some myths of psychotherapy research and the search for a paradigm. *Psychological Bulletin, 65,* 110–136.

Kirsch, I. (1997). Specifiying nonspecifics: Psychosocial mechanisms of placebo effects. In A. Harrington (Ed.), *The placebo effect: An interdisciplinary exploration* (pp. 166–186). Cambridge, MA: Harvard University Press.

Klein, D. F. (1996). Preventing hung juries about therapy studies. *Journal of Consulting and Clinical Psychology, 64,* 81–87.

Koch, S. (1985). The nature and limits of psychological knowledge. In S. Koch & D. E. Leary (Eds.), *A century of psychology as science* (pp. 75–97). Washington, DC: American Psychological Association.

Lambert, M. J., & Bergin, A. E. (1994). The effectiveness of psychotherapy. In S. Garfield & A. E. Bergin (Eds.), *Handbook of psychotherapy and behavior change* (pp. 143–189). New York: Wiley.

Luborsky, L. (1954). A note on Eysenck's article, "The effects of psychotherapy : An evaluation." *British Journal of Psychology, 45,* 129–131.

Luborsky, L., Crits-Christoph, P., McLellan, T., Woody, G., Piper, W., Imber, S. & Liberman, B. (1986). Do therapists vary much in their success? Findings from four outcome studies. *American Journal of Orthopsychiatry, 56,* 501–512.

Luborsky, L., McLellan, A. T., Diguer, L., Woody, G., & Seligman, D. A. (1997). The psychotherapist matters: Comparison of outcomes across twenty-two therapists and seven patient samples. *Clinical Psychology: Science and Practice, 4,* 53–65.

Lynn, S. J., & Garske, J. P. (1985). *Contemporary psychotherapies: Models and methods* (pp. 3–16). Columbus, OH: Merrill.

Mallinckrodt, B., & Nelson, M. L. (1991). Counselor training level and the formation of the psychotherapeutic working alliance. *Journal of Counseling Psychology, 38,* 135–138.

Martin, D. J., Garske, J. P., & Davis, M. K. (2000). Relation of the therapeutic alliance with outcome and other variables: A meta-analytic review. *Journal of Consulting and Clinical Psychology, 63,* 438–450.

Nathan, P. E., & Gorman, J. M. (1998). *A guide to treatments that work.* New York: Oxford University Press.

Ogles, B. M., Lambert, M. J., & Sawyer, J. D. (1995). Clinical significance of the National Institute of Mental Health Treatment of Depression Collaborative Research Program data. *Journal of Consulting and Clinical Psychology, 63*, 321–326.

Orlinsky, D. E. (1999). The master therapist: Ideal character or clinical fiction? Comments and questions on Jennings and Skovholt's "The cognitive, emotional, and relational characteristics of master therapists." *Journal of Counseling Psychology, 46*, 12–15.

Paul, G. L. (1966). *Effects of insight, desensitization, and attention placebo on the treatment of anxiety*. Stanford, CA: Stanford University Press.

Ricks, D. F., Thomas, A., & Roff, M. (1974). *Life history research in psychopathology: III*. Minneapolis: University of Minnesota Press.

Rosenzweig, S. (1936). Some implicit common factors in diverse methods of psychotherapy: "At last the Dodo said, 'Everybody has won and all must have prizes.' " *American Journal of Orthopsychiatry, 6*, 412–415.

Seligman, M. E. P. (1995). The effectiveness of psychotherapy: The *Consumer Reports* survey. *American Psychologist, 50*, 965–974.

Seligman, M. E. (1998). Afterword. In P. Nathan & J. Gorman (Eds.), *A guide to treatments that work* (pp. 568–572). New York: Oxford University Press.

Seligman, M. E. P., & Levant, R. F. (1998). Managed care policies rely on inadequate science. *Professional Psychology: Research and Practice, 29*, 211–212.

Sloane, R. B., Staples, F. R., Cristol, A. H., Yorkston, N. J., & Whipple, K. (1975). *Psychotherapy versus behavior therapy*. Cambridge, MA: Harvard University Press.

Smith, M. L., & Glass, G. V. (1977). Meta-analysis of psychotherapy outcome studies. *American Psychologist, 132*, 752–760.

Smith, M. L., Glass, G. V., & Miller, T. L. (1980). *The benefits of psychotherapy*. Baltimore: Johns Hopkins University Press.

Soldz, S. (1990). The therapeutic interaction. In R. A. Wells & V. J. Giannetti (Eds.), *Handbook of the brief psychotherapies* (pp. 27–53). New York: Plenum Press.

Stiles, W. B., Shapiro, D. A., & Elliott, R. (1986). Are all psychotherapies equivalent? *American Psychologist, 41*, 165–180.

Stricker, G. (1995). Failures in psychotherapy. *Journal of Psychotherapy Integration, 5*, 91–93.

Strupp, H. H., & Anderson, T. (1997). On the limitations of therapy manuals. *Clinical Psychology: Science and Practice, 4*, 76–82.

Strupp, H. H., & Hadley, S. W. (1979). Specific vs. nonspecific factors in psychotherapy. *Archives in General Psychiatry, 36*, 1125–1136.

Strupp, H. H., Hadley, S. W., & Gomes-Schwartz, B. (1977). *Psychotherapy for better or worse: An analysis of the problem of negative affects*. New York: Jason Aronson.

Tarrier, N., Kinney, C., McCarthy, E., Humphreys, L., Wittkowski, A., & Morris, J. (2000). Two-year follow-up of cognitive-behavioral therapy and supportive counseling in the treatment of persistent symptoms in chronic schizophrenia. *Journal of Consulting and Clinical Psychology, 68*, 917–922

Turner, S. M., & Hersen, M. (1997). *Adult psychopathology and diagnosis* (3rd ed.). New York: Wiley.

Wampold, B. E. (2001). *The great psychotherapy debate: Models, methods, and findings*. Mahwah, NJ: Erlbaum.

Wampold, B. E., Mondin, G. W., Moody, M., Stich, I., Benson, K., & Ahn, H. (1997). A meta-analysis of outcome studies comparing bona fide psychotherapies: Empirically "all must have prizes." *Psychological Bulletin, 122*, 203–215.

Westerman, M. A., Foote, J. P., & Winston, A. (1995). Change in coordination across phases of psychotherapy and outcome: Two mechanisms for the role played by patients' contribution to the alliance. *Journal of Consulting and Clinical Psychology, 63*, 672–675.

7

New Age Therapies

MARGARET THALER SINGER
ABRAHAM NIEVOD

ACCOUNTABILITY AS THE BASIS FOR
EVALUATION OF NEW AGE THERAPIES

In the last decades of the 20th century, "New Age therapies" have aroused much comment, led to many legal cases, and engendered public astonishment over their content. Such therapies have been built around inculcating clients and patients into believing that their psychological distress results from, for example, being molested by space aliens and satanists, invaded by "entities," having lived many past lives, and being fragmented into hundreds of personalities. "New Age therapies" have aroused bitter disagreements. Criticisms of the "New Age therapies" are viewed variously as internecine arguments among schools of psychotherapy based on succeeding generations of therapists, or among rival siblings within the psychology family. Criticism, either in the professional or popular literature, has been experienced as personalized. Many individual therapists experience their own sense of competence as either challenged or supported by being labeled a "New Age therapist." In the last decades therapeutic orientation for many therapists has come to define the boundaries of peer group relations, professional membership, employment opportunities, and financial security. It comes as no surprise that in an era in which providing therapeutic services to troubled clients is often limited by managed care, institutional decisions, or group service provider policies, some therapists defend their therapeutic approach with great tenacity and view criticism in a personalized manner.

A catalogue of New Age therapies is beyond the scope of this chapter.

The following examples have been chosen as representative, based on the New Age therapy's thematic concerns, the relationship between therapist and client, the therapeutic techniques employed, and the announced goals of the therapy:

- *Recovered memory therapy* (RMT): Therapists operate on the assumption that their client's psychological distress, lack of success, failed relationships, and so forth are due to traumatic experiences, typically under the control of their parents. RMT often involves the belief that the intensity of the childhood trauma was so great as to cause dissociative "splitting" into multiple personalities, now known as dissociative identity disorder (see Chapter 5). In RMT, the process of therapy often consists of diverse methods of recovering the "lost memories," including hypnotic induction, administration of "truth serum" (sodium pentathol), group therapy, guided fantasies, religious-based prayer, and assertions by therapists that the client's symptoms could only have been caused by a traumatic event (see Chapter 8, for a critique of these and related methods). Given a New Age therapist's belief in RMT, therapy becomes unending as the client is taken back into earlier past lives, additional alien abductions, and additional split-off personalities (known as "alters"; see Chapter 5). Alien abduction therapy, one variation of RMT, holds that extraterrestrials landed on earth and abducted and then molested the individual, thereby causing the past trauma. Past lives therapy, another variation of RMT, holds that all of life's travails are due having lived a series of past lives and having "unfinished business" from past lives invading one's current life.
- *Satanic ritual abuse (SRA) therapy*, another variation of RMT, holds that the client's trauma derived from having been molested by their parents, who were members of satanic cults. These parents forced their children to participate in satanic rituals that involved killing and eating babies, forced pregnancies, and bloodthirsty, egregious ritual sacrifices.
- *Evil entities or entities therapy* asserts that, at the time of death, the soul did not migrate to the next world, but instead invaded the client's life and remains as the cause of the client's present symptoms.
- *Rebirthing and reparenting therapy*, a variation of several of the aformentioned methods, holds that because the client was not "properly born," the therapy must offer the client an opportunity to be "reborn" or "reparented" (see also Chapter 1).

Apart from issues of internecine or sibling rivalries, the New Age therapies, as well as traditional approaches, must be evaluated using criteria that focus on issues of (1) accountability for the therapeutic approach and the therapist; and (2) quality of care for any treatment provided, regardless of theoretical approach.

Chodoff (1999) argued that psychiatrists are increasingly aware that they practice within a fairly well-defined ethical framework, with derelictions having professional consequences. Chodoff believes that this increased awareness comes as a result of the changing role of the psychiatrists in society and the severity of consequences. One factor in this change has been the pronounced shift away from the previously prevailing paternalistic model ("Father knows best—you should do what he tells you and not complain") of the doctor–patient relationship. A different model now prevails (at least theoretically), one in which the patient has moved away from being a subject of paternalism, toward what might be called a contractual relationship with the doctor, who will be held accountable for incompetent or unacceptable behavior. This means that, like anyone else engaging in activities sanctioned by society and which involve a certain degree of power, psychiatrists must be able to provide responsible answers to questions about the scope, legitimacy, and effectiveness of what they do, and provide machinery to redress errors or wrongs (Chodoff, 1999).

Although seen as a threat to private psychotherapists, the issues generated by a managed care system or the insurers of institutionally based health care services have also brought to the fore general issues of health care that hold promise for mental health professionals. The intense scrutiny being devoted to health care, in general, aids in focusing evaluative discussions as to the issues of accountability and quality of care.

THE "THIRD REVOLUTION"

Relman (1988) proclaimed three revolutions in medical care. The first occurred after World War II in the Era of Expansion—increased medical providers, hospitals, research programs, and government support of medical delivery programs, such as Medicare and Medicaid. The second revolution occurred in the 1970s and is the Era of Cost Containment, when the state and federal governments, private employers, and insurers responded to soaring medical costs by implementing measures that led to managed care, group service providers, and drastic budgeting of health care services by the government, employers, and insurers.

Global budget cutting led to concerns regarding the quality of health care. Thus, Relman's third revolution is the Era of Assessment and Accountability. Quality assessment has become a major theme in questions raised by consumers regarding the efficacy of managed care and group service provider organizations. As dissatisfactions with health care delivery systems have mounted, quality assessment and accountability for the quality of health services provided have been viewed by many as the two means to correct the cost-cutting extremes of the second revolution. To justify its place in a "leaner," "meaner" world of health care economics, psychotherapy will be assessed on the quality of services provided and will be held accountable for its methods and consequent results.

> If the first revolution was fueled by a therapeutic optimism borne of biomedical breakthroughs; and the second driven by financial anxiety at the cost of progress; the third is built on the hope that the tools of quality assessment will help separate the gold from the dross, the valuable health care from the useless. . . . If we can specify what constitutes good quality in health care, we can assess how closely current practice approximates that ideal, and then convey that data to all concerned. This "feedback loop" then has the potential to move practice closer to the ideal, or to catalyze interventions to do so. (Wolf, 1994, p. 107)

No longer will the only focus be among competing therapeutic methodologies based on academic, generational, or sibling rivals. Rather, New Age therapies will be held accountable on the quality of services provided on two levels: first, the degree to which the therapy is effective in ameliorating the presenting problem, that is, the degree to which a therapist provides quality care, and, second, the degree to which the therapist's professional conduct is ethical and comports with the standards of the profession. As Wolf (1994) wrote, "Quality assessment requires specification of what constitutes good quality, then the formulation of measures to gauge good quality, their application to generate data on how closely real practices approximate good quality, and reporting the data to allow feedback and change" (p. 106). Regulators, administrators, and those being regulated can determine through ongoing feedback how standards are (or are not) being implemented. Significantly, the range of people receiving data on practices within health plans would be expanded. In addition to administrators, regulators, and the health professionals themselves, patients and potential patients will be important recipients of accountability and quality of service data. The result would be that the entire process would have the potential to render health plans and professionals accountable to consumers directly (Wolf, 1994).

A new type of therapist–client relationship, based on direct access to efficacy evaluations and accountability, presents therapists with ethical issues that directly affect the nature of the therapeutic process itself and the intensity of scrutiny focused on them.

HISTORICAL CONTEXT OF NEW AGE THERAPIES

Psychology originated in the rational world of philosophy and science. Gradually psychology incorporated contributions from medicine, biology, sociology, anthropology, and education. A split arose between academic laboratory psychologists and clinicians (Watters & Ofshe, 1999). Psychol ogists whose primary focus was clinical practice emphasized providing psychotherapy to the community and left the laboratory and classrooms of academia. Clinical psychologists, counselors, and allied mental health providers—such as social workers; marriage, family, and child counselors; educational counselors; and pastoral counselors—became the providers of mental health care in the community. Each category of mental health provider became licensed in some, but not all, states.

Individuals with many backgrounds have stepped in to fill the ever-widening interest in the workings of the human mind and to offer help for all sorts of human worries, mental illnesses, and counsel the "walking worried." New Age therapies depart greatly from the methods and values of traditional rational rehabilitative therapies, and the merits of their new methods often are evaluated in the courts rather than in scientific circles.

The phrase "New Age" is a term, taken from astrology, that refers to the historical change from the Piscean Age to the Age of Aquarius. Two lines of development coalesced to establish the "New Age" as a contemporary social movement. First, the New Age movement had its beginnings in the United States in the 1960s and 1970s. Several streams of ideas merged that had their origin in, first, popular culture; second, political changes in the social fabric of society; and, third, the cyclical trends that shape "fashionable" experience. For example, popular culture brought together the publication of Marilyn Ferguson's (1980) book and the national publicity that occurred when such entertainment stars as Shirley MacLaine (MacLaine, 1985) popularized the term in print and on television.

Second, many Eastern religious groups and "cults" came into this country to recruit members during the 1960s and 1970s (Singer & Lalich, 1995). Such groups espoused a simplified belief system that can be characterized as "all is one." These groups used the religious practices of many different faiths to offer ready-made solutions to the individual's problems. Directing their message at cultural subgroups (such as college students, foreign travelers, and members of the 1960s "dropout" generation), these Eastern religious groups advertised that their movements could transform the individual into a person who is "one with the world of the spirit," "one with the energy of the universe," "one with Nature," or "one with alien beings from different universes or different spiritual and/or temporal realities." Directed toward the naive, uninitiated "seeker," these groups promised that the group's belief system and experiential regime would not rehabilitate but rather transform individuals—changing them into persons capable of achieving a desired state of "oneness with Nature," "a state of personal mastery," "living in a state of spirituality/ pure energy," "union with extraterrestrial beings," and so forth. Transformation was to be achieved through devotion to a prescribed belief system and adherence to the rules and dictates of the group's belief system (Singer & Lalich, 1996)

Alternative publications and, after a time, mainstream publications, were filled with advertisements by therapists conveying the promise of transformation couched in the language of the New Age therapies (Boylan & Boylan, 1994; Fiore, 1989; Goldberg, 1982; Hoyt & Yamamoto, 1987; Mack, 1994; MacLaine, 1985; Weiss, 1988, 1992; West & Singer, 1980). The general rule was that these groups guaranteed success if the seeker followed the dictates of the group or the therapist. By contrast, it is a given that ethical mental health professionals do not guarantee cures.

The older established psychotherapies were primarily rehabilitative and restorative, being based on therapeutic approaches that viewed psychotherapy as directed toward restoring the individual to a (prior) state of productivity and social involvement (Singer, 1997). One source for the rise in the importance of psychotherapy is the use made of therapy to treat soldiers during the World War II. The aim of military therapy was to rehabilitate and restore the soldier to an effective state. Similarly, the traditional, rehabilitation-model therapies were directed toward helping patients become more independent; to aid patients in inspecting their own values, motives, emotions, and behavior; and to help them develop appropriate means of functioning in the world. The goal was self- reliance and responsible participation in society. This rehabilitative/ restorative approach made no promises of "total fulfillment," creating a "new you," or similar goals that have become the hallmark of the New Age therapies.

A second major methodological approach to psychotherapy based on psychoanalytic or psychodynamic principles provided a context from which the New Therapies developed. Psychoanalysts and psychodynamic therapists placed emphasis on the etiology of the patient's present-day behavior. They generally interpreted a patient's problems as derivative of universal, transgenerational conflicts, flowing inevitably from the nature of the primary family unit. Given these universal, transgenerational sources for patients' problems, a psychodynamic therapist had little choice but to delve into the individual's "original psychological sin," believing that derivative problems would continue in one form or another until the etiological conflicts were made available for interpretation, appropriate abreaction permitted, and the nature of the conflict rendered conscious and understood. That such treatment often lasted many years was seen as a consequence of the "depth" of the problem and the cleverness of the unconscious in defending its drive-derivative, defensive formations.

"WHEREVER YOU GO, THERE YOU ARE"—YOGI BERRA

In the beginning of the New Age, the 1960s and 1970s, an escalating number of therapists began to search for etiological causes of mental disorders that were not necessarily based on psychoanalytic and psychodynamic models. These New Age therapists began to construct theories of behavior based on assumptions flowing from their idiosyncratic models. New Age therapies have been based on beliefs and assumptions that are imposed on the client as if an individual's problems derive from a single cause and can be cured by a single methodology (Singer & Lalich, 1996).

In general, their proponents promulgate New Age therapies without critical evaluation of their therapeutic methodologies by the scientific community. New Age therapy belief systems are imposed on clients as if the assumptions associated with their belief systems were accepted and agreed-upon single pathways to psychological cures. Some of the more common assumptions in typical New Age therapies fall within the following major themes:

1. Extraterrestrials exist and are abducting and experimenting on humans on a regular basis, and there is a government conspiracy to cover up this information.
2. All humans have lived one or more past lives, aspects of which interfere with our current life. A subtheme is that various "entities" (human and nonhuman)—spirit beings from "the other side"—reside within individuals and are the cause of difficulties in a person's life today.
3. Trauma and abuse experienced in early childhood is the root cause of all psychological and emotional problems. This includes having been subjected to incest and other forms of sexual abuse, having been raised by incompetent and "toxic" parents, and even having suffered through the trauma of birth itself. A subtheme is that childhood sexual abuse, including participation in intergenerational satanic ritual cults, is rampant.
4. It is possible to regress people to their moment of birth, then "rebirth" them and bring them up correctly.
5. Emptying out the emotion attached to past and present experiences will cure people. The idea is that catharsis brings cure, and especially that screaming out in anger or pain brings curative release, sort of like a purgative for the mind.
6. Reliving traumatic experiences will cure people. The idea is to revivify and relive the remembrance, whether real or imagined.
7. It is acceptable for therapists and patients to have sexual relations, as it makes patients feel better and is not harmful to them.
8. There is a human mental mechanism that prevents people who have suffered abuse and trauma from remembering this aspect of their lives, and certain techniques can help people to retrieve these blocked memories. As visions of specific events come forth in more detail, they become like a motion picture of the past abuse and are to be accepted as valid memories.

9. The world is full of certain magical powers. These powers can reside in spirit guides and angels, symbols, and archetypes, inanimate objects such as crystals and wands, and potions and herbal treatments. Special, gifted individuals can also have magical powers (Singer & Lalich, 1996).

The justification for each New Age therapy came to be based on the etiological model each espoused. As with psychoanalytic or psychodynamic therapies, the goal of New Age Therapies became to overcome etiology to free the individual from original psychological sin. The New Age therapists believed that a rehabilitative and/or restorative approach merely skimmed the surface of a deep pool of cultural, political, spiritual, and/or religious impediments to personal fulfillment. Therefore, New Age therapists placed only secondary or tertiary importance on fixing, repairing, or restoring clients to prior levels of functioning and responsible behavior (Singer, 1997).

One of the streams of thought feeding the infusion of New Age concepts into the general culture was the human potential movement, which gained cultural significance in the 1980s. Human potential movement practitioners, along with many mental health providers, characterized the individual's problems as caused by contemporary society, a society that made victims of individuals. The externalization of individual problems mirrored the depth of internalization in psychoanalytic reasoning. Blaming society for individual problems was adopted as a means of shifting responsibility to an objectified force outside the individual, by adopting a theme that "as long as we could find someone to blame, we could then change" (Singer & Lalich, 1996, pp. 201–202). As to the more immediate concerns raised by the rehabilitative/restorative approach, New Age therapies moved from rehabilitation to offering to make clients into a "reborn," "energized," "personally motivated," and "directed" human—"a new you" impervious to the external forces that were being blamed—whether those forces were parents, space aliens, entities, or whatever the therapist believed in.

Because of their reliance on idiosyncratic belief systems, the New Age therapies stand in contrast to most traditional psychotherapies, in which therapists have avoided inculcating new and untested theories of behavior into the belief systems of their patients. As an answer to the ills perpetrated by external powers (e.g., society, parents) the New Age therapies hold out the promise of re-creating the client as a whole new self, with totally new experiences. External powers had so corrupted the unconscious, the soul, the spirit, and/or the intellect that rehabilitation no longer was effective.

The New Age therapies teach individuals to overcome their problems by adopting and developing a belief in new cosmologies and belief systems. In so doing, therapists tend to create intense dependency in their clients.

Within this context, induced dependency often leads to (1) domination and control by therapists and (2) very long relationships between client and therapist (Singer & Lalich, 1996).

Examples of the new belief systems being taught patients include the belief that:

1. Space aliens have molested them.
2. They have lived many past lives and residuals from those past lives intrude into current life.
3. They need to be "rebirthed," or "reparented," so that therapy is a process wherein the client is "brought up right" by the therapist.
4. They have been invaded by evil "entities" that must be exorcised.
5. Spiritual entities from the client's present-day life or the client's spirit from a "past life" are available for communication through "channelers"/therapists. Channelers are the modern version of mediums. They supposedly contact spirits that live in a dimension other than the world we know or who exist in a world between life and death. The "channelers" contact these beings and allegedly transmit messages from presumed spiritual-world sources (Singer & Lalich, 1996).
6. They have been victims of satanic ritual abuse, having been molested by their parents, who were members of satanic cults. They are taught that they, too, were in the satanic group and participated in killing and eating babies.
7. As a result of the abuse associated with the preceding belief systems, such as satanic cults, patients have developed multiple personalities (see also Chapter 5). Therefore, the therapist must repeatedly delve into the patient's deepest core to discover more and more of the multiples created by the abuse (Acocella, 1999; de Rivera & Sarbin, 1988; Loftus & Ketcham, 1994; Ofshe & Singer, 1994; Ofshe & Waters, 1993a; Pendergrast, 1996; Piper, 1994, 1997; Spanos, 1996; Watters & Ofshe, 1999)

THE APPEAL OF NEW AGE THERAPIES

In general, individuals seek out New Age therapists for the same reasons that individuals seek out traditional therapists. The factors that bring individuals to any therapist create a psychological vulnerability that may be of short or long duration. Psychological vulnerability is characteristic of a period in anyone's life when specific personal and situational factors combine to create symptomatology. Vulnerability is increased when an individual is elderly or aged, very young, brain damaged, ill, drugged, drunk or alcoholic, frightened, stressed, fatigued, exhausted, rushed, distracted, dependent, lonely, unsophisticated, uncertain, indifferent, or uninformed. Vulnerability may be heightened when the individual is alone and without a meaningful social support system; is depressed or has other psychological disorders; is under increased levels of stress or fatigue; has undergone dramatic changes in lifestyle, such as after the end of an important relationship or the death of a family member; and has reached a point of feeling "helpless and hopeless." A common element underlying many if not all of these situations is that vulnerability is increased when a person's central self-concept is destabilized. As Ofshe and Singer (1986) used the term, the central self-concept encompasses "reality awareness, emotional control, and basic consciousness [that] are at the core of the self" (p. 4). Such vulnerability is often a precursor to seeking the "one cause–one cure" methods of New Age Therapies.

Tens of thousands of members of the general public find the "pitch" of New Age therapies appealing. This appeal may be based on a variety of foundational issues derived from (1) the manner in which contact is first made, (2) the nature of the activities required by the group, (3) the psychological state of the client, and (4) the degree to which that person believes he or she is in a critical moment of life. The appeal of many New Age therapies is that their structural methodologies and etiologically based ideologies provide point-by-point counters to problems critics and supporters have acknowledged as inherent in traditional psychotherapies. By seeming to offer point-by-point countermethods and externalizing etiological blame, the New Age therapies have gained in popularity and developed loyal adherents. The New Age Therapies, as contrasted with most traditional psychotherapies, find their appeal in providing various combinations of all or some of the following: (1) inclusion, (2) transformation, (3) purification, and (4) justification of decisions.

Inclusion versus Exclusion

In traditional therapy, a client "steps out of his or her everyday world" to seek help and guidance from a professional with whom the client has had no previous social or personal relationship. For many, this structural element of therapy takes on a psychological meaning that mirrors their internal problems. Phenomenologically, some clients experience the structural necessities of therapy as a tacit admission that their psychological problems have left them excluded from others. Therapy is seen as a means to overcome their feelings of exclusion. At another level, the structure of the therapeutic relationship, which tends to exclude external interdependencies, emphasizes the disparity of knowledge and experience of the therapist. The structure of the therapeutic relationship thereby enhances a sense of dependence of the client on the therapist.

In contrast, New Age therapies generally offer the client ready-made means of inclusion. Inclusion refers to an emphasis on breaking down the barriers that keep a person from being "included in" whatever social process, experience, identity group, or "epiphany" that is designated as the ideal. Often the process of the New Age therapy involves the individual being gradually submerged in programmed in-group experiences. There is an emphasis in these large group settings on joining the perceived group process—whether it be a group meditation, often done with the induction of hypnotic states; a group awareness training exercise, in which new behavior and identity are molded from the group exercises; or group spiritual experience, in which individuating characteristics are shucked off, as with old clothes, in favor of a spiritualism based on group emotional states that promote a sense of spiritual, religious, or psychological identity connected to the group ethos. The individual is kept unaware that many in the group are already experienced members who focus the group in the direction of the desired response. There is an appeal to experience inclusion by immersion in groupwide emotional or behavioral prescribed response sets. For example, many New Age therapies hold out the promise that the means of overcoming individual problems is through merging clients' identity with that of the group In many New Age therapies, the structure of the client experience is manipulated to produce feelings of well-being based on inclusion and reinforcement of sanctioned behavior. In some large group awareness training programs, lectures and exercises are arranged so that behavior advancing the "one cause–one solution" ethos of the group is first demonstrated by "shills" planted in the large group and reinforced in individual members by general group approval. Approved thinking and behavior are molded by the group leader, with reinforcement by the group, for the purpose of attaining inclusion within the group and being considered as acting in concert with the group's ethos.

A large percentage of clients become involved with a group without being told the true nature of the experience. Often the client is suffering from either psychological distress, such as mild to moderate depression, or involved in a transitional life circumstance, such as seeking changes in employment or career choices, when he or she chooses to consult a psychotherapist. Many believe they were not adequately informed that they entered into a form of nontraditional psychotherapy. Most New Age therapists do not inform clients that the therapy techniques are experimental and have not been scientifically validated. Frequently, clients who choose a New Age therapist have little understanding of the theoretical underpinnings of the therapist's methods prior to therapy. Clients in emotional distress tend to be naïve and uninformed regarding the nature of the therapeutic process and the multiple types of therapy available. Soon after entering into a therapeutic relationship, they feel that they must rely on a therapist's judgment concerning the proper procedures by which to conduct the "healing process." Inevitably, many clients feel "trapped" into specific procedures and techniques without adequate forewarning and without informed consent. Later, they often report that had they been adequately informed regarding the techniques and methodologies used, they would have withheld their consent.

Transformation

Many New Age therapies promise that client problems will be solved through transformation. The pitch is that by immersion into the New Age therapy's programmed set of experiences, problems will be overcome. Transformation often relies on simplistic techniques derived solely from the New Age therapy's basic assumptions. Implicit in these assumptions is that the treatment technique does all the "hard work" of bringing to the fore hidden experiences and/or feelings and that change occurs "naturally" as a result of the technique. Transformation is a product of a New Age therapy technique requiring only the client's compliance.

- *Example 1.* In the treatment technique associated with "rebirthing," the therapist urges the client to acknowledge that the client's family exerted a substantial adverse influence and that the client's mother was cold and unloving. Next, the therapist regresses the client to late gestation, and holds the client while the client is "reborn" in the arms of the therapist. The client puts on a diaper and drinks from a baby bottle that remains constantly in the client's possession. At the end of "rebirthing," the client expects to be better, if not cured.
- *Example 2.* In "past lives" therapy, a client is asked to relax and permit the therapist to induce hypnotic trance states. While in a trance state the client is "guided" to visualize a past life, complete with descriptions of time, setting, and actions. While in this state, the client is guided to finding the significant, traumatic event that took place during this other lifetime. After being brought back to the present, the client is expected to gain insight concerning how the trauma of a past life continues to influence and control present-day events.
- *Example 3.* In many large group awareness training programs, participants are instructed to return to the traumatic, real-life event that is the source of present-day troubles. The client is instructed to reexperience the traumatic event in as much emotional depth as possible. At the same time, the client is instructed to express every primitive idea, emotion, and/or impulse that emerges. The expectation is that reliving and releasing such trauma will make the individual spontaneous and free.

Purification

The desired state, signifying completion of the New Age therapy, is purification. The "taint" of whatever troubling forces controlled the client is removed during transformation. One hidden assumption is that the source of psychological problems is not internalized conflict, but rather an external force that has tainted the native purity of the individual. New Age therapies aim at removing this taint. Other individuals in large group awareness training, such as the leader or the therapist/spiritual guide/religious leader, are models of purification. Stages of purification are attained as the client models more and more appropriate behavior following the implicit directives of each technique.

Justification of Decisions

Many New Age therapies propel clients through a steady path of decision making. Yet the nature of the decisions being confronted and the options available are often dictated by the etiological assumptions at the heart of the New Age therapy belief system. Decision making occurs at two overlapping levels. The first set of decisions focuses on acceptance of the assumptions and beliefs associated with a particular brand of New Age therapy. Thus, in past lives therapy, one must decide that one has had a past life, that hypnotic regression is a viable means of experiencing that past life, that one had a specific identity in a past life, that one's past life trauma was significant, and that the past-life trauma continues to carry some disturbing valence for the present because one is inhabited by the spirits of these past lives.

The second set of decisions focuses on applying the same beliefs and assumptions to one's life. If a client is induced into accepting the assumptions of a given system, the next step is applying these etiological principles to everyday life. Therefore, if repeated hypnotic regression produces first-time "memories" of repeated abuse by parents or by a ring of satanists, to effect a cure the client must decide to treat his or her parent or relatives as abusers. Transformation and purification are based on implementing decisions to treat the world as consistent with New Age therapy etiological assumptions. Justification for decisions to implement etiological belief derives from the particular New Age therapy's techniques for reinforcing approved behavior. The tendency is for the locus of control for decisions to shift from internalized processes to externalized justification modeled and promoted by the New Age therapist.

ISSUES OF ACCOUNTABILITY AND QUALITY IN THE NEW AGE THERAPIES

Participation in traditional and New Age therapies is widespread. It is estimated that there are presently more than 250,000 accredited therapists in the United States presently. Moreover, approximately one in three Americans has visited a therapist at some point. In California alone, there are approximately 50,000 licensed psychologists, licensed clinical social workers, and licensed Marriage Family and Child Counselors. Individuals with training ranging from high school dropouts to doctoral degrees are offering the public a vast array of putative treatments for worry, misery, and psychological conditions based on 500 recognized psychotherapies. From the 1960s to the present, a plethora of psychotechnology gurus of the New Age arose.

Ethical and Legal Accountability

Psychotherapies began within academic psychology settings as procedures based on scientific knowledge, with a claim that their methods and findings be judged by the same standards by which any science is to be judged (Campbell, 1992, 1994; Crews, 1995,1998; Dawes, 1994). Because psychotherapy is a behavioral science, with an academic pedigree, the public expects it to be held to ethical and professional standards in keeping with its history and with the state governments' regulation of professional health care practitioners. Many New Age therapists have protested that because their brand of New Age therapy grew from different origins, such as spiritual, religious, or "other-worldly wisdom," New Age therapies should be judged by different standards, namely, those based on their own belief systems. These protests have generally failed. The law maintains a firm foundation for its jurisdiction based on the principle that when an individual or group holds itself out as providing services that affect the health or safety of the individual, the state government or the courts are a proper place to determine issues of accountability and quality of services provided. Therefore, the specific claims for effective care made by many of the New Age therapies have been tested in courtrooms.

Reviews of the efficacy of New Age therapies by scientific and professional organizations have been largely absent. Although each mental health discipline has developed ethical guidelines for its profession, these ethical guidelines do not carry sufficient regulatory power to monitor the quality of psychotherapy available to the public. The ability of various psychotherapy disciplines to police themselves has generally proven ineffective in maintaining a check on the quality of psychotherapy provided by therapists. The triers of fact, whether state court judge or civil jury, have moved into the position of judging the validity of therapeutic methodology. The civil litigation process, through trial or negotiated settlement, has become the unofficial arbitrator of accountability.

The means of regulating and policing therapy professionals is found in two separate but parallel legal jurisdictions. The first is the governmental authority held by state regulatory agencies that grant or rescind professional licenses under the state's duty to protect the health and safety of its citizens. Therapists whose conduct is judged either below standard or directly harmful to the public have their licenses revoked or suspended, or are actively monitored.

The second means of regulating the therapy professional is found in the power given by the legislature through statutes that grant the individual the right to seek compensation for the damages suffered as a result of a therapist's substandard or unethical conduct. The court system in general and the specific case law that has accumulated provide a measure of what the average citizen judges to be harmful professional conduct.

Civil lawsuits have consistently been used to determine whether a therapist has met the standards of professional practice. Thus, there are provisions within the statutes of every state authorizing individual lawsuits for tortious misconduct by all mental health professionals. Therapists have been sued on a wide range of legal grounds (Bloch, Chodoff, & Green, 1999; Chodoff, 1999; Conte & Karasu, 1990; McHugh, 1994; Slovenko, 1999). Misconduct has included: (1) therapists having sexual relations with clients (Bloom, Nadelson, & Notman, 1999; Hyams, 1992; McHugh, 1992; Simon, 1999), (2) misappropriation of client funds, (3) fraudulent misrepresentation of methods or qualifications (Slovenko, 1999), (4) failure to provide necessary treatment (Klerman, 1990; Stone, 1990), (5) failure to provide proper medication or the provision of improper medication (Klerman, 1990; Stone, 1990), (6) failure to warn a third party when a client makes a direct threat of harm to a specific target (Felthous, 1999; Slovenko, 1999), (7) using the therapeutic relationship to exploit the client for the therapist's personal gain (Conte & Karasu, 1990; Crews, 1995, 1998; Slovenko, 1999), (8) failure to obtain informed consent for a therapeutic intervention, such as medication or electroconvulsive therapy (ECT) (Walker-Singleton, 1999), (9) breaches of confidentiality (Walker-Singleton, 1999), and (10) failure to provide treatment (Klerman, 1990).

In addition, many state legislatures have established a statutory basis for licensure review by establishing an oversight agency controlling licensing of individual practitioners or institutions. Criminal indictment has also been used in some situations, such as assault charges, for the unwanted touching that accompanies sexual contact between therapists and client, or criminal fraud based on the misappropriation of client funds (Borruso, 1991). In a typical civil lawsuit, the trier of fact determines whether a therapist has "injured" the client through the use of questionable therapeutic methods or unethical practices while acting in the role of a professional. Civil injuries may be physical, emotional, or financial. The trier of fact then determines whether the questionable methods have injured the client and whether those injuries should be recompensed.

Traditional and New Age therapists are subject to the same liabilities within the civil litigation system. Misuse of the therapeutic relationship, for example, through the therapist having a sexual relationship, and misuse of psychotherapeutic methods can occur in both traditional and New

Age therapies. The use of questionable methodologies is a charge that the New Age therapies are particularly vulnerable to having upheld in court.

New Age Therapists Should Be Judged by Standards That Apply to Fiduciaries

Under the laws of most states, both licensed and unlicensed clinicians who hold themselves out to the general public as performing the functions of a therapist establish a relationship with their clients based on trust, confidence, and confidentiality. In the law, when a relationship occurs between individuals, based on trust and confidence, and one individual has greater knowledge, experience, training, and skill, than the other, then that relationship is generally considered in the eyes of the law to be a fiduciary relationship. In many states, therapists are considered fiduciaries. Because of their disproportionate knowledge, training, and experience, fiduciaries are held to a higher standard of care and responsibility for (1) the services provided to a client and (2) the appropriateness of the services to aid the client in overcoming problems.

We propose that all therapeutic relationships be considered fiduciary relationships and that the standard of care against which a therapist is judged be the standard applied to fiduciaries. That same standard should be applied to the New Age or traditional therapist regardless of espoused ideology.

Relative or Professionwide Standards of Accountability

In civil litigation, when a charge of professional malpractice is made, the professional is judged against the accepted standards of practice for that profession within the local community of professionals. When their methodology or practice is questioned, New Age therapists often maintain that they should only be judged by the standards of their New Age discipline. To do otherwise, they argue, would mean that they would be judged by traditional psychotherapy standards, which the New Age practitioners have typically shunned. New Age therapists often espouse a belief that traditional psychotherapy is (1) bankrupt of contemporary meaning, (2) based on an elitist view of human suffering, and/or (3) part of the external, social forces that have harmed the individual. Therefore, they believe that the only community capable of adequately judging their practice methods is their own.

Nevertheless case law has been clear that "community" cannot be so narrowly interpreted as to refer only to the individual's immediate peer group. Rather, the "standards of the community" yardstick represents a critical view of the professional and ethical standards of therapy drawn from

1. ethical principles of conduct and practice promoted by local and national professional organizations, such as the American Psychological Association, the American Psychiatric Association, and the American Medical Association (Bloch & Pargiter, 1999);
2. state licensing agencies' rules of conduct, whether adopted by vote of the governing administrative body or by direct legislation in the form of state and local statutes (Bloomberg, 2000; Hyams, 1992; Walker-Singleton, 1999); and
3. the rules of local professional associations, such as a state or county professional organization.

Established rules of professional conduct derived from these three sources have been admitted as evidence of "professional community standards" against which the conduct of New Age therapists can be judged. To do otherwise would produce ethical standards based on cultural trends, narrowly defined subpopulations, and exceptions.

Externalization of Accountability

Another argument frequently advanced by New Age therapists is that they are merely "counselors" who have been sought out by potential clients for advice. Thus, the therapist's services were obtained as a result of the client's free choice, and the client made that choice of methodology based on his or her needs and beliefs. Therefore, the argument goes, the therapist's conduct should be measured solely on the basis of the client's choices. By labeling themselves as "counselors," New Age therapists adopt the strategy of placing the counselor on the same plane of responsibility as the client or completely outside the circle of responsibility, in the role of a neutral advisor. Such an argument shifts the responsibility for choice of methodology from therapist to client.

Again, this argument would fail to remove the burden of professional responsibility from the New Age therapist under the professional standards discussed previously. First, as a fiduciary, the responsibility for choosing the proper therapeutic methodology must lie with the professional. Second, state regulatory statutes and the courts have found that anyone who performs acts that are of the same character as those performed by a licensed professional must be judged by the standards applied to the licensed therapist, whether or not the "therapist" holds himself or herself out to the public as a psychotherapist. That a client sought out a therapist with a particular orientation cannot shield the therapist from being scrutinized by the same professional standards as would be used to evaluate a licensed professional. The same liabilities that a professional would face if found to have fallen below the standard of his or her profession will be those used to evaluate the work of an unlicensed therapist.

Interviews with approximately 400 persons who had entered New Age therapies (Singer & Lalich, 1996) revealed that most therapists introduced their New Age ideas after the client had entered therapy. In contrast, other New Age therapists promote their services through national advertisements. Some have asserted that their programs have very long (e.g., 3,000 persons) waiting lists of individuals who wish to engage in past lives regression or other New Age techniques.

New Age Therapies and Legal Accountability

The most dramatic attacks on the New Age therapies have stemmed from litigation. The civil court system has become the arbiter of whether New Age therapies serve valuable societal purposes or are harmful. With the lack of national standards for accountability, a jury of 12 ordinary citizens, for the most part without training in psychology or "the healing arts," decides on issues of accountability, effectiveness of care, and ethical conduct. The virtue of this arrangement is that the 12 ordinary citizens are the actual or potential consumers of health care acting as representatives of the community. The jury thereby decides the limits of permissible conduct and the extent to which a client may have been injured by the therapist or the treatment.

R. Christopher Barden, PhD, JD, President of the National Association for Consumer Protection in Mental Health Practices, has proposed solutions to providing protections for the uninformed consumer (Barden, 1999). A group of nationally known psychiatrists and psychologists signed a document in 1994 urging legislative bodies to undertake the following action:

> To reduce the possibility of future, similar psychotherapy frauds, we suggest that the following language be included in all appropriate sections of relevant health care codes: No tax or tax exempt monies may be used for any form of health care treatment, including any form of psychotherapy, that has not been proven safe and effective by rigorous, valid and reliable scientific investigations and accepted as safe and effective by a substantial majority of the relevant scientific community. (Barden, 1999)

This group has been effective in bringing attention to the lack of informed consent for experimental, unproven psychotherapies. Fifteen state legislatures have enacted laws to protect consumers from experimental mental health practices.

It is difficult to estimate the number of legal cases that have grown out of New Age therapies. Barden, who developed and authored the Truth and Responsibility in Mental Health Practices Act Model Legislation, comments that "there is no way to know how many of these suits have been filed, but everyone seems quite certain there were hundreds. Many of these suits settled quietly before they are even filed. Others have strict secrecy provision in the settlement. The real number could be in the thousands" (personal communication, 1999). We interviewed insurance company representatives, who indicated that an estimated $60–100 million annually are paid for suits against psychologists alone—settlements, judgments, and legal costs for the suits.

Television talk shows did much to publicize "recovered memory therapy" and dissociative identity disorder, known formerly as multiple personality disorder or MPD (see Chapter 5). Oprah Winfrey's program publicized MPD as "the syndrome of the 90s." In late 1995, Geraldo Rivera apologized on his program for his contributions to the RMT and satanic ritual abuse epidemics (Acocella, 1999).

LEGAL CASES RELEVANT TO NEW AGE THERAPIES

Legal cases relevant to the New Age therapies have focused on a specific set of issues.

Informed Consent Cases

In many cases, the client or group participant enters treatment with a New Age therapist without being told explicitly about the types of therapeutic techniques used and/or the beliefs and assumptions on which the therapy is based. Often, New Age therapists fail to obtain informed consent for the administration of therapeutic techniques that are by definition experimental and unproven. From a legal and ethical standpoint, the New Age therapist offering alien abduction, channeling, past lives regression, and other idiosyncratic, belief-driven treatments is moving into the arena of experimentation.

State licensing agencies have adopted positions on the issues related to the use of untested treatment methods. For example, on May 3, 1999, Renee Fredrickson, PhD, LP, had her license placed on restricted and conditional status by an Order of the Board of Psychology of the State of Minnesota (Walker-Singleton, 1999). Dr. Fredrickson had gained national attention for her work on recovered memories of abuse (Fredrickson, 1992). The Board based its order on the following grounds:

> Since 1994, . . . Licensee [Dr. Fredrickson] . . . has demonstrated a number of practice deficiencies including, but not limited to: failing to adequately inform clients of Licensee's use of innovative or newly emerging services and techniques and their related risks; providing psychological services to clients when Licensee's objectivity and effectiveness were impaired; failing

to obtain written informed consent to share private information on clients. (Walker-Singleton, 1999, p. 1)

In part, the Board held that Dr. Fredrickson, who used hypnosis in her treatment, had failed to inform her clients "that hypnosis can sometimes result in very vivid memories which are false but which are still believed" (Walker-Singleton, 1999, p. 9; see Chapter 8).

The Minnesota Board of Psychology permanently restricted Dr. Fredrickson from providing therapy to clients whose therapy involves cult, ritual, or satanic abuse. Dr. Fredrickson was also restricted from providing hypnosis or guided imagery to clients except under conditions specified by the Board.

The following cases illustrate reasonably typical examples of some of the procedures used by New Age therapists that have resulted in traumatic harm to the clients and damage awards commensurate with the trier of fact's perception of the harm caused by the therapist.

Satanic Ritual Abuse: The Case of Patricia Burgus, the "Satanic Princess"

The most widely publicized case of SRA is that of Patricia Burgus, who won a $10.6 million settlement (Acocella, 1999; Ofshe & Waters, 1993b; Pendergrast, 1996). In 1995, *Frontline,* a national TV documentary, aired a program titled "The Search for Satan." The program chronicled Ms. Burgus's treatment with Dr. Bennett Braun. She originally sought treatment for postpartum depression, but was hospitalized for 3 years by Dr. Braun in the Dissociative Disorders unit of Rush-Presbyterian Hospital in Chicago. Ms. Burgus was labeled as a "satanic princess." At Braun's suggestion, her two sons, ages 4 and 5, were also hospitalized for over 3 years. Each son was told that he was a multiple personality (see Chapter 5), that he had been in his mother's satanic cult, that he had eaten babies, and that he had felt what it was like to bite into a baby while it was still alive. As part of therapy, both sons "learned" that they were practiced killers. Ms. Burgus was led to believe that she had molested them. While in treatment with Dr. Braun, she was led to believe that she (1) had 300 personalities, (2) had been raised in a satanic cult, and (3) was a "satanic princess" in charge of a nine-state region, and (4) had eaten more than 2,000 dead bodies per year in whole or part. Dr. Braun instructed her to have her husband bring a hamburger from a family picnic to the hospital so that it could be tested for human tissue. After 3 years, when her insurance was almost exhausted, she was released from the hospital. The insurance carrier paid over $3 million in hospitalization costs for Ms. Burgus and her two sons. Acocella (1999) indicates that other patients of Dr. Braun initiated similar lawsuits based on similar grounds.

Dr. Braun is a psychiatrist who has been highly active in the recovered memory movement (see also Chapter 8). The Illinois Department of Professional Regulation (IDPR) filed a complaint against Dr. Braun and two of his colleagues, based on the case of Patricia Burgus. As a result of a settlement agreement, Dr. Braun lost his medical license for 2 years, followed by a probation period of at least 5 years (Bloomberg, 2000). At the end of the 7-year period, Dr. Braun will need to apply to the IDPR to be removed from probation.

Dissociative Identity Disorder: The Case of Elizabeth Carlson

In Minneapolis, Elizabeth Carlson sought psychiatric care for depression from Dr. Diane Humenansky. Dr. Humenansky soon suggested that Ms. Carlson suffered from dissociative identity disorder (see Chapter 5) and started her on visualization exercises to "recall" and search for episodes of being molested by people in her family (Acocella, 1999). Through the use of guided imagery, Ms. Carlson came to "see" scenes in which she joined others in eating a dead baby. Dr. Humenansky eventually "discovered" countless alters within Carlson. Later, Dr. Humenansky stated that she "lost count after twenty five" (Acocella, 1999, p. 10). Eventually 10 other former patients sued Humenansky.

Space Aliens: Myra

Myra was referred to a psychologist for relaxation training by her treating physician. The referral was to a psychologist who specialized in pain relief. During Myra's initial visits, the psychologist took virtually no history. Nevertheless, after hypnosis, the psychologist informed Myra that her back problems were a result of her having been molested by her father. The psychologist further informed Myra that she mentioned visiting her favorite uncle while she was hypnotized. The psychologist shifted to saying that her uncle had molested her. While in a normal waking state, Myra had no memories of abuse, either by her father or her uncle and took issue with the therapist's claims of such abuse. At her next session, the therapist indicated that, during another hypnotically induced state, Myra had remembered being abducted by a UFO while at her uncle's home. The UFO descended into her uncle's backyard and had taken her onboard a spacecraft that looked like the white "inside of an eggshell." There, she was reported to have been sexually examined by aliens. This examination and subsequent examinations, performed while she was lying on an table, were the cause of her back problems. The psychologist hypnotized Myra in each of her sessions, maintaining that hypnosis was necessary with clients abducted by space aliens because the aliens hypnotized humans to force them to forget their alien encounters. Over the

next 3 years, the psychotherapist focused on uncovering all of Myra's alleged encounters with aliens. Myra felt that the therapist only seemed interested when she cooperated by producing information concerning these
purported encounters. She reported that she began "to feel foggy, tired
all the time, and out of touch with my feelings about anything." The
psychologist significantly enlarged the boundaries of the therapy, eventually seeing her in 3–4 hour sessions held 3 days a week. The psychologist
also forbade her from taking medications prescribed by her physician because the medications would interfere with her "recalling all the experiences on the UFOs which were central to the therapy." When Myra's
savings were depleted, she was forced to terminate therapy. After she reflected on what had occurred in her therapy, she sought out legal counsel. After a lawsuit was filed, the therapist settled out of court.

Multiple New Age Therapies: Ellen

Ellen entered therapy because she became mildly depressed over a relationship that had ended abruptly. Ellen believed that therapy would be of help
to relieve her depression and to learn more about relationships. She had
had a series of relationships with men that ended unsatisfactorily, each
time leaving her more depressed.

   During an interview with one of the authors (MTS), Ellen disclosed
that at her first therapy session, Ellen's therapist had her lie down in a re-
cliner and covered her with a blanket. The therapist softly played music in
the background and asked her to "drift with the music." After 10 years of
therapy, Ellen had (1) "discovered" that she repressed memories of her father and other family members abusing her during satanic rituals; (2) filed
suit against her father and severed all ties with her family; (3) uncovered
that she was a multiple personality with 159 alters; (4) been purportedly
held captive by extraterrestrials; and (5) become convinced that she had
been invaded by other-worldly "entities." Finally, two of Ellen's women
friends shared with her their observations regarding her therapy, telling her
that the course of her therapy had followed the "therapy fads" they had
seen on television talk shows, progressing from repressed memories, to
satanic ritual abuse, to extraterrestrial molestation, to being invaded by
"entities," to having multiple personalities. Her friends also told her that
her therapist had kept her "in bondage" and controlled her by persuading
her of each succeeding, newly discovered revelation. Ellen disclosed transcripts of her therapy session to her friends. Her therapist audiotaped each
session and often asked Ellen to transcribe the session, informing Ellen that
the material was intended for a book that the two would cowrite. After reviewing the transcripts, the friends understood the methods Ellen's therapist used to influence Ellen's thoughts. The following is a reconstruction of
a conversation between Ellen and her therapist, based on Ellen's explanation
to one author (MTS). It is not a direct quotation from these transcripts.

THERAPIST: Stay relaxed; just report whatever comes to mind. Trust your mind. Trust the pictures you see. See yourself out in a backyard. Look up at the sky. Do you see a light?

ELLEN: Yes.

THERAPIST: Tell me more about it.

ELLEN: It is a star, just a star in the sky.

THERAPIST: Is it coming closer? Can you move or not?

ELLEN: (*crying*) I can't move. It is coming close, it is getting brighter and close. I don't know. I can't move, I don't know.

THERAPIST: You are going to let yourself remember.

ELLEN: (*crying*)

THERAPIST: What do you see? Who is there? Are you lying down?

ELLEN: They said I should relax.

THERAPIST: Do you hear their voices or are they communicating directly into your mind?

ELLEN: It is in my mind, I don't hear words.

THERAPIST: What are they telling you that they are going to do to you?

ELLEN: That they are going to implant an electronic disc in the sole of my foot. (*crying, screaming*) I don't know, I don't know.

THERAPIST: You want to remember don't you? You came here to remember. You've remembered so much already. Just look around and describe for me what you see.

Eventually Ellen described the soft touch of a group of small gray personages with large black eyes together with her in a white, clean room. As she described the scene, the therapist interspersed such comments as "You are going to experience it as you did at the time. You are going to remember again all that happened."

As she recognized what had transpired through her decade of therapy, Ellen contacted other clients of her therapist who had left treatment prior to Ellen's realizations. A number of former clients filed lawsuits against the therapist. Each former client received a large settlement from the therapist and her insurance company.

When interviewed by one of the authors (MTS), Ellen stated:

"Therapy was never going to end. She [the therapist] kept finding more and more things wrong with me that I had to work on, she called it 'deep work.' I have not felt good about myself in 10 years. Now that I look back on the therapy I can't thank my friends enough for telling me their observations—I would have dragged on and on believing that I had had even worse things hidden in my mind from my past that I still had to 'dig deeper' and remember. . . . I really had no one but the therapist to talk with. She had forbidden me to reveal what went on in therapy saying it would 'dilute the impact' of our 'deep work.' "

Recent Professional Actions

Lilienfeld and Lohr (2000) wrote that many research-oriented psychologists "contend that the increasing proliferation of unvalidated treatment poses a serious threat to clients and to the scientific status of clinical psychology." They reported on two recent sanctions placed on the use of thought field therapy (TFT) the first by the Arizona Board of Psychology Examiners and the second by the American Psychology Association (APA) Continuing Education Committee.

TFT was invented in the early 1980s by Roger Callahan (see Chapter 9). It was touted as "The Five Minute Phobia Cure." TFT consists of clients imagining an anxiety-provoking event; tapping body parts in a predetermined order under the therapist's direction; moving their eyes in specific directions; counting to five; humming snatches of a tune; and again tapping body parts in a specified order. Another TFT technique is called "voice technology." In this method, an electronic device converts a client's voice into a visual display. Voice technology is claimed by TFT proponents to allow a therapist to diagnose "the client's energy blocks over the telephone and then prescribe a formal course of TFT treatment without ever having to meet the client in person."

The Arizona Board of Psychology Examiners placed a TFT therapist on probation, ordering him to refrain from administering TFT within the practice of psychology and informed the therapist that he would be monitored to determine whether he refrained from using this method. Among the prime reasons for the ruling was "the therapist's inability to substantiate his advertised claims of effectiveness." In addition, The APA Continuing Education Committee ruled that "the absence of any compelling scientific support for its efficacy rendered TFT an inappropriate subject for continuing education." Lilienfeld and Lohr (2000) noted that "these two recent actions herald a shift away from a laissez-faire approach to psychotherapeutic practice and toward heightened clinician accountability" (p. 5).

Psychotherapy Gone Awry

The preceding cases provide examples of "psychotherapy gone awry" (McHugh, 1994). McHugh (1992) described the "misadventures" that occur when therapists follow the lead of cultural fashions into false, even disastrous directions, as in the case of Ellen.

I have become familiar with how these fashions and their consequences caused psychiatry to lose its moorings. Roughly every ten years, from the mid-1960s on, psychiatric practice condoned some bizarre misdirections, proving how all too often the discipline has been the captive of culture. Each misdirection was the consequence of one of the three common medical mistakes—oversimplification, misplaced emphasis, or pure invention. (p. 498)

CONCLUSIONS

Psychotherapy, from its earliest inception, was intended as a method to assist persons to function capably in the world, act responsibly as citizens, and participate fully in life's opportunities. We have described recent therapeutic fads, foibles, and fashions that work against the potential for psychotherapy to serve these purposes. Approaches designated as New Age therapy have permitted therapists to unjustly (1) impose the therapist's will on the client, with the benefits of therapy aggrandizing the therapists instead of aiding the client; (2) induce the client into a prolonged and unnecessary dependence on the therapist; and (3) violate the fiduciary role of the therapist. Many New Age therapies run counter to psychotherapy's potential by actions that

1. misuse and abuse legitimate adjunctive procedures, such as hypnosis;
2. introduce methodologies that are idiosyncratic, untested, and not accepted by the community of professional therapists;
3. impose a distorted and unfounded belief in how human memory functions (see Chapter 8);
4. impose a therapist's "pet theory" of what lies behind human distress, based on the therapist's own momentary enthusiasm for a passing fashion;
5. avoid or disavow current scientific evidence that contradicts idiosyncratic beliefs, such as the inherent unreliability of memories recalled under hypnosis (which serve as the validation for the existence of extraterrestrials, conspiratorial satanic organizations, corporeal invasion by spiritual entities, and millennial histories of past lives); and
6. misuse or disavow scientific evidence of memories as a reconstructive process (see Chapter 8), instead clinging to an outdated belief that memory is an eidetic reservoir of perfectly preserved memories, which can be brought forth through the use of trance induction, guided fantasies, and/or direct suggestion.

The language of psychotherapy should be recast to eliminate jargon that obscures the fact that certain interpretations or interventions are based on idiosyncratic myth or "a therapist's pet theory." If diagnoses are made and serve as the basis of a treatment plan, they should comport with the diagnostic criteria accepted within the professional mental health community rather than appealing to speculative proposals of partisan groups.

Clients have the right to know in advance that they are being subjected to experimental approaches. Therapists have the fiduciary obligation of informing clients when such methods are used. Therapists have the further responsibility of informing the clients that alternative therapeutic approaches are available and that these approaches are based on methods commonly accepted within the professional psychological community. In another publication, one author of this chapter (MTS) has described general patterns found in therapists who have been inadequately trained or who may be "impaired professionals" (Singer & Lalich, 1996). As fiduciaries, therapists must ensure that psychotherapy furthers the aims and purposes of clients, rather than adding to the prestige, self-image, or feelings of power and control of the therapist. Finally, clients must be educated about whether a treatment methodology is based on accepted scientific research or the personal beliefs of the therapist.

GLOSSARY

Accountability: Therapists can be held accountable within a contractual relationship for incompetent and unacceptable behavior. First, they will be judged by the degree to which therapy is effective in ameliorating the client's presenting problem, that is, the degree to which a therapist provides quality care. Second, they will be judged by the degree to which the therapist's professional conduct is ethical and comports with professional standards. The law maintains that when individuals hold themselves out as providing services that affect the health or safety of the individual, the state government has the power to legislate rules of conduct, and the courts are the place to determine issues of accountability.

Etiology: The science or theory of causes. Etiology addresses the following question: What are the origins of this problem?

Fiduciary: In law, a specific type of relationship, often defined by statute or case law. In many states, a fiduciary relationship is characterized as (1) being between individuals, with one of the individuals having greater education, training, experience and knowledge than the other; (2) based on the less knowledgeable individual placing his or her trust and confidence in the more knowledgeable individual; (3) an agreement that the more knowledgeable individual will provide services or act on behalf of the less knowledgeable individual; and (4) based on the less knowledgeable person relying on the more knowledgeable person to provide either the needed services or to act on the other's behalf. Common fiduciary relationships are those between attorney and client, doctor and patient, and accountant and client.

Human potential movement: A group of diverse "therapies" with a common theme that treating individuals should move clients beyond restoration and rehabilitation to making the person into a "new me," for example, to be "reborn" or to move into a new era of personal or human development.

Inculcation, influence, indoctrination: May occur in a relationship when a person with more power uses his or her role, power, and/or knowledge to influence and persuade others to accept a set of ideas and/or belief system(s).

Rehabilitative/restorative therapy: A psychotherapy methodology emphasizing returning the client to functioning at his or her former level of competence. Emphasis is placed on acquiring skills to function in society as a responsible person and to make one's own choices and perform ethically in society.

Transformation: The belief held by certain therapists that therapy will "transform" the person into a new, changed individual (the "new me") with compliance but with little effort.

REFERENCES

Acocella, J. (1999). *Creating hysteria*. San Francisco: Jossey-Bass.

Barden, R. C. (1999, May 8). *Law, science and mental health: Protecting liberty and reforming the mental Health System*. Paper presented at the British False Memory Society, London. (Original work presented at the False Memory Syndrome Foundation/Johns Hopkins Medical School meeting, Baltimore, March 23, 1997)

Bloch, S., Chodoff, P., & Green, S. A. (Eds.). (1999). *Psychiatric ethics* (3rd ed.). Oxford: Oxford University Press.

Bloch, S., & Pargiter, R. (1999). Codes of ethics in psychiatry. In S. Bloch, P. Chodoff, & S. A. Green (Eds.), *Psychiatric ethics* (3rd ed., pp. 81–104). Oxford: Oxford University Press.

Bloom, J. D., Nadelson, C. C., & Notman, M. T. (Eds.). (1999). *Physician sexual misconduct*. Washington, DC: American Psychiatric Press.

Bloomberg, D. (2000). Bennett Braun case settled; Two-year loss of license, five years probation. *Skeptical Inquirer, 1*, 7–8.

Borruso, M. T. (1991). Note: Sexual abuse by psychotherapists: The call for a uniform criminal statute. *American Journal of Law and Medicine, 17*(3), 289–311.

Boylan, R. J., & Boylan, L. K. (1994). *Close extraterrestrial encounters: Positive experiences with mysterious visitors.* Tigard, OR: Wild Flower Press.

Campbell, T. W. (1992). Therapeutic relationships and iatrogenic outcomes: The blame and change maneuver in psychotherapy. *Psychotherapy, 29,* 474–480.

Campbell, T. W. (1994). *Beware the talking cure: Psychotherapy may be hazardous to your mental health.* Boca Raton, FL: Upton Books.

Chodoff, P. (1999). Misuse and abuse of psychiatry: An overview. In S. Bloch, P. Chodoff, & S. A. Green (Eds.), *Psychiatric ethics* (3rd ed., pp. 49–66). Oxford: Oxford University Press.

Conte, H. R., & Karasu, T. B. (1990). Malpractice in psychotherapy: An overview. *American Journal of Psychotherapy, 44*(1), 232–246.

Crews, F. C. (1995). The memory wars: Freud's legacy in dispute. New York: New York Review of Books.

Crews, F. C. (1998). *Unauthorized Freud.* New York: Viking Books.

Dawes, R. M. (1994). *House of cards: Psychology and psychotherapy built on myth.* New York: Free Press.

de Rivera, J., & Sarbin, T. R. (1988). *Believed-in imaginings: The narrative construction of reality.* Washington, DC: American Psychological Association.

Felthous, A. R. (1999). The clinician's duty to protect third parties. *Psychiatric Clinics of North America, 22*(1), 49–60.

Ferguson, M. (1980). *The Aquarian conspiracy.* Los Angeles, CA: J. P. Tarcher.

Fiore, E. (1989). *A psychologist reveals case studies of abductions by extraterrestrials.* New York: Ballantine Books.

Fredrickson, R. (1992). *Repressed memories: A guide to recovery from sexual abuse.* New York: Simon & Schuster.

Goldberg, B. (1982). *Past lives, future lives.* New York: Ballantine Books.

Hoyt, K., & Yamamoto, J. I. (1987). *The New Age rage.* Old Tappen, NJ: Fleming H. Revell.

Hyams, A. L. (1992). Expert psychiatric evidence in sexual misconduct cases before state medical boards. *American Journal of Law and Medicine, 18*(3), 171–201.

Klerman, G. L. (1990). The psychiatric patient's right to effective treatment: Implications of *Osheroff v. Chestnut Lodge. American Journal of Psychiatry, 147*(4), 409–418.

Lilienfeld, S. O., & Lohr, J. M. (2000, March/April). Thought field therapy practitioners and educators sanctioned. *Skeptical Inquirer,* p. 5.

Loftus, E., & Ketcham, K. (1994). *The myth of repressed memory.* New York: St. Martin's Press.

Mack, J. E. (1994). *Abduction: Human encounters with aliens.* New York: Scribner.

MacLaine, S. (1985). *Dancing in the light.* New York: Bantam Books.

McHugh, P. R. (1992). Psychiatric misadventures. *American Scholar, 61*(4), 497–510.

McHugh, P. R. (1994). Psychotherapy awry. *American Scholar, 63*(1), 17–30.

Ofshe, R., & Singer, M. T. (1986). Attacks on peripheral versus central elements of self and the impact of thought reform techniques. *Cultic Studies Journal, 3*(1), 3–24.

Ofshe, R., & Singer, M. T. (1994). Recovered memory therapy and robust repression: Influence and pseudomemories. *International Journal of Clinical and Experimental Hypnosis, 13*(4), 391–408.

Ofshe, R., & Waters, E. (1993a). Making monsters. *Society, 30*(3), 4–16.

Ofshe, R., & Waters, E. (1993b). *Making monsters: False memories, psychotherapy and sexual hysteria.* New York: Scribner.

Pendergrast, M. (1996). *Victims of memory: Sex abuse accusations and shattered lives* (2nd ed.). Hinesburg, VT: Upper Access.

Piper, A. (1994). Multiple personality disorders and criminal responsibility: Critique of a paper by Elyn Saks. *Journal of Psychiatry and Law, 22,* 7–49.

Piper, A. (1997). *Hoax and reality: The bizarre world of multiple personality disorder.* Northvale, NJ: Aronson.

Relman, A. S. (1988). Assessment and accountability: The third revolution in medical care. *New England Journal of Medicine, 319,* 1220.

Simon, R. I. (1999). Therapist–patient sex: From boundary violations to sexual misconduct. *Psychiatric Clinics of North America, 22*(1), 31–47.

Singer, M. T. (1997). From rehabilitation to etiology: Progress and pitfalls. In J. K. Zeig (Ed.), *The evolution of psychotherapy* (pp. 349–358). New York: Brunner/Mazel.

Singer, M. T., & Lalich, J. (1995). *Cults in our midst.* San Francisco: Jossey-Bass.

Singer, M. T., & Lalich, J. (1996). *Crazy therapies: What are they? Do they work?* San Francisco: Jossey-Bass.

Slovenko, R. (1999). Malpractice in psychotherapy: An overview. *Psychiatric Clinics of North America, 22*(1), 1–15.

Spanos, N. P. (1996). *Multiple identities and false memories.* Washington, DC: American Psychological Association.

Stone, A. A. (1990). Law, science, and psychiatric malpractice: A response to Klerman's indictment of psychoanalytic psychiatry. *American Journal of Psychiatry, 147*(4), 419–427.

Walker-Singleton, P. (Executive Director, Minnesota Board of Psychology). (1999). *In the matter of Renee Fredrickson, Ph.D., L.P.: Stipulation and consent order* [Stipulation and Consent Order]. Minnesota Board of Psychology.

Watters, E., & Ofshe, R. (1999). *Therapy's delusions: The myth of the unconscious and the exploitation of today's walking worried.* New York: Scribner.

Weiss, B. L. (1988). *Many lives, many masters.* New York: Fireside/Simon & Schuster.

Weiss, B. L. (1992). *Through time into healing.* New York: Simon & Schuster.

West, L. J., & Singer, M. T. (1980). Cults, quacks and the nonprofessional psychotherapies. In H. I. Kaplan, A. M. Freedman, & B. J. Saddock (Eds.), *Comprehensive textbook of psychiatry* (3rd ed., Vol. 3, pp. 3245–3258). Baltimore: Williams & Wilkins.

Wolf, S. M. (1994). Quality assessment of ethics of health care: The accountability revolution. *American Journal of Law and Medicine, 20*(1 & 2), 105–128.

8

The Remembrance of Things Past

Problematic Memory Recovery Techniques in Psychotherapy

STEVEN JAY LYNN
TIMOTHY LOCK
ELIZABETH F. LOFTUS
ELISA KRACKOW
SCOTT O. LILIENFELD

In 1997, Nadean Cool won a $2.4 million malpractice settlement against her therapist in which she alleged that he used a variety of techniques and suggestive procedures to convince her that she had suffered horrific abuse and harbored more than 130 personalities including demons, angels, children, and a duck (see also Chapter 5). According to Nadean, prior to therapy she had a few problems typical of many women, namely a history of bulimia and minor depression. She initiated therapy to deal with her feelings concerning the sexual assault of a family member. Her bulimia was reportedly under good control, and she no longer abused substances.

During 5 years of treatment in which her therapist allegedly insisted she could not improve unless she excavated traumatic past experiences, Nadean "recovered" what her therapist claimed were repressed memories of her having been in a satanic cult, of eating babies, of being raped, of having sex with animals, and of being forced to watch the murder of her 8-year-old friend. These memories surfaced after Nadean participated in repeated hypnotic age regression and guided imagery sessions, was subjected to an exorcism and 15-hour marathon therapy sessions, and charted her various supposed personalities and their dynamic interactions with one another. According to Nadean, as her therapy progressed and she became overwhelmed by frightening images of events she came to believe occurred in her past, her psychological equilibrium deteriorated apace. Eventually, Nadean began to have serious concerns about what had transpired in therapy, came to doubt that the memories she recovered were "real," terminated treatment with her therapist, and recouped much of the ground she had lost over the past 5 years.

Dramatic legal cases such as Nadean Cool's provide vivid and cautionary examples of how highly directive and coercive therapeutic approaches can shape a patient's history and sense of personal identity. Cases like Nadean's prompt two major questions. First, does the broader community of therapists use special techniques to enhance recall of traumatic events such as child abuse? Second, do these techniques do more than merely access memories but, instead, shape them and thereby instate a distorted personal history?

With respect to the first question, there is good reason to believe that the use of memory recovery techniques is not limited to rare yet highly publicized legal cases. Poole, Lindsay, Memon, and Bull (1995) surveyed 145 licensed U.S. doctoral-level psychotherapists who were randomly sampled from the National Register of Health Service Providers in Psychology in two studies, and 57 British psychologists who were sampled from the Register of Chartered Clinical Psychologists. They found that 25% of the respondents who conduct therapy with adult female patients believe that memory recovery is an important part of treatment, believe that they can identify patients with repressed or otherwise unavailable memories as early as the first session, and use two or more techniques such as hypnosis and guided imagery to facilitate the unearthing of repressed memories. Additionally, Poole and colleagues reported that over three quarters of the U.S. doctoral-level psychotherapists sampled in their study reported using at least one memory recovery technique to "help clients remember childhood sexual abuse."

The following year, Polusny and Follette (1996) conducted a survey of 1,000 psychologists who were randomly selected from Division 12 (Clinical) and Division 17 (Counseling) of the American Psychological Association. Of the sample of 223 individuals who ultimately completed the survey, 25% of therapists reported using guided imagery, dream interpretation, bibliotherapy regarding sexual abuse, and free association of childhood memories as memory retrieval techniques with clients who had no specific memories of childhood sexual abuse.

These survey findings are not particularly surprising when viewed in the light of ideas propounded by therapists (Bass & Davis, 1988; Frederickson, 1992) who accept most of what clients report as accurate, do not hold much stock in the notion that serious memory distortions arise as a function of psychotherapeutic procedures, and maintain that when clients suddenly recall memories of sexual abuse in treatment, the memories are likely to be reasonably accurate replicas of historical events. Memories of abuse that emerge in therapy are thought to spring to consciousness when trauma-related repression or dissociative barriers are lifted.

Given the apparent ubiquity of memory recovery techniques and the rationale that has been advanced for their use, it is imperative to address the second question of whether memory recovery techniques that are commonly used in therapy to recover childhood memories of abuse can distort patients' recollections of past events. In this chapter, we review research that bears on the impact of commonly used therapeutic procedures of symptom interpretation, hypnosis, and dream interpretation on memory.

CLINICAL TECHNIQUES

The term "memory work" has been used to refer to psychotherapy that focuses on retrieving "repressed" memories of childhood sexual abuse (Loftus, 1993). Many therapeutic techniques fall under this umbrella category, including hypnosis, guided imagery, journaling, age regression, and symptom interpretation. These techniques are used with two kinds of clients: those who remember abuse but wish to fill in more details, and those who suspect early childhood abuse but have no memories of maltreatment.

Some researchers have begun to question the validity of using these techniques to uncover memories of past sexual abuse as well as other memories, both traumatic and nontraumatic (e.g., Lindsay & Read, 1994; Loftus & Ketcham, 1994). These techniques are some of the same that are touted by others (e.g., Bass & Davis, 1988; Frederickson, 1992) as trustworthy tools for uncovering memories of childhood abuse. One important class of techniques that includes guided imagery, hypnosis, and age regression relies heavily on imagery and imagination to review past events.

Guided Imagery

Lindsay and Read (1994) described guided imagery as a technique whereby patients are instructed to relax, close their eyes, and imagine various scenarios described by the therapist. Survey research suggests that between 26% and 32% of U.S. psychotherapists use this technique in some capacity (Poole et al., 1995). However, guided imagery lacks a consensus definition in the field. Numerous techniques could be considered variants of guided imagery, including implosive therapy (i.e., therapist-directed fantasy imagery scenes designed to provoke anxiety; Stampfl & Levis, 1967) and prolonged exposure (i.e., client-directed imaginal reliving of traumatic experience; Foa & Rothbaum, 1998), even though relaxation is not a constituent of these procedures. If the definition of guided imagery is expanded to include any procedure in which a therapist guides or encourages a client's imaginal review of specific or nonspecific (e.g., "Imagine whatever comes to mind") events or experiences, it is likely that even more therapists than suggested by survey research incorporate some form of guided imagery into their clinical practice.

So long as imagery techniques focus on current problems and issues, as in visualizing pleasant scenes to develop relaxation skills, or when imaginal exposure is used to extinguish fears associated with recent corroborated events, there is probably little cause for concern about false memory creation. However, concerns have been expressed (Lindsay & Read, 1994; Loftus, 1993) about such highly controversial approaches as the use of imagery procedures in therapeutic settings to elicit recall of allegedly repressed or dissociated memories of childhood sexual abuse. For example, Roland (1993) proposed using a visualization technique for jogging "blocked" memories of sexual abuse, and a "reconstruction" technique for recovering repressed memories of abuse.

There is reason to believe that these approaches enjoy wide acceptance. Poole and colleagues (1995) found that a substantial number of practitioners use imagery procedures to help clients retrieve memories of abuse. They found that 32% of the U.S. practitioners in their sample reported using "imagery related to the abuse," and a disturbing 22% reported using liberal imagery strategies in which clients are given "free reign" to their imaginings.

A Source Monitoring Perspective

These statistics provide little comfort to researchers and clinicians who argue that imagery-based techniques may lead to increased confabulation when used to facilitate recall of childhood events (Lindsay & Read, 1994; Loftus & Ketcham, 1994). Trepidations regarding the use of imagery techniques are based in part on a sizable body of evidence that individuals frequently confuse real and imagined memories. For instance, Anderson (1984) asked adult subjects either to trace or to imagine tracing line drawings of common objects. On a later test subjects were asked to indicate if they had traced the items or if they had only imagined tracing them. Of the items that subjects indicated that they remembered tracing, 39% had only been imagined. Similar "source misattributions" have been demonstrated by many researchers (see Lindsay, Johnson, & Kwon, 1991).

How do such misattributions originate? Johnson and her colleagues (Johnson, Hashtroudi, & Lindsay, 1993; Johnson & Raye, 1981) have investigated how individuals identify the origins of their memories. Johnson, Foley, Suengas, and Raye (1989) distinguished between such internally generated sources as imagination, fantasies, and confabulation, and such externally generated sources as actual perceived events and information obtained from outside sources (e.g., others' recollections, newspaper stories). Johnson and Raye (1981) identified cues that help individuals infer the likely source of a memory. Compared with memories for imagined events, memories for perceived events tend to include more perceptual information (e.g., sound, color), contextual information (spatial, temporal), semantic detail, and affective information (e.g., emotional reactions), and relatively less information about cognitive operations (e.g., records of organizing, elaborating, retrieving, or identifying). Accordingly, a memory with a great deal of visual and spatial detail and contextual information would most often be judged as corresponding to an experience that was actually perceived (Johnson et al., 1989).

By and large, this decision strategy works well, and leads to accurate source monitoring in many situations. However, in situations in which the perceptual clarity of the memory for an imagined event is high (e.g., a vivid dream, nonrealistic events imagined vividly), and when few details can be recalled for a perceived event (e.g., due to distraction, stress, or other impairments), individuals may have a difficult time making this discrimination, resulting in confusion and a greater propensity for errors in source monitoring (Hirt, Lynn, Payne, Krackow, & McCrea, 1999). Moreover, both laboratory and field studies demonstrate that longer delays between experiencing an event and attempted recall compromise memory accuracy. The relatively large delays between childhood and adulthood would be expected to result in problems in determining the source of memories (i.e., real vs. imagined) and degradation of memory for those childhood experiences (DuBreuil et al., 1998). Studies of imagination inflation show that when adult participants imagine childhood events, the events are judged as more likely to have occurred than nonimagined events (Garry, Manning, Loftus, & Sherman, 1996; Heaps & Nash, 1999; Paddock et al., 1998, Study 1; but see Clancy, McNally, & Schacter, 1999, and Paddock et al., 1998, Study 2).

Problems in source monitoring can also lead to difficulties in distinguishing between events that actually occurred and events that were merely suggested by misinformation provided after an event. In some cases, subjects actually claim to remember in considerable detail the presentation of items in the original event when the items were in fact only mentioned in the postevent narrative (Payne, Neuschatz, Lampinen, & Lynn, 1997).

Our discussion implies that memory errors are likely to occur when memories are initially hazy, disjointed, or completely unavailable. However, memory errors are often not random. What is recalled at any given time seems to be highly dependent on current beliefs, inferences, "best guesses," and expectancies about what was experienced in the past (see Hirt et al., 1999, for a review). Moreover, suggestions about what occurred in the past can be influential determinants of memories, particularly when the suggested events could plausibly have occurred.

Suggesting False Memories

The research reviewed thus far suggests that providing information that falsely implies that an event occurred and that encourages a person to imagine or review the false event could lead to source monitoring difficulties and the production of false memories. Support for this hypothesis derives from research by Loftus and her colleagues (Loftus, 1993; Loftus & Ketcham, 1994; Loftus & Pickrell, 1995), which demonstrates that people can be led to integrate an entirely fabricated event into their personal histories. In Loftus's research, participants were asked by an older sibling to remember real and fictitious events (e.g., getting lost in a shopping mall). The older sibling initially provided a few details about the false event, such as where the event occurred. All subjects participated in interviews over several days. Subjects claimed to remember the false event and provided surprisingly detailed accounts of the event that they believed actually occurred.

Similar studies in other laboratories also found that a significant minority of people reported false events. For instance, Hyman, Husband, and Billings (1995) asked college students to recall childhood experiences that had been recounted by their parents. The researchers told the students that the study concerned the different ways that people remember shared experiences. In addition to actual events reported by parents, each participant was provided with a false event—either an overnight hospitalization for a high fever and a possible ear infection, or a birthday party with pizza and a clown—that purportedly occurred at about the age of 5. The parents confirmed that neither of these events actually took place. The researchers found that students recalled over 80% of the true events in both the first and second interviews. None of the participants recalled the false event during the first interview, but 20% said they remembered something about the false event in the second interview. One participant who had been exposed to the emergency hospitalization event later remembered a male doctor, a female nurse, and a friend from church who came to visit at the hospital.

In another study, along with true events, Hyman and colleagues (1995) presented different false events including accidentally spilling a bowl of punch on the parents of the bride at a wedding reception and having to evacuate a grocery store when the overhead sprinkler systems erroneously activated. Again, none of the participants recalled the false event during the first interview, but 18% remembered something about it in the second interview and 26% in the third interview.

In a third study by Hyman and Pentland (1996), participants who engaged in guided imagery reported more false memories of attending a wedding and knocking over a punchbowl than did individuals in a control group who received instructions to do their best to remember childhood events. Individuals were tested on three occasions for their recall of both true events and the false target event item of the spilled punch bowl. By the third recall trial, 9% of the control group reported the false event compared with 25% of the guided imagery group. Although these differences failed to reach statistical significance, when the definition of an implanted memory was broadened to include partial false memories or memories that included "consistent elaborations with some statements of remembering, but did not include memory of actually spilling the punchbowl" (p. 109), the guided imagery group reported significantly more memories than did the control group.

Porter, Yuille, and Lehman (1999) recently found that 26% of participants reported at least one "complete" (i.e., incorporated all misinformation into memory) false memory of six suggested emotional childhood events (serious animal attack, serious indoor accident, serious outdoor accident, getting lost, serious medical procedure, being injured by another child). The events were suggested in three different interviews over a 2-week period in which the interviewer attempted to elicit false memories using guided imagery, context reinstatement, mild social pressure, and encouraging repeated recall attempts. In addition to the substantial minority of participants who reported a "complete" false memory, another 30% of participants reported a "partial" false memory in which some of the information was recalled or the individual was uncertain about whether the memory was false. In short, more than half of individuals who are exposed to a variety of memory recovery techniques can be led to report an emotional false memory, with a substantial minority elaborating the memory in a detailed and confident manner.

A very different line of research provides support for the idea that people can genuinely believe in memories of traumatic events that are highly unlikely to have occurred in real life. Mulhern (1992) conducted a sociohistorical analysis of claims of satanic ritual abuse and concluded that there is virtually no evidence to suggest that memories of ritualistic torture and abuse are veridical (see also Lanning, 1989). Spanos, Burgess, and Burgess (1994) drew similar conclusions concerning the veracity of alien abduction and past-life reports, as we will now review in more detail.

Hypnosis

Like many guided imagery procedures used in clinical situations, hypnosis often involves eye closure and relaxation and, when used to recover memories, guided imagery or mental review of past events. Accordingly, many of the concerns that have been raised with respect to guided imagery apply to hypnosis. However, an added problem associated with hypnosis is the popular (Loftus & Loftus, 1980; Whitehouse, Dinges, Orne, & Orne, 1988) yet mistaken belief that hypnosis can improve recall. This belief can result in the tendency to overvalue the use of hypnosis for purposes of memory recovery. Survey research (Poole et al., 1995) reveals that approximately one third (29% and 34%) of psychologists in the United States who were sampled reported that they used hypnosis to help clients recall memories of sexual abuse. In contrast, this figure was only 5% among British therapists.

If hypnosis were able to retrieve forgotten memories accurately, then confidence in its use for recovering memories of abuse would be warranted. Hypnosis has received considerably more research attention than any of the other techniques we review. Although there still are strong proponents of the use of hypnosis for memory recovery (e.g., Brown, Scheflin, & Hammond, 1998; Hammond et al., 1995), we believe that the weight of evidence falls unambiguously on the side of those who caution against its use for this purpose. We contend that the following conclusions are justified by major reviews of the literature (Erdelyi, 1994; Lynn, Lock, Myers, & Payne, 1997; Lynn, Neuschatz, Fite, & Kirsch, 2000; Nash, 1987; Spanos, 1996; Steblay & Bothwell, 1994):

1. Hypnosis increases the sheer volume of recall, resulting in both more incorrect and correct information. When response productivity is statistically controlled, hypnotic recall is no more accurate than nonhypnotic recall (see Erdelyi's [1994] narrative review of 34 studies and Steblay and Bothwell's [1994] meta-analysis of 24 studies) and results in increased confidence for responses designated as "guesses" during a prior waking test (Whitehouse et al., 1988).

2. Hypnosis produces more recall errors, more intrusions of uncued errors, and higher levels of memories for false information (Steblay & Bothwell, 1994).

3. Hypnosis does not accurately reinstate experiences from the distant past (Nash, 1987).

4. False memories are associated with hypnotic responsiveness, although even relatively nonresponsive participants report false memories (Lynn, Myers, & Malinoski, 1997).

5. Hypnotized subjects are at least as likely as nonhypnotized participants to be misled in their recall by leading questions and sometimes exhibit recall deficits compared with nonhypnotized participants. There also are indications that highly hypnotizable persons are particularly prone to memory errors in response to misleading information (see Spanos, 1996; Steblay & Bothwell, 1994).

6. In general, hypnotized individuals are more confident about their recall accuracy than are nonhypnotized individuals (Steblay & Bothwell,

1994). Furthermore, an association between hypnotizability and confidence has been well documented, particularly in hypnotized participants (Steblay & Bothwell, 1994). Although confidence effects are not always present and are not universally large in magnitude, hypnosis by no means selectively increases confidence in accurate memories.

7. Contextual influences, particularly situational demand characteristics, influence the frequency and nature of pseudomemory reports.

8. Questions remain about the extent to which participants genuinely "believe" in the reality of suggested memories and how recalcitrant false memories are in clinical and experimental situations. However, even when participants are warned about possible memory problems associated with hypnotic recollections, they continue to report false memories during and after hypnosis, although some studies indicate that warnings have the potential to reduce the rate of pseudomemories in hypnotized and nonhypnotized individuals (Lynn, Neuschatz, et al., 2002).

9. Some defenders of the use of hypnosis for memory recovery have argued that this procedure is particularly useful in facilitating recall of emotional or traumatic memories (Brown et al., 1998; Hammond et al., 1995). However, contrary to this claim, eight studies (see Lynn, Myers, & Malinoski, 1997) that have compared hypnotic with nonhypnotic memory in the face of relatively emotionally arousing stimuli (e.g., films of shop accidents, depictions of fatal stabbings, a mock assassination, an actual murder videotaped serendipitously) have yielded two unambiguous conclusions: Hypnosis does not improve recall of emotionally arousing events and arousal level does not moderate hypnotic recall.

10. Hypnosis does not necessarily yield more false memories than nonhypnotic procedures that are highly suggestive in nature (Lynn, Myers, & Malinoski, 1997). Indeed, any memory recovery procedure that is either suggestive in nature or conveys the expectation that accurate memories can be easily recovered is likely to increase the sheer volume of memories, and bolster confidence in inaccurate as well as accurate memories. However, Scoboria, Mazzoni, Kirsch, and Milling (2002) found that hypnosis impaired recall relative to a waking condition independent of the degree of suggestibility of the procedures, which also had an additional independent effect on recall.

11. Although hypnosis can increase the raw number of accurate memories (with a trade-off in the number of recall errors), simply asking participants to focus on the task at hand and to do their best to recall specific events yields accurate recall comparable to hypnosis, but with fewer or comparable recall errors (see Lynn, Lock, et al., 1997).

Our dour assessment of the usefulness of hypnosis for recovering memories in psychotherapy has been echoed by several professional societies. For example, the American Psychological Association, Division 17

guidelines (1995) state that hypnosis should not be used for memory recovery, a conclusion also reached by the Canadian Psychiatric Association
(1996). The American Psychological Association (1995) recommended
that hypnosis not be used for clients who are attempting to retrieve or confirm recollections of histories of abuse, and the American Medical Association (AMA; 1994) asserted that hypnosis should be used only for investigative purposes in forensic contexts. However, it is worth mentioning that
even when hypnosis is used solely for investigative purposes, there may be
attendant risks. If hypnosis is conducted very early in an investigation, the
information obtained could lead investigators to pursue erroneous leads
and even to interpret subsequent leads as consistent with initial (and perhaps erroneous) hypnotically generated evidence (see Chapter 2 for a discussion of confirmatory bias in psychological assessment).

Searching for Early Memories

Many clinicians have long regarded the exploration of early memories as
crucial to the enterprise of psychotherapy (Bindler & Smokler, 1980;
Papanek, 1979). Adlerian clinicians (e.g., Adler, 1927; Weiland & Steisel,
1958) were the first to assert that the first reported memory holds particular significance and provides a window on current mental status and functioning. According to Adler (1931), "The first memory will show the individual's fundamental view of life; his first satisfactory crystallization of his
attitude. . . . I would never investigate a personality without asking for the
first memory" (p. 75). More recently, Olson (1979) articulated a belief
shared by many therapists (Papanek, 1979) that "[Early memories] when
correctly interpreted often reveal very quickly the basic core of one's personality, or life-style, and suggest important, bedrock themes with which
the therapist must currently deal in treating the client" (p. xvii).

Although certain early memories might well have special significance,
such memories are highly malleable. By examining early memory reports,
it is possible to study the influence of memory recovery techniques on implausible memories that cross the threshold of infantile amnesia of about 2
years of age. Most adults' earliest reported memories date back to between
36 and 60 months of age. Indeed, virtually all contemporary memory researchers agree that accurate memory reports of events that occur before
24 months of age extremely rare (see Malinoski, Lynn, & Sivec, 1998, for
a review). This inability to recall very early life events is attributable largely
to developmental changes that influence how children process, retrieve,
and share information.

Adults' memory reports from 24 months of age or earlier are likely to
represent confabulations, condensations, and constructions of early events,
as well as current concerns and stories heard about early events (Bruhn,
1984; Loftus, 1993). Spanos (1996) argued that "the phenomenon of in-

fantile amnesia is relevant to the topic of recovered memories in that it suggests that memories recovered in therapy, of abuse that supposedly occurred when the person was younger than 3 of so years of age, are very likely to be confabulations" (p. 80).

Very early memory reports, like reports of later childhood events, are vulnerable to subtle suggestive influences. Lynn, Malinoski, and Green (1999) used two different wordings to try to elicit early memories. In one version, the high expectancy case, the participants were told, "Tell me when you get an earlier memory." In the other version, the low expectancy case, participants were told, "If you don't remember, it's all right." The high expectancy version led to earlier memory reports: The high expectancy mean was 2.48 years, whereas the low expectancy mean was 3.45 years, a difference of nearly 1 full year. By the end of four recall trials, 43% of participants in the high expectancy condition reported a memory at or before 2 years of age, compared with 20% of participants in the low expectancy group.

If subtle suggestions that convey the expectation that earlier memories can be remembered result in marked changes in the age of earliest reported memory, what would be the effect of using memory recovery techniques to elicit early memories? Lynn and colleagues (1999) addressed this question in a study in which interviewers probed for increasingly early memories until participants twice denied any earlier memories. Participants then received a strong suggestion to promote earlier memory reports using "memory recovery techniques" similar to those promoted by some therapists (e.g., Farmer, 1989; Meiselman, 1990). Interviewers asked participants to close their eyes, see themselves "in their mind's eye" as a toddler or infant, and "get in touch" with memories of long ago. Interviewers also conveyed the expectation that it was possible to recall very early life events by informing participants that most young adults can retrieve memories of very early events—including their second birthday—if they "let themselves go" and try hard to visualize, focus, and concentrate. Interviewers then asked for subjects' memories of their second birthdays. Participants were complimented and otherwise reinforced for reporting increasingly early memories.

The mean age of the initial reported memory was 3.70 years. Only 11% of individuals reported initial memories at or before age 24 months, and 3% of the sample reported an initial memory from age 12 months or younger. However, after receiving the visualization instructions, 59% of the participants reported a memory of their second birthday.

After the birthday memory was solicited, interviewers pressed participants for even earlier memories. The mean age of the earliest memory reported was 1.60 years, fully 2 years earlier than their initial memory report. One of the most interesting findings was that 78.2% of the sample reported at least one memory that occurred at 24 months of age or earlier. Furthermore, more than half (56%) of the participants reported a memory between birth and 18 months of life, a third of the participants (33%) reported a memory that occurred at age 12 months or earlier, and 18% reported at least one memory of an event that occurred at 6 months or earlier, well outside the boundary of infantile amnesia. Finally, a remarkable 4% of the sample reported memories from the first week of life. It is worth underscoring that neither of these studies used particularly invasive methods for eliciting implausible memories. Nevertheless, it is clear that with increasing pressure, participants report increasingly implausible memories.

Based on our earlier review of the hypnosis literature, it should come as no surprise that hypnosis is associated with an increased rate of early implausible memories. Sivec, Lynn, and Malinoski (1997a) asked 40 hypnotized and 40 nonhypnotized participants about their earliest memories. The first time they were asked to report their earliest memory, only 3% of the nonhypnotized participants recalled a memory earlier than 2 years. However, 23% of the hypnotized participants reported a memory earlier than age 2, 20% reported a memory earlier than 18 months, 18% reported a memory earlier than a year, and 8% reported a memory of earlier than 6 months. The second time they were asked for an early memory, only 8% of the nonhypnotized participants reported a memory earlier than 2 years, and only 3% reported memories of 6 months or earlier. In contrast, 35% of hypnotized participants reported memories earlier than 18 months, 30% of participants reported memories earlier than a year, and 13% of participants reported a memory before 6 months.

In another study of hypnosis and early memories (Marmelstein & Lynn, 1999), participants reported earlier memories during hypnosis than they did both prior to hypnosis and prior to instructions to recover memories over a 2-week period. A third of the participants reported memories prior to the cutoff of infantile amnesia (i.e., age 2) after they received suggestions that they could recall earlier memories. However, during hypnosis, two thirds of participants reported such memories. Even after being debriefed and contacted by telephone outside the experimental context, more than a third (37%) of the participants continued to report memories prior to age 2.

Age Regression

In the studies we have just reviewed, participants were simply asked to recall early memories. In contrast to this rather straightforward procedure, age regression involves "regressing" a person back through time to an earlier life period. Subjects are typically given relaxation instructions and then asked to mentally re-create events that occurred at successively earlier periods in the person's life, or to focus on a particular event at a specific age, with suggestions that they are to fully relive the target event. Poole and colleagues (1995) found that 17% of their U.S. practitioner sample reported using age regression procedures with the explicit intention of retrieving memories of childhood abuse. Many popular self-help resources also recommend age regression procedures. For example, Bass and Davis (1992) indicated that one way to retrieve memories of childhood incest is by "going back" to earlier times using self- or therapist-guided regression. In one example they cite, a woman stated that in a particularly vivid age regression session,

> " . . . I felt like I was being sucked down a drain. And then I felt like a real baby. I started crying and clinging and saying, 'You can't go! You have to stay with me!' And I began to talk in a five-year-old's voice, using words and concepts that a five-year-old might use. All of a sudden I thought I was just going to throw up. I ran to the bathroom, and then I really started to sob. I saw lots of scenes from my childhood. Times I felt rejected flashed by me, almost in slides." (pp. 73–74)

Such anecdotes are often used to support the notion that the regressed person has actually returned psychologically to an earlier life period. Some regression aficionados further believe that because the individual has actually regressed to an earlier age, the regression experience accurately reflects what was experienced at that age. Proponents of this view point to cases like the aforementioned one and argue that the level of detail, the vividness of the recall, and apparent accuracy of regression experiences demonstrate that age regression is an effective memory retrieval technique. Of course, their argument deteriorates in the face of regression-prompted reports of prenatal, past life, and alien abduction memories. But let us put aside these bizarre reports and turn our attention to empirical issues. What does the research indicate about age regression?

The literature strongly suggests that the experiences of age-regressed individuals are contextually dependent and expectancy-driven social constructions. According to this empirically based view, age-regressed subjects behave according to cues they derive from the social situation and their knowledge and beliefs about age-relevant behaviors. After reviewing the relevant literature, Nash (1987) concluded that the behavior of age-regressed adults was substantially different from the behavior of children at the age to which adults are regressed. For example, adult participants age-regressed to childhood do not perform as expected on Piagetian (e.g., conservation) tasks, if one were to believe that they had truly assumed the psychological characteristics of children. In addition, age-regressed participants do not show the expected developmental patterns on either electroencephalograms (EEGs) or on visual illusions (e.g., the Ponzo or railroad tracks illusion). Nash argued that no matter how compelling "age-regressed experiences" appear to observers, they reflect participants' fantasies and beliefs and assumptions about childhood, and do not represent literal reinstatements of childhood experiences, behaviors, and feelings.

A televised documentary (Bikel, 1995) showed a group therapy session in which a woman was age regressed through childhood, to the womb, and eventually to being trapped in her mother's Fallopian tube. This case is not an isolated example of the kind of experience we consider extremely questionable. The mental health and counseling literature contains numerous case studies of prenatal remembering that are nearly, if not equally, unlikely (van Husen, 1988; Lawson, 1984).

Hypnotic Age Regression

Hypnosis is often used to facilitate the experience of age regression. However, if hypnosis is not a viable means of recovering memories of the recent past, then there is no reason to believe that it would be any more effective in recovering memories of childhood events. As mentioned earlier, Nash's (1987) review revealed that there is no special correspondence between the behavior and experience of hypnotized adults and that of actual children. In fact, as the following two studies indicate, hypnosis can contribute to memory distortions of early life events.

Nash, Drake, Wiley, Khalsa, and Lynn (1986) attempted to corroborate the memories of subjects who had participated in an earlier age regression experiment. This experiment involved age regressing hypnotized and role-playing (i.e., simulating) subjects to age 3 to a scene in which they were in the soothing presence of their mothers. During the experiment subjects reported the identity of their transitional objects (e.g., blankets, teddy bears). Third-party verification (parent report) of the accuracy of recall was obtained for 14 hypnotized subjects and 10 simulation control subjects. Despite the similarity to children in their means of relating to transitional objects, hypnotic subjects were less able than were control subjects to correctly identify the specific transitional objects actually used. Hypnotic subjects' hypnotic recollections, for example, matched their parent's reports only 21% of the time, whereas simulators' reports after hypnosis were corroborated by their parents 70% of the time. All recollections obtained during hypnosis were incorporated into posthypnotic recollections, regardless of accuracy.

Sivec, Lynn, and Malinoski (1997b) age-regressed participants to the age of 5 and suggested that girls play with a Cabbage Patch Doll and boys with a He-Man toy. An important aspect of this study was that these toys were not released until 2 or 3 years after the target time of the age regression suggestion. Half of the subjects received hypnotic age regression instructions and half of the subjects received suggestions to age regress that were not administered in a hypnotic context. Interestingly, none of the nonhypnotized persons was influenced by the suggestion. In contrast, 20% of the hypnotized subjects rated the memory of the experience as real and were confident that the event occurred at the age to which they were regressed.

Past Life Regression

The search for traumatic memories can extend to before birth (see Mills & Lynn, 2000). One type of therapy, known as "past life regression therapy," is based on the premise that traumas that occurred in previous lives influence a person's current psychological and physical symptoms (e.g., Woolger, 1988). For example, Weiss (1988) published a widely publicized series of cases focusing on patients who were hypnotized and age regressed to "go back to" the source or origin of a particular present-day problem. When the patients were regressed, they reported events that Weiss and his patients interpreted as having their source in previous lives.

When regressed persons have vivid, compelling, and seemingly realistic and detailed experiences during regression, they may seem very convincing to both patient and therapist. However, when Spanos, Menary, Gabora, DuBreuil, and Dewhirst (1991). examined past life reports for historical accuracy, they determined that the information participants gave about specific time periods during their hypnotic age regression enactments was almost "invariably incorrect" (p. 137). For example, one participant who was regressed to ancient times claimed to be Julius Caesar, emperor of Rome, in 50 BC, even though the designations of BC and AD were not adopted until centuries later, and even though Julius Caesar died decades prior to the first Roman emperor.

Additionally, it is possible to elicit and manipulate past life reports by structuring participants' expectancies about past life experiences. For example, in one study (Spanos et al., 1991, Study 2), participants were informed at the outset of the experiment that past life identities were likely to be of a different gender, culture, and race from that of the present personality. In contrast, other participants received no prehypnotic information about the characteristics of their past life identities. Spanos and his colleagues (1991) found that participants' past life experiences were not only quite elaborate but that they tended to conform to induced expectancies about the nature of past life identities. In another study, Spanos and his associates (Spanos et al., 1991, Study 3) showed that participants' past life reports during hypnotic age regression varied in terms of the prehypnotic information they received about whether children were frequently abused during past historical periods. Finally, Spanos and colleagues found that past life reports in hypnosis were associated with participants' prior beliefs in reincarnation.

Spanos (1996) concluded that hypnotically induced past life experiences are rule-governed, goal-directed fantasies that are context generated and sensitive to the demands of the hypnotic regression situation. Such imaginative scenarios are constructed from available cultural narratives about past lives and known or surmised details and facts regarding specific historical periods.

Symptom Interpretation

Therapists working with suspected abuse victims often inform them that the symptoms they experience are suggestive of a history of abuse (Bass & Davis, 1988; Blume, 1990; Fredrickson, 1992; Loftus, 1993). "Psychological symptom interpretation" is often followed by an explanation that abuse memories can be recovered because memory functions like a tape or video recorder. Treatment then focuses on recovering those memories for the purposes of healing past psychological wounds.

Many popular psychology self-help sources (e.g., Bass & Davis, 1992; Blume, 1990; Fredrickson, 1992) contain examples of symptom interpretation. Some popular self-help books on the topic of incest include lists of symptoms (e.g., "Do you have trouble knowing what you want?" "Do you use work or achievements to compensate for inadequate feelings in other parts of your life?"; see Loftus & Ketcham, 1994, for other examples) that are presented as possible or probable correlates of childhood incest.

Blume's Incest Survivors' Aftereffects Checklist consists of 34 such correlates. The scale instructions read: "Do you find many characteristics of yourself on this list? If so, you could be a survivor of incest." Blume also indicates that "clusters" of these items are significant predictors of childhood sexual abuse, and that "the more items endorsed by an individual the more likely that there is a history of incest."

The reader will note that many of the characteristics on such checklists are quite vague and seemingly applicable to many nonabused individuals. Much of the seeming "accuracy" of such checklists could stem from Barnum effects, or the tendency to believe that highly general statements that are true of many individuals in the population apply specifically to oneself (see Chapter 2 for a more detailed discussion of Barnum effects).

Researchers agree that there may be numerous personality and psychological correlates of sexual abuse (but see Rind, Tromovitch, & Bauserman, 1998, for a competing view). However, there is no known constellation of specific symptoms, let alone diagnosis, that is indicative of a history of abuse (Beitchman et al., 1992). Some genuine victims of childhood incest may experience many symptoms, others only some, and still others none. Moreover, nonvictims experience many of the same symptoms often associated with sexual abuse (Tavris, 1993). Nevertheless, Poole and colleagues (1995) found that therapists often view symptom interpretation as an important component of therapy aimed at recovering memories of suspected childhood sexual abuse. In fact, Poole and colleagues found that more than one third of the U.S. practitioners sampled reported that they used this technique.

Bogus Personality Interpretation

For ethical reasons, researchers have not directly tested the hypothesis that false memories of a history of abuse can be elicited by informing individuals that their personality characteristics are suggestive of such a history. However, a number of studies have shown that personality interpretation can indeed engender implausible or false memories. Spanos and his colleagues (Spanos, Burgess, Burgess, Samuels, & Blois, 1999) informed participants that their personality structure indicated that they had a certain experience during the first week of life. After participants completed a questionnaire, they were told that a personality profile that was generated by a computer based on their responses indicated they were "High Perceptual Cognitive Monitors." Participants were further informed that people with this profile had experienced special visual stimulation by a mobile within the first week of life. Participants were falsely told that the study was designed to recover memories in order to confirm the personality test scores. The participants were age regressed back to the crib; half of the participants were hypnotized and half received nonhypnotic age regression instructions.

In the nonhypnotic group, 95% of the participants reported infant memories and 56% reported the target mobile. However, all of these participants indicated that they thought the memories were fantasy constructions or they were unsure if the memories were real. In the hypnotic group, 79% of the participants reported infant memories, and 46% reported the target mobile. Forty-nine percent of these participants believed the memories were real, and only 16% classified the memories as fantasies.

DuBreuil, Garry, and Loftus (1998) extended Spanos and colleagues' (1999) research in a number of important respects. The researchers used the bogus personality interpretation paradigm and nonhypnotic age regression to implant memories of the second day of life (crib group) or the first day of kindergarten (kindergarten group). College students were administered a test that purportedly measured personality and were told that, based on their scores, they were likely to have participated in a nationwide program designed to enhance the development of personality and cognitive abilities by means of the use of red and green moving mobiles. The crib group was told that this enrichment occurred in the hospital immediately after their birth, and the kindergarten group was told that the mobiles were placed in kindergarten classrooms. Finally, participants were given the false information that memory functions "like a videotape recorder" and that memory retrieval techniques (e.g., nonhypnotic age regression) can access otherwise inaccessible memories.

Twenty participants in the crib condition and 16 participants in the kindergarten condition were age regressed (nonhypnotically) to the appropriate time period and given suggestions to visualize themselves at the target age. All of the kindergarten and 90% of the crib participants reported experiences consistent with the time period targeted by the regression suggestions. Twenty-five percent of the kindergarten group and 55% of the crib group reported the target memory. All kindergarten participants believed their memories corresponded to real events. In the crib group, 33% believed in the reality of their memories, 50% were unsure, and 17% of participants did not believe in the reality of their memories. Finally, a pretest questionnaire revealed that participants who believed that specific techniques could recover memories reported more suggested memories.

Dream Interpretation

With Freud (1900/1953, 1918/1955) as an influential and ardent proponent, dream interpretation became a staple in the panoply of psychoanalytic techniques that dominated psychotherapy until they were eclipsed by behavioral, humanistic, and cognitive approaches in the past two or three decades. Viewed as the "royal road to the unconscious," dreams have been used to provide a window on past experiences, including repressed traumatic events. For example, van der Kolk, Britz, Burr, Sherry, and Hartmann (1994) claimed that dreams can represent "exact replicas" of traumatic experiences (p. 188), a view not unlike that propounded by Fredrickson (1992), who argued that dreams are a vehicle by which "buried memories of abuse intrude into . . . consciousness" (p. 44).

Although the popularity of dream interpretation has, along with psychoanalysis, waned in recent years, survey research indicates that upwards of a third of psychotherapists (37–44%) in the United States still use this technique (see also Brenneis, 1997; Polusny & Follette, 1996). These statistics are of particular interest given Lindsay and Read's (1994) observation that no data exist to support the idea that dreams accurately reveal autobiographical memories that fall outside the purview of consciousness. When dreams are interpreted as indicative of a history of child sexual abuse (Bass & Davis, 1988; Fredrickson, 1992), the fact that the information is provided by an authority figure can constitute a strong suggestion that abuse, in fact, occurred in "real life."

Ethical constraints preclude studies that examine false memories in the context of child abuse. However, Mazzoni and her colleagues (Mazzoni, Lombardo, Malvagia, & Loftus, 1997) conducted a series of studies that attempted to simulate the effects of dream interpretation of non–abuse-related yet stressful life events. In their first study (Mazzoni et al., 1997), participants reported on their childhood experiences on two occasions, separated by 3–4 weeks. Between these sessions, some subjects were exposed to a brief-therapy simulation in which an expert clinician analyzed a dream report that they had brought to the session. No matter what the content of their dreams, the participants received the suggestion that their dream was indicative of having experienced, before age 3, certain events such as having been lost in a public place or abandoned by their parents. Although subjects had previously indicated that they had not experienced these critical events before age 3, this 30-minunte therapy simulation led many individuals to develop new beliefs about their past. Relative to controls who had not received the personalized suggestion, these "therapy" participants were far more likely to develop false beliefs that before age 3 that they had been lost in a public place, had felt lonely and lost in an unfamiliar place, and had been abandoned by their parents.

In a follow-up study using a similar procedure, Loftus and Mazzoni (1998) showed that subjects whose dreams were interpreted to indicate that they had experienced a very dangerous event before age 3 later reported an increased belief that the dangerous event had occurred. The new beliefs that were generated by the dream interpretation were maintained for at least 4 weeks.

In a third study, Mazzoni, Loftus, Seitz, and Lynn (1999) extended this research paradigm to a target memory of having been bullied as a child. Participants in the experimental condition were individually given specific feedback, based on the content of their dreams, suggesting that their dreams indicated that they had an interaction with a bully or had been lost in a public place. Control participants were either given a brief lecture about dreams by the "clinical psychologist" or simply did not attend the middle session. The authors found that the dream interpretation increased participants' confidence that the target event had occurred compared with control participants. Six of the 22 (27%) participants in the dream interpretation condition recalled the bullying event and 4 of the 5 (80%) participants in the dream interpretation condition recalled the getting-lost event. Overall, 10 out of 27 participants (37%) in the experimental condition reported the target memory, although the ages given for the target event tended to be over 3. In conclusion, a growing body of evidence demonstrates that it is possible to implant autobiographical childhood memories using a variety of strategies that involve personality and dream interpretation.

Physical Symptom Interpretation: Body Memories

A "body memory" can be defined as an unexplained physical symptom that is interpreted as the result of childhood sexual abuse (CSA) or other historic trauma (cf. Fredrickson, 1992; Levis, 1995). In van der Kolk's

(1994) words, "The body keeps the score." According to survey research, 36% of U.S. psychotherapists (Poole et al., 1995) interpret body pains or physical symptoms as indicative of a history of childhood sexual abuse.

Some surveys of women seeking medical services have found that abuse survivors do indeed report more frequent physical symptoms, visits to physicians, and more lifetime surgeries than women without an abuse history (Austin, 1995). Austin (1995) attempted to explore the correlations of location of physical symptoms in adult survivors of CSA with the location of the purported physical insults during the abuse. Although a significant correlation was found for gynecological symptoms in adult sexual abuse survivors (i.e., adult rape), this association was not evident for CSA survivors. Relatedly, there were no significant correlations for gastrointestinal, throat, or rectal bleeding symptoms in adult or childhood survivors of sexual abuse. Nevertheless, these findings were limited by a small sample size ($N = 14$). Hence, although the literature suggests a relative abundance of physical symptoms in CSA survivors, the limited available research does not reveal a correlation between location of abuse and physical symptoms, thereby providing no support for the "body memory" hypothesis.

At least one treatment approach is based on the notion of body memories. Levis (1995) instructs patients to focus on a particular physical sensation or pain, and to bridge the experience back in time to the etiology of the pain. This approach clearly implies that current physical problems have a historical psychological or physical etiology, and engenders clear expectancies regarding the antecedents of current problems based on symptom interpretation. It is notable that similar expectancy-altering information has elicited highly implausible memory reports (e.g., abuse in a "past life"; Spanos, 1996) in previous research. Studies that use the concept of "body memories" to suggest that individuals experienced specific early life events are clearly warranted to examine the effects of this interpretive set on the creation of false memories.

Bibliotherapy

Many therapists who treat patients with suspected abuse histories prescribe "survivor books" or self-help books (see also Chapter 14) written specifically for survivors of childhood abuse to provide "confirmation" that the individual's symptoms are due to past abuse (psychological symptom interpretation) and to provide a means of gaining access to memories. The books typically provide imaginative exercises and stories of other survivors' struggles (Lindsay & Read, 1994). Some of the most influential popular books of this genre include Bass and Davis's (1988) *The Courage to Heal*, Fredrickson's (1992) *Repressed Memories*, and Blume's (1990) *Secret Survivors: Uncovering Incest and Its Aftereffects in Women*. These books offer potential support for, and validation to, actual abuse survivors. However, the fact that the writers interpret current symptoms as indicative of an abuse history, invite readers to imaginatively review their past experiences, and include suggestive stories of survivors of abuse may increase the risk that readers incorporate false memories of abuse into their archive of personal memories.

Mazzoni, Loftus, and Kirsch (2001) provided a dramatic illustration of how reading material and psychological symptom interpretation can increase the plausibility of an initially implausible memory of witnessing a demonic possession. The authors conducted their study in Italy, where demonic possession is viewed as a more plausible occurrence than in the United States. However, in an initial testing session, all of the participants indicated that demonic possession was not only implausible, but that it was very unlikely that they had personally witnessed an occurrence of possession as children.

A month after the first session, participants in one group first read three short articles (in a packet of 12), which indicated that demonic possession is more common than is generally believed and that many children have witnessed such an event. These participants were compared with (1) individuals who read three short articles about choking and (2) individuals who received no manipulation. Individuals who received one of the manipulations returned to the laboratory the following week and, based on their responses to a fear questionnaire they completed, were informed (regardless of their actual responses) that their fear profile indicated that they had probably either witnessed a possession or had almost choked during early childhood.

When the students returned to the laboratory for a final session and completed the original questionnaires, they indicated that the two suggested events—witnessed possession and choking—were more real than before. Additionally, 18% of the participants indicated that they had probably witnessed possession. No changes in memories were evident in the control condition. These findings provide evidence that events that were not experienced during childhood and are initially thought to be highly implausible can, with sufficient credibility-enhancing information, come to be viewed as having plausibly occurred in real life. Clearly, therapists should exercise caution in implying that such events as abuse might have occurred on the basis of current symptoms alone.

INDIVIDUAL DIFFERENCES

The General Public: Popular Beliefs

It is unlikely that all individuals are equally susceptible to the potentially suggestive influences of memory recovery procedures. At the very least, subjects must believe, first, that at least some memories remain intact in definitely and are stored so that they can be retrieved, and, second, that memory recovery techniques enable them to retrieve these stored memories.

Lay people hold various misconceptions about how human memory works. Survey studies have shown that many people believe in the permanence of human memory (Garry, Loftus, & Brown, 1994; Loftus & Loftus, 1980) and in the ability of techniques such as hypnosis to assist in the recovery of early childhood memories (McConkey & Jupp, 1986). Additionally, a substantial proportion of subjects in Garry and colleagues (1994) believed in the veridicality of memories retrieved from the womb, and Yapko (1994) and Garry and colleagues both found that a substantial proportion of lay samples believed in the existence of past lives.

Practitioners

Some research shows that practitioners' beliefs about memory are not very different from those of lay people. Yapko (1994) found that 47% of professionals (the majority of whom were practitioners) had greater faith in the veridicality of hypnotic than nonhypnotic memories, and 31% believed that events recalled during hypnosis were likely to be accurate. Furthermore, 54% of his sample believed to some degree in the effectiveness of hypnosis for recovering memories as far back as birth, and 28% believed in its effectiveness for recovering memories from past lives. Fortunately, the majority of his sample (79%) also recognized that false memories could emerge using hypnosis. Nonetheless, a noteworthy percentage of his subjects endorsed assertions regarding hypnosis that are inconsistent with the research literature on hypnosis (e.g., hypnotized people cannot lie, hypnotized people can access memories as far back as birth).

Individual Difference Measures

A number of studies have provided evidence for small to moderate relations between dissociation (as measured by the Dissociative Experiences Scale [DES]; Bernstein & Putnam, 1986) and recall errors in studies that use a variety of different paradigms (e.g., DRM; Deese, 1959; Roediger & McDermott, 1995) (see Eisen & Lynn, 2001, for a review). In addition to dissociation, vividness of visualization has been found to be related to increased suggestibility and source monitoring difficulties (see Eisen and Lynn, 2001), as have compliance (Malinoski & Lynn, 1999), schizotypy (Clancy, McNally, Schacter, Lenzenweger, & Pitman, 2002), hypnotizability (see Lynn, Lock, et al., 1997), interrogative suggestibility (Malinoski & Lynn, 1999), and extraversion in interviewers and relatively low extraversion in interviewees (Porter, Birt, Yuille, & Lehman, 2000). The available evidence implies that clinicians should be especially vigilant to avoid leading interview procedures with clients who evince particularly vivid imagery and visualization abilities, high hypnotizability, and dissociative tendencies (see also Chapter 5).

CRITICISMS OF THE LITERATURE

There have been three major criticisms of the research we have reviewed. First, studies that rely on parents or siblings as a means of implanting memories have been criticized (Freyd, 1998; Pope, 1996; Pope & Brown, 1996) as inadequate analogues of what occurs in psychotherapy. Accordingly, critics suggest that studies such as the Lost-in-the-Mall study (i.e., Loftus & Pickrell, 1995) demonstrate the suggestive influence of siblings or parents who claim to be present at the time of the event, rather than the influence of therapists who were not present at the time of the event. However, this criticism does not apply to the studies we reviewed that did not use parents' or siblings' reports to lend credence to a false memory that was elicited, but nevertheless demonstrated that memories for a variety of implausible or impossible events (e.g., playing with toys that were not produced at the time, witnessing demonic possession) could be instated with a variety of memory recovery techniques.

A second criticism of some of the studies reviewed concerns whether the implanted memory is, in fact, false. Brown and colleagues (1998) claimed that the experimenter can never know if the target false event actually occurred; therefore, the "implanted false memory" may be real. Furthermore, Brown and colleagues argue that whereas the experimenter may initially obtain feedback from a parent by asking, for example, "Was your child ever lost in a mall at age 5?" studies have not attempted to corroborate the implanted "false" memory. That is, researchers have not attempted to corroborate the ostensibly false implanted memory with parents after the experiment terminated. Brown et al. suggested that discussing the content of the implanted memory with the parents may serve as a reminder cue to elicit parental recall. On the other hand, it would seem that this procedure presents a danger of implanting or altering parental memory reports due to blatant demand characteristics for parents to corroborate their children's memory report.

Using the imagination inflation paradigm, Goff and Roediger (1998) asked participants to perform a number of simple actions (e.g., flipping a coin, breaking a toothpick). Other simple actions were merely heard but not performed. In a second session, which ranged from either 10 minutes to 2 weeks later depending on the experimental condition, these participants were asked to imagine performing subsets of these actions either 0, 1, 3, or 5 times. When Goff and Roediger tested participants' memories in a third session, they found that as actions were imagined an increasing number of times, participants were increasingly likely to erroneously recall having performed actions that they did not actually perform. Goff and Roediger's findings provide an existence proof for the assertion that in at least certain cases, suggestive procedures (in this case imagination inflation) can lead to inaccurate memories of events that can be unambiguously documented as never having occurred.

Brown and colleagues (1998) have also suggested that parents' memory reports do not necessarily represent more accurate accounts of the past than participants' renditions of what occurred. Accordingly, the failure to corroborate a particular memory based on parental report provides no guarantee that the event the participant remembers did not occur. However, once again, these criticisms do not apply to the studies we reviewed that targeted impossible or unlikely events with a vanishingly small probability (e.g., witnessing a demonic possession) of having occurred in real life.

The third critique of the memory implantation literature is that it is difficult if not impossible to generalize the laboratory research that has been conducted to reports of abuse in clinical settings (Pope, 1996; Pope & Brown, 1996). Critics contend that a memory of being abused cannot be easily implanted. That is, abuse is a complex event that typically occurs repeatedly and would therefore be more difficult to implant (cf. Brewin, 1997; Brown et al., 1998; Olio, 1994). The critics do not offer a clear explanation of why this would be the case. Nevertheless, they raise an interesting question (e.g., Are complex repeated events more difficult to implant than relatively less complex, single occurrences?) that should be explored in future research.

Additionally, critics contend that laboratory research may not generalize to the real world because the events that are typically suggested do not approximate the degree of trauma experienced by actual survivors of childhood sexual abuse. Although critics assume that a highly traumatic memory such as abuse would be much more difficult to implant (Olio, 1994; Pope & Brown, 1996) than a less traumatic memory, they do not advance a clear rationale for this contention. The level of "trauma" or distress associated with target memories could be systematically manipulated in future research to determine whether there is an inverse relationship between the frequency of false memories and the degree of trauma of the suggested life event.

The critics of the research we have reviewed have correctly identified generalizability as an important issue. It is difficult to make informed comparisons regarding false memory rates in clinical versus laboratory contexts because the precise rates of false memories associated with the procedures we have reviewed in clinical situations are unknown. Indeed, in clinical situations, little is known about the rates of (1) false memories that arise spontaneously due to the vagaries of ordinary memory, (2) false memories that are elicited by memory recovery procedures, (3) accurate memories that arise spontaneously in the process of therapeutic discourse, and (4) accurate memories that are elicited by memory recovery procedures.

However, it seems plausible, if not likely, that expectancies, suggestive procedures, and demand characteristics play a far more significant role in therapeutic situations than in experimental contexts. The therapist's potential to exert social influence on a help-seeking, eager to please, vulnerable patient is likely much greater than the experimenter's influence on a subject participating in a "one shot" experiment for money or course credit. Accordingly, the effects of hypnosis, guided imagery, suggestion, and symptom interpretation on memory may be more, rather than less, pronounced in a clinical than in a laboratory context.

HYPOTHESIZED PATH OF FALSE MEMORY CREATION

We believe that imaginative narratives of sexual abuse that never occurred, past life reports, and alien abduction experiences can and do arise in the context of a treatment in which the patient comes to believe that the narrative provides a plausible explanation for current life difficulties. The narrative can achieve a high degree of plausibility due to a variety of factors we have delineated. The most important of these factors include the following:

1. cultural beliefs that link the idea of abuse, for example, with psychopathology;
2. the therapist's support or suggestion of this interpretation;
3. the failure to consider alternative explanations for problems in living presumed to be associated with abuse;
4. the search for confirmatory data (see also Chapter 2);
5. repeated unsuccessful attempts to recall past events, which lead to the perception of significant "amnesia" for the past and justifies the need for memory recovery procedures (Belli, Winkielman, Read, Schwartz, & Lynn, 1998);
6. the use of suggestive memory recovery techniques that increase the plausibility of abuse (Pezdek, Finger, & Hodge, 1997) and yield information and remembrances consistent with the idea that abuse occurred;
7. increasing commitment to the narrative on the part of the client and therapist, escalating dependence on the therapist, and anxiety reduction associated with ambiguity reduction;
8. the encouragement of a "conversion" or "coming out" experience by the therapist or supportive community (e.g., therapy group), which solidifies the role associated with the narrative (e.g.,"abuse

victim") and is accompanied by feelings of empowerment, which
constitute an additional source of positive reinforcement; and

9. the narrative's provision of a measure of continuity to the past and
the future, and a sense of comfort, belonging, and identity.

SHOULD THERAPISTS ENGAGE IN MEMORY RECOVERY?

The extant evidence provides little support for the use of memory recovery
techniques to uncover memories of abuse in psychotherapy. In fact, there
are a number of reasons for therapists to eschew these procedures.

1. "Recovered memory therapy ... is predicated on the trauma-
memory argument—that memories of traumatic events have special properties that distinguish them from ordinary memories of the sort usually
studied in the laboratory (p. 70). . . . Nothing about the clinical evidence
suggests that traumatic memories are special, or that special techniques are
required to recover them" (Shobe & Kihlstrom, 1997, p. 74; but see Nadel
& Jacobs, 1998, for a different view).

2. Most survivors of traumatic abuse past the age of 3 do not forget
their abuse. In fact, the literature points to the opposite conclusion: In general, memory following traumatic events is enhanced relative to memory
following nontraumatic events (see Shobe & Kihlstrom, 1997).

3. Even if a certain percentage of accurate memories can be recovered
in therapy, it may be unprofitable to do so. As Lindsay (1996) observed,
"numerous lines of evidence suggest that only a very small percentage of
psychotherapy clients have problems that are caused by non-remembered
histories of abuse" (p. 364). Certainly no empirical work reveals a causal
connection between nonremembered abuse and psychopathology.

4. There is no demonstrable benefit associated with the straightforward catharsis of emotional events in treatment. To the contrary, a review
of the literature (Littrell, 1998) on exposure therapies (which rely not on
memory recovery but rather on the reexperience of already remembered
events) reveals that the mere experience and expression of painful memories and emotions, when not grounded in attempts to engender positive
coping and mastery, can be harmful.

5. There is no empirical basis on which to argue that hypnotic or
nonhypnotic memory recovery procedures are more effective than present-
centered approaches in treating the presumed sequelae of trauma or psychological problems in general. Indeed, there is no empirically supported
psychotherapy or procedure that relies on the recovery of forgotten traumatic events to achieve a positive therapeutic outcome (Chambless &
Ollendick, 2001). Adshead (1997) has gone so far as to argue that if memory work with trauma patients is not effective, then "it would therefore be

just as unethical to use memory work for patients who could not use it or benefit by it, as it would be to prescribe the wrong medication, or employ a useless surgical technique" (p. 437).

We further contend that if therapists decide to use memory recovery techniques, then they should provide their clients with a written informed consent document that apprises them of (1) accurate, scientifically grounded information about the reconstructive nature of memory, (2) the fact that recovered memories must be corroborated before they can be given special credence, and (3) information regarding laboratory studies of memory pertinent to the techniques employed.

CONCLUSIONS

Let us be clear about what our findings do not mean as well as what they do mean. First, our findings do not imply that all memory recovery techniques are necessarily problematic. For example, the "cognitive interview" (Fisher & Geiselman, 1992), which incorporates a variety of basic techniques derived from experimental research on memory (e.g., providing subjects with appropriate retrieval cues, searching for additional memorial details), appears to hold promise as a method of enhancing memory in eyewitness contexts. Some of the techniques comprising this interview could ultimately prove helpful in the therapeutic context for enhancing memories of specific events. Thus, although we wish to warn practitioners against the use of certain suggestive procedures, such as hypnosis and guided imagery, to recover memories, we do not intend to throw out the baby with the bathwater. Certain techniques derived from the basic psychology of memory, such as the cognitive interview, may enhance recall of certain memories, and we encourage further investigation of such techniques in the therapeutic context.

Second, we do not wish to imply that all uses of hypnosis in psychotherapy are problematic. To the contrary, at least some controlled research evidence suggests that hypnosis may be a useful adjunct to cognitive-behavioral therapy, pain control procedures, obesity, and smoking cessation treatments (Lynn, Kirsch, Barabasz, Cardeña, & Patterson, 2000), although the extent to which hypnosis provides benefits above and beyond relaxation (and other nonspecific effects) in such cases remains unclear. In any case, we emphasize that the questionable scientific status of hypnosis as a memory recovery technique has no direct bearing on its therapeutic efficacy, which must ultimately be investigated and judged on its own merits.

Finally, we do not wish to claim that all memories recovered after years or decades of forgetting are necessarily false, although space constraints preclude us from discussing this fascinating issue in depth. Suffice it to say that several case reports are consistent with the possibility that people can sometimes recall old childhood experiences after long periods of non recall (Schooler, Ambadar, & Bendiksen, 1997; but see Loftus & Guyer, 2002). In some of these cases, there is evidence that such apparently unrecalled memories were previously recalled. Nevertheless, we remain open to the possibility that certain recovered childhood memories are veridical, although we believe that further research will be needed to document their existence and possible prevalence.

These important and unresolved issues notwithstanding, the conclusion that certain suggestive therapeutic practices, particularly those that we have discussed in this chapter, can foster false memories in some clients appears indisputable. We urge practitioners to exercise considerable caution when using these techniques in psychotherapy, and to base their memory-related therapeutic practices on the best available scientific evidence.

GLOSSARY

DRM paradigm: In the Deese/Roediger–McDermott (DRM; Roediger & McDermott, 1995; see also Deese, 1959) paradigm, participants are presented (auditorily) with a series of lists of thematically related words such as *bed*, *rest*, *wake*, *doze*, *dream*, and *pillow*, all of which are thematically related to such nonpresented words as *sleep*. They then are administered an oral recognition test consisting of the words actually presented in the experiment, "critical" nonpresented words that are thematically related to the presented words (e.g., sleep), and a series of nonpresented, thematically related, words. Using this paradigm, many participants (approximately 70%, on average) experience "memory illusions," that is, they falsely recognize thematically related nonpresented words with a high degree of confidence.

Hypnosis: The American Psychological Association, Division of Psychological Hypnosis, has adopted a consensus definition of hypnosis as a procedure during which a health professional or researcher suggests that a client, patient, or subject experience changes in sensations, perceptions, thoughts, or behavior. The hypnotic context is generally established by an induction procedure. Although there are many different hypnotic inductions, most include suggestions for relaxation, calmness, and well-being.

Hypnotizability: The degree or extent of responsiveness to suggestions administered in a situation that is defined as hypnosis. How people respond to hypnosis is dependent largely on their motivation to respond; their beliefs, attitudes, and expectancies about hypnosis and how they will respond; and their responsiveness to waking imaginative suggestions.

Infantile amnesia: Virtually all contemporary memory researchers agree that accurate memory reports of events that occur before 24 months of age are extremely rare. This inability to recall very early life events is known as "infantile amnesia," a phenomenon attributable to developmental changes that influence how children process, retrieve, and share information (see Malinoski et al., 1998).

Interrogative suggestibility: Interrogative suggestibility involves the tendency of an individual's account of events to be altered by misleading information and interpersonal pressure within an interview. The Gudjonsson Scale of Interrogative Suggestibility (GSS; Gudjonsson, 1984) was initially used to predict individual differences in susceptibility to highly suggestive and misleading questioning during a police interrogation, but it has been used widely in research on memory and suggestibility.

REFERENCES

Adler, A. (1927). *Understanding human nature.* New York: Greenberg.

Adler, A. (1931). *What life should mean to you.* Boston: Little, Brown.

Adshead, G. (1997). Seekers after truth: Ethical issues raised by the discussion of "false" and "recovered" memories. In J. D. Read & D. S. Lindsay (Eds.), *Recollections of trauma: Scientific evidence and clinical practice.* (pp. 435–440). New York: Plenum Press.

American Medical Association, Council on Scientific Affairs. (1994). *Memories of childhood abuse* (CSA Report No. 5-A-94). Washington, DC: American Medical Association.

American Psychological Association, Division 17 Committee on Women, Division 42 Trauma and Gender Issues Committee (1995, July 25). *Psychotherapy guidelines for working with clients who may have an abuse or trauma history.* Washington, DC: American Psychological Association.

Anderson, R. E. (1984). Did I do it or did I only imagine doing it? *Journal of Experimental Psychology: General, 113,* 594–613.

Austin, S. (1995). *Exploration of a conditioning model in understanding the manifestation of physical symptoms of sexual abuse survivors.* Unpublished doctoral dissertation, University of Denver.

Bass, E., & Davis, L. (1988). *The courage to heal.* New York: Harper & Row.

Beitchman, J. H., Zucker, K. J., Hood, J. E., da Costa, G. A., Akman, D., & Cassavia, E. (1992). A review of the long-term effects of child sexual abuse. *Child Abuse and Neglect, 16,* 101–118.

Belli, R. F., Winkielman, P., Read, J. D., Schwartz, N., & Lynn, S. J. (1998). Recalling more childhood events leads to judgments of poorer memory: Implications for the recovered/false memory debate. *Psychonomic Bulletin and Review, 5,* 318–323.

Bernstein, E. M., & Putnam, F. W. (1986). Development, reliability, and validity of a dissociation scale. *Journal of Nervous and Mental Diseases, 174,* 727–735.

Bikel, O. (Producer). (1995). Divided memories. In *Frontline.* New York: CBS.

Bindler, J. L., & Smokler, I. (1980). Early memories: A technical aid to focusing in time-limited dynamic psychotherapy. *Psychotherapy: Theory, Research and Practice, 17*, 52–62.

Blume, E. S. (1990). *Secret survivors: Uncovering incest and its aftereffects in women.* New York: Wiley.

Brenneis, C. B. (1997). *Recovered memories of trauma: Transferring the present to the past.* Madison, CT: International Universities Press.

Brewin, C. R. (1997). Commentary on dispatch from the (un)civil memory wars. In D. Read & S. Lindsay (Eds.), *Recollections of trauma: Scientific research and clinical practice* (pp. 194–196). New York: Plenum Press.

Brown, D., Scheflin, A. W., & Hammond, D. C. (1998). *Memory, trauma treatment, and the law.* New York: Norton.

Bruhn, A. R. (1984). The use of earliest memories as a projective technique. In P. McReynolds & C. J. Chelune (Eds.), *Advances in psychological assessment* (Vol. 6, pp. 109–150). San Francisco: Jossey-Bass.

Canadian Psychiatric Association. (1996, March 25). Position statement: Adult recovered memories of childhood sexual abuse. *Canadian Journal of Psychiatry, 41*, 305–306.

Chambless, D. L., & Ollendick, T. H. (2001). Empirically supported psychological interventions: Controversies and evidence. *Annual Review of Psychology, 52*, 685–716.

Clancy, S. A., McNally, R. J., & Schacter, D. L. (1999). Effects of guided imagery on memory distortion in women reporting recovered memories of childhood sexual abuse. *Journal of Traumatic Stress, 12*, 559–569.

Clancy, S. A., McNally, R. J., Schacter, D. L., Lenzenweger, M. F., & Pitman, R. K. (2002). Memory distortion in people reporting abduction by aliens. *Journal of Abnormal Psychology, 111*, 455–461.

Deese, J. (1959). Influence of inter-item associative strength upon immediate free recall. *Psychological Reports, 5*, 305–312.

DuBreuil, S. C., Garry, M., & Loftus, E. F. (1998). Tales from the crib: Age-regression and the creation of unlikely memories. In S. J. Lynn & K. M. McConkey (Eds.), *Truth in memory* (pp. 137–160). New York: Guilford Press.

Eisen, M., & Lynn, S. J. (2001). Memory, suggestibility, and dissociation in children and adults. *Applied Cognitive Psychology, 15*, 49–73.

Erdelyi, M. (1994). Hypnotic hypermnesia: The empty set of hypermnesia. *International Journal of Clinical and Experimental Hypnosis, 42*, 379–390.

Farmer, S. (1989). *Adult children of abusive parents: A healing program for those who have been physically, sexually, or emotionally abused.* Los Angeles, CA: Lowell House.

Fisher, R. P., & Geiselman, R. E. (1992). *Memory enhancement techniques for investigative interviewing.* Springfield, IL: Charles C Thomas.

Foa, E. B., & Rothbaum, B. O. (1998). *Treating the trauma of rape: Cognitive-behavioral therapy for PTSD.* New York: Guilford Press.

Frederickson, R. (1992). *Repressed memories.* New York: Fireside/Parkside.

Freud, S. (1953). The interpretation of dreams. In J. Strachey (Ed. & Trans.), *The standard edition of the complete psychological works of Sigmund Freud.* London: Hogarth Press. (Original work published 1900)

Freud, S. (1955). From the history of an infantile neurosis. In J. Strachey (Ed. &

Trans.), *The standard edition of the complete psychological works of Sigmund Freud*. London: Hogarth Press. (Original work published 1918)

Freyd, J. J. (1998). Science in the memory debate. *Ethics and Behavior, 8*, 101–113.

Garry, M., Loftus, E. F., & Brown, S. W. (1994). Memory: A river runs through it [Special issue: The recovered memory/false memory debate]. *Consciousness and Cognition: An International Journal, 3*, 438–451.

Garry, M., Manning, C., Loftus, E. F., & Sherman, S. J. (1996). Imagination inflation: Imagining a childhood event inflates confidence that it occurred. *Psychonomic Bulletin and Review, 3*, 208–214.

Goff, L. M., & Roediger, H. L. (1998). Imagination inflation for action events: Repeated imaginings lead to illusory recollections. *Memory and Cognition, 26*, 20–33.

Gudjonsson, G. H. (1984). A new Scale of Interrogative Suggestibility. *Personality and Individual Differences, 5*, 303–314.

Hammond, D. C., Garver, R. B., Mutter, C. B., Crasilneck, H. B., Frischholz, E., Gravitz, M. A., Hilber, N. S., Olson, J., Scheflin, A., Spiegel, H., & Wester, W. (1995). *Clinical hypnosis and memory: Guidelines for clinicians and for forensic hypnosis*. Des Plaines, IL: American Society of Clinical Hypnosis Press.

Heaps, C., & Nash, M. R. (1999). Individual differences in imagination inflation. *Psychonomic Bulletin and Review, 6*, 313–318.

Hirt, E. R., Lynn, S. J., Payne, D. G., Krackow, E., & McCrea, S. M. (1999). Expectancies and memory: Inferring the past from what must have been. In I. Kirsch (Ed.), *How expectancies shape experience* (pp. 93–124). Washington, DC: American Psychological Association.

Hyman, I. E., Jr., Husband, T. H., & Billings, F. J. (1995). False memories of childhood experiences. *Applied Cognitive Psychology, 9*, 181–197.

Hyman, I. E., Jr., & Pentland, J. (1996). The role of mental imagery in the creation of false childhood memories. *Journal of Memory and Language, 35*, 101–117.

Johnson, M. K., Foley, M. A., Suengas, A. G., & Raye, C. L. (1989). Phenomenal characteristics of memories for perceived and imagined autobiographical events. *Journal of Experimental Psychology: General, 117*, 371–376.

Johnson, M. K., Hashtroudi, S., & Lindsay, D. S. (1993). Source monitoring. *Psychological Bulletin, 114*, 3–28.

Johnson, M. K., & Raye, C. L. (1981). Reality monitoring. *Psychological Review, 88*, 67–85.

Lanning, K. V. (1989). Satanic, occult, and ritualistic crime: A law enforcement perspective. *Police Chief, 56*, 62–85.

Lawson, A. J. (1984). Perinatal imagery in UFO abduction reports. *Journal of Psychohistory, 12*, 211–239.

Levis, D. J. (1995). Decoding traumatic memory: Implosive theory of psychopathology. In W. O'Donohue & L. Krasner (Eds.), *Theories in behavior therapy* (pp. 173–207). Washington, DC: American Psychological Association.

Lindsay, D. (1996). Commentary on informed clinical practice and the standard of care: Proposed guidelines for the treatment of adults who report delayed memories of childhood trauma. In J. D. Read & D. S. Lindsay (Eds.), *Recollections of trauma: Scientific evidence and clinical practice* (pp. 361–370). New York: Plenum Press.

Lindsay, D. S., Johnson, M. K., & Kwon, P. (1991). Developmental changes in memory source monitoring. *Journal of Experimental Child Psychology, 52*, 297–318.

Lindsay, D. S., & Read, D. (1994). Psychotherapy and memories of childhood sexual abuse: A cognitive perspective. *Applied Cognitive Psychology, 8*, 281–338.

Littrell, J. (1998). Is the experience of painful emotion therapeutic? *Clinical Psychology Review, 18*, 71–102.

Loftus, E. F. (1993). The reality of repressed memories. *American Psychologist, 48*, 518–537.

Loftus, E. F., & Guyer, M. (2002). Who abused Jane Doe? The hazards of the single case history. *Skeptical Inquirer, 26*(3), 24–32.

Loftus, E. F., & Ketcham, K. (1994). *The myth of repressed memories.* New York: Plenum. Press.

Loftus, E. F., & Loftus, G. R. (1980). On the permanence of stored information in the brain. *American Psychologist, 35*, 409–420.

Loftus, E. F., & Mazzoni, G. (1998). Using imagination and personalized suggestion to change behavior. *Behavior Therapy, 29*, 691–708.

Loftus, E. F., & Pickrell, J. E. (1995). The formation of false memories. *Psychiatric Annals, 25*, 720–725.

Lynn, S. J., Kirsch, I., Barabasz, A., Cardeña, E., & Patterson, D. (2000). Hypnosis as an empirically supported adjunctive technique: The state of the evidence. *International Journal of Clinical and Experimental Hypnosis, 48*, 343–361.

Lynn, S. J., Lock, T. G., Myers, B., & Payne, D. G. (1997). Recalling the unrecallable: Should hypnosis be used to recover memories in psychotherapy? *Current Directions in Psychological Science, 6*, 79–83.

Lynn, S. J., Malinoski, P., & Green, J. (1999). *Early memory reports as a function of high versus low expectancy.* Unpublished manuscript, State University of New York at Binghamton.

Lynn, S. J., Myers, B., & Malinoski, P. (1997). Hypnosis, pseudomemories, and clinical guidelines: A sociocognitive perspective. In D. Read & S. Lindsay (Eds.), *Recollections of trauma: Scientific research and clinical practice* (pp. 305–331). New York: Plenum Press.

Lynn, S. J., Neuschatz, J., Fite, R., & Kirsch, I. (2000). Hypnosis in the forensic arena. *Journal of Forensic Practice, 1*, 113–122.

Lynn, S. J., Neuschatz, J., Fite, R., & Rhue, J. R. (2002). Hypnosis and memory: Implications for the courtroom and psychotherapy. In M. Eisen & G. Goodman (Eds.), *Memory and suggestibility in the forensic interview* (pp. 287–308). New York: Guilford Press.

Malinoski, P., & Lynn, S. J. (1999). The plasticity of very early memory reports: Social pressure, hypnotizability, compliance, and interrogative suggestibility. *International Journal of Clinical and Experimental Hypnosis, 47*, 320–345.

Malinoski, P., Lynn, S. J., & Sivec, H. (1998). The assessment, validity, and determinants of early memory reports: A critical review. In S. J. Lynn & K. M. McConkey (Eds.), *Truth in memory* (pp. 109–136). New York: Guilford Press.

Marmelstein, L., & Lynn, S. J. (1999). Expectancies, group, and hypnotic influences on early autobiographical memory reports. *International Journal of Clinical and Experimental Hypnosis, 47*, 301–319.

Mazzoni, G. A., Loftus, E. F., & Kirsch, I. (2001). Changing beliefs about implausible autobiographical events: A little plausibility goes a long way. *Journal of Experimental Psychology: Applied, 7,* 51–59.

Mazzoni, G. A., Loftus, E. F., Seitz, A., & Lynn, S. J. (1999). Creating a new childhood: Changing beliefs and memories through dream interpretation. *Applied Cognitive Psychology, 13,* 125–144.

Mazzoni, G. A., Lombardo, P., Malvagia, S., & Loftus, E. F. (1997). *Dream interpretation and false beliefs.* Unpublished manuscript, University of Florence and University of Washington.

Meiselman, K. (1990). *Resolving the trauma of incest: Reintegraton therapy with survivors.* San Francisco: Jossey-Bass.

Mills, A., & Lynn, S. J. (2000). Past-life experiences. In E. Cardeña, S. J. Lynn, & S. Krippner (Eds.), *The varieties of anomalous experience: Examining the scientific evidence* (pp. 283–314). Washington, DC: American Psychological Association.

Mulhern, S. (1992). Ritual abuse: Defining a syndrome versus defending a belief. *Journal of Psychology and Theology, 20,* 230–232.

Nadel, L., & Jacobs, J. W. (1998). Traumatic memory is special. *Current Directions in Psychological Science, 7,* 154–157.

Nash, M. R. (1987). What, if anything, is regressed about hypnotic age regression? A review of the empirical literature. *Psychological Bulletin, 102,* 42–52.

Nash, M. J., Drake, M., Wiley, R., Khalsa, S., & Lynn, S. J. (l986). The accuracy of recall of hypnotically age regressed subjects. *Journal of Abnormal Psychology, 95,* 298–300.

Olio, K. A. (1994). Truth in memory. *American Psychologist, 49,* 442–443.

Olson, H. A. (1979). The hypnotic retrieval of early recollections. In H. A. Olson (Ed.), *Early recollections: Their use in diagnosis and psychotherapy* (pp. 163–171). Springfield, IL: Charles C Thomas.

Paddock, R. J., Joseph, A. L., Chan, F. M., Terranova, S., Loftus, E. F., & Manning, C. (1998). When guided visualization procedures may backfire: Imagination inflation and predicting individual differences in suggestibility. *Applied Cognitive Psychology, 12,* 63–75.

Papanek, H. (1979). The use of early recollections in psychotherapy. In H. A. Olson (Ed.), *Early recollections: Their use in diagnosis and psychotherapy* (pp. 223–229). Springfield, IL: Charles C Thomas.

Payne, D. G., Neuschatz, J. S., Lampinen, J. M., & Lynn, S. J. (1997). Compelling memory illusions: The qualitative characteristics of false memories. *Current Directions in Psychological Science, 6,* 56–60.

Pezdek, K., Finger, K., & Hodge, D. (1997). Planting false childhood memories: The role of event plausibility. *Psychological Science, 8,* 437–441.

Polusny, M. A., & Follette, V. M. (1996). Remembering childhood sexual abuse: A national survey of psychologists' clinical practices, beliefs, and personal experiences. *Professional Psychology: Research and Practice, 27,* 41–52.

Poole, D. A., Lindsay, D. S., Memon, A., & Bull, R. (1995). Psychotherapists' opinions, practices, and experiences with recovery of memories of incestuous abuse. *Journal of Consulting and Clinical Psychology, 68,* 426–437.

Pope, K. S. (1996). Memory, abuse, and science: Questioning claims about the false memory syndrome epidemic. *American Psychologist, 51,* 957–974.

Pope, K. S., & Brown, L. S. (1996). *Recovered memories of abuse: Assessment, therapy, forensics.* Washington, DC: American Psychological Association.

Porter, S., Birt, A. R., Yuille, & Lehman, D. R. (2000). Negotiating false memories: Interviewer and rememberer characteristics relate to memory distortion. *Psychological Science, 11,* 507–510.

Porter, S., Yuille, J. C., & Lehman, D. R. (1999). The nature of real, implanted, and fabricated childhood emotional events: Implications for the recovered memory debate. *Law and Human Behavior, 23,* 517–537.

Rind, B., Tromovitch, P., & Bauserman, R. (1998). A meta-analytic examination of assumed properties of child sexual abuse using college samples. *Psychological Bulletin, 124,* 22–53.

Roediger, H. L. & McDermott, K. B. (1995). Creating false memories: Remembering words not presented in lists. *Journal of Experimental Psychology: Learning, Memory, and Cognition, 21,* 803–814.

Roland, C. B. (1993). Exploring childhood memories with adult survivors of sexual abuse: Concrete reconstruction and visualization techniques. *Journal of Mental Health Counseling, 15,* 363–372.

Schooler, J. W., Ambadar, Z., & Bendiksen, M. (1997). A cognitive corroborative case study approach for investigating discovered memories of sexual abuse. In J. D. Read & D. S. Lindsay (Eds.), *Recollections of trauma: Scientific research and clinical practice* (pp. 379–388). New York: Plenum Press.

Scoboria, A., Mazzoni, G., Kirsch, I., & Milling, L. S. (2002). Immediate and persisting effects of misleading questions and hypnosis on memory reports. *Journal of Experimental Psychology: Applied, 8,* 26–32.

Shobe, K. K., & Kihlstrom, J. F. (1997). Is traumatic memory special? *Current Directions in Psychological Science, 6,* 70–74.

Sivec, H. J., Lynn, S. J., & Malinoski, P. T. (1997a). *Early memory reports as a function of hypnotic and nonhypnotic age regression.* Unpublished manuscript, State University of New York at Binghamton.

Sivec, H. J., Lynn, S. J., & Malinoski, P. T. (1997b). *Hypnosis in the cabbage patch: Age regression with verifiable events.* Unpublished manuscript, State University of New York at Binghamton.

Spanos, N. P. (1996). *Multiple identities and false memories: A sociocognitive perspective.* Washington, DC: American Psychological Association.

Spanos, N. P., Burgess, C. A., & Burgess, M. F. (1994). Past life identities, UFO abductions, and satanic ritual abuse: The social construction of "memories. " *International Journal of Experimental and Clinical Hypnosis, 42,* 433–446.

Spanos, N. P., Burgess, C. A., Burgess, M. F., Samuels, C., & Blois, W. O. (1999). Creating false memories of infancy with hypnotic and nonhypnotic procedures. *Applied Cognitive Psychology, 13,* 201–218.

Spanos, N. P., Menary, E., Gabora, M. J., DuBreuil, S. C., & Dewhirst, B. (1991). Secondary identity enactments during hypnotic past-life regression: A sociocognitive perspective. *Journal of Personality and Social Psychology, 61,* 308–320.

Stampfl, T. G., & Levis, D. J. (1967). The essentials of implosive therapy: A learning-theory-based psychodynamic behavioral therapy. *Journal of Abnormal Psychology, 72,* 496–503.

Steblay, N. M., & Bothwell, R. K. (1994). Evidence for hypnotically refreshed testimony: The view from the laboratory. *Law and Human Behavior, 18*, 635–651.

Tavris, C. (1993, January 3). Beware the incest survivor machine. *New York Times Book Review*, pp. 1, 16–17.

van der Kolk, B. A. (1994). The body keeps the score: Memory and the evolving psychobiology of posttraumatic stress. *Harvard Review of Psychiatry, 1*, 253–265.

van der Kolk, B. A., Britz, R., Burr, W., Sherry, S., & Hartmann, E. (1994). Nightmares and trauma: A comparison of nightmares after combat with life-long nightmares in veterans. *American Journal of Psychiatry, 141*, 187–190.

van Husen, J. E. (1988). The development of fears, phobias, and restrictive patterns of adaptation following attempted abortions. *Pre- and Peri-Natal Psychology Journal, 2*, 179–185.

Weiland, I. H., & Steisel, I. M. (1958). An analysis of the manifest content of the earliest memories of children. *Journal of Genetic Psychology, 92*, 41–52.

Weiss, B. L. (1988). *Many lives, many masters*. New York: Simon & Schuster.

Whitehouse, W. G., Dinges, D. F., Orne, E. C., & Orne, M. T. (1988). Hypnotic hypermnesia: Enhanced memory accessibility or report bias? *Journal of Abnormal Psychology, 97*, 289–295.

Woolger, R. J. (1988). *Other lives, other selves: A Jungian psychotherapist discovers past lives*. New York: Bantam Books.

Yapko, M. D. (1994). Suggestibility and repressed memories of abuse: A survey of psychotherapists' beliefs. *American Journal of Clinical Hypnosis, 36*, 163–171.

PART III

CONTROVERSIES IN THE TREATMENT OF SPECIFIC ADULT DISORDERS

9

Novel and Controversial Treatments for Trauma-Related Stress Disorders

JEFFREY M. LOHR
WAYNE HOOKE
RICHARD GIST
DAVID F. TOLIN

The purpose of this chapter is to critically examine novel or controversial interventions for psychological trauma and its sequelae. Because the field of trauma treatment has recently witnessed a substantial increase in unusual treatments with questionable claims of efficacy, careful scrutiny of these treatments is warranted. We begin by discussing psychological trauma and its prevalence. We next describe the symptoms of posttraumatic stress disorder (PTSD), and discuss data concerning the risk of developing this disorder following a trauma. We outline current cognitive-behavioral theories of PTSD, and describe empirically supported treatments based on such theories. Finally, we describe a number of novel and controversial trauma interventions, including eye movement desensitization and reprocessing (EMDR), thought field therapy (TFT), and critical incident stress debriefing (CISD). We examine the theoretical and empirical bases of these three treatments and discuss the implications of their promotion for the field of clinical psychology.

TRAUMA AND ITS CONSEQUENCES

For purposes of the present review, we will define "trauma" according to Criterion A of the *Diagnostic and Statistical Manual of Mental Disorders*

243

(DSM-IV; American Psychiatric Association, 1994) criteria for PTSD. DSM-IV considers a person to have experienced a trauma when he or she: (1) experienced, witnessed, or was confronted with an event or events that involved actual or threatened death or serious injury, or a threat to the physical integrity of self or others, and (2) responded with intense fear, helplessness, or horror.

Epidemiological studies indicate that 50–70% of adults have experienced at least one such event in their lifetimes. The traumas experienced most frequently include violent death of a loved one, robbery, motor vehicle accidents, and physical assault (Breslau et al., 1998; Norris, 1992).

One potential consequence of traumatic experiences is PTSD. DSM-IV defines PTSD as consisting of the following core symptoms:

1. Mentally reexperiencing the traumatic event. Reexperiencing symptoms include recurrent and intrusive distressing recollections of the event, recurrent distressing dreams of the event, acting or feeling as if the event were happening again, or psychological or physiological distress when exposed to stimuli that remind the person of the traumatic event.

2. Avoidance of stimuli associated with the trauma, or numbing of general responsiveness. Symptoms in this category include efforts to avoid thoughts, feelings, or conversations associated with the trauma; efforts to avoid activities, places, or people that arouse recollections of the trauma; inability to recall an important aspect of the trauma; diminished interest in usual activities; feelings of detachment from others; restricted range of affect; and sense of a foreshortened future.

3. Increased arousal symptoms including sleep disturbance, irritability or anger outbursts, difficulty concentrating, hypervigilance, and exaggerated startle response.

In addition to these core symptoms, DSM-IV specifies that the symptoms must last at least 1 month and cause significant distress or functional impairment.

Studies of the general population indicate a lifetime prevalence of PTSD ranging from 1% (Davidson, Hughes, Blazer, & George, 1991) to 8% (Kessler, Sonnega, Bromet, Hughes, & Nelson, 1995). The conditional risk of developing PTSD following a trauma varies greatly, depending on the type of trauma. For males, combat and witnessing of violence are most likely to lead to PTSD; for females, rape and sexual molestation are most likely to lead to PTSD (Kessler et al., 1995).

COGNITIVE-BEHAVIORAL THEORIES OF PTSD

Although numerous psychosocial theories have been advanced to explain the etiology of PTSD, behavioral and cognitive models have the strongest empirical support and are more widely accepted in the scientific community than other models. The behavioral model of PTSD, as posited by Keane, Zimering, and Caddell (1985), suggests that traumatized individuals acquire conditioned fears of a wide assortment of trauma-related stimuli. Subsequently, they avoid these stimuli. Through the processes of higher-order conditioning and stimulus generalization, the number of feared stimuli continues to increase even after the trauma has occurred.

The cognitive model of PTSD articulated by Foa, Steketee, and Rothbaum (1989) holds that PTSD develops when the traumatic event reinforces negative beliefs concerning one's safety and competence. Individuals with PTSD may believe the world to be completely dangerous and therefore live in almost constant fear. They may also believe themselves to be incompetent and are reluctant to confront challenging situations. Other cognitive models focus on such basic cognitive processes such as attention and memory (e.g., Litz & Keane, 1989). According to these models, PTSD develops and/or is maintained when trauma- or threat-related information receives preferential information processing over less threatening information. This processing bias leads to distorted ways of perceiving and understanding the world.

TREATMENTS FOR PTSD BASED ON COGNITIVE-BEHAVIORAL THEORY

Cognitive and behavioral models of PTSD have informed several treatment approaches. We next describe those approaches with the strongest empirical support. We limit our literature review to randomized clinical trials (RCTs). These are efficacy studies in which research participants have been randomly assigned to treatment conditions, one of which is designed to control for possible artifacts of the treatment procedure. Although many different treatments have been described as "cognitive-behavioral," we limit our discussion to three broad classes of interventions: exposure therapy, cognitive therapy, and anxiety management training. These interventions have been subjected to the most empirical scrutiny, and have been identified by an expert consensus panel as treatments of choice for PTSD (Foa, Davidson, & Frances, 1999). For more thorough reviews of empirical studies of cognitive-behavioral therapy and other interventions, the reader is referred to Keane (1998) and Foa and Meadows (1997).

Exposure

Exposure-based treatments are predicated on the notion that exposure to feared stimuli facilitates habituation of conditioned fear. *Imaginal exposure* involves instructing the patient to imagine the traumatic event as vividly as possible. For example, a war veteran could be instructed to imagine his combat experiences in detail. In vivo exposure generally involves con structing a hierarchy of safe but avoided stimuli, and encouraging the patient to confront them gradually. For example, a rape victim who is afraid to stay home alone could be instructed to remain at home alone for progressively longer periods of time. Such terms as prolonged exposure or flooding are often used to describe imaginal and/or in vivo exposure exercises in which the exposure is applied for a prolonged period of time. *Systematic desensitization* pairs imaginal exposure with an anxiety-incompatible response, such as relaxation. Typically, the exposures in systematic desensitization are briefer than in imaginal exposure.

An early RCT of exposure for PTSD used imaginal exposure with combat veterans. Compared with a wait-list control condition, exposure produced greater reductions in PTSD symptom severity on both standardized measures and clinicians' ratings. Treatment gains were maintained at 6-month follow-up (Keane, Fairbank, Caddell, & Zimering, 1989). Similar results were reported by Brom, Kleber, and Defares (1989) using systematic desensitization for civilians who had undergone a variety of traumatic experiences. A treatment combining imaginal and in vivo exposure was also shown to be superior to supportive counseling and wait list, and marginally superior to anxiety management, for rape victims suffering from PTSD (Foa, Dancu, et al., 1999; Foa, Rothbaum, Riggs, & Murdock, 1991). In a mixed sample of civilians with PTSD, imaginal exposure was shown to be roughly equivalent to cognitive therapy (Tarrier et al., 1999). Combined imaginal and in vivo exposure was shown to be superior to wait list, comparable with cognitive therapy, and superior to relaxation training (Marks, Lovell, Noshirvani, Livanou, & Thrasher, 1998).

Cognitive Therapy

Cognitive therapy (CT) aims at modifying the dysfunctional beliefs associated with PTSD (e.g., Resick & Schnicke, 1992). Typically, the therapist engages patients in *Socratic dialogue*, through which patients learn to challenge the validity of their beliefs. For example, PTSD patients who believe that the world is completely dangerous might be encouraged to think of places and people that they consider safe. Often, *behavioral tests* are introduced to help determine whether the patient's beliefs are accurate. For example, patients who believe that they are incompetent could be encouraged to assume more responsibility. If they act in a competent manner, then this information is used to challenge their sense of personal incompetence.

CT has received less empirical investigation than has exposure, although two RCTs suggest that it can be efficacious for PTSD. Tarrier and colleagues (1999) compared CT with imaginal exposure for mixed civilian trauma; both groups showed significant and comparable symptom reduction. In another study, CT was shown to be superior to a wait list and to relaxation training, and comparable with combined imaginal and in vivo exposure (Marks et al., 1998).

Anxiety Management Training

Anxiety management training (AMT), also known as stress inoculation training, refers to an armamentarium of cognitive and behavioral strategies designed to reduce symptoms of anxiety, irritability, and hyperarousal. These techniques include *relaxation training*, in which patients are taught to reduce muscle tension; *breathing retraining*, which aims to prevent hyperventilation; *psychoeducation*, which involves teaching patients about normal responses to trauma; *self-instruction*, in which patients are taught to solve problems by "coaching" themselves mentally; *communication training*, which is aimed at improving social functioning; and *cognitive therapy*, which we described earlier. Some or all of these techniques could be included in a given AMT package.

AMT packages have been compared with exposure in two RCTs. Using a civilian sample of assault victims, Foa and colleagues (1991) showed that AMT reduced symptoms of PTSD, although the effects were slightly less than those produced by combined imaginal and in vivo exposure. In a later study, Foa, Dancu, and colleagues (1999) compared exposure, AMT, their combination, and a wait-list control using assault victims. AMT produced decreased symptoms of PTSD as shown by standardized measures, although exposure produced greater effects. Furthermore, combination therapy was no better than AMT and was less effective than exposure alone. This finding may have been due to the reduced number of exposure sessions in the combination treatment.

Summary and Conclusions

In summary, cognitive and behavioral models of PTSD have informed several specific treatments, including exposure, cognitive therapy, and anxiety management training. All three of these treatments have been demonstrated to reduce symptoms of PTSD compared with a wait-list control. Exposure and cognitive therapy have also been shown to be more efficacious than other treatments. For example, AMT's effects appear to be weaker than those of exposure and cognitive therapy. However, AMT may be useful in cases in which exposure and cognitive therapy are not feasible or contraindicated (e.g., with patients who are acutely suicidal or otherwise unstable), or as an adjunct to such treatments, provided that it does not replace more effective techniques.

RCTs comparing cognitive-behavioral interventions with control treatments are particularly informative, as they help differentiate the specific factors in cognitive-behavioral therapy from "nonspecific" factors (see

Chapter 6). Specific factors are those directly identified with the therapeutic intervention—for example, repeated exposure to trauma-related stimuli, cognitive restructuring, or the teaching of anxiety management strategies. In addition to these specific factors, however, all therapeutic interventions also contain nonspecific factors that are not associated with any single intervention, but may be common to several treatments and may have therapeutic effects of their own. Some nonspecific factors include the passage of time, deciding to seek professional help, receiving attention from a caring professional, and the expectation that one's personal problems will improve.

One kind of nonspecific factor effect is the "placebo" effect, which involves the belief that a specific intervention will cause a problem to improve (see Chapters 6 and 11). As with other nonspecific factors, the placebo effect can by itself be powerful. Strong placebo effects have been noted for psychological problems (Eysenck, 1994) and even for such ailments such as asthma, ulcers, and herpes (Roberts, Kewman, Mercier, & Hovell, 1993). Frequently, part of effective psychotherapy involves capitalizing on these nonspecific factors in order to maximize therapeutic benefit (e.g., Frank, 1974). However, in research, nonspecific factors and their effects often obscure the specific effects of a particular treatment, rendering it difficult to evaluate whether patients improved due to the treatment itself or other nonspecific factors. Comparisons with control conditions, such as those described in this section, help to support the conclusion that cognitive-behavioral interventions lead to improvements that cannot be attributed solely to nonspecific factors. That is, the interventions describe appear to be therapeutically potent (for a more complete discussion of nonspecific treatment factors and their psychotherapeutic effects, see Lohr, Lilienfeld, Tolin, & Herbert; 1999).

NOVEL TREATMENTS FOR ANXIETY AND TRAUMA

Several novel treatments vying for the attention of clinicians treating anxiety and trauma have been referred to as "power therapies" (Figley, 1997). This moniker derives from the claim that such treatments work much more efficiently than extant interventions for anxiety disorders and exert their effects through processes distinctly different from psychological insight or learning (Gallo, 1995, 1998). The power therapies include eye movement desensitization and reprocessing (EMDR; Shapiro, 1995), thought field therapy (TFT; R. Callahan, 1995b; Gallo, 1995, 1998), emotional freedom therapy (EFT; Craig, 1997), critical incident stress debriefing (CISD; Mitchell, 1983); traumatic incident reduction (TIR; Gerbode, 1995), and visual/kinesthetic dissociation (V/KD; Bandler & Grinder, 1979). Because of the virtually complete absence of research evidence for EFT, TIR, and V/

KD, we focus primarily on EMDR, TFT, and CISD (see Wylie, 1996, for descriptions of the procedures involved in TIR and V/KD).

EMDR

Treatment Description and Rationale

The most visible of these novel treatments is EMDR. In the 13 years since its inception (Shapiro, 1989), the commercialization of EMDR has been remarkably successful. According to Francine Shapiro (1998b), the developer of EMDR, over 30,000 mental health clinicians have been trained in this procedure. The EMDR Institute, Inc., maintains an extensive training schedule for two levels of training (www.emdr.org). In addition, the EMDR International Association (EMDRIA) holds numerous training and research conferences, and administers a worldwide humanitarian assistance program (www.emdria.org). In addition, EMDR has been directly publicized to the consuming public through trade books (Shapiro & Forrest, 1997). EMDR has also been the subject of numerous television programs, including ABC News' *20/20* (see Lilienfeld, 1996).

EMDR uses a structured, prescriptive intervention procedure that incorporates such general clinical components as history taking and verbal report of the nature and emotional consequences of the traumatic experience. In addition, the EMDR procedure requires the client to construct and maintain both an imaginal representation of a memory (or other image) and the physical sensations associated with the traumatic event. While maintaining the image, the therapist induces a series of side-to-side eye movements by asking the client to visually track the therapist's finger across the visual field. The client is asked to express the negative cognitions that accompany the affective distress, and to generate a more positive appraisal about the trauma and the client's experience with it. This component is referred to as "reprocessing" and is added to the desensitization that accompanies the imaginal exposure (Shapiro, 1991; see Tolin, Montgomery, Kleinknecht, & Lohr, 1995, for a more complete summary of the procedure).

EMDR is based on a set of theoretical conjectures that rely heavily on physiological concepts closely related to neurological processes. The nature of trauma pathology and its effective treatment is predicated on a model called accelerated information processing, which is ostensibly akin to a psychological immune system (Shapiro, 1995, p. 31). Healing is posited to occur after eye movements and other features of the clinical protocol "unlock" the pathological condition. The accelerated information processing model defines pathology as "dysfunctionally stored information that can be properly assimilated through a dynamically activated processing system" (Shapiro, 1995, p. 52). Although this neurophysiological speculation has superficial appeal, Keane (1998) noted that the theoretical formulation of EMDR bears little connection with existing models of psychopathology and psychotherapy, and is inconsistent with the body of knowledge gleaned from experimental psychology regarding the nature, acquisition, and modification of fear and anxiety.

Literature reviews of the efficacy of EMDR (Cahill, Carrigan, & Frueh, 1999; DeBell & Jones, 1997; Lohr, Tolin, & Lilienfeld, 1998; Lohr et al., 1999) have questioned the efficacy of EMDR in light of methodological limitations in studies that purported to show clinical effects (Shapiro, 1996). An examination of the methodological issues will aid in the evaluation of EMDR's efficacy for the sequelae of traumatic experience. There are several methodological issues to be considered, including the rigor of the control for procedural artifacts, the control for nonspecific factors, and component controls for the active ingredients of the treatment procedures.

Controls for Effects of Nonspecific Factors in Treatment

Nonspecific factors in an experimental treatment procedure include the incidental effects of treatment, such as measurement reactivity, credibility, expectation for improvement, experimental demand, therapist–experimenter enthusiasm, and therapist–experimenter allegiance. It is reasonable to presume that structured, prescriptive treatments that do not have empirical support for the disorders to which they are applied could serve as comparative control conditions to assess the substantive treatment effects of EMDR beyond shared nonspecific factors (Lohr et al., 1999).

EMDR has been compared with image habituation training and applied muscle relaxation (Vaughan et al., 1994), biofeedback and group-administered relaxation training (Silver, Brooks, & Obenchain, 1995), health management organization treatment (Marcus, Marquis, & Sakai, 1997), and routine Veterans Hospital care or biofeedback-assisted relaxation (Carlson, Chemtob, Rusnak, Hedlund, & Muraoka, 1998; Jensen, 1994). The same results were obtained when EMDR was compared with a credible attention control for the treatment of panic disorder (Goldstein, de Beurs, Chambless, & Wilson, 2000). These several studies provide little evidence that EMDR results in benefits beyond client expectation of improvement, therapeutic attention, nonspecific factors, and/or the imagery exposure that is incidental to EMDR (see Lohr, Kleinknecht, Tolin, & Barrett, 1995; Lohr et al., 1998, 1999, for more detailed critiques).

EMDR Component Controls

The theoretical conjectures underlying EMDR's efficacy are based on the importance of eye movements or other alternating/bilateral stimulation

such as finger taps. Shapiro (1994a, 1994b, 1995) suggested that other external stimulation has the same effect as induced eye movements, but has
not specified the neurophysiological mechanisms that make them function-
ally equivalent in activating the putative curative phenomenon of accelerated information processing. Nonetheless, the experimental analysis of
EMDR efficacy should take into account the possibility of such equivalence and include experimental control conditions that address the equivalence hypothesis.

The most important experimental controls for rigorous tests of treatment components rely on additive and subtractive experimental designs
(Cahill et al., 1999; Mahoney, 1978; Nezu, 1986; Nezu & Perri, 1989).
These "dismantling" designs are necessary to identify the components that
are specific to EMDR and the nonspecific factors (e.g., placebo effects) that
are common to all treatments or components that are specific to other effective treatments (Lohr et al., 1999; see also Chapter 6).

Boudewyns, Stwertka, Hyer, Albrecht, and Sperr (1993) randomly assigned Veterans Hospital patients to either EMDR, exposure control (EC),
or a hospital-milieu-only control. The EC group was procedurally similar
to the EMDR group except for eye movements. Standardized measures
showed no significant differential effects of treatment, and no form of
treatment appeared to affect scores on psychophysiological measures. Although therapist ratings of treatment responders versus nonresponders favored the EMDR group, assessors of treatment outcome were not blind to
treatment conditions.

Renfrey and Spates (1994) recruited 23 trauma victims, 21 of whom
met diagnostic criteria for PTSD. Participants were randomly assigned to
one of three conditions: standard EMDR, an EMDR analogue in which
eye movements were induced by an optical device alternating the position
of a light in the right and left peripheral visual field, and an EMDR analogue in which a light blinked in the center of the visual field. Dependent
variables included subjective ratings of discomfort, changes in heart rate,
and standardized measures of PTSD symptoms. After treatment, 5 of the
23 participants met criteria for PTSD and were roughly distributed evenly
across treatment groups. Analyses of heart rate and subjective ratings revealed significant main effects for repeated assessment but no interaction
between assessment and treatment condition. Analyses of the standardized
measures were not reported. Thus, it appears that the general EMDR procedure, rather than saccadic eye movements per se, are responsible for reductions in self-report indices and heart rate. However, the control conditions did not directly control for measurement reactivity or nonspecific
treatment factors.

Boudewyns and Hyer (1996) compared EMDR with a no-movement
imagery analogue (EC) and a no-imagery control (C) procedure in the

treatment of combat-related PTSD. All subjects received eight sessions of the standard inpatient or outpatient PTSD treatment program at a Veterans Administration hospital. Participants in the EMDR and EC groups received between five and eight sessions of EMDR. The EC subjects did not engage in eye movements during individual treatment but kept their eyes closed and engaged in imaginal exposure for the same period of time. Participants in the no-imagery control (C) condition received only the standard group treatment. Outcome measures included the Clinician Administered PTSD Scale (CAPS), Impact of Event Scale (IES) scores, Profile of Mood States—Anxiety (POMS-A), subjective distress ratings, and Heart Rate (HR) in response to a tape-recorded script of the participant's most disturbing memory. All measures were obtained before and after treatment by a clinician blind to experimental condition.

The statistical analyses revealed that the EMDR and the EC conditions showed greater change than the control condition on subjective distress ratings, POMS-A, and HR. Nevertheless, the EMDR and EC conditions did not differ from one another. In addition, the analyses indicated that the three groups showed equal change on the CAPS and that all groups showed no significant change on IES scores. Thus, it appears that neither eye movements nor any lateral stimulation was necessary for measured change, and that imagery exposure may be sufficient for change on some indices of PTSD.

Pitman and colleagues (1996) used a crossover design in which combat-related PTSD patients were randomly assigned to one of two treatment sequences using EMDR or a no-movement imagery analogue (fixed-eye) treatment. The analogue control procedure consisted of all EMDR components, including movement of the therapist's hand. The participant, however, maintained eye fixation and tapped one finger to correspond to therapist hand movement. Each treatment was applied for a maximum of six sessions once per week. Treatment efficacy variables included subjective distress ratings and four psychophysiological indices: HR, skin conductance, and two electromyographic measures. Treatment outcome measures included Impact of Events Scale (IES) Intrusion and Avoidance scores on two images, Mississippi-PTSD scores, Symptom CheckList–90–Revised (SCL-90-R) scores, Clinician-Administered PTSD Scale (CAPS) score, and a cued intrusive thought log.

Analyses of variance between treatment conditions showed no significant differences between treatment conditions on psychophysiological measures. The results showed that on outcome variables, there was limited change (only three of eight measures) within each of the procedures. The use of the control procedure suggests that eye movements confer no clear advantage over other forms of stimulation. Macklin and colleagues (2000) later reported that all of the participants exposed to EMDR had returned to pretreatment levels of PTSD symptomatology 5 years after the completion of treatment.

Devilly, Spence, and Rapee (1998) compared EMDR with a no-movement imagery analogue condition that was presented to participants as "reactive eye dilation desensitization and reprocessing," which involved the full EMDR protocol except that a flashing light was substituted for lateral eye movements. Both treatments were compared with a no extra treatment control condition that included the same assessment battery as the treatment conditions. Treatment outcome measures included standardized anxiety, depression, and PTSD scales, as well as HR and blood pressure. The results showed that both treatment groups improved by posttreatment, but that there was no significant difference between the two treatment conditions. Participants in the two treatment conditions did not differ significantly on standardized measures from the control condition, but did improve more than the control condition when the reliability change index on the Mississippi-PTSD scale was examined. Nevertheless, there was no statistical or clinical difference in symptoms from pretreatment to 6-month follow-up. The authors concluded that eye movements are not the agent of change and that other nonspecific factors are responsible for the high levels of efficacy reported in previous EMDR research conducted without adequate procedural controls.

One apparent exception to these findings is a study by Wilson, Silver, Covi, and Foster (1996), who reported evidence that eye movements contribute to EMDR's efficacy. However, this study was seriously flawed on methodological grounds, including assignment of subjects to treatment conditions, confounding of treatment conditions with the method of assessing efficacy, and inappropriate statistical analyses (see Lohr et al., 1998, pp. 140–142, for a more detailed critique).

Cusack and Spates (1999) recruited community members who reported the experience of a traumatic event and met diagnostic criteria for at least two of the three main symptom clusters for PTSD. Participants were randomly assigned to EMDR or to the same procedure without the cognitive reprocessing elements, namely, composition of a positive attribution regarding the traumatic event and its "installation" following eye movements. Analyses of standardized symptom measures revealed reductions in both groups but no significant differential effects between groups, indicating no additional effect of the reprocessing component.

The overall conclusion that can be drawn from the component-controlled efficacy studies is that eye movements, alternative stimulation, or cognitive reprocessing do not provide any incremental clinical efficacy. Thus, it is reasonable to conclude that any measurable change following EMDR is most likely a function of the imagery exposure that is incidental to EMDR (Muris & Merckelbach, 1997). The same shared process appears to be at work when comparing EMDR with in-vivo exposure (Muris, Merckelbach, Holdrinet, & Sijsenaar, 1998; Muris, Merckelbach, van Haaften, & Mayer, 1997).

Comparison with Validated Treatments or Components of Validated Treatments

Rogers and colleagues (1999) randomly assigned 12 veterans with combat-related PTSD to either one session of EMDR or one session of imaginal exposure (Lyons & Keane, 1989). The standardized outcome measure was IES score, and HR was included as a psychophysiological measure. Data analyses showed that total IES scores were reduced in both conditions following treatment but that those reductions did not achieve statistical significance at the $p > .05$ level. The same findings were obtained for IES Intrusion and Avoidance subscale scores. Although HR was reduced in both groups, there was no significant difference between groups.

Devilly and Spence (1999) compared EMDR with a cognitive-behavioral treatment (Foa et al., 1991) for PTSD. Participants diagnosed with PTSD were assessed for PTSD symptoms with self-report and clinician-administered questionnaires and then randomly assigned to either EMDR or cognitive-behavioral therapy (CBT), which consisted of prolonged imaginal exposure, stress inoculation training, and cognitive restructuring. All participants received nine sessions of treatment. Treatments were videotaped for treatment fidelity and participants were assessed before and immediately after treatment, as well as at a 1-year follow-up. The results showed that CBT was statistically and clinically more efficacious than EMDR at both posttreatment and follow-up. Although the two treatments were rated as equally distressing, CBT was rated as more credible and generated higher expectancies for change.

EMDR as a Novel and Distinct Treatment

The findings from the best available efficacy studies are clear: (1) The effects of EMDR as a distinct treatment are limited largely to verbal report indices; (2) the observed effects of EMDR are consistent with nonspecific factors; (3) eye movements and other methods of lateral stimulation are unnecessary for clinical improvement; and (4) any effects of EMDR may be the result of imagery exposure, which EMDR shares with standard behavioral treatments. Moreover, comparisons with effective treatment or effective treatment components show the relative effects of EMDR to be weak or negligible. The scientific status of the efficacy of eye movement desensitization and reprocessing has perhaps been best summarized by McNally (1999): "What is effective in EMDR is not new, and what is new is not effective" (p. 619).

In response to findings that eye movements are irrelevant to the efficacy of EMDR and the absence of compelling scientific evidence that EMDR is more efficacious than extant empirically supported techniques, some proponents of EMDR have made ad hoc modifications (see Chapter 1) to the hypothesized mechanisms of clinical change. For example,

Shapiro (personal communication, August 20, 1996) argued that eye movements are not necessary for EMDR's efficacy: "EMDR is not simply eye movement. Eye movement, or other stimulation is merely one component of a complex method that combines aspects of many of the major modalities. That is why behaviorists, cognitivists, psychodynamic [sic], etc. . . . are able to find EMDR useful. Remove the eye movement and there is still a very powerful method."

Such statements obfuscate the empirical and theoretical issues. If eye movements are not necessary for EMDR's efficacy, then it is incumbent on EMDR's proponents to specify the essential features of the treatment to permit the conduct of controlled experiments assessing the relative effects of procedural artifacts and the substantive clinical procedure (Grünbaum, 1985). Without a clear specification of the necessary (characteristic) features of treatment, any number of convenient ad hoc accounts can be advanced to explain away disconfirmatory evidence. Under such conditions, the theory may be difficult or impossible to test unless much more specific predictions are advanced (see Herbert et al., 2000, for a more complete discussion of these issues; see also Chapter 1).

Thought Field Therapy

Treatment Description

Thought field therapy (TFT), known previously as the "Callahan techniques" (R. Callahan, 1994), is a unique treatment that has been used for a variety of anxiety disorders and other emotional conditions. TFT has slowly attracted the attention of practitioners over the last 20 years (R. Callahan, 1981), but is now expanding at a more rapid rate due in part to promotion over Internet Websites and listserves. Much, but not all, of this attention comes from clinicians and researchers seeking more effective means of treating the aftermath of psychological trauma. TFT workshops are routinely offered in major American cities (American Psychological Association, 1996). As more practitioners have learned and applied the technique, it has come to the attention of researchers (Figley & Carbonell, 1999).

The "thought field" is posited to be both the locus of psychopathology and the vehicle for therapeutic change. It has been described thus (J. Callahan, 1998):

> A "field," in scientific terms, is defined as "an invisible sphere of influence"; magnetic fields and gravitational fields being familiar examples. In this case, when we *think* about a situation a Thought Field (a manifestation of the body's energy system) becomes active. Effectively, the Thought Field has been "tuned in" to that specific thought. The body responds to its influence by reproducing, to a greater or lesser extent, the nervous, hormonal, and cognitive activity that occurs when we are in the real situation.

If that Thought Field contains perturbations then the body response is in-appropriate." (p. 2)

The treatment protocol is directed at the removal of these perturbations. The TFT procedure combines the metacognition of thinking about a distressing problem with the palpation (tapping) of specific points on the body in order to eliminate psychological distress.

The technique is applied in conjunction with a number of procedural variations called "algorithms." The algorithms consist of a series of activities that are followed in prescriptive fashion, with different algorithms for different emotional problems. The algorithm for psychological trauma (R. Callahan, 1995b; C. R. Figley, personal communication, November 27, 1995) consists of a number of steps. First, the client "attunes" to the thought field. That is, the client is placed in the distressing situation or thinks about this situation. Clients then rate their self-perceived level of anxiety using a subjective units of distress scale (SUDs) rating on a 10-point Likert scale. Clients are then tapped with two fingertips (or tap themselves) on a variety of points on the face, hands, and body while remaining attuned to the thought field. Following the tapping, the individual takes a deep breath and provides another SUDs rating. The algorithm continues, adding tapping on a specific point on the back of the hand (referred to as the gamut spot) while performing a variety of activities, such as rolling the eyes, humming a happy tune, and counting. The algorithm ends by repeating the tapping and SUDs rating procedures. Normally, the algorithm is repeated at least four times. Other problems are treated by different algorithms that modify the order of the points that are tapped, and by tapping at different points.

TFT Rationale

The rationale for TFT is that negative emotions are caused not by neurochemical or cognitive processes, but by disruptions in the body's bioenergic system (R. Callahan, 1995b). The proponents of TFT contend that tapping on acupoints directly modifies a hypothetical bioenergic system by means of a transduction of the mechanical energy of the tapping directly into bioenergy (R. Callahan, personal communication, February 4, 1996; Gallo, 1995). The specific places on the face, limbs, and body that are tapped during the algorithms are said to be the traditional points needled by acupuncturists. Acupuncturists have explained the therapeutic effect of the needling of acupoints as a correction of the flow of chi (the energy of yin/yang) throughout the body. It is alleged that chi flows through the body along channels known as meridians. Although many acupuncture practitioners assume the existence of such meridians, no convincing scientific evidence has been found in support of their existence (Stux & Pomeranz,

1995). Nonetheless, the prescriptive algorithms require that tapping occur at the acupoints and in precise sequences (R. Callahan, 1995b).

The TFT rationale is based on four fundamental components: (1) the existence of meridians that act as a bioenergic bodily control system, (2) the tapping (palpation) of acupoints as a means of transducing mechanical/kinetic energy into the energy of the meridian system, (3) the existence of reversed electrical polarity within this system, and (4) the correction of this reversed polarity by means of psychological techniques. The theory asserts that small bioenergic perturbations (disturbances, blockages, or imbalances) at specific points along the energy meridians cause negative emotions. Tapping the acupoints provides the transformation of the meridian energy, which then removes or transforms the blockages, thereby eliminating the negative emotion and its corresponding pathology (R. Callahan & J. Callahan, 1996).

An additional construct derived from the bioenergic system is that of "psychological reversal." TFT practitioners sometimes report that tapping at the appropriate points along the meridians fails to correct the energy flow. Such failures are explained by an appeal to psychological reversal, which is a harmful condition in which the normal flow of energy in the meridian system is reversed. R. Callahan (1995a) suggested that psychological reversal is a pathological condition responsible for the development of such diverse phenomena as dyslexia, the supposed paradoxical response of children with attention-deficit/hyperactivity disorder to methylphenidate (see Chapter 12), and cancer. The broad application of a bioelectric hypothesis to such varied clinical phenomena must be viewed as highly speculative in the absence of direct evidence. There is no scientific evidence that extracellular bioelectric currents are pathological mechanisms of emotional disorder, nor is there evidence that TFT reverses such currents.

Summary of Efficacy Research

Although TFT has been promoted as an effective treatment for virtually every emotional disorder, including PTSD (J. Callahan, 1998), there is only one published study in which TFT has been applied to traumatic memories (but not to PTSD per se; Figley & Carbonell, 1999). The scientific claim of TFT's efficacy for all emotional disorders is based on four studies, one of which is available only from the authors (Wade, 1990), one of which is in a proprietary archive (R. Callahan, 1987), one of which is published in a TFT newsletter (Leonoff, 1995), and only one of which is published in a peer-reviewed journal (Figley & Carbonell, 1999). Callahan (1987) and Leonoff (1995) used callers to radio talk shows as participants and reported reductions in average self-reported SUD ratings following treatment. However, the method of sampling research participants allows for self-selection bias and fails to control for demand characteristics. The measurement of clinical effects is limited by the use of a nonstandardized outcome measure and the absence of any meaningful quantification of change, much less an acceptable statistical analysis with which to infer that change occurred. Finally, the absence of any control condition renders the reported results essentially uninterpretable.

An unpublished doctoral dissertation by Wade (1990) evaluated the effects of TFT on self-concept in the treatment of specific phobia. Participants were recruited from a university community and administered an unspecified rating scale of fear intensity. Potential participants were not formally assessed for phobic symptoms nor was there any formal diagnostic evaluation. Participants were nonrandomly assigned to a TFT condition that was administered in a group setting, and another series of participants underwent only the assessment procedure. Self-concept was assessed before and after treatment with two self-report questionnaires. Between-group by pre–post analyses of variance were conducted on seven self-concept scales.

The analyses revealed only two statistically significant interactions that are required for between-group comparisons following treatment. Subsequent analyses of the interactions revealed only 2 statistically significant differences in favor of TFT out of a total of 14 possible comparisons. Moreover, the serious limitations of the experimental and control procedure may have resulted in confounds that could account for the minimal statistical significance observed.

Figley and Carbonell (1999) reported an uncontrolled investigation of the clinical efficacy of TFT and EMDR, as well as two other techniques mentioned earlier, TIR and V/KD. Clients at a trauma treatment center were preselected to participate in the demonstration and were nonrandomly assigned to one of the four treatments based on the next available treatment practitioner. Although some participants may have met diagnostic criteria for PTSD, their inclusion in the treatment protocol did not require it. Twelve of 39 subjects were assigned to TFT and completed the protocol. Eight subjects were available for a 6-month follow-up assessment using standardized outcome measures. The authors reported that participants experienced reduced subjective reports of emotional discomfort and lower standardized questionnaire indices of PTSD symptoms following TFT. However, there were no formal statistical tests performed, and there was no control group with which to compare TFT.

It is evident that the scientific research on TFT is minimal in both quantity and quality despite the expansive claims of effectiveness for trauma symptoms made by its promoters (American Psychological Association, 1996; J. Callahan, 1998; Gallo, 1995). Moreover, this conclusion has been arrived at by other reviewers (Gaudiano & Herbert, 2000; Hooke, 1998). The scientific evidence for other "energy" techniques based loosely on TFT, such as emotional freedom technique (Craig, 1997), is even weaker.

The discrepancy between the promotional claims and the scientific evidence for TFT has prompted actions to improve the professional accountability of TFT promoters and practitioners (see also Chapter 7). The first was the action of a state licensing board (Arizona Board of Psychologist Examiners, 1999) that reprimanded a psychologist who used TFT as his principal therapeutic modality. Foremost among the reasons for the Board's action was the psychologist's inability to substantiate the advertised claims of effectiveness (American Psychological Association; 1996; see Lilienfeld & Lohr, 2000, for a more detailed discussion of the issues involved in the decision). The second was the action of the Continuing Professional Education Committee of the American Psychological Association in ruling that the absence of any compelling scientific support for TFT's efficacy rendered this treatment an inappropriate subject for continuing education (American Psychological Association, 1999).

Critical Incident Stress Debriefing

Intervention Rationale

Both EMDR and TFT are promoted as treatments for extant trauma-related symptoms and syndromes. However, there also exist psychosocial interventions that are intended to prevent the development of disorders following exposure to traumatic events among civilians in general, and among those who have a high probability of exposure to such events. These latter groups include fire, police, and emergency service personnel. The most widely promoted of these preventative interventions is critical incident stress debriefing (CISD; Mitchell, 1983, 1988b; Mitchell & Everly, 1993, 1995, 1998).

CISD is predicated on two basic assumptions: first, that exposure to traumatic life events is a sufficient precursor for the development of psychological symptoms that can readily grow to pathological proportions, and, second, that early and proximal intervention, often presumed to involve some element of emotional catharsis, is necessary for prevention of such sequelae and the amelioration of such sequelae should they occur. These propositions have spawned a movement toward aggressive attempts at mental health prophylaxis, typically through the importation of practitioner treatment teams to the scenes of disaster.

The notion of "psychological debriefing" entered the lexicon from several sources (see, e.g., Stuhlmiller & Dunning, 2000, for a historical overview of its various geneses). It was popularized by Mitchell (1983), a paramedic instructor, for application to members of the emergency services occupations as an immediate prophylactic response to prevent the presumed ill effects of occupational exposure to stressful career events. The original notions and techniques were variations of basic rubrics associated with crisis intervention center and suicide hotline programs of the 1970s (Echterling & Wylie, 1981; Gist & Woodall, 1995, 1999; Gist, Woodall, & Magenheimer, 1999).

CISD arose as an easily implemented remedy for a commonly perceived need within a readily defined group. The early renditions were disseminated principally through trade venues (e.g., conference presentations and, somewhat later, trade magazines) and evolved into proprietary training seminars, geared primarily toward "peer providers" but also including some mental health professionals. As the procedure became more widely promoted, so did the claims of its breadth of applicability, its clinical and preventative efficacy, and its purported empirical grounding (Mitchell, 1992). In the process, Mitchell (1988a, 1988b, 1992) promoted it as an indispensable preventive intervention for PTSD. He asserted that CISD is a tested and proven approach, that it is the only way to deliver the appropriate kind of help, and that other approaches might even engender harm (Mitchell, 1992).

Intervention Procedure

CISD is conducted in groups and is administered within 24–72 hours following a stressful event (Mitchell, 1983, 1988a, Mitchell & Bray, 1990; Mitchell & Everly, 1993, 1995). The intervention strategy is a version of standard group counseling (cf. Corsey, 1995) that is based on the premise that group disclosure produces beneficial effects (primarily, normalization). The CISD protocol follows seven steps: (1) introduction of the debriefing, (2) statement of facts regarding the nature of the traumatic event, (3) disclosure of thoughts regarding the event, (4) disclosure of emotional reactions (specifically focused on those with the strongest negative valence), (5) specification of possible symptoms, (6) education regarding consequences of trauma exposure, (7) planned reentry to the social context (Mitchell & Everly, 1993).

The intervention is conducted by a mental health provider with the help of trained peers. The group experience generally lasts from 2 to 3 hours. Attendance by emergency service personnel is frequently mandatory. More specifically, election to discontinue participation is actively discouraged, even to the point of retrieving by the peer facilitator those workers who choose to terminate participation in the debriefing.

Efficacy Research

Gist, Lubin, and Redburn (1998) investigated the structure and efficacy of debriefing following the crash of a wide-bodied airliner in Sioux City in which 112 of 296 passengers died. The findings of that study, including a nearly complete sample of career firefighters engaged in body recovery and related operations, showed no clinically significant impact on personnel at 2 years post-incident, no evidence of superior resolution for debriefed responders versus those who declined, a slight but statistically significant trend toward worsening in resolution indices for those accepting debriefing, and a clear preference for informal sources of support and assistance that correlated strongly with effective resolution. Other studies have reported similar findings (Alexander & Wells, 1991; Fullerton, Wright, Ursano, & McCarroll, 1993; Hytten & Hasle, 1989; McFarlane, 1988) and have drawn similar conclusions (Bisson, Jenkins, Alexander, & Bannister, 1997; Carlier, Lamberts, van Uchlen, & Gersons, 1998; Deahl, Gillham, Thomas, Dearle, & Strinivasan, 1994; Griffiths & Watts, 1992; Hobbs, Mayou, Harrison, & Worlock, 1996; Kenardy et al., 1996; Lee, Slade, & Lygo, 1996; Stephens, 1997).

The most recent peer-reviewed study (Mayou, Ehlers, & Hobbs, 2000) reported a 3-year follow-up from a randomized controlled trial of debriefing following motor vehicle accident injuries wherein patients who received the intervention fared worse on several measures. Most tellingly, those who initially had high levels of avoidance and intrusion symptoms remained symptomatic if they had received debriefing, but recovered if they had not. The authors of this study concluded that "psychological debriefing is ineffective and has adverse long-term effects. It is not an appropriate treatment for trauma victims" (p. 589).

Questions and concerns arising from the lack of empirical support to justify CISD's extensive promotion and the steady accumulation of data suggesting it to be inert at best and iatrogenic at worst have led to cautionary editorials and critical reviews in a number of venues (Avery & Orner, 1998; Bisson & Deahl, 1994; Deahl & Bisson, 1995; Foa & Meadows, 1997; Gist, 1996; Kenardy, 1998; Kenardy & Carr, 1996; Ostrow, 1996; Raphael, Meldrum, & McFarlane, 1995; Rose & Bisson, 1999). Although the promotion of CISD continues with little diminution, the debate in the scientific community is all but over. The prestigious Cochrane Reviews on the topic of psychological debriefing (Wessley, Rose, & Bisson, 2000) offered this decisive conclusion: "There is no current evidence that psychological debriefing is a useful treatment of posttraumatic stress disorder after traumatic incidents. Compulsory debriefing of victims of trauma should cease" (On-line, p. 1).

IMPLICATIONS

It is clear that there is insufficient empirical evidence to support the use of EMDR, TFT, or CISD as standard treatments for PTSD or trauma sequelae.

We believe the widespread application of these treatments can be partially accounted for by the pseudoscientific manner in which these treatments have been promoted to mental health practitioners and the consuming public.

The discrepancy between the meager research support and the extensive promotion of EMDR, TFT, and CISD may be due in part to improper allocation of the burden of proof. McFall (1991) argued that the burden of proof of positive effects should rest squarely on those who implement and promote novel therapies (see also Chapter 1). Thus, it is reasonable to expect proponents of new treatments to answer clearly and convincingly such questions as:

- "Does your treatment work better than no treatment?"
- "Does your treatment work better than a placebo?"
- "Does your treatment work better than standard treatments?"
- "Does your treatment work through the processes you claim it does?"

Affirmative answers to these questions require high-quality evidence, and the burden of proof ought not be placed on those who raise the questions. It is our opinion that the proponents of EMDR, TFT, and CISD have not met their reasonable burden of evidence, but have often acted as though they have (R. Callahan, 1995b; Mitchell, 1998; Mitchell & Everly, 1997, 1998; F. Shapiro, personal communication, August 20, 1996, and August 6, 1998; Shapiro, 1995, 1998).

If EMDR, TFT, and CISD were the only treatments being commercially promoted for trauma, the task of empirical evaluation would be large but not insurmountable. It would take time and professional resources to rectify the commercial excesses, but the effort would be worth the likely outcome. For example, several years elapsed following the introduction of facilitated communication for the treatment of severe autistic and developmental disorders before its empirical debunking was convincing (Delmolino & Romanczyck, 1995; Jacobson, Mulick, & Schwartz, 1995, see Chapter 13). There are, however, a large number of largely or entirely unvalidated therapies being actively marketed to those providing traumatology services (Deitrich et al., 2000). These interventions represent a cottage industry that is being actively promoted to the mental health profession through workshop training that is largely outside the context of substantive evaluation (C. R. Figley, personal communication, November 27, 1995; Figley, 1997; Figley & Carbonell, 1999).

How are clinical psychologists to understand the phenomena of EMDR, TFT, and CISD? We suggest that the field of psychotherapy has been insufficiently rigorous regarding the evidentiary credentials of psychotherapeutic procedures (Borkovec & Castonguay, 1998; Hazlett-

Stevens & Borkovec, 1998). The treatments discussed here appear to possess the outward form of science but little of its substance. The appearance of science, such as case studies reported in peer-reviewed journals, selective publicity of weak tests of effectiveness, scientific-sounding jargon, and seemingly cautious promotion ("only clinicians with sanctioned training should use it") serve to obscure their lack of scientific substance and have persuaded many of the scientific legitimacy of such treatments (see also Chapter 1). However, the professional evaluation of treatments must rest upon the substantive aspects of the scientific enterprise, rather than on superficial appearance. If pretensions to science are emphasized over substance, the process of inquiry itself risks becoming pseudoscientific.

We argue that the promotion of some novel trauma treatments are characterized by pseudoscientific practices (see also Herbert et al., 2000). Although these practices have resulted in substantial financial return for the promoters, we believe the costs of adopting pseudoscientific treatments have been substantial for both consumers and the profession.

Scientific research has revealed a number of efficacious treatment procedures for the amelioration of PTSD symptoms. Most are based in cognitive-behavioral theory and involve procedures that have withstood rigorous scientific scrutiny. By the same token, there are a number of trauma treatments that possess the trappings of science, but are not based on solid scientific theory and have failed to withstand strong scientific tests of their specific effects. Nonetheless, these treatments pose a strong challenge to the dissemination of empirically supported treatments. Treatments that purport to be novel or unique in their effects may adventitiously incorporate features of other effective treatments or capitalize on nonspecific factors common to psychosocial treatments or social influence processes.

If a procedure is extensively promoted through extraordinary claims, those claims must be accompanied by extraordinary evidence. The nature of the evidence must not be based on clinical testimony or on vivid case studies, as has often been the case in the promotion and marketing of EMDR, TFT, and CISD. The onus lies with the proponents of these treatments to demonstrate that their alleged effects are genuine and do not derive substantially from nonspecific factors or well-established mechanisms of change that are incidental to the theory and procedure. The evidence should rest on strong experimental tests using control conditions that can identify the effects of procedural artifacts and extraneous factors that provide only the appearance of efficacy. It is true that the attitude of scientific skepticism carries with it the necessary risk of delaying the implementation of new treatments. However, uncritical acceptance of psuedoscientific research and promotional tactics carries greater risks for both consumers and the profession of clinical psychology.

GLOSSARY

Anxiety management training (AMT): A set of cognitive-behavioral techniques designed to facilitate adaptive coping with stress. AMT components include relaxation training, breathing retraining, psychoeducation, self-instruction, communication training, and cognitive therapy. AMT as actually practiced may contain some or all of these components.

Cognitive-behavioral therapy (CBT): A set of therapeutic techniques based on cognitive and behavioral theories of psychopathology.

Cognitive therapy (CT): A form of psychotherapy that aims to modify dysfunctional beliefs or assumptions. CT techniques include Socratic questioning and behavioral tests.

Exposure: A cognitive-behavioral intervention for anxiety disorders. In exposure therapy, the patient either confronts previously avoided objects or situations in vivo, or confronts previously avoided thoughts or memories.

Measurement reactivity: The spurious effect of prior administration of an assessment procedure on the results of a second administration of the same assessment procedure. Measurement reactivity may make it appear that an intervening treatment has resulted in beneficial change when the difference is only an artifact of the measurement process. The possibility of measurement reactivity requires the inclusion of wait-list control condition to rule out procedural artifacts and reduce the probability of Type I error.

Meridians: Channels that purportedly traverse the body and act as transmitters of bioenergy (the Chinese concept of chi). There are twelve meridians associated with the twelve major organs of the body, as well as several other types of meridians. Symptoms experienced by a patient are often seen on a particular meridian. Modification of the function of meridians through palpation or needling is claimed by proponents to improve health and functioning.

Randomized clinical trial: An experiment in which research participants are randomly assigned to a group receiving the treatment to be tested or at least one control group that tests for the effects of procedural artifacts or the nonspecific factors of being treated with any procedure (see also Chapter 6).

Systematic desensitization: A behavioral treatment procedure that includes the training of relaxation that is paired with imaginal or in vivo exposure to feared stimuli in a stepped or graduated manner.

Perturbation: A disruption or anomaly in bioenergy at a particular point in the hypothetical meridian system. According to TFT proponents, it is the cause of emotional disturbance.

Psychological reversal: The hypothetical psychological correlate of reversed polarity in the body's meridian system. It is allegedly manifested as generalized impairment, verbal reversals (e.g., saying "up" when one means "down)," and is an explanation for failed TFT interventions.

Thought field: The energy field that purportedly represents mental events.

REFERENCES

Alexander, D.A., & Wells, A. (1991). Reactions of police officers to body handling after major disaster: A before and after comparison. *British Journal of Psychiatry*, *159*, 547–555.

American Psychiatric Association. (1994). *Diagnostic and statistical manual of mental disorders* (4th ed). Washington, DC: Author.

American Psychological Association. (1996). There is a cure [Paid advertisement]. *APA Monitor*, *27*, 14.

American Psychological Association. (1999). APA no longer approves CE sponsorship for thought field therapy. *APA Monitor, 30* [On-line]. Available: www.apa.org. monitor/dec1999nl10.html

Arizona Board of Psychologist Examiners. (1999). Board sanctions a psychologist for use of "thought field therapy." *Newsletter, 3*, 2.

Avery, A., & Orner, R. (1998). First report of psychological debriefing abandoned—the end of an era? *Traumatic Stress Points, 12* [On-line], 3. Available: www.istss.org/ Pubs/ TS/summer98frame.htm

Bandler, R., & Grinder, J. (1979). *Frogs into princes: Neuro-linguistic programming.* Moab,UT: Real People Press.

Bisson, J. I., & Deahl, M. P. (1994). Psychological debriefing and prevention of post traumatic stress: More research is needed. *British Journal of Psychiatry, 165*, 717–720.

Bisson, J. I., Jenkins, P. L., Alexander, J., & Bannister, C. (1997). A randomized controlled trial of psychological debriefing for victims of acute harm. *British Journal of Psychiatry, 171*, 78–81.

Borkovec, T. D., & Castonguay, L. G. (1998). What is the meaning of "empirically supported therapy?" *Journal of Consulting and Clinical Psychology, 66*, 136–142.

Boudewyns, P. A., & Hyer, L. A. (1996). Eye movement desensitization and reprocessing (EMDR) as treatment for post-traumatic stress disorder. *Clinical Psychology and Psychotherapy, 3*, 185–195.

Boudewyns, P. A., Stwertka, S. A., Hyer, L. A., Albrecht, J. W., & Sperr, E. V. (1993). Eye movement desensitization for PTSD of combat: A treatment outcome pilot study. *Behavior Therapist, 16*, 29–33.

Breslau, N., Kessler, R.C., Chilcoat, H. D., Schultz, L. R., Davis, G. C., & Andreski, P. (1998). Trauma and posttraumatic stress disorder in the community. *Archives of General Psychiatry, 55*, 626–632.

Brom, D., Kleber, R. J., & Defares, P. B. (1989). Brief psychotherapy for posttraumatic stress disorders. *Journal of Consulting and Clinical Psychology, 57*, 607–612.

Cahill, S. P., Carrigan, M. H., & Frueh, B. C. (1999). Does EMDR work? If so, Why?:

A critical review of controlled outcome and dismantling research. *Journal of Anxiety Disorders, 13,* 5–33.

Callahan, J. (1998). *Frequently asked questions* [On-line]. Available: http://homepages. enterprise.net/ig/faqs/html

Callahan, R. (1981). *A rapid treatment for phobias.* The Proceedings of the International College of Applied Kinesiology. Proprietary archive.

Callahan, R. (1987). *Successful psychotherapy by telephone and radio.* The Proceedings of the International College of Applied Kinesiology. Proprietary archive.

Callahan, R. (1994). *The Callahan techniques* [Promotional pamphlet]. Available from Callahan Techniques, Ltd. 45350 Vista Santa Rosa, Indian Wells, CA 92210.

Callahan, R. (1995a). *The successful rapid TFT treatment of "Lynn," a fourteen year old girl victim of a gang drive-by shooting: A video.* Available from Thought Field Therapy Training Center, 45350 Vista Santa Rosa, Indian Wells, CA 92210.

Callahan, R. (1995b, August). *A thought field therapy (TFT) algorithm for trauma: A reproducible experiment in psychotherapy.* Paper presented at the 105th Annual Convention of the American Psychological Association.

Callahan, R., & Callahan, J. (1996). *Thought field therapy (TFT) and trauma: Treatment and theory.* Available from Thought Field Therapy Training Center, 45350 Vista Santa Rosa, Indian Wells, CA 92210.

Carlier, I. V. E., Lamberts, R. G., van Uchlen, A. J., & Gersons, B. P. R. (1998). Disaster related post-traumatic stress in police officers: A field study of the impact of debriefing. *Stress Medicine, 14,* 143–148.

Carlson, J. G., Chemtob, C. M., Rusnak, K., Hedlund, N. L., & Muraoka, M. Y. (1998). Eye movement desensitization and reprocessing (EMDR) treatment for combat-related posttraumatic stress disorder. *Journal of Traumatic Stress, 11,* 3–24.

Corsey, G. (1995). *Theory and practice of group counseling* (4th ed.). Pacific Grove, CA: Brooks/Cole.

Craig, G. (Producer). (1997). *Six days at the VA: Using emotional freedom therapy* [Videotape]. (Available from Gary Craig, 1102 Redwood Blvd., Novato, CA 94947)

Cusack, K., & Spates, C. R. (1999). The cognitive dismantling of eye movement desensitization and reprocessing (EMDR) treatment of posttraumatic stress disorder (PTSD). *Journal of Anxiety Disorders, 13,* 87–99.

Davidson, J., Hughes, D., Blazer, D., & George, L. (1991). Post-traumatic stress disorder in the community: An epidemiological study. *Psychological Medicine, 21,* 713–722.

Deahl, M. P., & Bisson, J. I. (1995). Dealing with disasters: Does psychological debriefing work? *Journal of Accident and Emergency Medicine, 12,* 255–258.

Deahl, M. P., Gillham, A. B., Thomas, J., Dearle, M. M., & Strinivasan, M. (1994). Psychological sequelae following the Gulf war: Factors associated with subsequent morbidity and the effectiveness of psychological debriefing. *British Journal of Psychiatry, 165,* 60–65.

DeBell, C., & Jones, R. D. (1997). As good as it seems? A review of EMDR experimental research. *Professional Psychology: Research and Practice, 28,* 153–163.

Delmolino, L. M., & Romanczyck, R. G. (1995). Facilitated communication: A critical review. *Behavior Therapist, 18,* 27–30.

Deitrich, A. M., Baranowsky, A. B., Devich-Navarro, M., Gentry, J. E., Harris, C. J., & Figley, C. R. (2000). A review of alternative approaches to the treatment of post traumatic sequelae. *TRAUMATOLOGYe,* 6 [On-line]. Available: http://www.fsu.edu/~trauma/v6i4/v6i4a2.htm

Devilly, G. J., & Spence, S. H. (1999). The relative efficacy and treatment distress of EMDR and a cognitive behavioral trauma treatment protocol in the amelioration of Post Traumatic Stress Disorder. *Journal of Anxiety Disorders, 13,* 131–157.

Devilly, G. J., Spence, S., & Rapee, R. (1998). Statistical and reliable change with eye movement desensitization and reprocessing: Treating trauma within a veteran population. *Behavior Therapy, 26,* 435–455.

Echterling, L., & Wylie, M. L. (1981). Crisis centers: A social movement perspective. *Journal of Community Psychology, 9,* 342–346.

Eysenck, H. J. (1994). The outcome problem in psychotherapy: What have we learned? *Behaviour Research and Therapy, 32,* 477–495.

Figley, C. R. (1997, December). *The active ingredients of the power therapies.* Paper presented at the Conference for the Integrative and Innovative Use of EMDR, TFT, EFT, Advanced NLP, and TIR, Lakewood, CO.

Figley, C., & Carbonell, J. (1999). Promising treatment approaches. *TRAUMATOLOGYe,* 5 [On-line]. Available: http://www.fsu.edu/~trauma/promising.html

Foa, E. B., Dancu, C. V., Hembree, E. A., Jaycox, L. H., Meadows, E. A., & Street, G. P. (1999). A comparison of exposure therapy, stress inoculation training and their combination for reducing PTSD in female assault victims. *Journal of Consulting and Clinical Psychology, 67,* 194–200.

Foa, E. B., Davidson, J. R. T., & Frances, A. (1999). The expert consensus guideline series: Treatment of posttraumatic stress disorder. *Journal of Clinical Psychiatry, 60*(Suppl.), 2–76.

Foa, E. B., & Meadows, E. A. (1997). Psychosocial treatments for posttraumatic stress disorder: A critical review. *Annual Review of Psychology, 48,* 449–480.

Foa, E. B., Rothbaum, B. O., Riggs, D. S., & Murdock, T. B. (1991). Treatment of posttraumatic stress disorder in rape victims: A comparison between cognitive-behavioral procedures and counseling. *Journal of Consulting and Clinical Psychology, 59,* 715–723.

Foa, E. B., Steketee, G., & Rothbaum, B. O. (1989). Behavioral/cognitive conceptualizations of post-traumatic stress disorder. *Behavior Therapy, 20,* 155–176.

Frank, J. D. (1974). *Persuasion and healing* (Rev. ed.). New York: Schocken Books.

Fullerton, C. S., Wright, K. M., Ursano, R. J., & McCarroll, J. E. (1993). Social support for disaster workers after a mass-casualty disaster: Effects on the support provider. *Nordic Journal of Psychiatry, 47,* 315–324.

Gallo, F. P. (1995). Reflections on active ingredients in efficient treatments of PTSD, Part 1. *TRAUMATOLOGYe,* 1 [On-line]. Available: http://www.fsu.edu/~trauma/traumaj.html

Gallo, F. P. (1998). *Energy psychology: Explorations at the interface of energy, cognition, behavior, and health.* Boca Raton, FL: CRC Press.

Gaudiano, B. A., & Herbert, J. D. (2000). Can we really tap our problems away? A critical analysis of thought field therapy. *Skeptical Inquirer, 24,* 29–33, 36.

Gerbode, F. (1995, May). *Presentation on traumatic incident reduction.* Paper presented at the Active Ingredients in Efficient Treatments of PTSD Conference, Florida State University, Tallahassee.

Gist, R. (1996). Is CISD built on a foundation of sand? *Fire Chief, 48*(8), 38–42.

Gist, R., Lubin, B., & Redburn, B. G. (1998). Psychosocial, ecological, and community perspectives on disaster response. *Journal of Personal and Interpersonal Loss, 3,* 25–51.

Gist, R., & Woodall, S. J. (1995). Occupational stress in contemporary fire service. *Occupational Medicine: State of the Art Reviews, 10,* 763–787.

Gist, R., & Woodall, S. J. (1999). There are no simple solutions to complex problems: The rise and fall of critical incident stress debriefing as a response to occupational stress in the fire service. In R. Gist & B. Lubin (Eds.), *Response to disaster: Psychosocial, community, and ecological approaches* (pp. 211–235). Philadelphia: Brunner/Mazel.

Gist, R., Woodall, S. J., & Magenheimer, L. K. (1999). And then you do the Hokey-Pokey and you turn yourself around. . . . In R. Gist & B. Lubin (Eds.), *Response to disaster: Psychosocial, community, and ecological approaches* (pp. 269–290). Philadelphia: Brunner/Mazel.

Goldstein, A. J., de Beurs, E., Chambless, D. L., & Wilson, K. A. (2000). EMDR for panic disorder with agoraphobia: Comparison with waiting-list and credible attention-placebo control conditions. *Journal of Consulting and Clinical Psychology, 68,* 947–956.

Griffiths, J., & Watts, R. (1992). *The Kempsey and Grafton bus crashes: The aftermath.* East Linsmore, Australia: Instructional Design Solutions.

Grünbaum, A. (1985). Explication and implications of the placebo concept. In L. White, B. Tursky, & G. E. Schwartz (Eds.), *Placebo: Theory, research and mechanisms* (pp. 9–36). New York: Guilford Press.

Hazlett-Stevens, H., & Borkovec, T. D. (1998). Experimental design and methodology in between-group intervention research. In R. Schulz, M. P. Lawton, & G. Maddox (Eds.), *Annual review of gerontology and geriatrics: Vol. 18. Intervention research with older adults* (pp. 17–47). New York: Springer.

Herbert, J. D., Lilienfeld, S. O., Lohr, J. M., Montgomery, R. W., O'Donohue, W. T., Rosen, G. M., & Tolin, D. F. (2000). Science and pseudoscience in the development of eye movement desensitization and reprocessing: Implications for clinical psychology. *Clinical Psychology Review, 20,* 945–971.

Hobbs, M., Mayou, R., Harrison, B., & Worlock, P. (1996). A randomized controlled trial of psychological debriefing for victims of road traffic accidents. *British Medical Journal, 313,* 1438–1439.

Hooke, W. (1998). A review of thought field therapy. *Electronic Journal of Traumatology* [On-line], *3.* Available: http://www.fsu.edu/~trauma/contv3i2.html

Hytten, K., & Hasle, A. (1989). Firefighters: A study of stress and coping. *Acta Psychiatrica Scandinavia, 355*(Suppl.), 50–55.

Jacobson, J. W., Mulick, J. A., & Schwartz, A. A. (1995). A history of facilitated communication: Science, pseudoscience, and antiscience. *American Psychologist, 50,* 75–765.

Jensen, J. A. (1994). An investigation of eye movement desensitization and reprocessing (EMD/R) as a treatment of Posttraumatic Stress Disorder (PTSD) symptoms of Vietnam combat veterans. *Behavior Therapy, 25,* 311–325.

Keane, T. M. (1998). Psychological and behavioral treatment of posttraumatic stress disorder. In P. Nathan & J. Gorman (Eds.), *A guide to treatments that work* (pp. 398–407). Oxford: Oxford University Press.

Keane, T. M., Fairbank, J. A., Caddell, J. M., & Zimering, R. T. (1989). Implosive (flooding) therapy reduces symptoms of PTSD in Vietnam combat veterans. *Behavior Therapy, 20,* 245–260.

Keane, T. M., Zimering, R. T., & Caddell, J. M. (1985). A behavioral formulation of posttraumatic stress disorder in Vietnam veterans. *Behavior Therapist, 8,* 9–12.

Kenardy, J. A. (1998). Psychological (stress) debriefing: Where are we now? *Australasian Journal of Disaster and Trauma Studies, 1* [On-line]. Available: http://www.massey.ac.nz/~trauma

Kenardy, J. A., & Carr, V. (1996). Imbalance in the debriefing debate: What we don't know far outweighs what we do. *Bulletin of the Australian Psychological Society, 18,* 4–6.

Kenardy, J. A., Webster, R. A., Lewin, T. J., Carr, V. J., Hazell, P. L., & Carter, G. L. (1996). Stress debriefing and patterns of recovery following a natural disaster. *Journal of Traumatic Stress, 9,* 37–49.

Kessler, R. C., Sonnega, A., Bromet, E., Hughes, M., & Nelson, C. B. (1995). Posttraumatic stress disorder in the national comorbidity survey. *Archives of General Psychiatry, 52,* 1048–1060.

Lee, C., Slade, P., & Lygo, V. (1996). The influence of psychological debriefing on emotional adaptation in women following early miscarriage: A preliminary study. *British Journal of Medical Psychology, 69,* 47–58.

Leonoff, G. (1995). The successful treatment of phobias and anxiety by telephone and radio: A replication of Callahan's 1987 study. *TFT Newsletter, 1*(2), 1, 6.

Lilienfeld, S. O. (1996). Eye movement and desensitization for anxiety: Less than meets the eye? *Skeptical Inquirer, 20,* 25–31.

Lilienfeld, S. O., & Lohr, J. M. (2000). News and comment: Thought field therapy practitioners and educators sanctioned. *Skeptical Inquirer, 24,* 5.

Litz, B. T., & Keane, T. M. (1989). Information processing in anxiety disorders: Application to the understanding of post-traumatic stress disorder. *Clinical Psychology Review, 9,* 243–257.

Lohr, J. M., Kleinknecht, R. A., Tolin, D. F., & Barrett, R. H. (1995). The empirical status of the clinical application of eye movement desensitization and reprocessing. *Behavior Therapy and Experimental Psychiatry, 26,* 285–302.

Lohr, J. M., Lilienfeld, S. O., Tolin, D. F., & Herbert, J. D. (1999). Eye movement desensitization and reprocessing: An analysis of specific versus nonspecific treatment factors. *Journal of Anxiety Disorders, 13,* 185–207.

Lohr, J. M., Tolin, D. F., & Lilienfeld, S. O. (1998). Efficacy of eye movement desensitization and reprocessing. *Behavior Therapy, 26,* 123–156.

Lyons, J. A., & Keane, T. M. (1989). Implosive therapy for the treatment of combat-related PTSD. *Journal of Traumatic Stress, 2,* 137–152.

Macklin, M. L., Metzger, L. J., Lasko, N. B., Berry, N. J., Orr, S. P., & Pitman, R. K. (2000). Five-year follow-up of EMDR treatment for combat-related PTSD. *Comprehensive Psychiatry, 41,* 24–27.

Mahoney, M. J. (1978). Experimental methods and outcome evaluation. *Journal of Consulting and Clinical Psychology, 46,* 660–672.

Marcus, S. V., Marquis, P., & Sakai, C. (1997). Controlled study of treatment of PTSD using EMDR in an HMO setting. *Psychotherapy, 34,* 307–315.

Marks, I., Lovell, K., Noshirvani, H., Livanou, M., & Thrasher, S. (1998). Treatment of posttraumatic stress disorder by exposure and/or cognitive restructuring: A controlled study. *Archives of General Psychiatry, 55,* 317–325.

Mayou, R. A., Ehlers, A., & Hobbs, M. (2000). Psychological debriefing for road traffic accident victims. *British Journal of Psychiatry, 176,* 589–593.

McFall, R. M. (1991). Manifesto for a science of clinical psychology. *Clinical Psychologist, 44,* 7588.

McFarlane, A. C. (1988). The longitudinal course of posttraumatic morbidity: The range of outcomes and their predictors. *Journal of Nervous and Mental Disease, 176,* 30–39.

McNally, R. J. (1999). On eye movements and animal magnetism: A reply to Greenwald's defense of EMDR. *Journal of Anxiety Disorders, 13,* 617–620.

Mitchell, J. T. (1983). When disaster strikes . . . the critical incident stress debriefing process. *Journal of Emergency Medical Services, 8,* 36–39.

Mitchell, J. T. (1988a). Development and functions of a critical incident stress debriefing team. *Journal of Emergency Medical Services, 13,* 42–46.

Mitchell, J. T. (1988b). The history, status, and future of critical incident stress debriefing. *Journal of Emergency Medical Services, 13,* 49–52.

Mitchell, J. T. (1992). Protecting your people from critical incident stress. *Fire Chief, 36,* 61–67.

Mitchell, J. T. (1998). Development and functions of a critical incident stress debriefing team. *Journal of Emergency Medical Services, 13,* 42–46.

Mitchell, J. T., & Bray, G. (1990). *Emergency services stress.* Englewood Cliffs, NJ: Brady.

Mitchell, J. T., & Everly, G. S., Jr. (1993). *Critical incident stress debriefing: An operations manual. The prevention of traumatic stress among emergency services and disaster workers.* Ellicott City, MD: Chevron Publishing.

Mitchell, J. T., & Everly, G. S., Jr. (1995). Critical incident stress debriefing and the prevention of work related traumatic stress among high risk occupational groups. In G. S. Everly, Jr., & J. M. Lating (Eds.), *Psychotraumatology: Key papers and core concepts in post traumatic stress* (pp. 267–280). New York: Plenum Press.

Mitchell, J. T., & Everly, G. S., Jr. (1997). The scientific evidence for critical incident stress management. *Journal of Emergency Medical Services, 22,* 86–93.

Mitchell, J. T., & Everly, G. S., Jr. (1998). Critical incident stress management: A new era in crisis intervention. *Traumatic Stress Points, 12,* 6–11.

Muris, P., & Merckelbach, H. (1997). Treating spider phobics with eye-movement desensitization and reprocessing: A controlled study. *Behavioural and Cognitive Psychotherapy, 25,* 39–50.

Muris, P., Merckelbach, H., Holdrinet, I., & Sijsenaar, M. (1998). Treating phobic children: Effects of EMDR versus exposure. *Journal of Consulting and Clinical Psychology, 66,* 193–198.

Muris, P., Merckelbach, H., van Haaften, H., & Mayer, B. (1997). Eye movement desensitization and reprocessing versus exposure in vivo: A single session crossover study of spider-phobic children. *British Journal of Psychiatry, 171,* 82–86.

Nezu, A. (1986). Efficacy of a social problem-solving therapy approach to unipolar depression. *Journal of Consulting and Clinical Psychology*, 54, 196–202.

Nezu, A., & Perri, M. G. (1989). Social problem-solving therapy for unipolar depression: An initial dismantling investigation. *Journal of Consulting and Clinical Psychology*, 57, 408–413.

Norris, F. H. (1992). Epidemiology of trauma: Frequency and impact of potentially traumatic events on different demographic groups. *Journal of Consulting and Clinical Psychology*, 60, 409–418.

Ostrow, L. S. (1996). Critical incident stress management: Is it worth it? *Journal of Emergency Medical Services*, 21, 28–36.

Pitman, R. K., Orr, S. P., Altman, B., Longpre, R. E., Poire, R. E., & Macklin, M. L. (1996). Emotional reprocessing during eye movement desensitization and reprocessing (EMDR) therapy of Vietnam Veterans with post-traumatic stress disorder. *Comprehensive Psychiatry*, 37, 419–429.

Raphael, B., Meldrum, L., & McFarlane, A. C. (1995). Does debriefing after psychological trauma work? Time for randomized controlled trials. *British Journal of Psychiatry*, 310, 1479–1480.

Renfrey, G., & Spates, C. (1994). Eye movement desensitization: A partial dismantling study. *Journal of Behavior Therapy and Experimental Psychiatry*, 25, 231–239.

Resick, P. A., & Schnicke, M. K. (1992). Cognitive processing therapy for sexual assault victims. *Journal of Consulting and Clinical Psychology*, 60, 748–756.

Roberts, A. H., Kewman, D. G., Mercier, L., & Hovell, M. (1993). The power of nonspecific effects in healing: Implications for psychosocial and biological treatments. *Clinical Psychology Review*, 13, 375–391

Rogers, S., Silver, S. M., Goss, J., Obenchain, J., Willis, A., & Whitney, R. L. (1999). A single session, group study of exposure and eye movement desensitization and reprocessing in treating posttraumatic stress disorder among Vietnam veterans: Preliminary study. *Journal of Anxiety Disorders*, 13, 119–130.

Rose, S., & Bisson, J. (1999). Brief early psychological interventions following trauma: A systematic review of the literature. *Journal of Traumatic Stress*, 11, 679–710.

Shapiro, F. (1989). Efficacy of the eye movement desensitization procedure in the treatment of traumatic memories. *Journal of Traumatic Stress*, 2, 199–223.

Shapiro, F. (1991). Eye movement desensitization and reprocessing procedure: From EMD to EMD/R—A new treatment model for anxiety and related trauma. *Behavior Therapist*, 14, 128, 133–135.

Shapiro, F. (1994a). Alternative stimuli in the use of EMD(R). *Journal of Behavior Therapy and Experimental Psychiatry*, 25, 89.

Shapiro, F. (1994b). EMDR: In the eye of a paradigm shift. *Behavior Therapist*, 17, 153–156.

Shapiro, F. (1995). *Eye movement desensitization and reprocessing: Basic principles, protocols, and procedures*. New York: Guilford Press.

Shapiro, F. (1996). Eye movement desensitization and reprocessing (EMDR): Evaluation of controlled PTSD research. *Journal of Behavior Therapy and Experimental Psychiatry*, 27, 209–218.

Shapiro, F. (1998). *From the desk of Francine Shapiro*. (Available from the Eye Movement Desensitization and Reprocessing International Association, P.O. Box 141925, Austin, TX 78714–1925)

Shapiro, F., & Forrest, M. S. (1997). *EMDR: The breakthrough therapy for overcoming anxiety, stress, and trauma.* New York: Basic Books.

Silver, S. M., Brooks, A., & Obenchain, J. (1995). Treatment of Vietnam War veterans with PTSD: A comparison of eye movement desensitization and reprocessing, biofeedback, and relaxation training. *Journal of Traumatic Stress, 8,* 337–342.

Stephens, C. (1997). Debriefing, social support, and PTSD in the New Zealand police: Testing a multidimensional model of organizational traumatic stress. *Australasian Journal of Disaster and Trauma Studies, 1* [On-line]. Available: http://www.massey.ac.nz/~trauma

Stuhlmiller, C., & Dunning, C. (2000). Challenging the mainstream: From pathogenic to salutogenic models of posttrauma intervention. In J. M. Violanti, D. Paton, & C. Dunning (Eds.), *Posttraumatic stress intervention: Challenges, issues, and perspectives* (pp. 10–42). Springfield, IL: Charles C Thomas.

Stux, G., & Pomeranz, B. (1995). *Basics of acupuncture* (3rd ed.). New York: Springer.

Tarrier, N., Pilgrim, H., Sommerfield, C., Faragher, B., Reynolds, M., Graham, E., & Barrowclough, C. (1999). A randomized trial of cognitive therapy and imaginal exposure in the treatment of chronic posttraumatic stress disorder. *Journal of Consulting and Clinical Psychology, 67,* 13–18.

Tolin, D. F., Montgomery, R. W., Kleinknecht, R. A., & Lohr, J. M. (1995). An evaluation of eye movement desensitization and reprocessing (EMDR). In S. Knapp., L. van de Creek, & T. L. Jackson (Eds.), *Innovations in clinical practice: A source book* (Vol. 14, pp. 423–437). Sarasota, FL: Professional Resource Press.

Vaughan, K., Armstrong, M. S., Gold, R., O'Connor, N., Jenneke, W., & Tarrier, N. (1994). A trial of eye movement desensitization compared to image habituation training and applied muscle relaxation in post-traumatic stress disorder. *Journal of Behavior Therapy and Experimental Psychiatry, 25,* 283–291.

Wade, J. F. (1990). *The effects of the Callahan phobia treatment technique on self concept.* Unpublished doctoral dissertation, The Professional School of Psychological Studies, San Diego, CA.

Wessley, S., Rose, S., & Bisson, J. (2000). Brief psychological interventions ("debriefing") for trauma-related symptoms and the prevention of posttraumatic stress disorder (Cochrane Review). *The Cochrane Library, 4* [On-line]. Available: http://www.cochranelibrary.com/cochrane/cochrane-frame.html

Wilson, D. L., Silver, S. M., Covi, W. G., & Foster, S. (1996). Eye Movement Desensitization and Reprocessing: Effectiveness and autonomic correlates. *Journal of Behavior Therapy and Experimental Psychiatry, 27,* 219–229.

Wylie, M. S. (1996, July/August). Going for the cure. *Family Therapy Networker, 21–*37.

10

Controversial Treatments for Alcoholism

JAMES MacKILLOP
STEPHEN A. LISMAN
ALLISON WEINSTEIN
DEBORAH ROSENBAUM

Formal treatment programs and procedures for alcohol dependence (alcoholism) are relatively recent endeavors. For several hundred years, Americans viewed alcohol problems as evidence of weakened mental and moral capacities, and as reflecting a character defect or a lack of self-control (Levine, 1978). During that time, societal responses to alcoholics ranged from criminalization (e.g., fines, jail sentences, and religious sanctions) to such offers of assistance as shelter, food, and spiritual advice. An array of new conceptual models of alcoholism emerged in the late 19th and early 20th centuries (see Miller & Hester's [1995] review of 13 such models), spawning self-help group treatments (see also Chapter 14), such as the Washingtonians and, later, Alcoholics Anonymous. When the United States Congress passed the Comprehensive Alcohol Abuse and Alcoholism Prevention, Treatment, and Rehabilitation Act in 1970 and created the National Institute on Alcohol Abuse and Alcoholism (NIAAA) in 1971, alcoholism moved into the purview of the professional treatment establishment. By the 1980s, outpatient and inpatient clinics had begun to proliferate.

This all too brief history belies the development of a fragmented and fractious treatment community. Indeed, Kalb and Propper (1976) suggested that two distinct groups have emerged, which they designated "craftsman" and "scientist," that work in parallel to treat alcoholism from fundamentally different perspectives. According to this formulation, the craftsman is characterized by an anti intellectual and anti-research bias, which stems primarily from a lack of training in research methodology (Kalb & Propper, 1976). In addition, a substantial portion of these craftsmen are themselves recovered addicts, understandable advocates of the treatments from which they benefited. Scientifically trained clinicians are not beyond reproach, however, and have been criticized for being overly dogmatic and unable to consider the merits of treatments that are not empirically based (Chiauzzi & Liljegren, 1993). Moreover, the treatments offered by the scientific community have not been incontrovertibly effective, especially not in the early days of clinical treatment. Only in recent years has a legitimate selection of scientifically based treatments for problem drinking become available (Miller et al., 1995).

Thus, in the last two decades a variety of treatments have emerged, from both the scientific and lay communities, that vary dramatically in terms of their adherence to evidence-based practice. We believe that the distinction between the practices of lay and professional groups has become blurred, as both often employ approaches that lack research support. This is consistent with the report of Hayes, Barlow, and Nelson-Gray (1999) that many professionally trained practitioners often have serious and warranted reservations about attempting to apply research findings to a wide range of clinical problems.

The large gaps between the lay and scientific treatment communities and even within the clinical community itself have resulted in substantial controversy regarding treatment approaches to alcoholism. We apply the term "controversial" to treatments or procedures that have become widely adopted or have generated popular appeal, but that have been demonstrated by controlled research to be of questionable or even nonexistent efficacy. As used in this chapter, this term does not include treatments whose efficacy has not yet been studied. Rather, controversial treatments are those that, despite the lack of evidence for their efficacy, derive their support from a community of believers. In turn, these believers often embrace such characteristics as reliance on personal experience, appeal to authority, or a lack of interest in data. In this sense, at least some of these controversial treatments can be thought of as pseudoscientific according the criteria outlined by a number of philosophers of science (Bunge, 1984), and a discussion of several of these treatments comprises the first portion of this chapter. Specifically, we discuss the efficacy of Alcoholics Anonymous, the Johnson Intervention, disulfiram pharmacotherapy, the debates about moderation as a treatment goal, and Project DARE. By no means are these the only controversial issues regarding alcoholism or addiction. Chiauzzi and Liljegren (1993) reviewed 11 contemporary "taboos" or incongruities between traditional assumptions about addiction and actual research findings. However, the controversies considered in this chapter are only those directly germane to treatment issues.

The substantial gap between treatment researchers and practicing clinicians is a major contributor to the continued use of unsupported treatments, and a "greater dialogue" between these groups has been called for to bridge this gap (Sobell, Sobell, & Gavin, 1995). For this reason, the second portion of the chapter describes the theory, evidence, and procedures of a selection of evidence-based treatments. We conclude with a comment on what we optimistically perceive to be the increasing visibility and influence of the scientific perspective in alcoholism treatment.

ALCOHOLICS ANONYMOUS: DOES IT REALLY WORK?

Debate over the efficacy of Alcoholics Anonymous (AA) is perhaps the most acrimonious of all the controversies in the field of alcoholism treatment. Members of the AA community are often perceived as overly theistic and unaccepting of other perspectives (Ellis & Schoenfeld, 1990), as well as excessively confident in the efficacy of their treatment (Tournier, 1979). Conversely, research-trained clinicians have been criticized for being myopic and discounting the potential of AA and related self-help treatments (Chiauzzi & Liljegren, 1993). Thus, we regard the question of the efficacy of AA an excellent illustrative controversy for discussion. It is reflective of the disconnection between society at large and the scientific clinical community, and reconcilable to some degree for both sides given a nonpartisan consideration of the literature (McCrady, 1995).

Founded in 1935, AA is probably the largest self-help group in the world (see also Chapter 14, for a discussion of self-help programs). In 1990, AA reported 87,000 groups worldwide and over 1.7 million members (Alcoholics Anonymous, 1990). Although it is easily the most prominent treatment for alcoholism in the United States, Miller (1986) observed that in no other part of the world does it wield such influence. Despite its size, AA is remarkably "flat" in its structure. The governing body is hierarchically only one level above the individual chapters, and cannot make decisions that affect AA as a whole. For this reason, AA remains both ideologically and organizationally very close to its grassroots origins.

In terms of treatment, AA's well known "12 steps" engage members in a regimen of spiritual and interpersonal rehabilitation. A religious component, although nondenominational, is nevertheless central to AA: Seven of the steps refer specifically to God, a "Higher Power," or Him. Despite specification of 12 steps, the form of treatment an individual receives when attending AA is highly variable. This is a direct result of the general heterogeneity across all AA groups; all that is required for an AA group is that two or more alcoholics meet together for the purpose of achieving sobriety (McCrady & Delaney, 1995).

The general format of AA is broadly known. Individuals meet and verbalize past experiences with alcohol, and often a "sponsorship" system is in place in which a neophyte is paired with a stable senior member to facilitate the process of recovery. Newcomers are advised to immerse themselves by attending a meeting each night for the first 90 days, although there is no enforcement of this recommendation.

The interpretation of outcome studies is complicated by the heterogeneity of AA groups and the length and nature of individuals' involvement. For example, AA does not specify who is a member or when treatment ends. By virtue of this and other such vague criteria, Bebbington's (1976) methodological critique concluded that it is impossible to operationalize an individual's involvement with AA, and consequently very difficult to assess AA's efficacy. Furthermore, an implicit level of motivation and spirituality is intrinsic to any individual who independently seeks AA's help (Ogborne, 1989), and fundamentally compromises random assignment, generally considered a prerequisite to internally valid treatment outcome research. Thus, assigning individuals to an AA treatment would not replicate the actual pathway that leads to participation and has the potential to create a negatively predisposed group of subjects (McCrady & Delaney, 1995).

These methodological problems are evident in the empirical literature. Three randomized trials of AA have been undertaken involving populations mandated to attend AA. None of these studies has shown AA to be more effective than an alternative treatment (Brandsma, Maultsby, & Welsh, 1980; Dittman, Crawford, Forgy, Moskowitz, & MacAndrew, 1967; Walsh et al., 1991). An exemplar of these studies is that of Walsh and colleagues (1991), who assigned 227 alcohol-abusing employees to one of three treatment conditions: inpatient treatment with compulsory AA follow-up, compulsory AA attendance only, and a selection of options. The inpatient group was found to exhibit significantly reduced alcohol and drug use, whereas the AA-only group fared worst, both on measures of alcohol and drug use and likelihood of subsequent inpatient treatment. Most recently, mandated AA attendance was included as an adjunctive component to alcohol-focused behavioral marital therapy and was found to make no significant difference in outcome (McCrady, Epstein, & Hirsch, 1996).

Studies of AA using quasi-experimental designs have been more supportive of AA's efficacy. Smith (1985, 1986) found striking differences in self-reported rates of abstinence after residential treatment; 79% of women and 61% of men in the AA group reported abstinence compared with 3% and 5% of the respective comparison groups. However, these findings were based on a comprehensive inpatient treatment that involved daily AA meetings as but one component, and has been subjected to other methodological criticisms (see McCrady & Delaney, 1995). A meta-analysis of nonrandomized studies indicated that AA showed significantly more positive outcomes than no-treatment conditions, and that individuals who attended more meetings experienced better outcomes than those who attended fewer (Kownacki & Shadish, 1999). However, a variety of unmeasured variables, such as premorbid psychological functioning, may have contributed to these results. Most recently, Timko, Moos, Finney, and Lesar (2000) studied the outcome of 248 problem drinkers who self-selected either AA, formal treatment, formal treatment and AA, or no treatment at all. Unsurprisingly, those who chose no treatment fared the worst. The AA-only and combined AA/formal treatment groups fared better than the formal treatment group alone at 1 and 3 years, although all three groups were equivalent at 8 years.

A project called Matching Alcohol Treatments to Client Heterogeneity (Project MATCH) comprised a multisite clinical trial of psychotherapeutic treatments for alcoholism, and entailed the random assignment of 1,726 clients to 12-step facilitation therapy (TSF), cognitive-behavioral coping skills therapy (CBT) and a motivational enhancement therapy (MET). TSF was conceptually grounded in the tenets of AA and other 12-step groups and attempted to foster a commitment to participate in AA (Project MATCH Research Group, 1997). The three treatments produced comparable outcomes (Project MATCH Research Group, 1998). Although the TSF intervention was explicitly not a test of AA as a treatment, the lack of outcome differences and retention rates among the three treatment conditions is noteworthy. Tellingly, subsequent analyses revealed that client ratings of the conceptual and spiritual underpinnings of AA predicted AA meeting attendance, engagement in AA practices, and greater abstinence (Tonigan, Miller, & Connors, 2000). This outcome certainly supports our earlier emphasis on the role of individual differences as predictors of success with AA.

Although some of these findings may be encouraging at first blush, they fail to address most of Bebbington's (1976) trenchant critique and other concerns articulated in the research literature. For example, Emrick (1987) noted that AA members who are studied (1) are typically the most active, (2) receive or have often received professional treatment, and (3) drop out at rates as high as 68% prior to 10 weeks. Further, quasi-experimental studies do not permit cause-and-effect inferences, and the Project MATCH findings do not speak directly to the efficacy of AA.

An important final point is that AA is by no means the only self-help group for alcoholism. Among these other organizations are groups with greater emphasis on specific religions, such as Overcomers Outreach and Calix, which are oriented to Christian interpretations of the 12 steps; Women For Sobriety, which evolved its secular orientation from the belief that some of the tenets of AA are countertherapeutic for women; Moderation Management, which attempts to assist individuals who want to reduce their drinking but not necessarily abstain; and Rational Recovery, an analogue of AA based on Albert Ellis's Rational Emotive Behavior Therapy. Nevertheless, in contrast to AA, many of these other groups are not readily found outside of major metropolitan areas or are still in early stages of development. These limitations contribute to the public perception of AA as the only viable choice for self-help.

In summary, "For whom and under what circumstances might AA prove helpful?" is probably a more reasonable question than this section's provocative subtitle, "Does it really work?" McCrady and Delaney (1995) provided practice guidelines for integrating self-help groups into professional treatment, and suggested that clinicians familiarize themselves with the ideologies, language, and practices of these groups and make literature available to clients. For example, the conduciveness of a client's social environment to drinking has been demonstrated as a positive matching characteristic for 12-step programs (Project MATCH, 1998) and should be integrated into active clinical practice. We urge that clinicians consider AA as one of many therapeutic approaches, inasmuch as it may complement an empirically supported treatment or even stand alone. This idea is congruent with evidence that individuals who are provided with the opportunity to select treatment pathways have better outcomes (Sanchez-Craig & Lei, 1986), as well as evidence of a positive association between AA attendance during and after professional treatment and drinking outcomes (Emrick, Tonigan, Montgomery, & Little, 1993). Thus, perhaps the most propitious approach for clinicians appears to be integrative, taking advantage of AA's tremendous proliferation and role in the cultural conception of alcoholism, but doing so in ways that are informed by research.

THE JOHNSON INTERVENTION

There is little evidence that "denial" of one's problems plays a larger role in alcoholism than in any other psychological disorder (Chiauzzi & Liljegren, 1993). Nevertheless, denial has often been considered a hallmark of alcoholism and, in a largely tautological fashion, an explanation for some problem drinkers' refusal to initiate treatment. In addition, one problem in viewing AA as the sole or primary source of treatment and recovery is that anyone with a drinking problem who disagrees with its philosophy or procedures may be highly reluctant to initiate treatment. Until recently, the prevailing answers to the distress of concerned family members regarding the problem drinker who refuses treatment have been to either urge attendance at Al-Anon, which emphasizes acceptance of powerlessness and the need for "loving detachment" by family, or to undertake an "Intervention." This term was used by the Johnson Institute to describe the process of supportive confrontation of problem drinkers by family and friends— typically by ruse or surprise—and was developed as a means to break down the drinkers' so-called denial, motivate them for treatment, and initiate the referral and treatment process immediately (Johnson, 1986).

Backed by undocumented claims of 97% success (Royce, 1989), "Interventions" have become sufficiently popular to be featured on national television dramas (e.g., *Beverly Hills 90210* and *Party of Five*).

However, from the perspective of controlled research, Johnson Interventions are not robustly supported. For example, Liepman, Nirenberg, and Begin (1989) reported a high rate of entry into detoxification or rehabilitation programs following an Intervention, but these authors also acknowledged an extremely high rate of families who failed to complete the Intervention, the nonrandom assignment of participants, and the low number of subjects overall. Additionally, although Loneck, Garrett, and Banks (1996a) reported that individuals who underwent a Johnson Intervention were more likely to enter treatment than were individuals who underwent four other treatment initiation strategies, their method was retrospective, and represented only the cases in which motivated family members enacted an Intervention. Moreover, upon further analysis of these groups, the Johnson Intervention group was found to be more likely to relapse than three of the four comparison groups (Loneck, Garrett, & Banks, 1996b). An alternative, empirically derived method for motivating individuals who are reluctant to initiate treatment will be described in detail later in the chapter.

This negligible research support, emphasis on immediate hospitalization to prevent resumption of patterns of denial, and concerns about clinical and family dynamics suggest great caution in advocating Intervention. Galanter (1993) warned that such coercive techniques often appear to confront individuals with "cataclysmic consequences" (e.g., loss of marriage) as the only alternative to treatment, often at the risk of ignoring the impact of such comorbid conditions as depression, panic disorder, or delusional disorder, which may foster self-destructive behavior or the breakdown of family ties.

Thus, despite the growing popular prominence of the Johnson Intervention, this method of initiating treatment falls short in terms of evidence of its efficacy, and for this reason remains controversial.

DISULFIRAM PHARMACOTHERAPY

Since 1948, the most common pharmacological agents for treating alcohol dependence have been *antidipsotropics*, medications that induce unpleasant reactions following ingestion of alcohol. The most commonly used of these aversive agents is disulfiram (commercial name, Antabuse), which has the effect of rendering the body unable to metabolize alcohol. This effect in turn leads to such intense physical symptoms as flushing, a rapid or irregular heartbeat, nausea, and vomiting. The rationale underlying antidipsotropics is punishment or aversive conditioning: By pairing an aversive experience with the act of drinking, it is anticipated that drinking, as well as attendant urges, will extinguish. However, despite decades of availability and use, disulfiram remains controversial because the weight of evidence from controlled studies does not support its efficacy.

Many early clinical trials were supportive of the efficacy of disulfiram, but these trials occurred prior to contemporary standards for controlled outcome studies and are methodologically unsound (Lundwall & Baekeland, 1971; Mottin, 1973). More rigorous treatment outcome studies have since been completed, but the results have been disheartening. Two multisite, placebo-controlled, clinical trials were undertaken in which men receiving care from a Veterans Administration (VA) hospital underwent a multidisciplinary treatment program including medical treatment, psychotherapeutic counseling, and differing levels of disulfiram or placebo (Fuller & Roth, 1979; Fuller et al., 1986). Neither of these trials yielded positive results; there were no differences between groups in terms of either abstinence or latency to resume drinking, although the active disulfiram treatment group had significantly fewer drinking days. Another positive finding that emerged was that older and more socially stable patients drank significantly less frequently after disulfiram treatment (Fuller et al., 1986). However, this result must be weighed against the overall findings of the VA trials and of two earlier studies that included appropriate control groups (Gallant et al., 1968; Gerrein, Rosenberg, & Manohar, 1973). All found that disulfiram was not successful in increasing abstinence or latency to resumption of drinking.

These weak overall results have been attributed to very low compliance, that is, poor adherence to a medication regimen. Quite simply, because compliant individuals expect to experience negative side effects when they drink alcohol, they typically stop taking disulfiram, rather than stop drinking. For example, in the larger of the two VA clinical trials, only 20% of the 577 completed patients were deemed compliant (Fuller et al., 1986). Efforts to improve compliance have resulted in a reduction in alcohol consumption when disulfiram is administered in a supervised fashion (Azrin, Sisson, Meyers, & Godley, 1982; Chick et al., 1992). One such example is the marital treatment program described by O'Farrell (1995), during which the spouse monitored disulfiram administration to maintain compliance and as a means of becoming engaged in treatment. For the alcoholic, compliance demonstrates a show of good faith and commitment to recovery. Although promising, studies of supervised disulfiram administration have yielded mixed findings (Keane, Foy, Nunn, & Rychtarik, 1984; O'Farrell, Choquette, Cutter, & Henry, 1998). Moreover, because these studies do not speak to standard clinical conditions, in which compliance is ultimately determined by the patient, an appropriately rigorous clinical trial comparing supervised with unsupervised use is necessary (Heather, 1989). Furthermore, these attempts to improve compliance have been seriously criticized in terms of their research design, including improper placebo conditions, failure to determine disulfiram blood levels across time intervals, and imprecise measures of alcohol use (Allen & Litten, 1992). More extreme approaches for improving compliance have been explored, such as subcutaneous implantation of disulfiram in the stomach wall, but they have met with limited success (Johnsen & Morland, 1991; Wilson, Davidson, & Blanchard, 1980). In addition, clinical accounts exist of alcoholics who have continued to drink despite taking disulfiram, having become tolerant of the aversive effects (Ewing, 1982). In summary, with the possible exceptions of older, more stable alcoholics and administration under supervision, disulfiram appears to provide no appreciable benefit to alcoholism treatment.

MODERATION TRAINING AND CONTROLLED DRINKING

As described at the outset of the chapter, the controversial treatments we review meet the criteria of being in widespread use as well as having been researched and shown to have doubtful or negligible efficacy. One controversial treatment for alcoholism does not meet these criteria. However, controlled drinking warrants our discussion by virtue of its history and the extent to which it divided not only the scientific and lay communities, but also the scientific community itself.

Most definitions of controlled drinking include some limit on the amount and frequency of consumption, as well as avoidance of legal, social, and physical problems. As a treatment goal, controlled drinking refers to assisting individuals with drinking problems to establish or reestablish control or moderation in drinking. Although at first glance this goal might not seem particularly controversial, in the late 1960s and 1970s (when psychological research first suggested the possibility of controlled drinking), the premise that some individuals could return to social drinking was antithetical to the ideology of AA and much of the alcoholism treatment establishment. For this reason, interventions with controlled drinking as their long-term goal have led to some of most acrimonious and public debates in the history of alcoholism treatment.

The onset of the contemporary controversy regarding controlled drinking can be marked by the report of British physician D. L. Davies (1962), who presented his follow-up of 93 alcoholics 7–11 years post-treatment, including 7 who had resumed nonabusive drinking. Although there had been earlier reports that some problem drinkers had successfully returned to social drinking, Davies was the first to cast this finding not as a mere anomaly, but as a basis for reexamining the premise of abstinence as a requirement for treatment. However, the controversy did not truly become a flashpoint for alcoholism research until two publications became widely publicized and attacked from scientific, political, and even ethical perspectives by those advocating abstinence as the only viable treatment goal. The first study and its follow-up reports by Mark and Linda Sobell (1973, 1976) described the favorable outcome of a treatment program to train hospitalized alcoholics to drink in a controlled fashion. The second study, a national survey of individuals treated in federally funded treatment centers, was conducted by the Rand Corporation in collaboration with the Stanford Research Institute (Armor, Polich, & Stambul, 1976), and reported the presence of "normal" drinkers in the follow-up samples. In both cases, it was difficult to dismiss the data as anomalous because of the systematic effort of the Sobells to train moderate drinking skills as well as the surprising percentages revealed in the Rand data: 12% normal drinkers at 6 months after treatment and 22% at 18 months.

Nonetheless, as recounted in various comprehensive narratives (e.g., Hunt, 1999; Marlatt, 1983; Roizen, 1987) an enormous effort to discredit and even suppress these findings ensued, including lawsuits, sensational media coverage, and the formation of independent investigative groups. As Roizen (1987) contended, these controversies served notice of the failure of scientific research in alcoholism, to that time, to have significantly advanced the treatment of alcoholism beyond its earliest beginnings.

The chilling effects of such virulent opposition certainly affected the initiation of new treatment outcome studies on moderation. Even into the 1990s, a survey of 196 treatment programs found that 75% viewed controlled drinking as an unacceptable treatment goal (Rosenberg & Davis, 1994). Nonetheless, over the past 25 years, reports of non–problem drinking by formerly alcohol-dependent or abusing individuals have continued to emerge, from treatment outcome studies, reports of self-treatment or natural recovery (Sobell, Cunningham, & Sobell, 1996), and longitudinal studies (e.g., Vaillant, 1996). Consequently, these data have become harder for the public to ignore, despite continued opposition. For example, the Institute of Medicine (1990) and the Ninth Special Report to Congress on Alcohol and Health (U.S. Department of Health and Human Services, 1997) describe moderation as a reasonable treatment goal for some problem drinkers. The recent publication of a popular text, *Sober for Good* (Fletcher, 2001), detailed the success stories of 222 "masters," individuals who have successfully overcome alcohol dependence. Interestingly, 56% resolved their drinking problems independent of 12-step programs, and approximately 10% reported that they drink occasionally. Because most of the latter group developed their own strategies for moderation, it remains unknown if more would have succeeded had formal training been accessible.

Despite the implications of research on controlled drinking and the beginnings of a change in the societal perception of controlled drinking, important questions remain unanswered, namely, "For whom is controlled drinking a viable treatment goal?" and "What are the most efficacious means of facilitating controlled drinking?" Rosenberg (1993) provided some answers to the former question in a comprehensive review of research on variables that predict successful controlled drinking. He concluded that although no single factor was consistently predictive of moderation, the following predictors emerged: lower severity of dependence, a belief that moderation is possible, employment, younger age, psychological and social stability, and female gender. Other studies reveal better outcome, both for moderation and for abstinence, when problem drinkers are allowed to select their treatment pathway (e.g., Orford & Keddie, 1986; Sanchez-Craig & Lei, 1986). In the face of these data, it would seem to be myopic for clinicians to disregard controlled drinking procedures as a treatment option for some alcoholics.

As for methods to facilitate controlled drinking, the selection of available procedures currently includes an array of manuals and programs, succinctly summarized by Heather (1995). In the face of an ever-increasing research base for controlled drinking, cleaving to an outmoded status quo of abstinence as the only acceptable goal of treatment maintains what we fear to be a self-fulfilling prophecy, and an artificial limitation on the range of outcomes possible for some drinkers.

PROJECT DARE

Although this chapter is oriented toward treatments of alcoholism, a contemporary controversy that significantly illustrates the gap between craftsman and professional is related not to treatment, but to prevention, namely, the efficacy of Project DARE (Drug Abuse and Resistance Education). Part of our decision to review this prevention program is motivated by its high profile; Project DARE is quite widespread in the United States and is used by approximately 50% of local school districts nationwide (Ringwalt & Greene, 1993).

Developed by the Los Angeles Police Department in 1983, Project DARE uses uniformed police officers to teach a drug abuse prevention program that focuses on negative aspects of substance abuse and emphasizes the positive aspects of a healthy lifestyle (Koch, 1994). The core curriculum is delivered to fifth- and sixth-grade students in 1-hour sessions for 17 consecutive weeks. Other components have been developed for students beginning from kindergarten through high school, creating a comprehensive developmental prevention program (Koch, 1994). Despite its widespread adoption, there is a fundamental absence of evidence that DARE has any appreciable effect on preventing substance use. A number of outcome studies have been conducted on Project DARE with remarkably consistent results. Rosenbaum, Flewelling, Bailey, Ringwalt, and Wilkinson (1994) found that for 1,584 fifth and sixth graders, there were no statisti-

cally significant differences on alcohol or cigarette use, or on school per
formance during the year following participation in the DARE program. A
similar study of 36 schools in Illinois indicated negligible impact on student drug use immediately following the intervention, as well as after 1 or
2 years (Ennett, Tobler, Ringwalt, & Flewelling, 1994). Additionally, no
significant impact on self-esteem, resistance to peer pressure, delay of experimentation with drugs, or drug use was found in a study of ninth-grade
students from 21 elementary schools who received the DARE program in
the sixth grade (Dukes, Ullman, & Stein, 1996).

In terms of extended outcome, a 6-year follow-up of 1,798 students
found Project DARE to exert no long-term beneficial effects on substance
use (Rosenbaum & Hanson, 1998). Moreover, in a 10-year follow-up of
1,002 individuals who participated in DARE in sixth grade, no significant
effect on substance use was found (Lynam et al., 1999). In addition, a
meta-analysis of eight outcome studies indicated negligible effect sizes of
DARE programs on multiple outcome measures, including alcohol and
drug use (Ennett et al., 1994).

Project DARE is an exemplar of a largely pseudoscientific program:
Its success lies primarily in its intuitive appeal and its "feel-good" approach (Clayton, Leukefeld, Harrington, & Cattarello, 1996) as well as
the political climate of the "Just Say No" post-Reagan era. DARE has been
shown to be popular with both parents and administrators (Donnermeyer,
2000; Donnermeyer & Wurschmidt, 1997). Together these factors have
built a sociopolitical monolith (Wysong, Aniskiewicz, & Wright, 1994)
propelled by its own momentum.

Although it is beyond the scope of this chapter, research evidence exists supporting alternate prevention programs, both in the short- and long-
term (Coombs & Ziedonis, 1995). Given these alternatives, the most serious implication is that, whether in terms of dollars or hours spent on
DARE instruction, community resources are being squandered on a program that does not work in lieu of potentially efficacious curricula (Ennett
et al., 1994).

EFFECTIVE TREATMENTS FOR ALCOHOLISM:
THE STATE OF THE SCIENCE

Because the gulf between contemporary clinical practice and scientific research serves to sustain controversial treatments, dissemination of research
findings and practice guidelines is critical to their integration. For this reason, in the second portion of the chapter we describe the theory, evidence,
and procedures of a selection of evidence-based treatments.

In this section, we describe psychotherapeutic interventions shown to
be efficacious treatments for drinking problems (dependence and abuse),

and review their theoretical and empirical bases. Our criteria for including these treatments are scientifically broad: The interventions discussed must be theory based and data driven. That is, designated interventions must reflect a theory couched in previous research and also be supported by empirically based outcome studies.

These criteria are intentionally broad enough to include an array of scientific treatments. Unsurprisingly, this group includes several treatments for drinking problems identified by the Task Force of the American Psychological Association (Chambless et al., 1998) in their list of empirically supported treatments (ESTs; see also Chapter 6) and overlaps with several of the successful major treatment modalities noted by Miller et al. (1995) in their extensive methodological analysis of alcohol treatment research.

SOCIAL LEARNING THEORY: COGNITIVE/SOCIAL SKILLS TRAINING

An underlying premise for several treatments of alcohol dependence derives from social learning theory (SLT), a broad theoretical approach that describes human behavior via an integration of principles of operant and classical conditioning, cognitive psychology, and observational learning (Bandura, 1969). SLT focused initially on stress reduction as the primary pharmacological action of alcohol, whereby alcohol provides negative reinforcement, or the removal of an aversive experience. In turn, alcohol dependence is a consequence of an inability to use an adaptive, alternative means of removing aversive stimuli and the excessive use of alcohol to do so. Recent versions of SLT (e.g., Wilson, 1988) incorporate principles of modeling, rehearsal, attribution theory, and self-efficacy. More specifically, SLT proposes that an individual lacks important coping skills for daily living and that deficits related to these domains contribute significantly to substance dependence problems and relapse.

Various findings support this hypothesized etiological deficit. First, there is evidence that alcoholics have inferior coping skills compared with nonalcoholics (Monti, Abrams, Kadden, & Rohsenow, 1989), especially in such diverse circumstances as interpersonal conflict or celebratory social gatherings. Skill levels also predict treatment outcome: Skills developed to deal with high-risk circumstances over the course of treatment predict positive outcome (Monti et al., 1990) and low skill levels measured during treatment follow-up predict relapse (Miller, Westerberg, Harris, & Tonigan, 1996). Specific capabilities that are treated via skills training, such as modulating affective states or tolerating negative emotions, have also been shown to be related to relapse (Marlatt & Gordon, 1985; Monti, Rohsenow, Colby, & Abrams, 1995), further supporting the possibility that assistance in these contexts could be significantly ameliorative.

This evidence of skills deficits has led to the development of several skills training programs, based primarily on cognitive and behavioral psychotherapeutic principles. One of the most thoroughly researched of these treatments is coping/social skills training (CSST; Monti et al., 1989).

CSST describes four primary themes, or domains, in which the problem drinker displays a dysfunctional interactional style: (1) interpersonal skills for building better relationships, (2) cognitive-emotional coping for mood regulation, (3) skills for improving daily living and dealing with stressful life events, and (4) coping in the context of substance use cues (Monti et al., 1995). Clearly, each of these themes focuses on the development of skills to replace problem drinking.

Although manualized forms of CSST exist, the treatment is highly idiographic and begins with an assessment of each patient's domains of vulnerability (Monti et al., 1995). These problem areas can be gleaned from several instruments, specifically the Situational Competency Test (Chaney, O'Leary & Marlatt, 1978), the Adaptive Skills Battery (Jones & Lanyon, 1981), and the Alcohol-Specific Role-Play Test (Abrams et al., 1991). Having developed a framework of vulnerabilities, the individual is introduced to a group setting within which the fundamental goal is to engage in behavioral rehearsal of role plays, with members using situations specific to themselves and modules designed to address general high-risk situations. These modules include Drink Refusal Skills, Receiving Criticism about Drinking/Drug Use, Developing Sober Supports, and Conflict Resolution Skills (Monti et al., 1989).

Considerable research attests to the effectiveness of CSST. Clinical trials have shown CSST to be more efficacious than systematic desensitization, covert sensitization, aversion therapy (Hedberg & Campbell, 1974), traditional supportive therapy (Oei & Jackson, 1980, 1982), human relations training (Ferrell & Galassi, 1981), discussion groups (Chaney et al., 1978), mood management treatment (Monti et al., 1990), and group discussion (Eriksen, Bjornstad, & Gotestam, 1986), as well as no-treatment control conditions (Chaney et al., 1978).

Although not all treatment outcome studies have provided unequivocally positive results, CSST has been shown to be of comparable efficacy to other treatment conditions. For example, CSST alone has been found comparable to CSST with additional therapeutic components, such as relaxation therapy or bibliotherapy (Miller, Taylor, & West, 1980). As mentioned earlier, this was also the case in Project MATCH, in which an enhanced version of CSST constituted the cognitive-behavioral treatment and was shown to be equally effective to motivational enhancement therapy and 12-step facilitation treatment (Project MATCH Research Group, 1998). Taken together, the evidence in support of CSST is among the most compelling in the literature.

The fourth domain of CSST, that of coping in contexts associated with alcohol, has a different theoretical foundation than social learning theory and has evolved into a separate treatment in its own right. Conditioning models of dependence are the basis for this domain and posit that classically conditioned associates of substance use can acquire motivational properties that influence behavior (Cunningham, 1998). As a consequence, reconditioning must take place to reduce the individual's association of the substance with various environmental factors.

This technique is referred to as cue exposure treatment (CET) and relies on extinction, that is, exposure to conditioned cues until previous associations are weakened and new associations strengthened. The standard procedure for this technique is to expose alcohol-dependent individuals to the sight and smell of alcohol. Via multiple exposures without consumption, the associated craving to drink ebbs, and similar urges are reduced when the patient is in social situations in which alcohol is present.

This component of CSST has been robustly supported. CSST with CET has resulted in patients being more likely to remain completely abstinent, having more abstinent days, and imbibing fewer drinks than control patients (Monti et al., 1993). Drummond and Glautier (1994) compared a CET group with a relaxation control group, and reported a more favorable outcome for the former in terms of latency to relapse and total alcohol consumption. Additionally, Sitharthan, Sitharthan, Hough, and Kavanagh (1997) compared CET with cognitive-behavioral strategies in attaining moderation in drinking, and found significant reductions in drinking quantity and frequency for the CET group compared with the cognitive-behavioral group.

Despite these positive findings, a recent meta-analysis of cue exposure therapy across substances of dependence has criticized the extent of therapeutic impact of CET and lamented its failure to utilize procedures and findings from contemporary animal research on extinction (Conklin & Tiffany, 2002). Although Drummond (2002) has cogently disagreed with some of the procedures and conclusions of this meta-analysis, it is clear that continued empirical research is necessary to refine this technique.

RELAPSE PREVENTION

A second major form of cognitive-behavioral skills training is relapse prevention (RP; Marlatt & Gordon, 1985). The most common outcome after treatment for any addiction is relapse: Approximately 60% resume substance use within 90 days of treatment, the majority within the first month (Dimeff & Marlatt, 1995). A major premise of RP is that following an initial lapse or slip, defined as a brief return to drinking with no adverse effects, one can implement an array of strategies to preclude a transition to heavy drinking. Such strategies directly address the "abstinence violation effect" (Marlatt & Gordon, 1985), which describes the impact of a slip on an abstinent individual who may then experience shame, guilt, and the belief that a relapse is inevitable, and proceed to continue drinking. RP is a systematic form of therapy designed to prepare for a possible relapse and to incorporate it into the recovery process in a positive way.

Procedurally, RP begins with an idiographic assessment that delineates two basic components of risk for relapse: proximal determinants, or circumstances that can precipitate relapse, and potential covert antecedents, or less obvious circumstances that can influence the relapse process (Larimer, Palmer, & Marlatt, 1999). Proximal determinants are variables that directly influence relapse, including such high-risk situations as social pressure or negative emotional states. In contrast, covert antecedents precede situations in which the individual is unprepared and thereby susceptible to relapse, including driving by a favorite bar or spending time with certain people. As in CSST, a functional analysis of the client's behavior leads to identification of the individual's precipitants, and skills training is used to cope with these circumstances.

A considerable body of research literature supports the efficacy of RP treatment. Recent meta-analyses of treatments using either RP alone or as an adjunct to other treatment found that RP was effective in reducing the frequency and intensity of relapse (Irvin, Bowers, Dunn, & Wang, 1999), although it was not associated with higher overall abstinence rates (Carroll, 1996; Irvin et al., 1999). However, RP has shown "delayed emergence effects" or significant improvements found only at later follow-up points (Carroll, 1996). These benefits of RP over standard clinical management are speculated to be a result of RP's more didactic approach and emphasis on reducing exposure to situations of increased risk for substance abuse (Carroll et al., 1994). Overall, findings suggest robust efficacy for RP interventions in the treatment of alcohol dependence, either adjunctively or as a stand-alone treatment.

OPERANT CONDITIONING:
THE COMMUNITY-REINFORCEMENT APPROACH

An exemplar of treatments derived from principles of operant conditioning is the community-reinforcement approach (CRA), developed by Hunt and Azrin (1973). Operant conditioning describes the interaction of organisms with their environments according to contingencies of reinforcement and punishment; reinforced behaviors are displayed more frequently, and punished behaviors are decreased or suppressed (Skinner, 1938). Alcohol (or any drug) can be a strong reinforcer, and addicted individuals often forgo socially acceptable reinforcers, such as interpersonal relationships or vocational efforts, to seek and consume excessive amounts of alcohol.

Treatment based on the CRA attempts to restructure the environmental contingencies in a person's life so that abstinence becomes more rewarding than drinking. This daunting goal typically entails a multifaceted rearrangement of the individual's vocational, social, recreational, and familial dynamics, and may even include monitored administration of disulfiram (Meyers & Smith, 1995).

The form of a CRA intervention is shaped by these multiple domains and, like CSST and RP, begins with an idiographic assessment of the environmental contingencies that shape an individual's behavior. Use of a structured protocol facilitates identification of external factors, such as where, when, and with whom an individual drinks; internal triggers, such as cognitions, emotions, or physiological experiences that precede drinking; and antecedents and consequents of both drinking and nondrinking behaviors (Smith & Meyers, 1995). Based on this assessment, different modules from a menu of treatment options are selected, all of which are intended to increase the amount of positive reinforcement from nondrinking sources. For example, because the course of alcoholism often leads to loss of employment, a common source of deficient reinforcement is vocational. Therefore, one module is called the "Job-Club," which focuses on improving skills to secure and maintain work.

Considerable empirical support exists for the CRA. Hunt and Azrin (1973) found that CRA clients spent significantly less time drinking or hospitalized than controls, and significantly more time working and being with their families. These findings were supported by a follow-up study including adjunctive disulfiram treatment (Azrin, 1976). In this case, the treatment condition drank an average of only 2% of posttreatment days, compared with 55% of days for the control group. These gains were sustained when assessed at a 2-year follow-up: 90% of the CRA group was still abstinent (Azrin, 1976). In the case of outpatient CRA plus disulfiram treatment, significant improvement was found compared with traditional 12-step treatment and a medication-only condition. Six months following the treatment, 97% of participants in the CRA group remained abstinent, compared with 45% and 74% in the other treatments, respectively (Azrin et al., 1982).

An innovative extension of the CRA has recently been developed to address the problem, described earlier, of problem drinkers who resist seeking treatment. Sisson and Azrin (1986) applied CRA principles to the development of training for families, as a means to motivate alcoholics to initiate treatment. Meyers and his colleagues (e.g., Meyers, Miller, Hill, & Tonigan, 1999; Meyers & Smith, 1997) developed a program that extended the principles of the CRA to community reinforcement and family training (CRAFT). The goal of CRAFT is to teach concerned significant others (CSOs) behavioral principles that could reduce their loved one's drinking and concurrently motivate the drinker to seek treatment. The promise inherent in the empirical bases of this new approach has met with initial success, according to the striking results of a recently published controlled outcome study. Miller, Meyers, and Tonigan (1999) conducted a randomized clinical trial in which 130 CSOs underwent counseling via one of three different approaches—Al-Anon facilitation, CRAFT, or a Johnson Intervention—to prepare for a family confrontation of the drinker. Using the criterion of moving initially unmotivated drinkers into treatment, success rates were 13% for CSOs who participated in the Al-Anon group, 30% for those in the Johnson Intervention group, and 64% for those enrolled in CRAFT. Future studies may clarify whether CRAFT sets the stage for an increased likelihood of successful subsequent treatment once the drinker has taken the initial steps.

MOTIVATIONAL ENHANCEMENT THERAPY

Community reinforcement approaches manipulate environmental contingencies to reengage and strengthen behaviors that lead to alternatives to drinking. However, these treatments rely on the influence of reinforcers that possess sufficient value to the person.

In complementary fashion, motivational enhancement therapy (MET) focuses on psychotherapeutic techniques to recalibrate individuals' motivation toward their environments, and in particular to stimulate motivation toward goals incongruent with ongoing abuse (DiClemente, Carbonari, & Velasquez, 1992; Miller & Rollnick, 1991; Miller, Zweben, DiClemente, & Rychtarik, 1992).

Individuals seeking treatment for alcohol (or other drug addiction) differ significantly in their levels of motivation for change, and these differences are related to treatment outcome (Carney & Kivlahan, 1995; DiClemente & Hughes, 1990). Studies have shown that high motivation is associated with high treatment retention, and that low motivation predicts worse outcomes (Ryan, Plant, & O'Malley, 1995).

One goal of MET is to help individuals progress through a series of stages that characterize the process of psychotherapeutic change (DiClemente & Velasquez, 2002). A recent version of this model of change (Prochaska, DiClemente, & Norcross, 1992) depicts five stages in a spiral, suggesting a nonlinear change process. First is a precontemplative stage, in which quitting is not even considered. This is followed by a contemplation stage in which the possibility of changing one's habits is broached, but with some ambivalence. Third is the preparation stage, in which self-regulation may increase as a decision to change is made, followed by action, the fourth stage and the one in which a strategy for change is engaged, and then maintained in the fifth stage. Although critics of the stages model have raised serious concerns about validity and measurement issues (e.g.,

Davidson, 1998; Littell & Girvin, 2002), most agree that it has provided both heuristic and practical benefits, such as providing a context in which practitioners develop motivational enhancement strategies.

The therapeutic form of MET is based on five principles (Miller & Rollnick, 1991). First, the therapist expresses empathy via reflective listening and clarification to communicate acceptance. This interactive process is intended to be the antithesis of the confrontational or didactic stance that many problem drinkers have experienced from family and professionals, and it paradoxically helps the client to become the agent of change. The second principle is the most central: The therapist facilitates clients' development of discrepancies between their drinking and their life goals. One might assume that the many negative consequences of drinking that led to the initiation of treatment have already highlighted these discrepancies. But this is often not the case; the problem drinker's ambivalence and counterarguments maintain inertia, whereas the safe environment of therapy can facilitate exploration of the pros and cons of personal change, free of outside judgment or coercion (Miller, 1995). Following efforts to develop discrepancies, the three remaining principles—namely, avoiding argumentation, "rolling" with resistance, and supporting self-efficacy—comprise the basis for changing drinkers' motivations and fostering their progress toward change.

In terms of outcome research, the most substantial trial of MET took place in Project MATCH, in which each treatment produced long-lasting results, and no treatment was substantially more effective than any other (Project MATCH Research Group, 1998). However, MET included only half of the therapist interactions (four sessions) as did the other two treatments. Subsequent analyses indicated that motivated patients were more likely to experience a better client–therapist relationship and better posttreatment drinking outcomes across treatments (DiClemente, Carbonari, Zweben, Morrel, & Lee, 2001). Project MATCH data also revealed that patients characterized by high levels of trait anger had a better outcome in MET than in 12-step facilitation or coping skills treatments (Project MATCH Research Group, 1998). Finally, considerable research evidence has accumulated to support the use of motivational treatments in brief interventions, which we will subsequently discuss in further detail.

MARITAL AND FAMILY THERAPY

One commonality of the previously discussed treatments has been a prevailing focus on the individual as the primary medium through which change is effected. Interest by the alcohol treatment community in marital and family therapy (MFT) evolved from field and laboratory observations of the problem drinker's interpersonal systems (e.g., Jacob & Seilhamer,

1987; Steinglass, 1981) and various findings indicating that marital dissatisfaction and alcoholism are intimately related. Not surprisingly, many alcoholics experience extensive marital and family problems (O'Farrell & Birchler, 1987), and successful treatment outcome, particularly posttreatment maintenance, is associated with better marital and family relationships (Moos, Finney, & Cronkite, 1990). The relationship between alcoholism and marital satisfaction appears to be bidirectional. That is, alcohol dependence affects the marriage and family, which in turn affect the alcoholic's drinking behavior and treatment prognosis. Evidence supports this reciprocal relationship: Marital and family conflicts may often exacerbate problems or precipitate renewed drinking in abstinent alcoholics (Maisto, O'Farrell, Connors, McKay, & Pelcovits, 1988).

MFT for alcoholism has two main agendas: first, acutely reducing abusive drinking and, second, rendering the family environment more conducive to sobriety (O'Farrell, 1995). The first goal employs a variety of strategies, including written behavioral contracts, structured discussions about drinking, and decreasing family members' behaviors that instigate drinking. In addition, a component of MFT for short-term alcohol-use reduction can include contracting to regularly take disulfiram, which O'Farrell (1995) has shown can generate high rates of compliance. In terms of making the marriage conducive to successful abstinence or reduction, MFT attempts to reengage the couple in a generally fulfilling relationship. This can be a difficult task, as often the alcoholic period(s) may have left remaining scars, both emotional and tangible (e.g., joblessness, debts). Once the alcoholic has begun to regain abstinence and the couple has begun to address any relationship-based triggers and reinforcers for drinking, in many respects MFT primarily comprises efforts to enhance the quality of the marital relationship (Noel & McCrady, 1993). Relevant strategies include increasing positive interchanges, problem solving, conflict resolution, planning shared recreational/leisure activities, training in communication skills, and behavior change agreements.

Outcome research attests to the benefits of enhancing the marital relationship in effecting change. Smith (1969) showed that the alcoholic husbands of wives who attended groups to increase understanding of alcoholism and their role in alcoholism significantly improved and had more days abstinent than did a control group. But for the most part, little outcome research has been conducted to support the efficacy of most of the prevailing popular methods that involve couples and families in the treatment of problem drinkers. The benefits that have been consistently demonstrated by outcome research have emerged primarily from investigations that used variations of behavioral-marital therapy for alcoholic couples. These variations include the Project for Alcoholic Couples' Treatment (PACT), described in a series of publications by McCrady and her colleagues (e.g., McCrady et al., 1986), and a project Counseling for

Alcoholic Marriages (CALM), directed by O'Farrell (e.g., O'Farrell, Cutter, & Floyd, 1985).

CALM uses both behavioral techniques and spousal monitoring of disulfiram administration. Compared with couples administered either no-treatment, interpersonal counseling, or unsupervised disulfiram, couples involved with MFT/disulfiram improved significantly on various follow-up measures of marital adjustment. These results were sustained at a 2-year follow-up (O'Farrell, Cutter, Choquette, Floyd, & Bayog, 1992). Of note, however, is that no significant differences were found among groups in terms of reductions in drinking either at immediate or 2-year follow-up. Encouragingly, a subsequent study of MFT revealed that the addition of a relapse prevention component resulted in significantly more days abstinent and higher disulfiram compliance for the experimental group (O'Farrell, Choquette, Cutter, & Brown, 1993). Because follow-up studies over several years reveal a variety of changes in these outcome measures, there is still much to learn about how marital therapy facilitates the problem drinker's recovery. Nonetheless, the results of MFT appear promising and the overall literature has been interpreted as supportive by both the APA Task Force (Chambless et al., 1998) and the Ninth Special Report to Congress (U.S. Dept. of Health and Human Services, 1997).

BRIEF INTERVENTIONS

A final form of treatment relevant to this discussion includes a variety of "brief" interventions. These interventions comprise a range of time-limited treatments, from 5 minutes of advice (e.g., urging individuals to cut down on their drinking or suggesting that their level of consumption could result in health problems) to several counseling sessions, implemented in a variety of settings, and used with a variety of dependent and abusive drinkers (Heather, 1995).

Brief interventions have evolved from Chafetz's (1961) report indicating that of 1,200 alcoholic patients admitted to the emergency room and advised to seek treatment, only 5% did so. However, following a brief empathic counseling session, 65% of a similar group of alcoholic patients attended a follow-up appointment for treatment. This and substantial subsequent research led to the widespread implementation of interventions of this sort in community-based initiatives, or "opportunistic" settings (e.g., the office of one's primary care physician) to which clients typically have not come to discuss alcohol use (Heather, 1995).

Although these studies primarily describe interventions by physicians to facilitate initiation of treatment, brief psychological interventions have been shown to be efficacious in and of themselves. Indeed, research has supported these interventions in a variety of settings and provided considerable evidence for their efficacy (Bien, Miller, & Tonigan, 1993; Kahan, Wilson, & Becker, 1995; Moyer, Finney, Swearingen, & Vergun, 2002; Wilk, Jensen, & Havighurst, 1997).

Since Edwards and colleagues (1977) demonstrated that a single session of "advice" was as effective as four sessions of treatment for alcoholics, brief interventions have become substantially more prevalent. A recent example is that of Marlatt and colleagues (Marlatt, Baer, & Larimer, 1995; Marlatt et al., 1998), who identified heavy drinkers in high school and provided a brief treatment using a single motivational interview. Follow-up assessments over a 2-year period showed reductions in drinking rates and harmful consequences from drinking.

Despite the implicit uniformity of the term, brief treatments are quite heterogeneous. For example, it is unclear what the ideal extent of treatment is, or for whom. Research has indicated that 5 minutes of simple advice may be as effective as more extensive counseling (World Health Organization, 1996) and, perhaps paradoxically, that a more extensive intervention may be superior (Israel et al., 1996). For these reasons, Drummond (1997) suggested that until research isolates the "effective ingredients" of brief interventions and the appropriate populations that benefit from them, health care providers should embrace them only cautiously. Nonetheless, the demonstrable benefits of brief interventions make them worthy of consideration by clinicians as a low-cost treatment of first resort.

CONCLUSIONS

In this chapter, we have focused on several controversial approaches to the treatment and prevention of alcohol problems, and we have also contrasted these questionable or ineffective strategies with others that have been found to be more useful by virtue of systematic outcome data. Although numerous psychological treatments can document a long history of controversy about the accuracy of their premises and consistency of positive findings, treatments for addictions seem particularly noteworthy for the acrimony and public visibility in which they have been engulfed. In many respects, this situation reflects the degree to which the treatment of substance abusers, particularly alcoholics, has been dominated by individuals with a personal stake in its outcome—addicts themselves, family, and concerned citizens. Thus, controversial treatment issues in the addictions reflect not only the usual inter- and intranecine battles among professionals and scientists that occur in various disciplines, but also contentions that pit scientists as adversaries to a politicized and determined lay public and nonscientific clinicians. The controversial treatments we highlighted have proceeded to advance despite the lack of strong evidence of their efficacy, often accompanied by their adherents' notable hostility toward those who seek such evidence. How these circumstances arose is germane to an under-standing of numerous critical aspects of controversial treatments in the ad-dictions, such as what maintains their vitality, how alternatives are pro-mulgated, and the problem of dissemination of research-based treatment innovations.

Nevertheless, we are cautiously optimistic about the foothold that evidence-based treatments are staking out for the future, as it is becoming apparent that successful treatment providers will need to adopt an increas-ingly flexible, scientifically "informed eclecticism" (Miller & Hester, 1995). For example, it is no longer uncommon to find that mainstream treatment programs include psychoeducational components comprising aspects of coping skills and relapse prevention.

Continued progress in replacing questionable therapies with well-validated treatments may hinge on researchers' awareness of the need for systematic and skillful dissemination of their findings. One inspiring illus-tration is a report by Sobell (1996) of her team's innovative and successful efforts to promulgate an evidence-based approach to problem drinking in the program repertoire of numerous treatment agencies in a large Cana-dian province. Another is the recent effort by Read, Kahler, and Stevenson (2001) to bridge the science–practice gap by publishing a review of effec-tive treatments in a journal widely read by practitioners. Indeed, these ini-tiatives are converging with pressure from managed health care to adopt evidence-based treatment, and with recent efforts by federal agencies both to fund science-based prevention and treatment programs and to develop better dissemination of research findings. We hope that these activities con-stitute the boosts that science-based treatments require to overcome the uncritical acceptance of treatments that merely "feel" right or reflect little more than clinical tradition.

GLOSSARY

Alcoholics Anonymous (AA): Founded in 1935, AA is a nonprofit, grassroots lay treatment for alcoholism. Core tenets include a chronic disease model of alcoholism, treatable only by total abstinence, adherence to its 12-step ideology, including an emphasis on nondenominational spirituality and the use of fellowship among alcoholics to maintain abstinence.

Antidipsotropic: Any medication whose administration induces illness follow-ing ingestion of alcohol; often used as part of aversive conditioning.

Community-Reinforcement Approach (CRA): A psychotherapeutic interven-tion based on operant conditioning that attempts to reduce drinking behavior by restructuring the individual's reinforcement contingencies to increase the value of nondrinking behaviors.

Coping/Social Skills Training (CSST): A psychotherapeutic form of treatment for alcohol dependence from the perspective of Social Learning Theory. CSST attempts to reduce drinking by improving individuals' ability to cope with relationships, events in their lives, and their own negative moods, often in the context of alcohol cues.

Cue Exposure Treatment (CET): Both a component of CSST and a stand-alone treatment, CET is based on a classical conditioning model of alcoholism and leads to drinking reduction or abstinence by exposing the alcoholic to alcohol-related cues.

Disulfiram (commercial name, Antabuse): The most common antidipsotropic medication, disulfiram induces flushing, rapid or irregular heartbeat, sweating, nausea, and dizziness by preventing the release of aldehyde dehydrogenase, a liver enzyme required to break down alcohol.

Marital and Family Therapy (MFT): A psychotherapeutic treatment that uses the marital relationship as the forum for reducing drinking behavior. Clinically, couples may learn improved communication skills, develop problem solving for conflict resolution, and address intimacy issues. One premise of these efforts its that improvement in the marital relationship will decrease the appeal of alcohol. Another is that spousal engagement will help problem drinkers to develop and maintain their treatment goals.

Motivational Enhancement Therapy (MET): A clinical intervention that identifies discrete stages of change and attempts to facilitate the client's progress through these stages toward abstinence or a reduction in drinking.

Relapse Prevention (RP): A form of psychotherapeutic intervention based on Social Learning Theory that focuses on incorporating plans for probable relapse into the treatment process. RP uses skills training and cognitive techniques to reduce the likelihood and severity of relapse.

Social Learning Theory (SLT): A broad theoretical approach to human behavior that incorporates principles of classical and operant conditioning, cognitive psychology, and observational learning. In applications to drinking problems, SLT provides the basis for strategies that include coping skills, modeling, rehearsal, attribution, and the enhancement of self-efficacy.

REFERENCES

Abrams, D. B., Binkoff, J. A., Zwick, W. R., Liepman, M. R., Nirenberg, T. D., Munroe, S. M., & Monti, P. M. (1991). Alcohol abusers' and social drinkers' responses to alcohol-relevant and general situations. *Journal of Studies on Alcohol, 52,* 409–414.

Alcoholics Anonymous. (1990). *Alcoholics Anonymous 1989 membership survey.* New York: Alcoholics Anonymous World Services.

Allen, J. P., & Litten, R. Z (1992). Techniques to enhance compliance with disulfiram. *Alcoholism: Clinical and Experimental Research, 16*, 1035–1041.

Armor, D . J., Polich, J. M., & Stambul, H. B. (1976). *Alcoholism and treatment.* Santa Monica, CA: Rand Corporation.

Azrin, N. H. (1976). Improvements in the community reinforcement approach to alcoholism. *Behaviour Research and Therapy, 14*, 339–348.

Azrin, N. H., Sisson, W., Myers, R., & Godley, M. (1982). Alcoholism treatment by disulfiram and community reinforcement therapy. *Journal of Behavior Therapy and Experimental Psychiatry, 13*, 105–112.

Bandura, A. (1969) *Principles of behavior modifcation.* New York: Holt, Rinehart & Winston.

Bebbington, P. E. (1976). The efficacy of Alcoholics Anonymous: The elusiveness of hard data. *British Journal of Psychiatry, 128*, 572–580.

Bien, T. H., Miller, W. R., & Tonigan, J. S. (1993). Brief interventions for alcohol problems: A review. *Addiction, 88*, 315–336.

Brandsma, J. M., Maultsby, M. C., & Welsh, R. J. (1980). Alcoholics Anonymous: An empirical outcome study. *Addictive Behaviors, 5*, 359–370.

Bunge, M. (1984). What is pseudoscience? *Skeptical Inquirer, 9*, 36–46.

Carney, M. M., & Kivlahan, D. R. (1995). Motivational subtypes among veterans seeking substance abuse treatment: Profiles based on stages of change. *Psychology of Addictive Behaviors, 9*, 135–142.

Carroll, K. M. (1996) Relapse prevention as a psychosocial treatment: A review of controlled clinical trials. *Experimental and Clinical Psychopharmacology, 4*, 46–54.

Carroll, K. M., Rounsaville, B. J., Gordon, L. T., Nich, C., Jatlow, P. M., Bisighini, R. M., & Gatwin, F. H. (1994). Psychotherapy and pharmacotherapy for ambulatory cocaine abusers. *Archives of General Psychiatry, 51*, 177–187.

Chafetz, M. E. (1961). A procedure for establishing therapeutic contact with the alcoholic. *Quarterly Journal of Studies on Alcohol, 22*, 325–328.

Chambless, D. L., Baker, M. J., Baucom, D. H., Beutler, L. E., Calhoun, K. S., Crits-Cristoph, P., Daluto, A., Derubeis, R., Detweiller, J., Haaga, D. A. F., Johnson, S. B., McCurry, S., Musser, K. T., Pope, K. S., Sanderson, W. C., Shoham, V., Stickle, T., Williams, D. A., & Woody, S. R. (1998). Update on empirically supported therapies II. *Clinical Psychologist, 51*, 3–16.

Chaney, E. F., O'Leary, M. R., & Marlatt, G. A. (1978). Skill training with alcoholics. *Journal of Consulting and Clinical Psychology, 46*, 1092–1104.

Chiauzzi, E. J., & Liljegren, S. (1993). Taboo topics in addiction treatment: An empirical review of folklore. *Journal of Substance Abuse Treatment, 10*, 303–316.

Chick, J., Gough, K., Falkowski, W., Kershaw, P., Hore, B., Mehta, B., Ritson, B., Popner, R., & Torley, R. (1992). Disulfiram treatment of alcoholism. *British Journal of Psychiatry, 161*, 84–89.

Clayton, R. R., Leukefeld, C. G., Harrington, N. G., & Cattarello, A. (1996). DARE (Drug Abuse Resistance Education): Very popular but not very effective. In C. B. McCoy, L. R. Metsch, & J. A. Inciardi (Eds.), *Intervening with drug-involved youth* (pp. 101–109). Thousand Oaks, CA: Sage.

Conklin, C. A., & Tiffany, S. T. (2002). Applying extinction research and theory to cue exposure addiction treatments. *Addiction, 97*, 155–167.

Coombs, R. H., & Ziedonis, D. (1995). *Handbook on drug abuse prevention.* Boston: Allyn & Bacon.

Cunningham, C. L. (1998). Drug conditioning and drug seeking behavior. In W. T. O'Donohue (Ed.), *Learning and behavior therapy* (pp. 518–544). Needham Heights, MA: Allyn & Bacon.

Davidson, R. (1998). The Transtheoretical Model: An overview. In W. R. Miller & N. Heather (Eds.), *Treating addictive behaviors* (2nd ed., pp. 25–38). New York: Plenum Press.

Davies, D. L. (1962). Normal drinking in recovered alcohol addicts. *Quarterly Journal of Studies on Alcohol, 23,* 94–104.

DiClemente, C. C, Carbonari, J. P., & Velasquez, M. M. (1992). Alcoholism treatment from a process of change perspective. In R. R. Watson (Ed.), *Alcohol abuse treatment* (pp. 115–142). Totowa, NJ: Humana Press.

DiClemente, C. C., Carbonari, J., Zweben, A., Morrel, T., & Lee, R. E. (2001). Motivation hypothesis causal chain analysis. In R. Longabaugh & P. W. Wirtz (Eds.), *Project MATCH hypotheses: Results and causal chain analyses* (NIAAA Project MATCH monograph series, Vol. 8, pp. 206–223). Washington, DC: Government Printing Office.

DiClemente, C. C., & Hughes, S. O. (1990). Stages of change profiles in outpatient alcoholism treatment. *Journal of Substance Abuse, 2,* 217–235.

DiClemente, C. C., & Velasquez, M. M. (2002). Motivation interviewing and the stages of change. In W. R. Miller & S. Rollnick (Eds.), *Motivational interviewing: Preparing people for change* (2nd ed., pp. 201–216). New York: Guilford Press.

Dimeff, L. A., & Marlatt, G. A. (1995). Relapse prevention. In R. K. Hester & W. R. Miller (Eds.), *Handbook of alcoholism treatment approaches: Effective alternatives* (2nd ed., pp. 176–194). Boston: Allyn & Bacon

Dittman, K. S., Crawford, G. C., Forgy, E. W., Moskowitz, H., & MacAndrew, C. (1967). A controlled experiment on the use of court probation for drunk arrests. *American Journal of Psychiatry, 124,* 160–163.

Donnermeyer, J. F. (2000). Parents' perceptions of a school-based prevention education program. *Journal of Drug Education, 30,* 325–342.

Donnermeyer, J. F., & Wurschmidt, T. N. (1997). Educators' perceptions of the D.A.R.E. program. *Journal of Drug Education, 27,* 259–276.

Drummond, D. C. (1997). Alcohol interventions: Do the best things come in small packages? *Addiction, 92,* 375–379.

Drummond, D. C. (2002). Is cue exposure *cure* exposure? *Addiction, 97,* 357–359.

Drummond. D. C., & Glautier, S. T. (1994). A controlled trial of cue exposure treatment in alcohol dependence. *Journal of Consulting and Clinical Psychology, 62,* 809–817.

Dukes, R. L., Ullman, J. B., & Stein, J. A. (1996). Three-year follow-up of drug abuse resistance education (D.A.R.E.). *Evaluation Review, 20,* 49–66.

Edwards, G., Orford, J., Egert, S., Guthrie, S., Hawkwer, A., Hensmen, C., Mitcheson, M., Oppenheimer, E., & Taylor, C. (1977). Alcoholism: A controlled trial of "treatment" and "advice." *Journal of Studies on Alcohol, 38,* 1004–1031.

Ellis, A., & Schoenfeld, E. (1990). Divine intervention and the treatment of chemical dependency. *Journal of Substance Abuse, 2,* 459–469.

Emrick, C. D. (1987). Alcoholics Anonymous: Affiliation processes and effectiveness as treatment. *Alcoholism: Clinical and Experimental Research, 11*, 416–423.

Emrick, C. D., Tonigan, S., Montgomery, H., & Little, L. (1993). Alcoholics Anonymous: What is currently known? In B. S. McCrady & W. R. Miller (Eds.), *Research on Alcoholics Anonymous: Opportunities and alternatives* (pp. 41–79). New Brunswick, NJ: Alcohol Research Documentation, Rutgers University.

Ennett, S. T., Tobler, N. S., Ringwalt, C. L., & Flewelling, R. L. (1994). How effective is drug abuse resistance education? A meta-analysis of Project DARE outcome evaluations. *American Journal of Public Health, 84*, 1394–1401.

Eriksen, L., Bjornstad, S., & Gotestam, K. G. (1986). Social skills training in groups for alcoholics: One year treatment outcome for groups and individuals. *Addictive Behaviors, 11*, 309–329.

Ewing, J. A. (1982) Disulfiram and other deterrent drugs. In E. M. Pattison & E. Kaufman (Eds.), *Encyclopedic handbook of alcoholism* (pp. 1033–1042). New York: Gardner Press.

Ferrell, W. L., & Galassi, J. P. (1981). Assertion training and human relations training in the treatment of chronic alcoholics. *International Journal of Addictions, 16*, 959–968.

Fletcher, A. (2001). *Sober for good.* New York: Houghton-Mifflin.

Fuller, R. K., Branchey, L., Brightwell, D. R., Derman, R. M., Iber, F. L., James, K., Lacoursiere, R. B., Lee, K. K., Lowenstam, I., Manny, I., Neiderheiser, D., Nocks, J. J., & Shaw, S. (1986). Disulfiram treatment of alcoholism: A Veterans Administration cooperative study. *Journal of the American Medical Association, 256*, 1449–1455.

Fuller, R. K., & Roth, H. P. (1979). Disulfiram for the treatment of alcoholism: an evaluation in 128 men. *Annals of Internal Medicine, 90*, 901–904.

Galanter, M. (1993). *Network therapy for alcohol and drug abuse.* New York: Basic Books.

Gallant, D. M., Bishop, M. P., Falkner, M. A., Simpson, L., Cooper, A., Lathrop, D., Brisolara, W. M., & Bossetta, J. B. (1968). A comparative evaluation of compulsory group therapy and /or Antabuse and voluntary treatment of the chronic alcoholic municipal court offender. *Psychosomatics, 9*, 306–310.

Gerrein, J. R., Rosenberg, C. M., & Manohar, V. (1973). Disulfiram maintenance in outpatient treatment of alcoholism. *Archives of General Psychiatry, 28*, 798–802.

Hayes, S. C., Barlow, D. H., & Nelson-Gray, R. O. (1999). *The scientist practitioner: Research and accountability in the age of managed care* (2nd ed.). Needham Heights, MA: Allyn & Bacon.

Heather, N. (1989). Disulfiram treatment for alcoholism. *British Medical Journal, 299*, 471–472.

Heather, N. (1995). Brief intervention strategies. In R. K. Hester & W. R. Miller (Eds.), *Handbook of alcoholism treatment approaches: Effective alternatives* (2nd ed., pp. 105–123). Boston: Allyn & Bacon.

Hedberg, A. G., & Campbell, L. (1974). A comparison of four behavioral treatments of alcoholism. *Journal of Behavior Therapy and Experimental Psychiatry, 5*, 251–256.

Hunt, G. M., & Azrin, N. H. (1973). A community-reinforcement approach to alcoholism. *Behavior Research and Therapy, 11*, 91–104.

Hunt, M. L. (1999). *The new know-nothings: The political foes of the scientific study of human nature.* New Brunswick, NJ: Transaction.

Institute of Medicine. (1990). *Broadening the base of treatment for alcohol problems.* Washington, DC: National Academy Press.

Irvin, J. E, Bowers, C. A., Dunn, M. E., & Wang, M. C., (1999). Efficacy of Relapse prevention: A meta-analytic review. *Journal of Consulting and Clinical Psychology, 67,* 563–570.

Israel, Y., Hollander, O., Sanchez-Craig, M., Booker, S., Miller, V., Gingrich, R., & Rankin, J. G. (1996). Screening for problem drinking and counseling by primary care physician-nurse team. *Alcoholism: Clinical and Experimental Research, 20,* 1143–1450.

Jacob, T., & Seilhamer, R. A. (1987). Alcoholism and family interaction. In T. Jacob (Ed.), *Family interaction and psychopathology* (pp. 535–580). New York: Plenum Press.

Johnsen, J., & Morland, J. (1991). Disulfiram implant: A double blind placebo controlled follow-up on treatment outcome. *Alcoholism: Clinical and Experimental Research, 15,* 532–536.

Johnson, V. E. (1986). *Intervention: How to help someone who doesn't want help.* Minneapolis, MN: Johnson Institute Books.

Jones, S. L., & Lanyon, R. I. (1981). Relationship between adaptive skills and outcome of alcoholism treatment. *Journal of Studies on Alcohol, 42,* 521–525.

Kahan, M., Wilson, L., & Becker, L. (1995). Effectiveness of physician-based interventions with problem drinkers: A review. *Canadian Medical Association Journal, 152,* 851–859.

Kalb, M., & Propper, M. S. (1976). The future of alcohology: Craft or science? *American Journal of Psychiatry, 133,* 641–645.

Keane, T. M., Foy, D. W., Nunn, B., & Rychtarik, R. G. (1984). Spouse contracting to increase Antabuse compliance in alcoholic veterans. *Journal of Clinical Psychology, 40,* 340–344.

Koch, K. A. (1994). The D.A.R.E. (Drug Abuse Resistance Education) Program. In J. A. Lewis (Ed.), *Addictions: Concepts and strategies for treatment* (pp. 359–364). Gaithersburg, MD: Aspen.

Kownacki, R. J., & Shadish, W. R. (1999). Does Alcoholics Anonymous work? The results from a meta-analysis of controlled experiments. *Substance Abuse and Misuse, 34,* 1987–1916.

Larimer, M. E., Palmer, R. S., & Marlatt, G. A. (1999). Relapse prevention: An overview of Marlatt's cognitive behavioral model. *Alcohol Research and Health, 23,* 151–160.

Levine, H. (1978). The discovery of addiction. *Journal of Studies on Alcohol, 40,* 143–173.

Liepman, M. R., Nirenberg, T. D., & Begin, A. M. (1989). Evaluation of a program designed to help family and significant others to motivate resistant alcoholics into recovery. *American Journal of Drug and Alcohol Abuse, 15,* 209–221.

Littell, J. H., & Girvin, H. (2002). Stages of change: A critique. *Behavior Modification, 26,* 223–273.

Loneck, B., Garrett, S. A., & Banks, M. (1996a). A comparison of the Johnson intervention with four other methods of referral to outpatient treatment. *American Journal of Drug and Alcohol Abuse, 22,* 233–246.

Loneck, B., Garrett, S. A., & Banks, M. (1996b). The Johnson intervention and re-
    lapse during outpatient treatment. *American Journal of Drug and Alcohol
    Abuse, 22,* 363–365.

Lundwall, L., & Baekeland, F. (1971). Disulfiram treatment of alcoholism. *Journal of
    Nervous and Mental Disease, 153,* 381–394.

Lynam, D. R., Milich, R., Zimmerman, R., Novak, S. P., Logan, T. K., Martin, C.,
    Leukefeld, C., & Clayton, R. (1999). Project DARE: No effects at 10-year fol-
    low-up. *Journal of Consulting and Clinical Psychology, 67,* 590–593.

Maisto, S. A., O'Farrell, T. J., Connors, G. J., McKay, J., & Pelcovits, M. A. (1988).
    Alcoholics' attributions of factors affecting their relapse to drinking and reasons
    for terminating relapse events. *Addictive Behaviors, 13,* 79–83.

Marlatt, G. A. (1983). The controlled-drinking controversy: A commentary. *Ameri-
    can Psychologist, 38,* 1097–1110.

Marlatt, G. A, Baer, J. S., Kivlahan, D. R., Dimeff, L. A., Larimer, M. E., Quigly, L. A.,
    Somers, J. M., & Williams, E. (1998). Screening and brief intervention for high
    risk college student drinkers: Results from a two year follow-up study. *Journal
    of Consulting and Clinical Psychology, 66,* 604–615.

Marlatt, G. A., Baer, J. S., & Larimer, M. (1995). Preventing alcohol abuse in college
    students: A harm-reduction approach. In G. M. Boyd, J. Howard, & R. A.
    Zucker (Eds.), *Alcohol problems among adolescents: Current directions in pre-
    ventive research* (pp. 147–172). Hillsdale, NJ: Erlbaum.

Marlatt, G. A., & Gordon, J. R. (Eds.). (1985). *Relapse prevention: Maintenance
    strategies in the treatment of addictive behaviors.* New York: Guilford Press.

McCrady, B. S. (1995). Alcoholics Anonymous and behavior therapy: Can habits be
    treated as diseases? Can diseases be treated as habits? *Journal of Consulting and
    Clinical Psychology, 62,* 1159–1166.

McCrady, B. S., & Delany, S. A. (1995). Self-help groups. In R. K. Hester & W. R.
    Miller (Eds.), *Handbook of alcoholism treatment approaches: Effective alterna-
    tives* (2nd ed., pp. 160–175). Boston: Allyn & Bacon.

McCrady, B. S., Epstein, E. E., & Hirsch, L. S. (1999). Maintaining change after con-
    joint behavioral alcohol treatment for men: Outcomes at 6 months. *Addiction,
    94,* 1381–1396.

McCrady, B. S., Noel, N. E., Abrams, N. E., Stout, R., Nelson, H., & Hay, W.
    (1986). Comparative effectiveness of three types of spouse involvement in
    outpatient behavioral alcoholism treatment. *Journal of Studies on Alcohol,
    47,* 459–467.

Meyers, R. J., Miller, W. R., Hill, D. E., & Tonigan, J. S. (1999). Community rein-
    forcement and family training (CRAFT): Engaging unmotivated drug users in
    treatment. *Journal of Substance Abuse, 10,* 291–308.

Meyers, R. J., & Smith, J. E. (1995). *Clinical guide to alcohol treatment: The commu-
    nity reinforcement approach.* New York: Guilford Press.

Meyers, R. J., & Smith, J. E. (1997). Getting off the fence: Procedures to engage treat-
    ment-resistant drinkers. *Journal of Substance Abuse Treatment, 14,* 467–472.

Miller, W. R. (1986). Haunted by the zeitgeist: Reflections on contrasting treatment
    goals and concepts of alcoholism in Europe and the United States. In T. F. Babor
    (Ed.), *Alcohol and culture: Comparative perspectives from Europe and America*
    (pp. 110–129). New York: New York Academy of Sciences.

Miller, W. R. (1995). Increasing motivation for change. In R. K. Hester & W. R.

Miller (Eds.), *Handbook of alcoholism treatment approaches: Effective alternatives* (2nd ed., pp. 89–104). Boston: Allyn & Bacon.

Miller, W. R., Brown, J. M., Simpson, T. L., Handmaker, N. S., Bien, T. H., Luckie, L. F., Montgomery, H. A., Hester, R. K., & Tonigan, J. S. (1995). What works? A methodological analysis of the alcohol treatment outcome literature. In R. K. Hester & W. R. Miller (Eds.), *Handbook of alcoholism treatment approaches: Effective alternatives* (2nd ed., pp. 12–45). Boston: Allyn & Bacon.

Miller, W. R., & Hester, R. K. (1995). Treatment for alcohol problems: Toward an informed eclecticism. In R. K. Hester & W. R. Miller (Eds.), *Handbook of alcoholism treatment approaches: Effective alternatives* (2nd ed., pp. 1–12). Boston: Allyn & Bacon.

Miller, W. R., Meyers, R. J., & Tonigan, J. S. (1999). Engaging the unmotivated in treatment for alcohol problems: A comparison of three strategies for intervention through family members. *Journal of Consulting and Clinical Psychology, 67,* 688–697.

Miller, W. R., & Rollnick, S. (1991). *Motivational interviewing: Preparing people to change addictive behavior.* New York: Guilford Press.

Miller, W. R., Taylor, C. A., & West, J. C., (1980). Focused versus broad-spectrum treatment for problem drinkers. *Journal of Consulting and Clinical Psychology, 48,* 590–601.

Miller, W. R., Westerberg, V. S., Harris, R. J., & Tonigan, J. S. (1996). What predicts relapse: Prospective testing of antecedent models. *Addiction, 91,* S155–S171.

Miller, W. R., Zweben, A., DiClemente, C. C., & Rychtarik, R. G. (1992) *Motivational enhancement therapy manual: A clinical research guide for therapists treating individuals with alcohol abuse and dependence* (NIAAA Project MATCH monograph series, Vol. 2; DHHS Publication No. [ADM] 92-1894). Washington, DC: Government Printing Office.

Monti, P. M., Abrams, D. B., Binkoff, J. A., Zwick, W. R., Liepman, M. R., Nirenberg, T. D., Rohsenow, D. J. (1990). Communication skills training, communication skills training with family and cognitive behavioral mood management training for alcoholics. *Journal of Studies on Alcohol, 51,* 263–270.

Monti, P. M., Abrams, D. B., Kadden, R. M., & Rohsenow, D. J. (1989). *Treating alcohol dependence: A coping skills training guide.* New York: Guilford Press.

Monti, P. M., Rohsenow, D. J., Colby, S. M., & Abrams, D. B. (1995). Coping and social skills training. In R. K. Hester & W. R. Miller (Eds.), *Handbook of alcoholism treatment approaches: Effective alternatives* (2nd ed., pp. 221–241). Boston: Allyn & Bacon.

Monti, P. M., Rohsenow, D. J., Rubonis, A., Niaura, R., Sirota, A., Colby, S., Goddard, P., & Abrams, D. B. (1993). Cue exposure with coping skills treatment for male alcoholics: A preliminary investigation. *Journal of Consulting and Clinical Psychology, 61,* 1011–1019.

Mottin, J. L. (1973). Drug-induced attenuation of alcohol consumption: A review and evaluation of claimed, potential or current therapies. *Quarterly Journal of Studies on Alcohol, 34,* 444–472.

Moos, R. H., Finney, I. W., & Cronkite, R. C. (1990). *Alcoholism treatment: Context, process and outcome.* New York: Oxford University Press.

Moyer, A., Finney, J. W., Swearingen, C. E., & Vergun, P. (2002). Brief interventions for alcohol problems: A meta-analytic review of controlled investigations in treatment-seeking and non-treatment-seeking populations. *Addiction, 97,* 279–292.

Noel, N. E., & McCrady, B. S. (1993). Alcohol-focused spouse involvement with behavioral marital therapy. In T. J. O'Farrell (Ed.), *Treating alcohol problems: Marital and family interventions* (pp. 210–235). New York: Guilford Press.

Oei, T. P. S., & Jackson, P. R. (1980). Long-term effects of social skills training with alcoholics. *Addictive Behaviors, 5,* 129–136.

Oei, T. P. S., & Jackson, P. R. (1982). Social skills and cognitive behavioral approaches to the treatment of problem drinking. *Journal of Studies on Alcohol, 43,* 532–547.

O'Farrell, T. J. (1995). Marital and family therapy. In R. K. Hester & W. R. Miller (Eds.), *Handbook of alcoholism treatment approaches: Effective alternatives* (2nd ed., pp. 195–221). Boston: Allyn & Bacon.

O'Farrell, T. J., & Birchler, G. R. (1987). Marital relationships of alcoholic, conflicted and nonconflicted couples. *Journal of Marital and Family Therapy, 13,* 259–274.

O'Farrell, T. J., Choquette, K. A., Cutter, H. S., & Brown, E. D. (1993). Behavioral marital therapy with and without additional couples relapse prevention sessions for alcoholics and their wives. *Journal of Studies on Alcohol, 54,* 652–666.

O'Farrell, T. J., Choquette, K. A., Cutter, H. S. G., & Henry, S. G. (1998). Couples relapse prevention sessions after behavioral marital therapy for male alcoholics: Outcomes during the three years after starting treatment. *Journal of Studies on Alcohol, 59,* 357–370.

O'Farrell, T. J., Cutter, H. S., Choquette, K. A., Floyd, F. J., & Bayog, R. D. (1992). Behavioral marital therapy for male alcoholics: Marital and drinking adjustment during the two years after treatment. *Behavior Therapy, 23,* 529–549.

O'Farrell, T. J., Cutter, H. S., & Floyd, F. J. (1985). Evaluating behavioral marital therapy for male alcoholics: Effects on marital adjustment and communication from before to after treatment. *Behavior Therapy, 16,* 147–167.

Ogborne, A. C. (1989). Some limitations of Alcoholics Anonymous. In M. Galanter (Ed.), *Recent developments in alcoholism* (Vol. 7, pp. 55–65). New York: Plenum Press.

Orford, J., & Keddie, A. (1986). Abstinence or controlled drinking in clinical practice: A test of the dependence and persuasion hypotheses. *British Journal of Addiction, 81,* 495–504.

Prochaska, J. O., & DiClemente, C. C. (1982). Transtheoretical therapy: Toward a more integrative model of change. *Psychotherapy: Theory, Research and Practice, 19,* 276–288.

Prochaska, J. O., DiClemente, C. C., & Norcross, J. C. (1992). In search of how people change: Applications to addictive behaviors. *American Psychologist, 47,* 1102–1114.

Project MATCH Research Group. (1997). Matching alcoholism treatments to client heterogeneity: Project MATCH posttreatment drinking outcomes. *Journal of Studies, 58,* 7–29.

Project MATCH Research Group (1998). Matching alcoholism treatments to client heterogeneity: Project MATCH three-year drinking outcomes. *Alcoholism: Clinical and Experimental Research, 22,* 1300–1311.

Read, J. P., Kahler, C. W., & Stevenson, C. F. (2001). Bridging the gap between alcoholism treatment research and practice: Identifying what works and why. *Professional Psychology: Research and Practice, 32*, 227–238.

Ringwalt, C. L., & Greene, J. M. (1993, March). *Results of school districts' drug prevention coordinators survey.* Paper presented at the Alcohol, Tobacco, and Other Drugs Conference on Evaluating School-Linked Prevention Strategies, San Diego, CA.

Roizen, R. (1987). The great controlled-drinking controversy. In M. Galanter (Ed.), *Recent developments in alcoholism* (Vol. 5, pp. 245—279). New York: Plenum Press.

Rosenbaum, D. P., Flewelling, R. L., Bailey, S. L., Ringwalt, C. L., & Wilkinson, D. L. (1994). Cops in the classroom: A longitudinal evaluation of drug abuse resistance education (DARE). *Journal of Research in Crime and Delinquency, 31,* 3–31.

Rosenbaum, D. P., & Hanson, G. S. (1998). Assessing the effects of school-based drug education: A six-year multilevel analysis of Project D.A.R.E. (1998). *Journal of Research in Crime and Delinquency, 35*, 381–412.

Rosenberg, H. (1993). Prediction of controlled drinking by alcoholics and problem drinkers. *Psychological Bulletin, 113*, 129–139.

Rosenberg, H., & Davis, L. A. (1994). Acceptance of moderate drinking by alcohol treatment services in the United States. *Journal of Studies on Alcohol, 55*, 167–172.

Royce, J. E. (1989). *Alcohol problems and alcoholism: A comprehensive survey* (Rev. ed.). New York: Free Press.

Ryan, R. M., Plant, R. W., & O'Malley, S. (1995). Initial motivations for alcohol treatment: relations with patient characteristics, treatment involvement, and dropout. *Addictive Behaviors, 20*, 279–297.

Sanchez-Craig, M., & Lei, H. (1986). Disadvantages of imposing the goal of abstinence on problem drinkers: An empirical study. *British Journal of Addiction, 81*, 505–512.

Sisson, R. W., & Azrin, N. H. (1986). Family-member involvement to initiate and promote treatment of problem drinkers. *Journal of Behavior Therapy and Experimental Psychiatry, 17*, 15–21.

Sitharthan, T., Sitharthan, G., Hough, M. J., & Kavanagh, D. J. (1997). Cue exposure in moderation drinking: A comparison with cognitive-behavior therapy. *Journal of Consulting and Clinical Psychology, 62*, 620–626.

Skinner, B. F. (1938). *The behavior of organisms.* New York: Appleton-Century-Crofts.

Smith, C. G. (1969). Alcoholics: Their treatment and their wives. *British Journal of Psychiatry, 115*, 1039–1042.

Smith, D. I. (1985). Evaluation of a residential AA program for women. *Alcohol and Alcoholism, 20*, 315–327.

Smith, D. I. (1986). Evaluation of a residential AA program. *International Journal of the Addictions, 21*, 33–49.

Smith, J. E., & Meyers, R. J. (1995). The community reinforcement approach. In R. K. Hester & W. R. Miller (Eds.), *Handbook of alcoholism treatment approaches: Effective alternatives* (2nd ed., pp. 251–266). Boston: Allyn & Bacon.

Sobell, L. (1996). Bridging the gap between scientists and practitioners: The challenge before us. *Behavior Therapy, 27*, 297–320.

Sobell, L. C., Cunningham, J. A., & Sobell, M. B. (1996). Recovery from alcohol problems with and without treatment: Prevalence in two population surveys. *American Journal of Public Health, 86*, 966–972.

Sobell, M. B., & Sobell, L. C. (1973). Alcoholics treated by individualized behavior therapy: One year treatment outcome. *Behaviour Research and Therapy, 11*, 599–618.

Sobell, M. B., & Sobell, L. C. (1976). Second year treatment outcome of alcoholics treated by individualized behavior therapy: Results. *Behaviour Research and Therapy, 14*, 195–215.

Sobell, M. B., Sobell, L. C., & Gavin, D. R. (1995). Portraying alcohol treatment outcomes: Different yardsticks of success. *Behavior Therapy, 26*, 643–669.

Steinglass, P. (1981). The alcoholic family at home: Patterns of interaction in wet, dry, and transitional phases of alcoholism. *Archives of General Psychiatry, 38*, 578–584.

Timko, C., Moos, R. H., Finney, J. W., & Lesar, M. D. (2000). Long-term outcomes of alcohol use disorders: Comparing untreated individuals with those in Alcoholics Anonymous, and formal treatment. *Journal of Studies on Alcohol, 61*, 529–540.

Tonigan, J. S., Miller, W. R., & Connors, G. J. (2000). Project MATCH client impressions about Alcoholics Anonymous: Measurement issues and relationship to treatment outcome. *Alcoholism Treatment Quarterly, 18*, 25–41.

Tournier, R. . E. (1979). Alcoholics Anonymous as treatment and as ideology. *Journal of Studies on Alcohol, 40*, 230–239.

Vaillant, G. E. (1996). A long-term follow-up of male alcohol abuse. *Archives of General Psychiatry, 53*, 243–249.

United States Department of Health and Human Services. (1997). *Ninth special report to the U.S. Congress on alcohol and health*. (NIH Publication No. 97-4017). Washington, DC: Author.

Walsh, D. C, Hingson, R. W., Merrigan, D. M., Levenson, S. M., Cupples, L. A., Heeren, T., Coffman, G. A., Becker, C. A., Barker, T. A., Hamilton, S. K., McGuire, T. G., & Kelly, C. A. (1991). A randomized trial of treatment options for alcohol abusing workers. *New England Journal of Medicine, 325*, 775–782.

Wilk, A. L., Jensen, N. M., & Havighurst, T. C. (1997). Meta-analysis of randomized controlled trials addressing brief interventions in heavy alcohol drinkers. *Journal of General Internal Medicine, 12*, 274–283.

Wilson, A., Davidson, W. J., & Blanchard, R. (1980). Disulfiram implantation: A trial using placebo implants and two types of controls. *Journal of Studies on Alcohol, 41*, 429–436.

Wilson, G. T. (1988). Alcohol use and abuse: A social learning analysis. In C. D. Chaudron & D. A. Wilkinson (Eds.), *Theories on alcoholism* (pp. 239–287). Toronto: Addiction Research Foundation.

World Health Organization (WHO) Brief Intervention Study Group. (1996). A cross-national trial of brief interventions with heavy drinkers. *American Journal of Public Health, 86*, 948–958.

Wysong, E., Aniskiewicz, R., & Wright, D. (1994). Truth and DARE: Tracking drug education to graduation and as symbolic politics. *Social Problems, 41*, 448–472.

11

Herbal Treatments and Antidepressant Medication

Similar Data, Divergent Conclusions

HARALD WALACH
IRVING KIRSCH

Depression is one of the most widespread of all psychological disorders. The cost of depression is estimated at $16 billion per year in the United States alone, one third of which is treatment cost, and the rest of which are costs of loss of work and function. Its prevalence is estimated to be between 3% and 13%, with 20–50% of the population having a history of depression and at least 20% experiencing some depressive symptoms during their lives (Antonuccio, Danton, DeNelsky, Greenberg, & Gordon, 1999). These symptoms include, among others, sadness or depressed affect, loss of energy and appetite, loss of interest in activities and life in general, feelings of guilt and worthlessness, and thoughts about suicide. The recurrence rate of depression is high: 50% with one episode suffer a recurrence, and up to 90% with three episodes will have recurrences. Mortality from suicide may be as high as 15% among the chronically depressed.

Over the past 20 years antidepressant prescriptions have risen steadily. Meanwhile, prescriptions of selective serotonin reuptake inhibitors (SSRIs) account for approximately half of all psychiatrists' prescriptions (Anderson, 2000). More recently, a controversy has developed regarding the efficacy of SSRIs and other antidepressant medications. Although a strong positive response to antidepressive medication is undeniable, clinical trials suggest that much of this response is duplicated by inert placebos. This finding has led some authors to question whether antidepressants are much more than active placebos.

Paralleling the development of new pharmacological treatments for depression, there has been an increased interest in some of the oldest treatments for physical and psychological disorders. As part of a more general interest in alternative and complementary medicines, the use of herbal remedies has recently attracted the attention of consumers and researchers.

In this chapter, we review the data on antidepressant medications and herbal remedies for psychological disorders, with particular (although not exclusive) focus on depression. Specifically, we address the issue of the degree to which the effects of these treatments are due to their physical properties and the degree to which they can be explained as placebo effects.

ANTIDEPRESSANT MEDICATION

Hopelessness is at the core of depression. Hopelessness is also an expectation. It is an expectancy that an intolerable situation will not improve. This being the case, one would expect depression to be very reactive to the placebo effect. Placebos instill an expectancy for improvement, and expectancy addresses a core feature of depression.

Placebos are typically used to control for the psychological effects of administering a treatment. To that end, articles reporting clinical trials and reviews of the literature typically focus on the difference between the response to placebo and the response to active treatment. The question that is conventionally addressed is whether this difference is statistically significant. The magnitude of the difference is less frequently considered, and scant attention is typically accorded to the magnitude of the response to placebo.

In contrast to conventional reviews, Kirsch and Sapirstein (1998, 1999) reported a meta-analysis of antidepressant medications, in which both the drug effect and the placebo effect were evaluated. Computer searches of Medline and PsychLit, supplemented by studies identified in prior reviews, yielded 19 published, placebo-controlled, randomized clinical trials of the acute effects of antidepressants on patients with a clear-cut primary diagnosis of depression. Taken together, these studies contained 2,318 participants, of whom 1,460 received medication and 858 received placebo.

Drug effects are generally assessed by comparing clinical outcomes in patients given medications with outcomes in patients given placebo. The drug effect is taken to be the difference between the response to the drug and the response to the placebo. Just as one needs to control for the placebo effect to evaluate the drug effect, one needs to control for natural history effects (e.g., spontaneous remission and regression to the mean) to evaluate placebo effects. To that end, Kirsch and Sapirstein (1998, 1999) conducted a second search to identify studies in which changes in depression were reported for patients assigned to no-treatment or wait-list control groups. This search produced an additional 19 studies containing 244 patients who had been assigned to wait-list or no-treatment control groups. Changes in depression among these patients were used as a baseline against which the response to placebo could be compared. Analyses of patient characteristics indicated that participants in the two groups of studies were comparable in terms of age, duration of treatment (or length of time between assessments for the no-treatment groups), and pretreatment scores on the Hamilton Rating Scale for depression and the Beck Depression Inventory.

The effect size (Cohen's d) for pretreatment to posttreatment changes in depression was evaluated for each of these three groups of patients (those randomized to active antidepressant, those randomized to placebo, and those randomized to no-treatment or wait-list control). In studies reporting multiple measures of depression, an effect size was calculated for each measure and these effect sizes were then averaged. In studies reporting the effects of two drugs, a single mean effect size for both was calculated. Thus, there were 19 effect sizes for each condition (drug, placebo, and no-treatment).

The pre–post effect size for antidepressant drugs (d) was 1.55 standard deviations. This is a very large effect (Cohen, 1988), and it indicates that administration of an antidepressant medication is followed by substantial clinical improvement. However, the pre–post effect size (d) for response to placebo was 1.16. This finding indicates that approximately 75% of the effect of antidepressant medication can be duplicated by administration of a chemically inert placebo. In contrast, analysis of the course of untreated depression over the same time period indicated an effect size (d) of only 0.37 standard deviations. Taken together, these effect sizes suggest that about 25% of the response to antidepressant medication may be a true drug effect, another 25% may be due to the natural history of the condition, and about 50% is likely an expectancy effect.

Despite the magnitude of the placebo effect, the data in the Kirsch and Sapirstein (1998, 1999) meta-analyses indicate a reasonably sizable advantage for the active drug over placebo. However, there is reason to believe that some of this difference might be due to expectancy rather than to the pharmacological properties of the drugs. Kirsch and Sapirstein reported that the correlation between response to medication and response to placebos across studies was $r = .90$. In an effort to track down the reason for this substantial correlation, they subdivided the set of studies by type of medication (e.g., tricyclics, SSRIs, monoamine oxidase inhibitors [MAOIs]). They found that the pretreatment to posttreatment effect size was fairly consistent across drug type. More remarkable, the proportion of the effect size duplicated by placebo was virtually identical across medication type (range = 74% to 76%). The biggest surprise, however, came when Kirsch and Sapirstein examined the effect size for a subset of studies in which the active drugs (amylobarbitone, lithium, liothyronine, and adinazolam) were not standard antidepressants for acute use, but sedatives, tranquilizers, or preventive medications. The effect of these drugs on depression (d = 1.69) was as large as that of antidepressants, and again an inactive placebo duplicated 76% of this effect. A recent analysis using all data submitted to the FDA for approval of new SSRIs (Kirsch, Moore, Scoboria, & Nicholls, 2002) found the same result: There is a small difference between placebo and the most frequently used SSRIs on the Hamilton Depression Rating Scale of 1.8 points on average, and between 68% and 89% of the effect is duplicated by placebo. A different meta-analysis, using all data submitted to the Dutch health authorities for approval of tricyclic antidepressants, reached virtually identical conclusions (Storosum et al., 2001): Of 32 studies in altogether 4,314 patients, only 10 were independently significant, while the pooled effect of the treatment groups was superior to placebo. The effect, however, was small: Improvement from baseline to end of treatment was 42% on the Hamilton Depression Rating Scale with treatment, and 31% with placebo. Again, 70% of the treatment effect was duplicated by placebo. Thus, tricyclic antidepressants, which are considered standard therapy for depression, show only a modest effect, which is difficult to separate from placebo.

It is possible that amylobarbitone, lithium, liothyronine, and adinazolam are in fact antidepressants, with pharmacological effects as large as those of tricyclics, SSRIs, MAOIs, and other standard antidepressants. Alternatively, it is possible that all of these drugs function as active placebos. An active placebo is an active medication that does not possess specific activity for the condition being treated, but that mimics the side effects of the active drug. Greenberg and Fisher (1989) summarized data indicating that the effect of antidepressant medication is smaller when it is compared with an active placebo than when compared with an inert placebo. In contrast, Quitkin, Rabkin, Gerald, Davis, and Klein (2000) reanalyzed these data and came to an opposite conclusion. In fact, relatively few studies have assessed this possibility, and no studies have assessed it in relation to the more recent antidepressants (e.g., the SSRIs).

The active placebo hypothesis is based on the idea that patients randomized to the active arm of clinical trials are able to deduce that they have been assigned to the drug condition, because the active drugs produce more side effects than inert placebos. The ability of patients and physicians to detect assignment to the drug condition has been well established, not only for antidepressants (Blashki, Mowbray, & Davies, 1971; Fisher & Greenberg, 1993; Rabkin et al., 1986), but also other medications (Quitkin et al., 2000). The penetration of the double blind may produce an enhanced placebo effect in drug conditions and a diminished placebo effect in placebo groups. Thus, the apparent drug effect of antidepressants may in part be a placebo effect, magnified by differences in experienced side effects and patients' subsequent recognition of the condition to which they have been assigned. Some support for this interpretation is provided by a meta-analysis of fluoxetine (Prozac), in which a correlation of $r = .85$ was found between the therapeutic effect of the drug and the percentage of patients reporting side effects (Greenberg, Bornstein, Zborowski, Fisher, & Greenberg, 1994).

Given these data, it is not surprising that the Kirsch and Sapirstein meta-analysis generated considerable controversy. One criticism was generic: Meta-analyses are limited both by the scope of the original studies that were included as well as by the studies that were excluded. The latter studies, of course, were not retrieved or not published in the first place. Thus, the results of meta-analyses should always be considered preliminary and open to revision depending on new and possibly conflicting evidence. In addition, it is at present unclear whether a series of smaller trials combined in a meta-analysis or single "mega-trials" are better for estimating true medication effects. Apart from these methodological questions, critics raised concerns about (1) the relatively small number of studies evaluated, considering the large body of literature evaluating antidepressant medication and (2) various aspects of the statistical analyses (e.g., Dawes, 1998; Klein, 1998). However, other meta-analyses (Gerson, Belin, Kaufman, Mintz, & Jarvik, 1999; Joffe, Sokolov, & Streiner, 1996; Kahn, Warner, & Brown, 2000; Walach & Maidhof, 1999), conducted by different authors on different sets of studies and using different statistical procedures, revealed pre–post drug and placebo effect sizes very similar to those reported by Kirsch and Sapirstein (1998, 1999). The close correspondence in the results of these independently conducted meta-analyses, despite little or no overlap in the studies included in them (only two studies were included in both the Joffe et al. meta-analysis and the Kirsch and Sapirstein meta-analysis), suggest that their findings and conclusions are robust.

The Kirsch and Sapirstein (1998, 1999) meta-analysis was limited to studies of the acute affects of antidepressant drugs and placebos (the mean duration of the studies was 5 weeks). Walach and Maidhof (1999) extended these findings to long-term effects (6 months to 3 years). In the most stringent analysis of their data (reported in Kirsch, 1998), which was confined to studies in which dropouts were analyzed as treatment failures, the results were virtually identical to those of Kirsch and Sapirstein. These findings indicated that 73% of the long-term improvement among patients treated with antidepressants was duplicated in patients treated by placebo, and that the correlation between the proportion of patients responding to antidepressants and the proportion of patients responding to placebos was $r = .93$.

A methodological feature of the Walach and Maidhof (1999) meta-analysis provides further information concerning the relative advantage of active medication compared with inert placebo. Instead of using standardized mean improvement scores, as had been done in the other meta-analyses, Walach and Maidhof based their calculations on the number of patients showing long-term clinically significant improvement in the drug and placebo conditions. With dropouts categorized as treatment failures, 63% of the patients in the drug groups improved, compared with 46% of patients in the placebo groups—a difference of 17% (Kirsch, 1998). Thus, only one in six patients showed long-term clinical improvement following medication who would not have done so following placebo.

The design of clinical trials is based on the assumption that drug effects and placebo effects are additive. That is, the drug effect is presumed to add to the placebo effect, so that it can be calculated as the difference between the response to the drug and the response to the placebo. It is possible, however, that the effects of antidepressant drugs and antidepressant placebos are not additive (Dawes, 1998; Kirsch, 1998, 2000). It is possible, for example, that placebos duplicate effects that are produced pharmacologically by antidepressant medication. At this point, there are no data directly addressing this issue. Thus, although the efficacy of antidepressants per se has been demonstrated in clinical trials, the magnitude of the effect and the clinical usefulness of these substances, as well as (1) their long-term benefits versus their costs, (2) their long-term side effects, and (3) the efficacy of other treatment options require clarification. The current data suggest that widespread claims that antidepressants possess very high levels of efficacy for major depression may not be warranted, although it is quite likely that antidepressants do possess true active effects.

Despite complex data that lend themselves to multiple interpretations, the received wisdom of the health industry is that antidepressant medication is exceptionally effective in the treatment of mood disorders. A careful examination of the research literature, we contend, yields a considerably more ambiguous and multifaceted picture. In the second part of this chapter we turn to another set of somatic treatments—herbal remedies—for which similar data have led to very different conclusions.

HERBAL TREATMENTS FOR PSYCHOLOGICAL DISORDERS

Among unconventional or complementary and alternative medicines, herbal treatments (phytotherapeutics) are increasingly popular (Chrubasik, Junck, Zappe, & Stutzke, 1998; LaFrance et al., 2000; Pirotta, Cohen, Kotsirilos, & Farish, 2000; Sparber et al., 2000). Phytotherapeutics have long been used in Germany, where they have a specific legal status. The pharmaceuticals derived from plants or with contents derived from plants cover about 20–30% of the market in Germany, which translates into $1.5–2 billion. In the United States, herbal treatments are second among alternative therapies. They are used by 12% of the U.S. population, with a sixfold rise in use since 1990. A conservative estimate of the total expenditure for alternative medicines is $27 billion, with $5.1 billion for herbal treatments (Eisenberg et al., 1998; but see Gorski, 1999, for a critique of these findings).

The preparation with the highest sale in prescriptions and over-the-counter sales in Germany is a phytotherapeutic remedy made from ginkgo biloba, which is discussed later (Rosslenbroich & Saller, 1992). From there, phytotherapeutics have made their way into drug stores and pharmacies around the world, including the United States, and are now major parts of the rising business of complementary and alternative medicine (Mills, 2001).

The increasing popularity of herbal medicines can be seen as part of a public trend toward natural, holistic, and ecological approaches to life in general and to health care in particular (Furnham & Kirkcaldy, 1996). By these approaches we mean orientations in life that opt for the integration of mind and body, honor the awareness that the well-being of humans is dependent on the well-being of other species and the whole planet, and posit that scientific approaches should cover analyses not only of wholes into constituent parts but also the knowledge of how those constituents interact synergistically to produce behavior.

These attitudes seem to reflect a subtle shift in lay perceptions about life and values in general, or that is, the *zeitgeist*. In some respects, they reflect the expression of disillusion with the technological and scientific approach to life in general and health in particular. Many people have become afraid that the "high tech" medical approach of Western countries might sacrifice the "human" aspects of care and the whole person, and focus only on diseased organs and mechanisms. If not really consciously reflected on, this ecological stance or a worldview expressing appreciation for nature and her intricate interconnectedness can evolve into a mindset that has aptly been called the "natural commonplace" (Pratkanis, 1995). This term denotes the prejudice that everything that is natural is good, that nature is better than culture, and that technology per se is an enemy to life.

The fitting together of belief systems in patients and therapists is part and parcel of maximizing nonspecific treatment factors (Frank, 1987). Thus, people subscribing to an ecological and holistic worldview are likely to seek out treatments consistent with those views. For instance, people who believe that the universe is permeated by an invisible life force are likely to be attracted to acupuncture or traditional Chinese medicine with its teaching that life is upheld by the flow and balance of *qi*. Similarly, someone who is convinced that well-being is dependent on the intimate functioning and interconnection of mental and bodily systems will likely be attracted to the system of homeopathy with its taking into account not only of physical symptoms of the present disease, but also the individuals' psychological symptoms and personality. Recent data indicate that patients who seek out complementary and alternative treatments are not necessarily dissatisfied with the outcomes of conventional medical treatments. Instead, it is primarily the ideological underpinnings of complementary and alternative treatments that seem attractive to these patients (Astin, 1998). In addition, the side effects that are common in effective conventional treatments are often cited as reasons for seeking out alternatives (Walach & Güthlin, 2000).

Thus the turn toward naturopathic treatments, and among them phytotherapeutic medicines, is a logical consequence of the turn toward nature in the zeitgeist. The same is true not only for patients, but for doctors: Those doctors who are younger, who have been treated by alternative and complementary medical approaches themselves, and who adhere to a more holistic view of medicine are likely to attribute more power to naturopathic interventions (Easthope, Tranter, & Gill, 2001).

Phytotherapeutic approaches are often seen as harmless and imbued with fewer side effects than traditional approaches, which probably is an extension of the widely held, albeit mistaken, assumption that everything that is natural is good and harmless, the "natural commonplace" (Pratkanis, 1995). In some scientific circles the inverse of the natural commonplace is popular: Everything that is "natural" is likely to have small effects. Both assumptions may be mistaken in two senses. First, because phytotherapeutic interventions fit some patients' worldviews better, they may be more likely to trigger positive expectancy effects. Often labeled as placebo effects, these expectancy effects are frequently dismissed and ignored, but they can be of substantial benefit. As discussed earlier, they have been reported to account for between 60% and 80% of the variance of pharmacological treatment effects in depression (Kirsch & Sapirstein, 1998, 1999; Kirsch et al., 2002; Walach & Maidhof, 1999) and some other disorders as well (Maidhof, Dehm, & Walach, 2000), thus potentially contributing considerably to the efficacy of pharmacological treatment. Second, placebo-controlled trials have shown that at least some of the more widely used phytotherapeutic methods exert specific effects over and above those attributable to placebo.

Hypericum

Preparations made of St. John's wort (hypericum) were used by traditional German naturopaths as treatments for depression. Hypericum is presently one of the most widely used phytotherapeutic compounds in Germany for the treatment of depression. More recently, it has seen widespread use in the United States and other countries. It has been used in folk medicines since the Middle Ages against bruises (as a bandage with the flowers preserved in oil or fat) or as a decoction in the form of tea against depression. Pharmacological research has determined that the effective components of St. John's wort, among them the flavonoids hypericin and hyperforin, show a variety of effects comparable with those of SSRIs (Greeson, Sanford, & Monti, 2001; Singer, Wonnemann, & Müller, 1999). In contrast to artificially manufactured SSRIs, hypericin does not inhibit the reuptake of serotonin. Instead, it may induce an expression of 5-HT receptors centrally and peripherally. The latter effects could, incidentally, explain the use of hypericum in folk medicine for cuts, bruises, and lacerations. An enhanced peripheral action of 5-HT would certainly explain pain killing and perhaps also immunological effects. Peripheral 5-HT receptors and/or enhanced availability of serotonin play an important role in the mediation of inflammation and pain perception. Nearly every immunocompetent cell can express 5-HT receptors. In this way, serotonin mediates immune responses. On the other hand, cytokines, which are the substances used by the immune system to communicate with itself and with other parts of the organism and that are produced when infections occur, induce higher bioavailability of serotonin in some parts of the brain (Mössner & Lesch, 1998).

One problem common to all phytotherapeutic medications has been researched extensively with hypericum preparations: depending on the time of harvest, the origin of plants and the method of extraction, the active compounds vary greatly in quality and quantity. This finding may explain, at least in part, the divergent results of clinical trials using different dosages (Laakmann, Schüle, Baghai, & Kieser, 1998).

One of the major tasks of phytopharmacology is to identify and analyze active ingredients, to determine the best means of extracting them, and to ascertain their efficacy. Until recently, this had been done through clinical experience, rather than systematic empirical study. In the case of hypericum, however, there have been considerable recent advances. A series of meta-analyses have confirmed the likelihood of a specific antidepressant action of St. John's wort (Field, Monti, Greeson, & Kunkel, 2000).

One of the first meta-analyses concluded that hypericum extracts are effective for mild to moderate depression, and that their therapeutic effects are superior to those of placebo and comparable with those of tricyclics, but with fewer side effects (Linde et al., 1996). This study included 23 randomized trials in 1,757 outpatients with mild to moderate depression. Fifteen of those trials compared hypericum with a placebo, and eight with active medication. The main outcome measure of the meta-analysis was a pooled responder rate ratio (RR; this is an effect size measure expressed as a ratio of responders in the group treated by responders in the control group). The analysis yielded a significant RR of 2.67 against placebo and a

RR of 1.10 with single or 1.52 with combination preparations of hypericum against conventional medications. In a recent update of their original review, now published as a Cochrane review following the strict criteria of the Cochrane collaboration, Linde and Mulrow (2001) found 27 randomized controlled trials meeting the inclusion criteria, 17 of which were placebo controlled and 10 of which compared hypericum with conventional drugs. Hypericum preparations were significantly superior to placebo (RR 2.47; 95% confidence interval (CI) 1.69 to 3.61) and about equally effective as standard antidepressants (single preparations RR 1.01; CI, 0.87 to 1.16; combinations RR 1.52; CI, 0.78 to 2.94). The proportions of patients reporting side effects were 26.3% for hypericum single preparations versus 44.7% for standard antidepressants (RR 0.57; CI, 0.47 to 0.69), and 14.6% for combinations versus 26.5% with amitriptyline or desipramine (RR 0.49; CI, 0.23 to 1.04). The authors concluded that the superiority of hypericum over placebo has been established, but that the evidence regarding hypericum's efficacy relative to conventional drugs is inconclusive, because the studies were too short and because extensive comparisons with SSRIs are absent.

One recent study (Woelk et al., 2000) randomized 324 patients to either receive hypericum or imipramine for 6 weeks. Patients in both groups improved significantly, with no significant between-group differences in therapeutic benefit. However, side effects were significantly more common among patients given imipramine. Side effects were reported by 63% of the patients in the imipramine group, compared with 39% of the patients in the hypericum group. Similar results were reported by Philipp, Kohnen, and Hiller (1999). Hypericum produced a mean improvement of 15.4 points on the Hamilton depression scale (HAM-D), compared with 14.2 points for imipramine and 12.1 points for placebo. In contrast, the incidence of side effects was only 0.5 events per patient for hypericum, which was not significantly different from that reported in the placebo group (0.6 events) and significantly less than that reported following imipramine (1.2 events). Hypericum preparations also may have fewer side effects than SSRIs (Schulz, 2000), although this possibility has not yet been tested sufficiently (Stevinson & Ernst, 1999).

Although there are fewer side effects with hypericum extracts than with some conventional antidepressants, certain serious side effects have been observed. Among these effects is photosensitization, which has led some researchers to caution against the simple equation of "natural equals harmless." Recently, the German regulatory agency posted a caveat against interactions with other pharmaceuticals (Bundesinstitut für Arzneimittel und Medizinprodukte, 2000). Most side effects, however, have been observed with dosages considerably higher than standard doses and rarely of the same severity as those of conventional preparations. Moreover, it is interesting to note that adverse effects are much more frequently seen in

316 CONTROVERSIES IN THE TREATMENT OF SPECIFIC ADULT DISORDERS

comparison trials with SSRIs (30–50%) than in placebo-controlled trials (3%; Greeson et al., 2001). This difference may be due, at least in part, to a greater expectancy for side effects when a conventional medication is included in the study, but it could also be due to dosage differences in the respective trials.

In a recent study accorded substantial coverage in the media, Shelton and colleagues (2001) reported a failure to find a significant difference between hypericum and placebo in 200 severely depressed patients. A positive response to hypericum was seen in 27% of the patients, whereas a positive response to placebo was seen in 19% of the patients. Thus, the treatment response was 42% greater than the response to placebo, which is comparable with that reported in meta-analyses of conventional antidepressants (e.g., Kirsch & Sapirstein, 1998, 1999). There were, however, significantly more patients who experienced complete remission with hypericum (14.3%), than with placebo (4.9%; $p = .02$). Side effects occurred in 10% or more of the patients in both groups, the most prominent of which were headaches and abdominal discomfort. There was a significant difference in headaches between groups: 41% of hypericum patients reported headaches, compared with 25% of the placebo group ($p = .02$). Based on these data, it can be concluded that the number of patients needed to treat to achieve one remission with hypericum in severe depression is 11, or that a sample size of 100 per group is needed to show a significant difference. When considering this result, two issues should be borne in mind (Berner, 2001). First, in contrast to other studies, in this study rather severely depressed patients were treated. The cutoff point on the Hamilton scale was 20 (instead of 18, which is conventionally used to define mild to moderate depression). Second, in this study the percentage of chronically relapsing patients was 64%, and thus rather high.

The results of this trial suggest that hypericum has a comparatively small effect size when used with more severely depressed patients or rather late in the course of a clinical depression. Nevertheless, the absence of a significant difference in this trial may have been due partially to a lack of sufficient statistical power. Similarly nonsignificant results have been reported in some clinical trials of conventional antidepressants, particularly with severely depressed patients.

Thus, the bulk of the data indicate a significant benefit for hypericum, at least for people with mild and moderate levels of depression. The efficacy of hypericum for severely depressed patients remains to be ascertained. Moreover, the lower incidence of side effects may make hypericum especially useful for some patients, as it is not uncommon for 30–40% of participants to discontinue their medication during clinical trials of conventional medication.

Following the reasoning that the experience of side effects creates the expectancy of being treated with active components, the occurrence of fewer side effects should diminish the effectiveness of a drug. One could perhaps argue that the lower incidence of side effects makes the superiority of hypericum to placebo more convincing than the superiority of conventional antidepressants to placebo. Participants in clinical trials of hypericum may be less likely to perceive that they have been randomized to the active drug condition. Thus, given the comparability of hypericum side effects and placebo side effects, it is perhaps more likely that drug–placebo differences in hypericum trials reflect a genuine pharmacological effect. It should be pointed out, however, that the replicated body of research supporting the efficacy of hypericum is considerably smaller than that supporting the efficacy of standard antidepressants. As a consequence, further research on hypericum's efficacy, especially in severely depressed patients, is necessary.

Although meta-analyses by and large support the efficacy of hypericum, its efficacy relative to conventional drugs, especially SSRIs, remains to be ascertained. Although SSRIs have often been hailed as more effective than traditional drugs, a recent meta-analysis did not substantiate this claim (Anderson, 2000). It will be important to determine how hypericum fares against one of the new drugs of the SSRI family.

The most recent and largest trial on the efficacy of hypericum preparations was the one commissioned by the Office of Alternative Medicine at the National Institutes of Health (Hypericum Depression Trial Study Group, 2002). In this trial, 340 patients with moderate to severe depression were either treated with hypericum ($n = 113$), with placebo ($n = 116$), or with sertraline ($n = 111$), an established antidepressant as active comparator. The study was conducted as a double-blind, double-dummy study over the course of 8 weeks, with prolongation possible for responders up to 18 weeks. This means that patients received either hypericum and a sertraline placebo, sertraline and a hypericum placebo, or two placebos. Main outcome measure was Hamilton Depression Rating Scale (HAM-D) scores from baseline to 8 weeks and rates of full response. All groups improved significantly, but no difference was found between any of the groups. Improvements varied between 9.2 HAM-D scores for placebo (CI, 10.5 to 7.9), 8.7 for hypericum (CI, 10.0 to 7.3), and 10.5 for sertraline (CI, 11.9 to 9.1). Full response occurred in 32% of patients treated with placebo, 24% of patients treated with hypericum, and 25% treated with sertraline. Side effect profiles were different, and side effects more prominent in the sertraline group. The authors conclude that hypericum was not shown to be significantly different from placebo in this patient population with moderate to severe depression; neither was sertraline. This trial thus confirms other data and the empirical wisdom that hypericum is not really helpful in patients with more severe depression who also have a longer history of depression. Thirty-four percent of the patients in the hypericum group had a depression of duration longer than 24 months (placebo, 28%;

sertraline, 33%). It is an altogether puzzling fact that an already established treatment, sertraline as an active comparator, could itself not show superiority over placebo or hypericum. This makes the results of this trial difficult to interpret. Certainly hypericum was not shown to be effective compared to placebo. On the other hand, hypericum was similarly effective as sertraline, which was not different from placebo either. In a double-dummy study all patients typically receive two medications. While they, theoretically, know that one of them is placebo, it is very likely that some of them forget or believe they receive two active medications, which again is bound to enhance the placebo component of the treatment.

Be this as it may, there is a mixed bag of results concerning hypericum: While it appears to be effective in European trials, which tend to include some patients who were better managed from a psychiatric point of view and who were less severely depressed (Berner, 2001), hypericum does not seem to be an effective option for patients with a more severe depression and a longer history of depression, as testified by the two recent U.S. trials. Thus the final word on hypericum is yet to be spoken, possibly by some future trials taking more care of patient selection, or a series of trials addressing the question of differential indications.

Ginkgo Biloba

Ginkgo biloba, a preparation made from the fresh leaves of the ginkgo tree, is another traditional phytotherapeutic drug. It is claimed to be invigorating, to slow down the aging process, and to diminish the cognitive deficits of old age (i.e., memory loss and dementia symptoms). The ginkgo tree is a "fossil" among plants, because it does not have a living relative among other plants and is said to be a unique species of tree, midway between leaf-bearing trees and needle trees. The ginkgolides, which belong to the family of terpenoids and are part of the extracts, are singular in the plant kingdom and contained only in ginkgo leaves. Ginkgo has been used for these indications in Asian cultures, and has conquered the Western market with what is probably the single most widely sold phytotherapeutic over-the-counter preparation (Kleijnen & Knipschild, 1992a; Rosslenbroich & Saller, 1992).

Ginkgo's widespread use and popularity stand in sharp contrast to the comparative scarcity of solid scientific data concerning its efficacy (see also Gold, Cahill, & Wenk, 2002, for similarly mixed conclusions regarding the effects of ginkgo on general cognitive functioning). In the first reviews on the efficacy of ginkgo for intermittent claudication (a reduction of blood flow in the peripheral and central blood vessels) and cerebral insufficiency (Kleijnen & Knipschild, 1992a, 1992b), systematic searches produced 15 controlled trials of intermittent claudication and 38 trials of cerebral insufficiency. Two of the intermittent claudication trials were reasonably well performed, that is, randomized, double-blind, and of otherwise good methodological quality, as were eight of the cerebral insufficiency studies. These studies were all significantly positive in favor of ginkgo. However, publication bias could not be excluded, and the authors concluded that although there was preliminary evidence for the efficacy of ginkgo in cerebral insufficiency and intermittent claudication, more and larger trials were necessary.

More recent trials of ginkgo in dementia were reviewed by Fugh-Berman and Cott (1999) and by Ott and Owens (1998). These more recent trials, which were placebo-controlled, randomized, and conducted in patients with well-established diagnoses of either Alzheimer's disease or other forms of memory impairment, provided further evidence of the efficacy of ginkgo for dementia (see also Gold et al., 2002). A recent, rigorous meta-analysis (Oken, Storzbach, & Kaye, 1998) found more than 50 studies, 4 of which fulfilled all inclusion criteria, among them having a clearly stated diagnosis of Alzheimer's disease, a placebo-controlled randomized design, a standardized extract of ginkgo, and objective outcome measures. Most studies failed to meet these criteria because diagnoses were insufficiently established. Three of the four studies showed significant effects. The pooled standardized mean difference was $d = 0.4$, which is a small to medium effect (Cohen, 1988), and significantly different from zero ($p < .0001$). Side effects were scarce; two cases of bleeding difficulties were reported. Based on this result, the authors concluded that ginkgo exerts a clear but modest effect on Alzheimer's disease.

As Gold and colleagues (2002) note, however, the effects of ginkgo may be limited primarily to current cognitive processes and may not extend to the chronic symptoms of dementia. Moreover, Gold and colleagues point out that ginkgo has been actually found to impair cognitive performance in some studies.

A more recent review of ginkgo in coronary artery disease identified eight randomized, placebo-controlled trials, four of which showed a significant difference in the increase of pain-free walking distance (in a brisk walking test normally carried out over a distance of 100 meters until pain occurs) in favor of ginkgo, with a weighted mean difference of 36.6 meters (Gundling & Ernst, 1999). A systematic review of trials of ginkgo in patients with tinnitus identified five randomized studies, four of which were placebo-controlled (Ernst & Stevenson, 1999). Only one of those trials reported negative results, which might have been due to suboptimal doses. The other trials showed superior effects of ginkgo to placebo. The authors of the review concluded that ginkgo seems to be an effective treatment for tinnitus, but that more and larger scale trials are needed. The common denominator regarding the mechanisms of action of ginkgo seems to be that it increases capillary blood flow in the brain and other organs.

Kava Kava

Kava kava, or piper methysticum, is a plant derived from the islands of the Pacific, where it is used in ritualistic contexts, such as harvesting festival or group prayers (Chrubasik, 1997). It was also used as a traditional relaxant, and in the United States is among the top-selling herbal preparations, with an approximate annual expenditure of $8 million (Pittler & Ernst, 2000). It has shown anxiolytic and antistress effects (Fugh-Berman & Cott, 1999). Pittler and Ernst (2000) conducted a systematic review of the efficacy of kava in anxiety disorders and identified seven trials that met the preset inclusion criteria of being randomized, double-blind, placebo-controlled studies using kava mono-preparations (i.e., preparations that did not contain other ingredients or mixtures of chemical drugs with kava). Three of these trials reported results suitable for meta-analysis as defined by the authors, that is, a common outcome measure (Hamilton Rating Scale for Anxiety). The weighted mean difference was $d= 9.69$ (confidence interval 3.54–15.83), with a wide variation of effect sizes between $d = 5.0$ and $d = 18.0$. This huge variation of effect sizes, and the remarkably high effect size of a nearly 10 standard deviations difference between kava and placebo, certainly necessitates close scrutiny. In addition, the trials were not flawless. Among the criticisms raised by Pittler and Ernst were the small sample sizes included in the trials, failures to describe how the randomization process was performed, and unclear methods of achieving double blinding.

A possible mechanism for kava's apparent efficacy is not known. However, kava seems to be another example of a traditional pharmacological substance, the use of which was based only on folklore and unsystematic experience, which may ultimately come to be vindicated by modern research. Nevertheless, it should be noted that the manufacturing of pharmaceuticals from plant extracts can be a cumbersome process compared with the synthesizing of chemical agents. This may be why until recently the production of phytotherapeutics was typically the purview of small family-owned businesses with little pressure and few funds to carry out research.

A series of reports on liver damage and liver failures related to long-term use of kava kava preparations (Escher, Desmeules, Giostra, & Mentha, 2001; Kraft et al., 2001) has recently led German authorities to prohibit its use. Although the probability of such severe damage does not appear to be very high, the decision was made against the background of limited evidence concerning kava's efficacy and usefulness and lack of systematic data on side effects. These cases provide evidence of the necessity to study phytotherapeutic preparations more thoroughly in long-term observational studies. One has to be aware here that those cases of liver damage and failure could also be related to the concurrent use of other substances, like other drugs or alcohol, but are certainly due to the fact that phytotherapeutic substances are frequently not considered pharmaceuticals. Hence their self-medicated use is often not reported to doctors, or doctors do not monitor them as thoroughly as they would conventional medications.

Phytopharmacy for Pain

Some phytotherapeuticals, among them harpagophytum (devil's claw), salix (willow), urtica (stinging nettle), and populus (poplar), have traditionally been used for pain problems in different cultures. Modern phytopharmacological research on the efficacy of these plants has only recently begun to investigate the truth of folklore ascribing painkilling properties to these herbs. Ernst and Chrubasik (2000) published an overview of randomized, placebo-controlled, double-blind trials of herbal preparations for pain conditions in rheumatoid problems. Four trials are available on devil's claw in patients with acute low back pain or osteoarthritis. Three trials showed significant improvement in pain scores in favor of the experimental treatment, one a nonsignificant trend. The largest and methodologically most sophisticated of these trials (Chrubasik, Junck, Breitschwerdt, Conradt, & Zappe, 1999) confirms this overview. In this trial, 197 patients with chronic low back pain were randomized to either receive a harpagophytum extract or placebo in a double-blind fashion. The principal outcome measure was number of patients who were pain free for at least 5 days without rescue medication after 3 weeks of treatment. This outcome measure significantly favored harpagophytum. Five percent of placebo patients, 9% of patients treated with 600 mg dosage, and 15% of patients treated with 1200 mg were free of pain for 5 days in the last week of the trial ($p = .027$).

Another promising substance with some initial research support is salix, the willow bark (Chrubasik & Eisenberg, 1998). Acetylsalicylic acid (ASA, commonly known as aspirin), which has an anti-inflammatory effect, was originally derived from the bark of the willow tree (Schonauer, 1994), thereby suggesting a possible mode of action of the plant substance salix. This possibility has been suggested by six randomized trials of willow bark preparations in patients with osteoarthritis (Chrubasik & Eisenberg, 1998). All trials were blinded and randomized. One was placebo-controlled and showed significant effects over placebo in 36 patients per group. One trial used another phytotherapeutic substance, poplar extract, as the comparison substance and found comparable effects. Four trials used standard medications, such as diclofenac, piroxicam, or indomethacin as comparison substances. Three of those trials, with Ns ranging from 72 to 417, showed comparable effects. In one trial, however, the control was superior. These trials suggest a possible place for willow-bark extracts in pain treatment, but additional research is clearly necessary.

The remedies mentioned here are those with comparatively good research records. Many other preparations are still used on the basis of open, uncontrolled trials. For these preparations, the available evidence is well below what is standard in conventional practice. This fact reflects the situation that research in the domain of phytotherapy has until recently received no public sponsoring. Because most of the preparations are licensed in European countries or in Germany, and many are sold as food or dietary supplements in the United States, there was no pressure for private sponsors to support research for marketing or licensing reasons. We hope that the increasing use of these preparations by the public will engender comparable research efforts that will answer crucial questions regarding their safety and efficacy, which remain unresolved with most of these substances.

Bach-Flower Remedies

Bach-flower remedies were introduced by the homeopathic physician Edward Bach (1886–1936) (Barnard, 1919). Bach postulated that by placing flowers from certain local shrubs, trees, flowers, and bushes in crystal plates that were covered with clear spring water and exposed to the sun, healing qualities would be transferred to the water. This water, in turn, can purportedly be used as a medical remedy. These stocks of flower essences are distributed by a commercial network and sold in drugstores. They are usually preserved with ethanol, brandy, or clear spirits, and are diluted with water for the purpose of application. Bach-flower remedies are completely unregulated, because they do not fulfill the criteria for drugs and medicinal substances. Anyone can purchase them over-the-counter in a drugstore. Application of the remedies is facilitated by self-help books, which contain commonplace descriptions and recipe-like combinations.

We studied the effect of Bach-flower remedies for test anxiety in a recent study (Walach, Rilling & Engelke, 2001). We recruited 61 participants who suffered from self-reported test anxiety and were about to undergo two exams within a 2-week period. The study was double-blind and placebo-controlled, with partial crossover. In the first half of the trial 32 participants received Bach-flower remedies (a mixture of 10 flowers: impatiens, mimulus, gentiana, chestnut bud, rock rose, larch, cherry plum, white chestnut, scleranthus, and elm). Twenty-nine participants received placebo. After the first part of the trial, all subjects received Bach-flower remedies. None of the participants knew when placebo would be distributed. We administered a battery of measures validated for test anxiety. A 2×3 factorial repeated measure analysis of variance revealed a significant effect of time, $F(2,102) = 5.8$; $p = .0042$, but no significant group or inter-action effect. All subjects exhibited markedly decreased test anxiety from 2 weeks before the test to the time immediately before the first test. Although in the second half of the trial both groups received Bach-flower remedies, test anxiety returned nearly to baseline level.

What we observed, namely a strong nonspecific or placebo effect of Bach-flower remedies, is characteristic of many unconventional interventions. It is very difficult outside of phytomedicine to demonstrate specific intervention effects, because the placebo component of these interventions seems to be substantial. This strong nonspecific component of Bach-flower remedies and other unconventional interventions, such as acupuncture or homeopathy, may be the reason why these interventions are highly re-garded by the public. If we consider that the promise of cure is high and the therapeutic ritual (which accompanies most of these unconventional in-terventions) is quite complicated, we can easily understand why they are a good vehicle for transporting expectations, hope, and attributional effects.

It is part of the art of a good therapist to interpret chance fluctuations in any baseline variable that point in a positive direction. This attribution could then install the belief in a subject undergoing this treatment that a positive change has begun. If that occurs, a positive expectation for change that may be self-reinforcing has set in. The therapeutic rationale of many of these unconventional interventions, including Bach-flower remedies, supports this type of strategy. Instead of regarding this as a defect because no true pharmacological agent can be isolated, it would seem more appro-priate to consider it a nonspecific effect typical of some psychotherapeutic strategies.

PARALLELS BETWEEN ANTIDEPRESSANT MEDICATION AND HERBAL REMEDIES

There is an important parallel in what is known and what remains un-known about conventional antidepressants and herbal treatments. In both cases, it is difficult to verify specific effects over and above placebo effects in randomized controlled trials. This is typically not because of a weak re-sponse to these treatments, but rather because of frequently large therapeu-tic responses to placebo. For example, many of the clinical trials sponsored by the manufacturers of SSRIs have yielded nonsignificant differences be-tween drug and placebo, but substantial improvement in patients assigned to either condition.

The relatively small differences between active substances and place-bos have created the prejudice that herbal treatments are "nothing but pla-cebos." Yet a similar set of data has left the reputation of conventional an-tidepressants largely intact. One reason for this divergence may be the difficulty involved in understanding the possible modes of action and molecular mechanisms of herbal treatments. Many of the compounds are extremely complex. This complexity renders it difficult to analyze all of their components, let alone to determine their effects on specific enzymatic or hormone systems. In addition, the compound may exert different (e.g., synergistic) effects than do the individual components. However, the mode of action of antidepressants is not well understood either, and it is likely that the divergence in the interpretations of similar data are partly due to ideological reasons. Ideological issues aside, it should be borne in mind that scientific research on herbal remedies is relatively recent. Many more trials have been conducted on standard medications than on phytotherapeutics, and the data concerning the efficacy and safety of phyotherapeutic substances require replications on a larger scale. Still, there seems to be sufficient similarity between the two bodies of literature to warrant a comparison.

For both antidepressants and herbal remedies, the relatively small differences between placebo and active substances do not necessarily mean that these treatments are of little value. If we define the usefulness of a treatment only in terms of (1) the difference between this treatment and placebo and (2) the direct and indirect costs of the treatment versus the costs of the untreated disease, as is implied by the conventional definitions of efficacy and utility, then some could conclude that both antidepressants and phytotherapeutic substances are only of relatively modest value. However, what matters is not only the relative size of the effect, but also the absolute size compared with baseline, or, in other words, the magnitude of specific and nonspecific effects combined. The provision of a good explanatory myth and a convincing therapeutic ritual are among the common factors of all efficacious therapies (Frank, 1987). Hence we can hypothesize that for certain people, the potential for nonspecific effects is greater in herbal treatments than in standard treatments. This is particularly true of people who have a worldview compatible with the application of "natural" products and who have a belief system favoring complementary and alternative treatments. For others, who subscribe to a more rational and mechanistic approach to diseases, conventional medical treatments are likely to be more effective. For still others, psychotherapy might elicit the greatest expectancy effects, and thereby the greatest therapeutic benefit.

It would be intriguing to determine whether patients requesting an herbal treatment experience greater benefits than do those who are either opposed or indifferent to this treatment. Our prediction is that the difference would be statistically and clinically significant, precisely because the nonspecific effects can be better harnessed in believers. Indeed, this effect has been demonstrated in a comparison of the use of hypnosis versus nonhypnotic treatment with clients who either did or did not request hypnotic treatment (Lazarus, 1973).

Herbal treatments provide a stimulus that counters dualistic thinking in terms of specific versus nonspecific effects. They invite us to think of specific effects sitting on top of nonspecific effects. In the Middle Ages, modern thinkers were seen as dwarfs sitting on the shoulders of giants and thereby able to see further (Klibansky, 1936). We would like to reinterpret this metaphor: In some cases, specific effects may be dwarfs sitting on the shoulder of nonspecific effects, and this is why they work so well.

GLOSSARY

Antidepressants: A heterogeneous grouping of different chemical substances, including tricyclics, SSRIs, and MAO inhibitors, that are used for the pharmacological treatment of depression. Antidepressants are considered the first line of intervention in acute and chronic episodes of depression.

Effect size: The primary statistic used in meta-analysis. It is often calculated by dividing the mean difference between a treated group and a control group by the standard deviation of the control group.

Monoamine oxidase inhibitors: Also known as MAO inhibitors, these substances inhibit the enzyme monoamine oxidase, which degrades serotonin and other monoamines, thereby prolonging the life of these amines and their availability. MAO inhibitors are commonly used as antidepressants, although they are associated with certain severe dietary restrictions.

Phytotherapeutics: Pharmaceutical substances made of plants or extracts from plants. These can be standardized liquid or dried extracts, which guarantee the same amount of active components. In some cases they can be made as decoctions in herbal teas.

Placebo: Of Latin origin, literally, "I will please, I will be a pleasure." In the prepharmaceutical era of the 19th and beginning of the 20th century the term placebo was used to denote a treatment with no known efficacy that was given to please a patient. Placebos were later introduced as control substances in trials. In that sense they are physically (but not necessarily psychologically) inert substances—corn flour, lactose, glycerin, and the like—that are packed, colored, and prepared to resemble the test substance.

Selective serotonin reuptake inhibitors (SSRIs): Since the 1970s new antidepressants based on the serotonin hypothesis of depression have been developed. They are called selective serotonin reuptake inhibitors (SSRIs) because they inhibit pharmacologically the process by which serotonin released by neurons is taken back into these neurons. The most widely used of these substances is fluoxetine, better known by the brand name Prozac.

Tricyclics: The older antidepressants are known as tricyclics, the most widely used of which are amitryptiline and imipramine, which are standard reference substances in controlled studies of depression.

REFERENCES

Anderson, I. M. (2000). Selective serotonin reuptake inhibitorsy versus tricyclic antidepressants: A meta-analysis of efficacy and tolerability. *Journal of Affective Disorders, 58*, 19–36.

Antonuccio, D. O., Danton, W. G., DeNelsky, G. Y., Greenberg, R. P., & Gordon, J. S. (1999). Raising questions about antidepressants. *Psychotherapy and Psychosomatics, 68*, 3–14.

Astin, J. A. (1998). Why patients use alternative medicine: Results of a national study. *Journal of the American Medical Association, 279*, 1548–1553.

Barnard, J. (Ed.). (1919). *Collected writings of Edward Bach.* Hereford, England: Bach Educational Programme.

Berner, M. (2001). Kommentar zu Shelton et al. (2001): Hypericum bei Depression [Commentary on Shelton et al. (2001): Hypericum in depression]. *Forschende Komplementärmedizin/Research in Complementary and Classical Natural Medicine 8*, 307–309.

Blashki, T. G., Mowbray, R., & Davies, B. (1971). Controlled trial of amitryptiline in general practice. *British Medical Journal, 1*(741), 133–138.

Bundesinstitut für Arzneimittel und Medizinprodukte. (2000). Bekanntmachung über die Registrierung, Zulassung und Nachzulassung von Arzneimitteln: Abwehr von Arzneimittelrisiken, Anhörung, Stufe II: Johanniskrauthaltige (Hypericum) Humanarzneimittel zur innerlichen Anwendung vom 24. März 2000 [Notice on registration, and admission of medicines: Defence of risks from medicines, hearing #2: Hypericum containing drugs for humans as inward applications, March 24, 2000]. *Bundesanzeiger, 52*, 6009–6010.

Chrubasik, S. (1997). Klinisch geprüfte Wirksamkeit bei nervösen Angst-, Spannungs- und Unruhezuständen. *Der Allgemeinarzt, 18*, 1683–1687.

Chrubasik, S., & Eisenberg, E. (1998). Treatment of rheumatic pain with herbal medicine in Europe. *Pain Digest, 8*, 231–236.

Chrubasik, S., Junck, H., Breitschwerdt, H., Conradt, C., & Zappe, H. (1999). Effectiveness of harpagophytum extract WS 1531 in the treatment of exacerbation of low back pain: A randomized, placebo-controlled, double-blind study. *European Journal of Anaestesiology, 16*, 118–129.

Chrubasik, S., Junck, H., Zappe, H., & Stutzke, O. (1998). A survey on pain complaints and health care utilization in a German population sample. *European Journal of Anaestesiology, 15*, 397–408.

Cohen, J. (1988). *Statistical power analysis for the behavioral sciences.* Hillsdale, NJ: Erlbaum.

Dawes, R. M. (1998). Commentary on Kirsch and Saperstein. *Prevention and Treatment, 1* [Online], Article 0005c. Available: http://journals.apa.org/prevention/volume1/pre0010005c.html

Easthope, G., Tranter, B., & Gill, G. (2001). General practitioners' attitudes toward complementary therapies. *Social Science and Medicine, 51*, 1555–1561.

Eisenberg, D. M., Davis, R. B., Ettner, S. L., Appel, S., Wilkey, S., Van Rompay, M., & Kessler, R. C. (1998) Trends in alternative medicine use in the United States, 1990–1997. Results of a follow-up national survey. *Journal of the American Medical Association, 280,* 1569–1575.

Ernst, E., & Chrubasik, S. (2000). Phyto-anti-inflammatories: A systematic review of randomized, placebo-controlled, double-blind trials. *Rheumatic Disease Clinics of North America, 26,* 13–27.

Ernst, E., & Stevenson, C. (1999). Ginkgo biloba for tinnitus: A review. *Clinical Otolaryngology, 24,* 164–167.

Escher, M., Desmeules, J., Giostra, E., & Mentha, G. (2001). Hepatitis associated with Kava, a herbal remedy for anxiety. *British Medical Journal, 322,* 139.

Field, H. L., Monti, D. A., Greeson, J. M., & Kunkel, E. J. S. (2000). St. John's wort. *International Journal of Psychiatry in Medicine, 30,* 203–219.

Fisher, S., & Greenberg, R. P. (1993). How sound is the double-blind design for evaluating psychotropic drugs? *Journal of Nervous and Mental Diseases, 181,* 345–350.

Frank, J. D. (1987). Therapeutic components shared by all psychotherapies. In J. H. Harvey & M. M. Parks (Eds.), *Psychotherapy research and behavior change* (pp. 73–122). Washington, DC: American Psychological Association.

Fugh-Berman, A., & Cott, J. (1999). Dietary supplements and natural products as psychotherapeutic agents. *Psychosomatic Medicine, 61,* 712–728.

Furnham, A., & Kirkcaldy, B. (1996). The health beliefs and behaviours of orthodox and complementary medicine clients. *British Journal of Clinical Psychology, 35,* 49–61.

Gerson, S., Belin, T. R., Kaufman, A., Mintz, J., & Jarvik, L. (1999). Pharmacological and psychological treatments for depressed older patients: A meta-analysis and overview of recent findings. *Harvard Review of Psychiatry, 7,* 1–28.

Gold, P. E., Cahill, L., & Wenk, G. L. (2002). Ginkgo biloba: A cognitive enhancer. *Psychological Science in the Public Interest, 3,* 2–11.

Gorski, T. (1999). Does the Eisenberg data hold up? *Scientific Review of Alternative Medicine, 3,* 62–69.

Greenberg, R. P., Bornstein, R. F., Zborowski, M. J., Fisher, S., & Greenberg, M. D. (1994). A meta-analysis of fluoxetine outcome in treatment of depression. *Journal of Nervous and Mental Diseases, 182,* 547–551.

Greenberg, R. P., & Fisher, S. (1989). Examining anti-depressant effectiveness: Findings, ambiguities, and some vexing puzzles. In S. Fisher & R. P. Greenberg (Eds.), *The limits of biological treatments for psychological distress: Comparisons with psychotherapy and placebo* (pp. 1–37). Hillsdale, NJ: Erlbaum.

Greeson, J. M., Sanford, B., & Monti, D. A. (2001). St. John's wort (hypericum perforatum): A review of the current pharmacological, toxicological, and clinical literature. *Psychopharmacology, 153,* 402–414.

Gundling, K., & Ernst, E. (1999). Complementary and alternative medicine in cardiovascular disease: What is the evidence it works? *Western Journal of Medicine, 171,* 191–194.

Hypericum Depression Trial Study Group. (2002). Effect of hypericum perforatum (St. John's wort) in major depressive disorder: A randomized controlled trial. *Journal of the American Medical Association, 287,* 1807–1814.

Joffe, R., Sokolov, S., & Streiner, D. (1996). Antidepressant treatment of depression: A meta-analysis. *Canadian Journal of Psychiatry, 41,* 613–616.

Kahn, A., Warner, H. A., & Brown, W. A. (2000). Symptom reduction and suicide risk in patients treated with placebo in antidepressant clinical trials: An analysis of the Food and Drug Administration database. *Archives of General Psychiatry, 57*, 311–317.

Kirsch, I. (1998). Reducing noise and hearing placebo more clearly. *Prevention and Treatment, 1* [Online], Article 0007r. Available: http://journals.apa.org/prevention/volume1/pre0010007a.html

Kirsch, I. (2000). Are drug and placebo effects in depression additive? *Biological Psychiatry, 47*, 733–735.

Kirsch, I., Moore, T. J., Scoboria, A., & Nicholls, S. S. (2002). The emperor's new drugs: An analysis of antidepressant medication data submitted to the U.S. Food and Drug Administration. *Prevention and Treatment, 5* [Online], 23. Available: http://journals.apa.org/prevention

Kirsch, I., & Sapirstein, G. (1998). Listening to Prozac but hearing placebo: A meta-analysis of antidepressant medication. *Prevention and Treatment, 1* [Online] Article 0002a. Available: http://www.journals.apa.org/prevention/volume1/pre0010002a.html

Kirsch, I., & Sapirstein, G. (1999). Listening to Prozac but hearing placebo: A meta-analysis of antidepressant medications. In I. Kirsch (Ed.), *Expectancy, experience, and behavior* (pp. 303–320). Washington, DC: American Psychological Association.

Klein, D. F. (1998). Listening to meta-analysis but hearing bias. *Prevention and Treatment, 1* [Online], Article 0006c. Available: http://journals.apa.org/prevention/volume1/pre0010006c.html

Kleijnen, J., & Knipschild, P. (1992a). Ginkgo biloba. *Lancet, 340*, 1136–1139.

Kleijnen, J., & Knipschild, P. (1992b). Ginkgo biloba for cerebral insufficiency. *British Journal of Clinical Pharmacology 34*, 352–358.

Klibansky, R. (1936). Standing on the shoulders of the giants. *Isis, 26*, 147–149.

Kraft, M., Spahn, T. W., Menzel, J., Senninger, N., Dietl, K.-H., Herbst, H., Domschke, W., & Lerch, M. M. (2001). Fulminantes Leberversagen nach Einnahme des pflanzlichen Antidepressivums Kava-Kava [Liver failure after ingestion of a phytotherapeuticals antidepressant kava-kava]. *Deutsche Medizinische Wochenschrift, 126*, 970–972.

Laakmann, G., Schüle, C., Baghai, T., & Kieser, M. (1998). St. John's wort in mild to moderate depression: The relevance of hyperforin for the clinical efficacy. *Pharmacopsychiatry, 31*, 54–59.

LaFrance, W. C., Lauterbach, E. C., Coffey, C. E., Salloway, S. P., Kaufer, D. I., Reeve, A., Royall, D. R., Aylward, E., Rummans, T. A., & Lovell, M. R. (2000). The use of herbal alternative medicines in neuropsychiatry: A report of the ANPA Committee on Research. *Journal of Neuropsychiatry and Clinical Neurosciences, 12*, 177–192.

Lazarus, A. A. (1973). "Hypnosis" as a facilitator in behavior therapy. *International Journal of Clinical and Experimental Hypnosis, 21*, 25–31.

Linde, K., Ramirez, G., Mulrow, C. D., Pauls, A., Weidenhammer, W., & Melchart, D. (1996). St John's wort for depression—an overview and meta-analysis of randomized clinical trials. *British Medical Journal, 313*, 253–258.

Linde, K., & Mulrow, C. D. (2001). St John's wort for depression (Cochrane Review). In *The Cochrane Library*, Issue 3. Oxford: Update Software.

Maidhof, C., Dehm, C., & Walach, H. (2000). Placebo response rates in clinical trials. A meta-analysis [Abstract]. *International Journal of Psychology, 35,* 224.

Mills, S. (2002). Herbal medicine. In G. Lewith, W. B. Jonas, & H. Walach (Eds.), *Clinical research for complementary medicine: Principles, problems, solutions* (pp. 211–227). London: Churchill Livingstone.

Mössner, R., & Lesch, K.-P. (1998). Role of serotonin in the immune system and in neuroimmune interactions. *Brain, Behavior, and Immunity, 12,* 249–271.

Oken, B. S, Storzbach, D. M., & Kaye, J. A. (1998). The efficacy of Ginkgo biloba on cognitive function in Alzheimer disease. *Archives of Neurology, 55,* 1409–1415.

Ott, B. R., & Owens, N. J. (1998). Complementary and alternative medicines for Alzheimer's disease. *Journal of Geriatric Psychiatry and Neurology, 11,* 163–173.

Philipp, M., Kohnen, R., & Hiller, K. O. (1999). Hypericum extract versus imipramine or placebo in patients with moderate depression: randomized multicentre study of treatment for eight weeks. *British Medical Journal, 319,* 1534–1539.

Pirotta, M. V., Cohen, M. M., Kotsirilos, V., & Farish, S. J. (2000). Complementary therapies: Have they become accepted in general practice? *Medical Journal of Australia, 172,* 105–109.

Pittler, M. H., & Ernst, E. (2000). Efficacy of Kava extract for treating anxiety: Systematic review and meta-analysis. *Journal of Clinical Psychopharmacology, 20,* 84–89.

Pratkanis, A. R. (1995, July/August). How to sell a pseudoscience. *Skeptical Inquirer, 19,* 19–25.

Quitkin, F. M., Rabkin, J. G., Gerald, J., Davis, J. M., & Klein, D. F. (2000). Validity of clinical trials of antidepressants. *American Journal of Psychiatry, 157,* 327–337.

Rabkin, J. G., Markowitz, J. S., Stewart, J. W., McGrath, P. J., Harrison, W., Quitkin, F. M., & Klein, D. F. (1986). How blind is blind? Assessment of patient and doctor medication guesses in a placebo-controlled trial of imipramine and phenelzine. *Psychiatry Research, 19,* 75–86.

Rosslenbroich, B ., & Saller, R. (1992). Phytotherapie im Überblick [A review on phytotherapeutics]. In M. Bühring & F. H. Kemper (Eds.), *Naturheilverfahren und unkonventionelle medizinische Richtungen [Naturopathic therapies and unconventional medical practices].* Berlin: SpringerLoseblattSysteme, section 8.01.

Schonauer, K. (1994). *Semiotic foundation of drug therapy: The placebo problem in a new perspective.* Berlin: Mouton de Gruyter.

Schulz, V. (2000). The psychodynamic and pharmacodynamic effects of drugs: A differentiated evaluation of the efficacy of phytotherapy. *Phytomedicine, 7,* 73–81.

Shelton, R. C., Keller, M. B., Gelenberg, A., Dunner, D. L., Hirschfeld, R., Thase, M. E., Russell, J., Lydiard, R. B., Crits-Cristoph, P., Gallop, R., Todd, L., Hellerstein, D., Goodnick, P., Keitner, G., Stahl, S. M., & Halbreich, U. (2001). Effectiveness of St. John's Wort in major depression. A randomized controlled trial. *Journal of the American Medical Association, 285,* 1978–1986.

Singer, A., Wonnemann, M., & Müller, W. E. (1999). Hyperforin, a major antidepressant constituent of St. John's Wort, inhibits serotonin uptake by elevating free intracellular Na+. *Journal of Pharmacology and Experimental Therapeutics, 290,* 1363–1368.

Sparber, A., Wootton, J. C., Bauer, L., Curt, G., Eisenberg, D., Levin, T., & Steinberg,

S. M. (2000). Use of complementary medicine by adult patients participating in HIV/AIDS clinical trials. *Journal of Alternative and Complementary Medicine, 5,* 415–422.

Stevinson, C., & Ernst, E. (1999). Hypericum for depression. An update of the clinical evidence. *European Neuropsychopharmacology, 9,* 501–505.

Storosum, J. G., Elferink, A. J. A., van Zwieten, B. J., van den Brink, W., Gersons, B. P. R., van Strik, R., & Broekmans, A. W. (2001). Short-term efficacy of tricyclic antidepressants revisited: A meta-analytic study. *European Neuropsychopharmacology, 11,* 173 180.

Walach, H., & Güthlin, C. (2000). Effects of acupuncture and homeopathy: A prospective documentation. Intermediate results. *British Homeopathic Journal, 89,* 31–34.

Walach, H., & Maidhof, C. (1999). Is the placebo effect dependent on time? In I. Kirsch (Ed.), *Expectancy, experience, and behavior* (pp. 321–332). Washington, DC: American Psychological Association.

Walach, H., Rilling, C., & Engelke, U. (2001). Efficacy of Bach-flower remedies in test anxiety: A double-blind, placebo-controlled, randomized trial with partial crossover. *Journal of Anxiety Disorders, 15,* 359–366.

Woelk, H., for the Remotiv/Imipramine Study Group. (2000). Comparison of St. John's wort and imipramine for treating depression: randomized controlled trial. *British Medical Journal, 321,* 536–539.

PART IV

CONTROVERSIES IN THE TREATMENT OF SPECIFIC CHILD DISORDERS

12

Empirically Supported, Promising, and Unsupported Treatments for Children with Attention-Deficit/ Hyperactivity Disorder

DANIEL A. WASCHBUSCH
G. PERRY HILL

Attention-deficit/hyperactivity disorder (ADHD) is a chronic disorder of childhood characterized by abnormally high levels of inattention, impulsivity, and overactivity (American Psychiatric Association, 1994). ADHD is a common mental health problem of childhood, affecting an estimated 3–5% of the elementary-age population (Anderson, Williams, McGee, & Silva, 1987), and is among the most common reasons for referrals to mental health clinics (Cantwell, 1996). ADHD is associated with serious impairment in many domains of daily functioning. For example, children with ADHD are often rejected by their peers, experience more negative interactions with parents, and frequently experience classroom and academic problems (Hinshaw, 1994). ADHD in childhood also predicts the development of serious problems in adolescence and adulthood, including school and vocational failure, disruptions in interpersonal relationships, criminal behavior, mental health problems, and alcohol or other substance abuse (Ingram, Hechtman, & Morgenstern, 1999), with the most severe out-

---

Each of the authors contributed equally to this chapter. Order of authorship was determined by a coin toss.

comes associated with the co-occurrence of ADHD and conduct problems (Lilienfeld & Waldman, 1990; Waschbusch, 2002). The costs associated with these difficulties are likely to be substantial not only for individual children, but also for their families, teachers, and peers. Thus, identification of effective treatments for ADHD has major public health implications.

A wide variety of treatments have been used with ADHD, perhaps more so than for any other form of child psychopathology. Purported treatments range from medication to restrictive or supplemental diets, allergy treatments, biofeedback, homeopathic remedies, and others. The wide variety and prevalence of treatments raises questions as to which treatments for ADHD work, which do not, and how to tell the difference between them. This chapter will address these questions by reviewing the empirical research literature. We will first review treatments that have substantial empirical support. Second, promising treatments for ADHD, defined as those that have limited empirical support, will be identified. Finally, treatments with no empirical support—both those that have evidence against them and those that have been suggested for use with ADHD but have not been researched—will be discussed. Criteria used to classify treatments into these categories will also be discussed. We will conclude the chapter with a discussion of concerns regarding controversial treatments for ADHD.

EMPIRICALLY SUPPORTED TREATMENTS

During the last half of the 1990s, considerable effort was exerted toward determining the evidential base of psychosocial treatments for mental health problems. Of special note is the Task Force that proposed that adult (Chambless et al., 1996) and child (Lonigan, Elbert, & Johnson, 1998) psychosocial treatments can be considered well supported by research if they are shown to be superior to placebo treatments (assuming the comparison has adequate statistical power; see Chapter 6). This can be accomplished in either of two ways: (1) using at least two group-design studies that are conducted by a different set of investigators, or (2) using at least 10 single-case studies. In addition, the treatments must be manualized and the samples used to research the treatment must be clearly specified.

Having established these criteria, experts in specific mental health problems were recruited to review the existing literature on child psychosocial treatments and apply these criteria. Among the areas reviewed was an evaluation of treatments for ADHD (Pelham, Wheeler, & Chronis, 1998). This review concluded that there are currently three types of treatments for ADHD that have been supported in the empirical literature:

(1) medications, (2) behavior modification, and (3) the combination of these two. Arguments for and against each of these treatments were well articulated in the Pelham and colleagues (1998) review, so we will only briefly summarize the same information here. We also present information on the Multisite Treatment of ADHD (MTA) study, as the results are directly relevant to the topic of empirically supported treatment of ADHD.

Psychostimulant Medications

Medication is the most common treatment for ADHD, with estimates indicating that 90% of children with ADHD are treated with medication at some point in their elementary school years (Safer & Krager, 1994). Although a variety of medications have been used to treat ADHD, only psychostimulants have a sufficient research base to be classified as empirically supported. Stimulant medication has been repeatedly shown to produce improvements in the core symptoms associated with ADHD, namely, inattention, impulsivity, and overactivity (see Swanson, McBurnett, Christian, & Wigal, 1995, for a review). There is also evidence that stimulants produce improvements in other associated features of ADHD, such as social behaviors, academic productivity, and classroom behavior (Brown & Sawyer, 1998). These changes are seen across multiple measures, including parent and teacher ratings, observational measures, and performance tasks (e.g., attention and inhibitory control tasks). Furthermore, these improvements are often immediate and meaningful, and are usually obtained with few side effects. Because of these benefits, as well as their ease of use and widespread availability, stimulant medication has become the most widely used treatment for ADHD (Safer & Krager, 1988, 1994).

Various types and preparations of psychostimulants are used to treat ADHD, including methylphenidate (Ritalin), d-amphetamine (Dexedrine), pemoline (Cylert), and more recently, d,l-amphetamine (Adderall) and methylphenidate HCl (Concerta). There is very little research comparing these different forms of psychostimulants. The limited evidence available suggests that although they share many important properties, they also have unique effects. That is, different stimulants, different doses of the same stimulant, and different preparations of the same stimulant may have unpredictable effects both between children and within children (Pelham & Milich, 1991). As a consequence, effective treatment of ADHD with psychostimulant medication must include a double-blind, placebo-controlled trial that objectively determines the most therapeutic stimulant preparation and dosage for that child's area(s) of difficulty (see Pelham, 1993, for details of how to conduct such a trial).

Despite the large base of empirical support for the use of stimulant medications in the treatment of ADHD, there are important limits to this type of treatment. First, treatment gains are maintained only as long as the child is actively taking the medication (e.g., Brown & Sawyer, 1998; Swanson et al., 1995). Second, not all children with ADHD respond favorably to stimulant medication. Best estimates suggest that about 70–80% of children with ADHD will show a positive response to psychostimulants, but the remaining 20–30% show either an adverse response or no response (Swanson et al., 1995). Furthermore, of those children who respond positively, only a minority show sufficient improvement for their behavior to fall entirely within the normal range. The remaining children are improved, but their behavior is not normalized.

Perhaps the most important limitation is the lack of evidence that treatment with stimulant medication results in long-term improvement. Studies that have followed children treated with psychostimulant medication for periods up to 5 years have failed to document any improvements in long-term prognosis (e.g., Weiss & Hechtman, 1993). Although methodological considerations require that these findings be interpreted cautiously (e.g., lack of random assignment to treatment condition, lack of information about treatment compliance), beneficial treatment effects of stimulant medications do not appear to yield substantially improved long-term outcomes for most children with ADHD. Additional research is needed to clarify the possible role of such factors as inconsistency of administration and termination of medication treatment in these studies.

Behavior Modification

Behavior modification has been used as a treatment for ADHD for more than 20 years (e.g., O'Leary, Pelham, Rosenbaum, & Price, 1976). In addition, many early studies of behavioral treatment for children with conduct problems or disruptive behaviors included children who were diagnosed with ADHD (e.g., Patterson, 1974). Thus, there is an extensive literature on behavioral treatments for ADHD.

The difficulties associated with ADHD are typically observed in multiple settings, especially in the child's home and at school. As a result, behavioral treatments for ADHD have been studied in both of these settings, and the Task Force review examined this research separately (Pelham et al., 1998). Both behavioral parent training and classroom contingency management programs met the Task Force criteria for empirically supported treatments. As was the case with stimulant medication treatments, behavioral interventions are typically effective in reducing the core symptoms of ADHD and in reducing related problems (such as academic productivity). This seems to be true regardless of the specific form of behavioral intervention that is used. That is, Pelham and colleagues (1998) examined whether their behavior management and contingency management procedures were differentially effective in treating ADHD. Behavior management procedures were described as those treatments that involve teaching parents to apply behavior management principles to their children with ADHD. Contingency management procedures were described as more intensive interventions that, although employing the same general techniques found in behavior management procedures, are implemented directly by a behavior modification expert (e.g., clinician or expert teacher) rather than by a parent or teacher who is coached from afar. Results of the review supported the efficacy of both these approaches, with relatively greater treatment effects attributed to contingency management procedures. Thus, research indicates that behavior modification is an effective treatment for ADHD, and that this is true whether the treatment is delivered at home or at school or is delivered by experts, parents, or teachers.

The limitations of behavioral treatments for ADHD parallel those of stimulant medication. First, although behavioral treatments frequently improve the behavioral functioning of children with ADHD, rarely are treatment effects sufficient to "normalize" children. Second, the effects of behavioral treatments appear to be short-term, with treatment gains limited to the period during which treatment programs are actually in effect. It is worth emphasizing that this is true for all current treatments of ADHD, including medication, a circumstance that has led some to suggest that ADHD should be conceptualized as a chronic condition that requires "chronic" treatment (Cantwell, 1996; Waschbusch, Kipp, & Pelham, 1998). Third, not all children with ADHD respond positively to behavioral treatments. Failure to respond positively may be attributable to factors that are external to the child, such as an inability or unwillingness of parents or teachers to implement the treatment program or a lack of knowledge or skills on the part of the therapists. In addition, the most effective behavioral treatment programs are often the most comprehensive and intensive and therefore the most difficult to implement consistently and continually. These factors suggest that even though behavioral programs are not effective for all children with ADHD, some of this can be explained by the fact that the child is not actually receiving the treatment, is not receiving the treatment consistently, or is not receiving an adequate form of the treatment. Such situations are akin to receiving medication at nontherapeutic dosage levels or receiving medication inconsistently.

A final limitation of current behavioral treatments for ADHD—again similar to limitations of stimulant treatments—is the lack of evidence for long-term effectiveness. No studies have yet been conducted to examine the effects of behavioral treatments in children with ADHD over extended periods of time. Demonstrating maintenance of effects of behavioral treatments over time is a major concern, especially given the chronic nature of

the disorder. Research examining long-term effects of behavioral treat
ments for ADHD is needed.

Combined Stimulant and Behavioral Treatments

A number of arguments can be made in favor of combining stimulant medication and behavioral approaches to treat ADHD. First, combined behavioral and stimulant treatments may show complementary effects, with each
addressing the weaknesses of the other. For example, behavioral treatments
can be used 24 hours a day, whereas medication treatments are typically
not used for at least part of the day (e.g., evening and weekends). Similarly,
medication treatments may address problems that occur in the absence of
adult authority figures or that occur at a low rate, whereas behavioral
treatments are often ineffective with these difficulties (Hinshaw, Heller, &
McHale, 1992; Hinshaw, Henker, Whalen, Erhardt, & Dunnington, 1989).
Second, combining behavioral and medication interventions may amplify
each other's effects. Indeed, some evidence shows that behavioral interventions are more effective when combined with medication, and that less
medication is needed to show positive effects on children's behavior when
combined with behavioral interventions (Pelham et al., 1993). Third, combined treatments may result in more cost-effective treatments because less
complex behavioral programs (thereby requiring less therapist attention) are
often needed to achieve the same effects in combined treatment interventions.

Despite this strong rationale, there are far fewer studies of combined
stimulant and behavior modification treatments for ADHD than there are
studies of each treatment alone. The research that is available supports the
efficacy of combined treatments for ADHD (Pelham & Murphy, 1986; Pelham & Waschbusch, 1999). For example, a review by Pelham and Murphy
(1986) showed that combined treatments were superior to behavioral or
medication treatments alone on at least one dependent measure (which included measures of classroom, motor, or social behavior) in 13 of 19 studies (68%). Furthermore, almost no studies showed that behavioral or pharmacological treatments alone were superior to their combination. Finally,
as discussed in the next section, some of the results from the recent National Institute of Mental Health funded multisite treatment study of
ADHD also suggest that combined treatments are superior to either behavioral or medication treatments alone (Pelham, 1999).

Despite these promising findings, several caveats and limitations
should be noted. First, combined stimulant and behavioral interventions
are relatively unstudied. Second, the incremental benefits of combined
treatments do not appear to persist when either component is withdrawn
or discontinued (Pelham et al., 1988). Third, existing studies of combined
treatments have focused on acute effects rather than long-term maintenance. No controlled, long-term studies have yet been conducted.

Multisite Treatment for ADHD (MTA) Study

As already noted, there is clear evidence supporting the efficacy of behavioral, medication, and combined treatment approaches to treating ADHD. However, the relative efficacy of these treatments remains largely unexamined. In other words, there is strong evidence that medication treatments, behavioral treatments, and the combination of the two treatments are an effective approach to treating ADHD, but there is relatively little evidence to determine whether one of these three approaches is superior to the other.

To address this issue, the National Institute of Mental Health (and other similar agencies) funded the largest clinical trial ever conducted on a treatment of psychopathology (Richters et al., 1995). The study included 579 boys and girls with ADHD, ages 7.0 to 9.9, who were assessed and treated at seven different locations across North America (Hinshaw et al., 1997). Children were randomly assigned to one of four treatment conditions: (1) medication only, (2) behavioral only, (3) both medication and behavioral, and (4) standard community care. These treatments were provided for 14 months, after which outcomes were evaluated in numerous domains. The main questions of interest were the following:

1. What are the relative efficacies of behavioral and pharmacological treatments?
2. What is the incremental benefit of combining these treatments over either treatment alone?
3. How do these evidenced-based treatments compare to treatments routinely given in the community? (MTA Cooperative Group, 1999a)

Although the majority of data from this study are still being analyzed, preliminary results have been published. These results suggested that medication treatments are superior to behavioral treatments, with little benefit added when combined with behavioral approaches (MTA Cooperative Group, 1999a). Furthermore, these effects were not moderated by age, comorbidity, or other potentially important factors (MTA Cooperative Group, 1999b).

On the other hand, not all data were consistent with the conclusion that medication treatments were superior to other treatments in the MTA study (Pelham, 1999, 2000). First, although the medication-only and combined medication/behavioral treatment conditions produced superior outcomes on measures of ADHD symptoms, behavior-only treatments produced equivalent effects on measures of impairment. These include observations of classroom behavior, parent and teacher ratings of social skills, parent ratings of parent–child relationships, peer sociometric ratings, and academic achievement measures. Second, the greatest improvements on all measures was produced by the combination of behavioral and medication treatment, although the differences between combined and other treatments were not always significant. Third, when the level of behavioral treatment provided was intensive, behavior-only treatment resulted in outcomes similar to combined behavioral/medication outcomes (Pelham et al., 2000). Thus, it can be persuasively argued that the MTA study provided evidence supporting behavior-only, medication-only, and combined treatment approaches, with no clear "winner" among them. Whether these treatments produce differing long-term improvements remains unclear.

PROMISING TREATMENTS

Recent years have seen increased efforts to investigate other treatments for ADHD, due in part to the limitations of established treatments. For purposes of the present discussion, criteria used to identify promising treatments were similar to Task Force criteria used to identify empirically supported treatments, except that we required fewer studies to meet criteria. The following criteria were used to identify treatments for inclusion in this section:

- At least one group design study that includes a no-treatment, placebo, and/or alternative treatment condition and that reports superior effects for the treatment of interest.
- Three to eight single-case design studies that compare a treatment with an alternative treatment or to a no-treatment condition and that report superior effects.

Some of the treatments identified in this section are more strongly supported than others. For example, some appear to have usefulness in treatment of ADHD, but only within certain parameters or under certain conditions. Others are not yet well-enough researched to determine their effectiveness, but enjoy a sufficient amount of empirical support to warrant further examination as well as consideration as adjunctive treatments for ADHD.

Nonstimulant Medications

Alternatives to psychostimulant medications for ADHD (especially antidepressants and antihypertensives) have received increased attention during the past decade. These treatments seem to be used primarily for children who do not respond to stimulant medications alone. Although these nonstimulant medications may prove effective in this capacity, it is worth noting that behavioral treatments, or combined behavioral and stimulant treatments, may be an effective alternative for children who do not respond to stimulants alone.

Chief among these alternative medications for ADHD are antidepressants, especially the class of tricyclic antidepressants (TCAs) that include amitriptyline (Elavil), nortriptyline (Pamelor), imipramine (Tofranil), desipramine (Norpramin), and clomipramine (Anafranil). Another class of antidepressants (selective serotonin reuptake inhibitors, or SSRIs) has not been systematically evaluated in the treatment of ADHD and was not endorsed as a treatment for ADHD in a recent review (National Institute of Mental Health, 1996). Monoamine oxidase inhibitor (MAOIs) antidepressants are rarely used with children because of their potential for severe adverse side effects and drug–drug interactions.

A growing body of research evidence demonstrates the efficacy of TCAs in reducing overt behavioral symptoms of childhood ADHD (e.g., Biederman, Baldessarini, Wright, Knee, & Harmatz, 1989). However, studies comparing the effectiveness of TCAs and stimulants on behaviors associated with ADHD have yielded mixed results. Specifically, some studies have reported superior behavioral response to stimulants (e.g., Gittleman-Klein, 1974), others have shown equal effects of TCAs and stimulants on behaviors associated with ADHD (e.g., Rapport, Carlson, Kelly, & Pataki, 1993), and still other studies (although far fewer) have reported superior response to TCAs in comparison with stimulants (e.g., Werry, 1980). In contrast to behavioral measures, studies are consistent in suggesting that TCAs are less effective than stimulants in improving the cognitive functioning of children with ADHD. Given that TCAs are potentially more toxic than stimulants, these results provide little rationale for using TCAs as a frontline treatment for ADHD.

TCAs may be a useful treatment for those children with ADHD who do not respond to stimulant medications. This possibility was demonstrated by Beiderman and colleagues (1989) who reported "dramatic improvement" in behavioral and classroom functioning in almost 70% of children with ADHD who were treated with desipramine, the majority of whom had previously shown no response or adverse response to stimulant medications. As would be expected, subjects also showed noticeable improvement in symptoms of depression, suggesting that desipramine may be useful in treatment of ADHD with comorbid depression or anxiety. Preliminary findings indicate good maintenance of therapeutic benefits with TCAs for up to 2 years (e.g., Biederman, Gastfriend, & Jellinek, 1986), provided that medication treatment remained in place. The long-term effects of TCAs on ADHD are unknown. Sustained improvements of ADHD symptoms with TCAs typically depend upon periodic upward adjustments in dosage, and it is unclear whether relatively higher dosage levels are necessary for positive response (Spencer, Biederman, & Wilens, 1998).

Antihypertensives, especially clonidine, have also been examined as an alternative medication treatment for ADHD. Much of the empirical evidence on effectiveness of clonidine with ADHD is lacking in methodological rigor. However, one double-blind study reported improvement in parent- and teacher-completed ratings of hyperactivity, impulsiveness, and aggression in youth with ADHD treated with clonidine as compared to youth in a placebo condition (Hunt, Minderaa, & Cohen, 1985). No studies have demonstrated improvement in cognitive impairments associated with ADHD, and there are also no studies of the long-term effects of clonidine on ADHD.

This cursory review indicates great potential for nonstimulant medications in the treatment of ADHD, but also reflects the sparse knowledge base of the use of these substances with ADHD in comparison with stimulant medications. There is evidence that antidepressants (especially tricyclic antidepressants) may be quite useful in treating children with ADHD who do not respond favorably to stimulant medications, and that they may also be useful in treating ADHD with comorbid depression or anxiety. Similarly, clonidine may be useful in cases where there is no favorable response to other, more well-established treatments (e.g., stimulant medications, behavioral treatments) or in the unusual case where use of other medications is contraindicated. However, given the limited empirical support for nonstimulant medication treatment for ADHD, it should be emphasized that both antidepressants and antihypertensives should be considered a secondline treatment.

Intensive Behavioral Treatment Programs

Several authors have suggested that regular outpatient treatments are not sufficient for children with ADHD and other disruptive behavior disorders and that intensive, community-based treatment programs represent a promising alternative (e.g., Henggeler, Melton, & Smith, 1992). Intensive treatments, as compared with traditional outpatient treatments, are characterized by frequent and ongoing therapeutic contacts, delivery in community rather than office settings, and targeting of the treatments toward functional daily activities. Thus, there is a strong rationale for intensive treatments.

Intensive behavioral treatments for ADHD have been offered in summer camp settings (Pelham et al., 1996; Pelham & Hoza, 1996) and in full-day school settings (Swanson, 1992). The children treated in these settings experience treatment the same as do children in more typical summer camp (e.g., playing soccer, going swimming, art and academic classrooms) or school settings, and it is in these contexts that the behavioral treatments are delivered and stimulant medications are assessed. This approach emphasizes improvement of peer relationships through participation in academic and recreational group activities. Early indications suggest that intensive treatments are effective (Pelham & Hoza, 1996). For example, intensive behavioral treatment provided as part of the MTA study resulted in treatment gains that were of the same magnitude as the combination of behavioral treatment and stimulant medication (Pelham et al., 2000). However, there are as yet no carefully controlled studies on the efficacy of such intensive treatment programs as the summer camp program. In addition, the initial costs of implementing such programs (including facilities and personnel) are quite high, even though the long-term financial savings are likely to be substantial (Pelham, 1999).

Classroom-Based Interventions

In addition to contingency management programs, other classroom-based interventions have been used in the treatment of ADHD, including educational strategies, peer-directed strategies, and self-management strategies. These treatments have addressed both social and academic performance problems associated with ADHD, and are designed to prevent, attenuate, or manage ADHD symptoms. Educational and instructional interventions manipulate classroom organization and instructional methodology in ways that prevent or minimize the occurrence of ADHD symptoms. This approach is consistent with the view that these problems can and should be addressed as instructional problems (Colvin & Sugai, 1988), and are compatible with applied behavior analysis procedures that emphasize functional assessment and antecedent control of ADHD symptoms (DuPaul & Ervin, 1996).

Examples of this treatment strategy include recent descriptions by Zentall (1993) regarding the timely use of instructional materials to increase stimulation to ADHD students during academic tasks to enhance attention and improve performance. Most classroom-based treatments for ADHD are teacher-directed. However, peers sometimes assume roles as behavior change agents by monitoring and reinforcing desirable social and academic behaviors of students with ADHD, prompting appropriate behavior, or serving as tutors for remediating specific academic skills. DuPaul and Stoner (1994) argued that peer tutor interventions target important skills typically unaffected by traditional contingency management programs and satisfy the learning needs of many students with ADHD by providing frequent, immediate feedback on important aspects of educational functioning. A recent study by DuPaul and Henningson (1993) reported improvements in both classroom behavior and academic performance in students with ADHD using a carefully designed and implemented peer tutor intervention.

Self-monitoring and self-reinforcement interventions involve having children monitor and evaluate their own social or academic performance according to prescribed criteria, then rewarding themselves based upon those self-evaluations. These treatment techniques have been used with students with ADHD to increase on-task behavior during individual seatwork (Barkley, Copeland, & Sivage, 1980), improve reading comprehension (Edwards et al., 1995), and increase cooperative play interactions (Hinshaw, Henker, & Whalen, 1984). Positive effects of self-monitoring treatments are generally not as strong as those obtained through contingency management procedures. However, these interventions may be useful in facilitating partial fading of token reinforcement programs, and they may have value in targeting specific skills or behaviors unaffected by traditional behavioral treatments.

UNSUPPORTED TREATMENTS

Popular interest in ADHD has resulted in a multitude of proposed treatments for this disorder, but few critical appraisals of these treatments have been published (Arnold, 1999; Goldstein & Ingersoll, 1993). In this section we summarize extant data for many of these proposed treatments. Treatments are grouped as either ineffective or largely unresearched and were identified through review of both professional and lay literature, as well as media sources (including Web search).

Ineffective Treatments

Criteria for inclusion in this category required that the purported treatment has been evaluated and found to have no effect in comparison with no treatment in at least two group studies or in six or more single-case design studies. Treatments were also included if previously judged ineffective in at least two published literature reviews by different authors.

Cognitive Training Programs

Cognitive-behavioral therapy for children with ADHD was first proposed almost 30 years ago (Meichenbaum & Goodman, 1971). Many types of cognitive treatments (also called cognitive-behavioral treatments) have been applied to children with ADHD, including training in verbal self-instruction, problem-solving strategies, cognitive modeling, self-monitoring, self-evaluation, and self-reinforcement (Abikoff, 1987, 1991; Braswell & Bloomquist, 1991). The rationale for these treatments is the belief that behavioral self-control can be increased by enhancing specific cognitive or meta-cognitive skills that are believed to underlie and promote impulse control, goal-directed behavior, or both. Because the seeming absence or inefficiency of such internal mediators appears to characterize children with ADHD, cognitive treatments enjoy a strong intuitive appeal and would appear to offer a natural remedy. Nevertheless, controlled studies have not supported their effectiveness.

Numerous studies have examined the effects of cognitive treatments for ADHD. For example, Abikoff and colleagues (1988) administered 16 weeks of intensive cognitive training to children with ADHD and found no differences on multiple academic, cognitive, and behavioral measures in comparison with attention control (i.e., providing support but no active intervention) and no-training groups. A number of other studies (e.g., Bloomquist, August, Cohen, Doyle, & Everhart, 1997; Brown, Borden, Wynne, Spunt, & Clingerman, 1987) are remarkably consistent in demonstrating that cognitive treatment for ADHD generally results in no clinically important changes in the academic or behavioral performance of children with ADHD, even though there has been demonstrated efficacy of cognitive training programs for other childhood disorders (e.g., Dujovne, Barnard, & Rapoff, 1995; Kendall & Gosch, 1994; Lochman, 1992). Braswell (1998) recently discussed the disappointing findings regarding cognitive treatments with children with ADHD and offered suggestions regarding possible but highly limited clinical applications of self-monitoring, self-reinforcement, and self-instructional training programs.

It is important to note there may be several exceptional circumstances under which cognitive training programs have some clinical usefulness in the treatment of ADHD, especially when combined with intensive, multi-component treatment packages. First, cognitive training that focuses on improving social skills and that is adjunctive to operant behavioral or clinical behavioral interventions may be beneficial (Pelham & Hoza, 1996; Pelham et al., 1988). Second, anger control training in the context of intensive behavioral interventions may also be useful (Hinshaw, Buhrmester, & Heller, 1989; Hinshaw et al., 1984). Third, problem-solving training may be helpful for children with ADHD who have comorbid aggression, especially if cognitive training is combined with parent training (Kazdin, Esveldt-Dawson, French, & Unis, 1987; Lochman, 1992; Lochman & Lenhart, 1993). In general, then, cognitive interventions might show adjunctive value by enhancing maintenance and generalization of clinical gains in the context of an intensive, combined behavioral and pharmacological treatment program, although this hypothesis has not been adequately tested to allow for firm conclusions.

Dietary Management

A number of naturally occurring and manufactured food substances have been hypothesized to act as allergens or toxins that result in ADHD (see also Chapter 13, for a review of dietary treatments for autism). This supposition has generated much popular interest and heated debate. The rationale for dietary management of ADHD is simple: Remove or restrict the offending substance(s) from the diet and ADHD symptoms will remit. We will review two dietary management treatments for ADHD that have been closely studied, namely the Feingold Diet and sugar elimination strategies.

Perhaps more than any other individual, Feingold (1973, 1975a, 1975b, 1976) popularized the notion that the occurrence of ADHD symptoms results from a toxic reaction to certain low molecular weight chemicals (called salycilates) through the diet. Salycilates occur naturally in some foods and artificially in food colors and flavorings. Feingold suggested that elimination of these substances through dietary restriction would result in improved behavioral and cognitive functioning for up to 60% of children with ADHD (Feingold, 1975a). Though his writings never fully delineated the precise mechanisms by which supposed toxic reactions occurred, Feingold's early (1975b) statements were quite emphatic, generating much debate and a flurry of research activity that continued for over a decade.

The first controlled investigation of dietary management used a counterbalanced design to compare the Feingold diet (i.e., a diet that excludes offending substances specified by Feingold) with a control exclusionary diet (Conners, Goyette, Southwick, Lees, & Andrulonis, 1976). Results were mixed, showing a modicum of support for the Feingold Diet and suggesting that continued investigation of effects of the diet on children with ADHD was warranted. The mixed results of the Conners and colleagues (1976) study foreshadowed findings from experimental studies during the next several years. Some studies (e.g., Cook & Woodhill, 1976; Holborow, Elkins, & Berry, 1981; Rapp, 1978) reported positive effects of the Feingold Diet in reducing hyperactive behavior. Other studies (e.g., Conners, 1980; Mattes & Gittleman-Klein, 1978; Stine, 1976) reported either minimal or no effects of the diet in reducing such hyperactive behavior.

These initial studies were characterized by a number of methodological problems. For example, improvements in ADHD symptoms following the Feingold Diet were typically detected only on rating measures by parents (many of whom were not blind to the treatment conditions) and were probably attributable to placebo or expectancy effects (Baker, 1980; see Chapter 11 for a discussion of placebo effects). Furthermore, reviews of research that accounted for these methodological difficulties concluded that research evidence did not support the dramatic effects of diet treatment reported anecdotally by Feingold and others and that well-controlled studies were unable to demonstrate clinically meaningful gains (Harley & Matthews, 1978; Kavale & Forness, 1983; Mattes, 1983). Several rebuttals to these reviews (Rimland, 1983; Weiss, 1982) were generally unconvincing in addressing methodological concerns and the lack of objective findings.

Results of more recent studies employing more stringent experimental procedures (Rowe, 1988; Rowe & Rowe, 1994) suggest that a very small percentage of children with ADHD (probably less than 10%) may respond positively to diet management as a treatment for ADHD. At present, however, there are no data available to assist in identifying these children on an a priori basis or to describe what risks and benefits they might enjoy from a restrictive diet. Furthermore, even for the responders, it is not clear that the restrictive diet is more effective than well-established treatment (e.g., behavioral and stimulant treatments). Thus, the Feingold Diet should be considered an ineffective treatment for ADHD.

Whereas the Feingold Diet implicates an entire class of food substances in the occurrence of ADHD, refined sugar is a specific substance presumed to cause hyperactivity and other child behavior problems (Smith, 1975). Despite the popular support for this proposition among parents, teachers, and some mental health professionals, well-controlled studies have not demonstrated an effect of sugar on children's behavior.

Milich, Wolraich, and Lindgren (1986) reviewed studies and found no consistent, significant effects of sugar on a variety of behavioral measures across studies, even among subjects who were thought to be "sugar sensitive." Similar conclusions have been reported in controlled studies of aspartame on behavior. As one example, Wolraich and colleagues (Wolraich, 1988; Wolraich et al., 1994) compared three controlled diets (high sucrose–low sweetener, low sucrose–high sweetener, and placebo) in two groups of children presumed to be especially vulnerable to the effects of sugar ingestion (i.e., preschool and school-age children nominated by parents as highly adverse to sugar). The diets were presented in 3-week blocks using a counterbalanced, double-blind, crossover design. Results showed no differences among the three diets on any of almost 40 behavioral and cognitive measures. Shaywitz and colleagues (1994) also found no effect on cognitive or behavioral measures with children with ADHD who consumed unusually high amounts of aspartame over a 4-week period. There is little evidence, then, that either sugar or aspartame ingestion have appreciable effects on children's behavior.

Nutritional and Dietary Supplements

Unlike alleged food allergens and toxins, which are argued to be related to ADHD because of their presence, nutritional and dietary supplements are hypothesized to be related to ADHD either because of their absence, or because they do not occur in optimum quantities or at critical levels in one's natural diet. If so, adding these nutrients to the diet might correct the hypothesized nutritional deficit or imbalance, thereby ameliorating the symptoms of ADHD.

Amino acids are one dietary supplement proposed as a treatment for ADHD. This proposal comes from observations that hyperactive boys and matched normal boys may differ in protein synthesis even though they have similar diets (Stein & Sammaritano, 1984). However, controlled studies examining amino acid treatments have shown inconsistent effects. When effects are found, they appear to dissipate quickly, presumably due to acquired tolerance to the supplement (Nemzer, Arnold, Votolato, & McConnell, 1986; Wood, Reimherr, & Wender, 1985; Zametkin, Karoum, & Rapoport, 1987). Furthermore, any gains resulting from amino acid supplements are offset by a risk for neurotoxicity (Sternberg, 1996).

Effects of combinations of vitamins at megadosage levels (multivitamin therapy) on ADHD have been investigated in several controlled studies. None of the studies has shown consistent positive results (Arnold, 1978; Kershner & Hawke, 1979).

Largely Unresearched Treatments

A variety of purported treatments for ADHD can be identified for which there exists little or no empirical evidence. Many enjoy only testimonial support and some present no theoretical or logical connection to current knowledge regarding ADHD that would recommend their serious consideration in the absence of otherwise compelling evidence. Some treatments may eventually prove helpful, but the absence of convincing objective evidence precludes any endorsement at present.

Psychological Treatments

Tinker and Wilson (1999) advocated the use of eye movement desensitization and reprocessing (EMDR) for treatment of ADHD. This technique was developed as a trauma-based therapeutic procedure (Shapiro, 1989, 1995) and denotes a process by which the aversive subjective experience of the trauma event is attenuated. However, EMDR has been harshly criticized on both conceptual and procedural grounds (e.g., Keane, 1997; Lohr, Tolin, & Lilienfeld, 1998; see also Chapter 9, this volume), and it is difficult to conceptualize how or why such an approach would be an effective treatment for ADHD. Not surprisingly, there is no empirical support for the use of EMDR in treating children with ADHD.

Play therapy has been suggested as a treatment for ADHD and a description of clinical application to ADHD has been provided (Kaduson, 1997). However, there is no evidence that play therapy is an effective treatment for ADHD.

Neurological Treatments

Electroencephalographic (EEG) biofeedback (sometimes called neurofeedback) is undoubtedly the best-known example of a neurological treatment for ADHD. In fact, EEG biofeedback has been touted as a treatment for ADHD for nearly 30 years. This treatment attempts to reduce hyperactivity, inattention, and impulsivity by training children with ADHD to increase brainwave activity that is associated with sustained attention and to decrease brainwave activity that is associated with inattention and daydreaming (Lubar & Shouse, 1977).

Proponents of EEG biofeedback have often made strong claims for its effectiveness as a treatment for ADHD. This has been particularly true in popular media outlets. In a recent article published in *Psychology Today* (Robins, 1998), EEG treatments for ADHD (as well as EEG treatments for epilepsy, closed head injury, chronic substance abuse, and posttraumatic stress disorder) were described as effective and supported by research. The author illustrated these claims by providing case study examples of how EEG has been successfully used to treat ADHD. Of note is Robins's (1998) report that EEG neurofeedback is currently being used as the primary treatment for ADHD by 22 schools in New York: "So far, neurofeedback [in these schools] has kept twenty students out of expensive special-education classrooms and thereby saved the district an estimated $500,000" (p. 42). The author went on to describe his own positive experiences with EEG. He will presumably discuss each of these topics in more detail in a book on EEG that the article indicates he is publishing.

Despite these and other similar claims, there is reason for caution in evaluating the positive effects of EEG treatments for ADHD. Specifically, studies that claim positive results of EEG biofeedback as a treatment for ADHD are characterized by such methodological problems as confounded treatments (Boyd & Campbell, 1998), inconsistent use of dependent measures among subjects (Rossiter & LaVaque, 1995), absence of clinically meaningful dependent measures of ADHD (Wadhwani, Radvanski, & Carmody, 1998), and nonstandardized collection of posttreatment measures anywhere from 0 to 12 months following cessation of treatment (Alhambra, Fowler, & Alhambra, 1995). In a recent review, Kline, Brann, and Loney (2002) have similarly concluded that the evidence for the efficacy of neurofeedback on ADHD is wanting and highly inconsistent across studies.

Furthermore, authors of many of these studies often draw conclusions that go well beyond supporting data. For example, many of these authors point to changes in laboratory measures of ADHD as proof that ADHD has been successfully treated. However, there is no satisfactory demonstration that changes on laboratory measures of ADHD correspond with changes in the behavioral, cognitive, or social correlates of ADHD as they occur in real-life settings (Barkley, 1991; Nichols & Waschbusch, 2002). It is particularly troubling that these methodological shortcomings continue to characterize the research on EEG treatments despite the fact that suggestions for improving the quality of research in this area have been published (Barkley, 1993).

Lead toxicity compromises neurological functioning and is a known etiology for ADHD, although it is estimated to account for less than 5% of all diagnosed cases among children (Fergusson, Fergusson, Horwood, & Kinzett, 1988). It is increasingly rare as a treatment for ADHD, no doubt largely due to mandated efforts to eliminate sources of lead toxins and lead exposure in the environment. Although de-leading is by no means a standard treatment for ADHD, it should certainly be performed whenever medically indicated (Arnold, 1999).

Sensorimotor integration therapy (SIT) is essentially neurophysiological in nature and has been suggested for use with children with ADHD. SIT is based upon the premise that sensory and motor input is processed and interpreted in faulty ways, resulting in inappropriate responses to sensory stimuli, as well as behavioral disturbance and disorganization (Ayers, 1979; see also Chapter 13, this volume). Sensory stimulation therapy activities (usually conducted by an occupational therapist) are used as a modality for correcting the presumed underlying neurological dysfunction and facilitating improved behavioral functioning. Interventions may also include compensatory strategies, such as altering or avoiding certain stimulus characteristics of the physical environment (e.g., decreasing aversive touch). Such strategies will be familiar to applied behavior analysts in cases in which functional relationships between environmental stimuli and aberrant behavior have been established. Claims of relatively high rates of sensory integrative dysfunction among persons with ADHD have been made (Cermak, 1988); however, no studies demonstrate the effectiveness of SIT in children with ADHD. In addition, this approach conceptualizes the central problem of ADHD as an "input" problem, which is contradictory to multiple lines of evidence and current theory indicating that ADHD is an "output" problem occurring downstream from cognitive processes that interpret basic input about the environment (Barkley, 1997). In this respect, SIT approaches differ considerably from similar compensatory strategies discussed in earlier sections, as these strategies make no statements or inferences regarding the role of sensory organizational processes that occur at lower brain levels.

Nutritional Approaches

Specific nutritional substances that have been proposed as treatments for ADHD but which await adequate documentation of their effectiveness include essential fatty acids, glyconutritional supplements (saccharides), and mineral supplements (magnesium, iron, and zinc). One recent study reported improvement in parent and teacher ratings for severity of ADHD symptoms in 17 children after a 6-week administration of a glyconutritional supplement (Dykman & Dykman, 1998). However, methodological considerations, including inappropriate control groups and lack of double-blind designs, limit the interpretation of these results and demonstrate a need for additional research. Furthermore, many of the claims for the effectiveness of nutritional approaches to ADHD have no empirical basis, as demonstrated by recent actions taken by the U.S. Food and Drug Administration against companies making such false claims (Reuter Media News, 2000). Some nutritional substances may also be associated with a risk of toxicity (Arnold, 1999).

Physiological Treatments

Proposed treatments for ADHD that appear to share a physiological basis for their rationale include acupuncture, candida yeast treatments, anti-motion sickness medications, and thyroid treatment, although specific proposed mechanisms for each of these treatments varies. There are currently no published controlled studies on any of these treatments for ADHD.

Homeopathic Remedies

A host of homeopathic treatments have been touted for use with ADHD (Reichenberg-Ullman, & Ullman, 1996). Chief among these (at least in terms of marketing effort) is pycnogenol, an organically based substance that originated in Europe and has been widely promoted within the United States in recent years. Although there does not appear to be any clear rationale for its application to ADHD, some of the claims for this substance are astounding. In addition to relieving symptoms of ADHD, it is purported to provide relief for physical and health problems as diverse as tennis elbow, acne, and blood clots. One Web site states that pycnogenol works "just as well as the commonly prescribed stimulants, including Ritalin" when used to treat ADHD (Carper, 1998). This claim was based on unspecified laboratory measures with no data reported and no references. This site offered a link to a list of references that examined the effects of pycnogenol on disorders other than ADHD, but all references were in European journals, and the great majority of those were in foreign languages, rendering availability of data for consumer use and independent review extremely difficult. There are also no data available regarding the safety and potential side effects of most homeopathic substances.

CHALLENGES AND PROBLEMS
WITH UNSUPPORTED TREATMENTS

Our review identified a number of proposed but unsupported treatments for ADHD as alternatives to established treatments. Curiosity and interest

in alternative treatments remains high, despite a lack of evidence supporting their efficacy. There are a number of reasons for this problematic state
of affairs.

First, some parents and professionals hold negative attitudes and beliefs regarding the desirability of established treatments even before trying
these treatments. A priori negative attitudes seem to be especially widespread for medication treatment. Such negative attitudes toward stimulant
medication treatment may be more common among parents than among
professionals (such as classroom teachers). For example, in the MTA study,
parents gave higher consumer satisfaction ratings to treatments that included behavioral components, whereas this same trend was not found for
teachers (Pelham, 1999). These different attitudes toward treatment could
lead to considerable tension, potentially undermining the effectiveness of
any treatment that is administered. A more fruitful approach would be for
both parents and teachers to suspend their a priori beliefs about empirically supported treatments for ADHD and let the child's own response
make the determination about treatment.

Second, even when such attitudes or beliefs are absent prior to treatment, the limitations of established treatments discussed earlier often arise
once treatments are implemented. Side effects of stimulants are mild but
common, and behavioral treatments can require considerable effort and
organization to be effective. These factors can lead parents to become dis-
enchanted with empirically supported treatments, thereby spurring interest
in alternative treatments.

Third, there seem to be different methods of delivering information
about empirically supported treatments as compared with controversial or
unsupported treatments. Proponents of empirically supported treatments
tend to be scientifically oriented professionals who are (to greater or lesser
degrees) trained to be skeptical and cautious in their claims of treatment effectiveness. In contrast, advocates of other treatments often do not have
such constraints and may be financially or otherwise motivated to make
exaggerated claims of treatment effects. For example, following the shoot-
ings at Columbine High School in Colorado, the Cable Network News
(CNN) repeatedly broadcast interviews with an "expert" who argued that
Ritalin was linked to school violence (Seay, 1999). What CNN apparently
neglected to report was that this "expert" had authored a book arguing
against the use of Ritalin (she has also authored a book arguing against the
use of amoxicillin), that the research she was basing her claims on was a
collection of anecdotal stories, and that the institute she directed was originally founded by the Church of Scientology, a group well known for its
opposition to Ritalin (Seay, 1999).

The result of these different attitudes about describing treatments for
ADHD is that parents with no formal training or knowledge about ADHD
may be in the position of selecting among treatments that they perceive as

(1) entailing a great deal of work (behavioral treatment) and (2) having a significant cost (side effects and monetary costs of stimulants), or choosing (3) one that has neither of these limitations and that promises to cure ADHD. One reason consumers are faced with this situation is that there is little or no regulation of nonmedication treatments for mental health problems, whereas the same is not true for most medical procedures or for most medications (Weisz, 2000).

Fourth, if available longitudinal studies are accurate in their suggestion that stimulants have little effect on long-term outcome, some parents and treatment providers may try controversial treatments because they become desperate. Given that ADHD is a chronic disorder, it is not difficult to imagine cases in which stimulants, behavioral modification, or both are used effectively in childhood but not in adolescence due to factors such as refusal to take stimulants or lack of parental control over the contingencies that motivate the youth. In such cases, alternative treatments could offer parents hope that established treatments no longer provide.

Almost all treatments for ADHD (whether empirically supported or not) require considerable investment of resources (time, energy, and/or money). Because these resources are limited, ethical considerations require that they be used judiciously and applied to intervention efforts with known risks and benefits. As collaborators in treatment decision making, professionals have both an opportunity and an obligation to (1) present parents with accurate information regarding various treatments for ADHD, (2) base their own decisions and recommendations about treatment options on empirical evidence (rather than on anecdotal stories or their own clinical intuition/experience), and (3) advocate strongly for the treatments that are most likely to benefit the child (i.e., empirically supported treatments).

Given these obligations, a major challenge to professionals is to stay abreast of new findings regarding established treatments for ADHD, not to mention findings regarding newly explored or promising but unestablished treatments. In addition, information regarding alternative treatments for ADHD often lies outside of the academic domain, requiring one to divide attention among various information sources and databases. Such challenges are difficult to meet but are fundamental to the advocacy role required of competent professionals.

CONCLUSIONS

ADHD is a chronic condition characterized by dysfunctions in impulse control and attention and associated with serious impairment in interpersonal, academic, and behavioral performance. Substantial empirical evidence supports the use of stimulant medication, classroom behavior interventions, and parent behavior management training as effective treatments for ADHD. Other treatments for ADHD enjoy limited but encouraging empirical support, and still other treatments have simply not been researched or have been shown to be ineffective. Because of the extensive body of knowledge that exists regarding well-established treatments for ADHD, those who would propose new, alternative treatments bear a "burden of proof" to provide convincing evidence of the benefits, costs, and risks of proposed treatments as compared with empirically established treatments.

There are a number of key questions concerning treatments for ADHD that remain to be addressed in future research. First, although empirically supported treatments for ADHD have considerable research backing, little is known about the underlying mechanisms that account for their effectiveness. What aspects of behavioral treatments and stimulants are effective for what aspects of ADHD? Answering these questions would not only greatly advance the effectiveness of treatments, but would also lead to important advances in our understanding of ADHD (Kazdin, 1999).

Second, more research is needed on promising treatments for ADHD. As described by our criteria for categorizing these treatments, such treatments seem to be effective in preliminary research, but there is currently insufficient evidence to render a decision on their efficacy.

Third, there is a need for studies examining whether treatments are moderated by factors such as age, gender, or comorbid disorders.

Fourth and finally, research is needed on long-term effects of treatment. Current information about the maintenance and generalization of treatment effects in children with ADHD is (by and large) based on methodologically poor studies. Further investigation of the long-term outcome of various types and combinations of treatment for ADHD is sorely needed.

GLOSSARY

Attention control: An experimental procedure used commonly in psychosocial treatment research that consists of providing clients with social support but no active intervention. Used to control for placebo effects due to simply interacting with a therapist.

Attention-deficit/hyperactivity disorder (ADHD): A disorder characterized by developmentally inappropriate levels of inattention, impulsivity, and/or hyperactivity. Also referred to attention deficit disorder (ADD) or childhood hyperactivity.

Behavior therapy: A treatment approach that relies on learning principles to effect behavior change.

Clonidine: An antihypertensive medication sometimes used to treat ADHD or conduct problems.

Fading: Gradually changing a stimulus that controls a response so that the response transfers to a new stimulus. Often used to help generalize the effects of treatment into the naturalistic environment.

Homeopathic treatment: A treatment approach that uses natural materials (e.g., plants, animals) to stimulate the body's own defenses.

Meta-cognitive skill: A higher-order mental process that consists of an awareness of one's own thought process. Sometimes referred to as "thinking about thinking."

Multisite treatment of ADHD (MTA) study: A large-scale research study funded by the National Institute of Mental Health to compare the efficacy of stimulant medication, behavior therapy, and the combination of these two treatments for ADHD.

Neurofeedback: A treatment approach that allows individuals to monitor their own brain waves in an effort to alter their behaviors.

Stimulant medications: Drugs that act on the central nervous system, and in particular the frontal-striatal region of the brain, by influencing neurotransmitters. Stimulant medications include methylphenidate (Ritalin) and dextroamphetamine (Dexadrine), which are commonly used to treat ADHD.

REFERENCES

Abikoff, H. (1987). An evaluation of cognitive behavior therapy for hyperactive children. In B. B. Lahey & A. E. Kazdin (Eds.), *Advances in clinical child psychology* (Vol. 10, pp. 171–216). New York: Plenum Press.

Abikoff, H. (1991). Cognitive training in ADHD children: Less to it than meets the eye. *Journal of Learning Disabilities, 24*(4), 205–209.

Abikoff, H., Ganeles, D., Reiter, G., Blum, C., Foley, C., & Klein, R. G. (1988). Cognitive training in academically deficient boys receiving stimulant medication. *Journal of Abnormal Child Psychology, 16*, 411–432.

Alhambra, M. A., Fowler, T. P., & Alhambra, A. A. (1995). EEG Biofeedback: A new treatment option for ADD/ADHD. *Journal of Neurotherapy, 1*, 39–43.

American Psychiatric Association. (1994). *Diagnostic and statistical manual of mental disorders* (4th ed.). Washington, DC: Author.

Anderson, J. C., Williams, S., McGee, R., & Silva, P. A. (1987). DSM-III disorders in preadolescent children: Prevalence in a large sample from the general population. *Archives of General Psychiatry, 44*, 69–76.

Arnold, L. E. (1978). Megavitamins for MBD: A placebo-controlled study. *Journal of the American Medical Association, 20*, 24.

Arnold, L. E. (1999). Treatment alternatives for attention-deficit/hyperactivity disorder (ADHD). *Journal of Attention Disorders, 3*(1), 30–48.

Ayers, A. J. (1979). *Sensory integration and the child*. Los Angeles, CA: Western Psychological Services.

Baker, A. M. (1980). The efficacy of the Feingold K-P diet: A review of pertinent empirical investigations. *Behavior Disorders, 6,* 32–35.

Barkley, R. A. (1991). The ecological validity of laboratory and analogue assessment methods of ADHD symptoms. *Journal of Abnormal Child Psychology, 19,* 149–178.

Barkley, R. A. (1993). Continuing concerns about EEG biofeedback/neurofeedback. *ADHD Report, 1*(3), 1–3.

Barkley, R. A. (1997). *ADHD and the nature of self-control.* New York: Guilford Press.

Barkley, R. A., Copeland, A., & Sivage, C. (1980). A self-control classroom for hyperactive children. *Journal of Autism and Developmental Disorders, 10,* 75–89.

Biederman, J., Baldessarini, R. J., Wright, V., Knee, D., & Harmatz, J. (1989). A double-blind placebo controlled study of desipramine in the treatment of attention deficit disorder: I. Efficacy. *Journal of the American Academy of Child and Adolescent Psychiatry, 28,* 777–784.

Beiderman, J., Gastfriend, D. R., & Jellinek, M. S. (1986). Desipramine in the treatment of children with attention deficit disorder. *Journal of Clinical Psychopharmacology, 6,* 359–363.

Bloomquist, M. L., August, G. J., Cohen, C., Doyle, A., & Everhart, K. (1997). Social problem solving in hyperactive-aggressive children: How and what they think in conditions of automatic and controlled processing. *Journal of Clinical Child Psychology, 26*(2), 172–180.

Boyd, W. D., & Campbell, S. E. (1998). EEG biofeedback in the schools: The use of EEG biofeedback to treat ADHD in a school setting. *Journal of Neurotherapy, 2,* 65–70.

Braswell, L. (1998). Self-regulation training for children with ADHD: Response to Harris and Schmidt. *ADHD Report, 1*(6), 1–3.

Braswell, L., & Bloomquist, M. L. (1991). *Cognitive-behavioral therapy with ADHD children: Child, family, and school interventions.* New York: Guilford Press.

Brown, R. T., Borden, K. A., Wynne, M. E., Spunt, A. L., & Clingerman, S. R. (1987). Compliance with pharmacological and cognitive treatment for attention deficit disorder. *Journal of the American Academy of Child and Adolescent Psychiatry, 26,* 521–526.

Brown, R. T., & Sawyer, M. G. (1998). *Medications for school-age children: Effects on learning and behavior.* New York: Guilford Press.

Cantwell, D. P. (1996). Attention deficit disorder: A review of the past 10 years. *Journal of the American Academy of Child and Adolescent Psychiatry, 35,* 978–987.

Carper, J. (1998). *Miracle cures: Dramatic new scientific discoveries revealing the healing powers of herbs, vitamins, and other natural remedies* [On-line]. Available: http://lifeplussupplements.securenow.com/link_attention_support.html

Cermak, S. A. (1988). The relationship between attention deficit and sensory integration disorders (Part 1). *Sensory Integration Special Interest Section Newsletter, 11,* 1–4.

Chambless, D. L., Sanderson, W. C., Shoham, V., Johnson, S. B., Pope, K. S., Crits-Christoph, P., Baker, M., Johnson, B., Woods, S. R., Sue, S., Beutler, L., Wil-

liams, D. A., & McCurry, S. (1996). An update on empirically validated therapies. *Clinical Psychologist, 49*, 5–18.

Colvin, G. T., & Sugai, G. M. (1988). Proactive strategies for managing social behavior problems: An instructional approach. *Education and Treatment of Children,
11*(4), 341–348.

Conners, C. K. (1980). *Food additives and hyperactive children.* London: Plenum
Press.

Conners, C. K., Goyette, C. H., Southwick, D. A., Lees, J. M., & Andrulonis, P. A.
(1976). Food additives and hyperkinesis: A controlled double-blind experiment.
Pediatrics, 58, 154–166.

Cook, P. S., & Woodhill, J. M. (1976). The Feingold dietary treatment of the
hyperkinetic syndrome. *Medical Journal of Australia, 2*, 85–90.

Dujovne, V. F., Barnard, M. U., & Rapoff, M. A. (1995). Pharmacological and cognitive-behavioral approaches in the treatment of childhood depression: A review
and critique. *Clinical Psychology Review, 15*, 589–611.

DuPaul, G. J., & Ervin, R. A. (1996). Functional assessment of behaviors related to
attention deficit hyperactivity disorder: Linking assessment to intervention design. *Behavior Therapy, 27*, 601–622.

DuPaul, G. J., & Henningson, P. N. (1993). Peer tutoring effects on the classroom
performance of children with attention deficit hyperactivity disorder. *School
Psychology Review, 22*, 134–143.

DuPaul, G. J., & Stoner, G. (1994). *ADHD in the schools: Assessment and intervention strategies.* New York: Guilford Press.

Dykman, K. D., & Dykman, R. A. (1998). Effect of nutritional supplements on attention-deficit hyperactivity disorder. *Integrative Physiological and Behavioral Science, 33*(1), 49–60.

Edwards, L., Salant, V., Howard, V. F., Brougher, J., & McLaughlin, T. F. (1995). Effectiveness of self-management on attentional behavior and reading comprehension for children with attention deficit disorder. *Child and Family Behavior
Therapy, 17*(2), 1–17.

Feingold, B. F. (1973). *Introduction to clinical allergy.* Springfield, IL: Charles C
Thomas.

Feingold, B. F. (1975a). Hyperkinesis and learning disabilities linked to artificial food
flavors and colors. *American Journal of Nursing, 75*, 797–803.

Feingold, B. F. (1975b). *Why your child is hyperactive.* New York: Random House.

Feingold, B. F. (1976). Hyperkinesis and learning disabilities linked to the ingestion of
artificial food colors and flavors. *Journal of Learning Disabilities, 9*, 19–27.

Fergusson, D. M., Fergusson, I. E., Horwood, L. J., & Kinzett, N. G. (1988). A longitudinal study of dentine lead levels, intelligence, school performance, and behaviour. *Journal of Child Psychology and Psychiatry, 29*, 811–824.

Gittleman-Klein, R. (1974). Pilot clinical trial of imipramine in hyperkinetic children.
In C. K. Conners (Ed.), *Clinical use of stimulant drugs in children* (pp. 192–
201). The Hague, Netherlands: Excerpta Medica.

Goldstein, S., & Ingersoll, B. (1993). Controversial treatments for children with
ADHD and impulse disorders. In L. F. Koziol & C. E. Stout (Eds.), *Handbook of
childhood impulse disorders and ADHD: Theory and practice* (pp. 144–160).
Springfield, IL: Charles C Thomas.

Harley, J. P., & Matthews, C. G. (1978). The Feingold hypothesis: Current studies. *Contemporary Nutrition, 3*, 171–173.

Henggeler, S. W., Melton, G. B., & Smith, L. A. (1992). Family preservation using multisystemic therapy: An effective alternative to incarcerating serious juvenile offenders. *Journal of Consulting and Clinical Psychology, 60*, 953–961.

Hinshaw, S. P. (1994). *Attention deficits and hyperactivity in children* (Vol. 29). Thousand Oaks, CA: Sage.

Hinshaw, S. P., Buhrmester, D., & Heller, T. (1989). Anger control in response to verbal provocation: Effects of stimulant medication for boys with ADHD. *Journal of Abnormal Child Psychology, 17*(4), 393–407.

Hinshaw, S. P., Heller, T., & McHale, J. P. (1992). Covert antisocial behavior in boys with attention deficit hyperactivity disorder: External validation and effects of methylphenidate. *Journal of Consulting and Clinical Psychology, 60*, 274–281.

Hinshaw, S. P., Henker, B., & Whalen, C. K. (1984). Self-control in hyperactive boys in anger-inducing situations: Effects of cognitive-behavioral training and of methylphenidate. *Journal of Abnormal Child Psychology, 12*(1), 55–77.

Hinshaw, S. P., Henker, B., Whalen, C. K., Erhardt, D., & Dunnington, R. E. (1989). Aggressive, prosocial, and nonsocial behavior in hyperactive boys: Dose effects of methylphenidate in naturalistic settings. *Journal of Consulting and Clinical Psychology, 57*, 636–643.

Hinshaw, S. P., March, J. S., Abikoff, H., Arnold, L. W., Cantwell, D. P., Conners, G. K., Elliott, G. R., Halperin, J., Greenhill, L. L., Hechtman, L. T., Hoza, B., Jensen, P. S., Newcorn, J. H., McBurnett, K., Pelham, W. E., Richters, J. E., Severe, J. B., Schiller, E., Swanson, J., Vereen, D., Wells, K., & Wigal, T. (1997). Comprehensive assessment of childhood attention-deficit hyperactivity disorder in the context of a multisite, multimodal clinical trial. *Journal of Attention Disorders, 1*, 217–234.

Holborow, P., Elkins, J., & Berry, P. (1981). The effect of the Feingold diet on "normal" school children. *Journal of Learning Disabilities, 14*, 143–147.

Hunt, R. D., Minderaa, R. B., & Cohen, D. J. (1985). Clonidine benefits children with attention deficit disorder and hyperactivity: Report of a double-blind placebo-crossover therapeutic trial. *Journal of the American Academy of Child and Adolescent Psychiatry, 24*, 617–629.

Ingram, S., Hechtman, L., & Morgenstern, G. (1999). Outcome issues in ADHD: Adolescent and adult long-term outcome. *Mental Retardation and Developmental Disabilities Research Reviews, 5*, 243–250.

Kaduson, H. G. (1997). Play therapy for children with attention-deficit hyperactivity disorder. In H. Kaduson (Ed.), *The playing cure: Individualized play therapy for specific childhood problems* (pp. 197–227). Northvale, NJ: Aronson.

Kavale, K. A., & Forness, S. R. (1983). Hyperactivity and diet treatment: A meta-analysis of the Feingold hypothesis. *Journal of Learning Disabilities, 16*, 324–330.

Kazdin A. E. (1999). Current (lack of) status of theory in child and adolescent psychotherapy research. *Journal of Clinical Child Psychology, 28*, 533–543.

Kazdin, A. E., Esveldt-Dawson, K., French, N. H., & Unis, A. S. (1987). Effects of parent management training and problem-solving skills training combined in the treatment of antisocial child behavior. *Journal of the American Academy of Child and Adolescent Psychiatry, 26*, 416–424.

Keane, T. M. (1997). Psychological and behavioral treatment of post-traumatic stress disorder (PTSD). In P. Nathan & J. Gorman (Eds.), *Guide to treatments that work* (pp. 398–407). Oxford: Oxford University Press.

Kendall, P. C., & Gosch, E. A. (1994). Cognitive-behavioral interventions. In T. H. Ollendick, N. J. King, & W. Yule (Eds.), *International handbook of phobic and anxiety disorders in children and adolescents* (pp. 415–438). New York: Plenum Press.

Kershner, J., & Hawke, W. (1979). Megavitamins and learning disorders: A controlled double-blind experiment. *Journal of Nutrition, 159,* 819–826.

Kline, J. P., Brann, C. N., & Loney, B. R. (2002). A cacophony in the brainwaves: A critical appraisal of neurotherapy for attention-deficit disorders. *Scientific Review of Mental Health Practice, 1,* 44–54.

Lilienfeld, S. O., & Waldman, I. D. (1990). The relation of childhood attention-deficit hyperactivity disorder and adult antisocial behavior reexamined: The problem of heterogeneity. *Clinical Psychology Review, 10,* 699–725.

Lochman, J. E. (1992). Cognitive-behavioral intervention with aggressive boys: Three-year follow up and preventive effects. *Journal of Consulting and Clinical Psychology, 60,* 426–432.

Lochman, J. E., & Lenhart, L. A. (1993). Anger coping intervention for aggressive children: Conceptual models and outcome effects. *Clinical Psychology Review, 13,* 785–805.

Lohr, J. M., Tolin, D. F., & Lilienfeld, S. O. (1998). Efficacy of eye movement desensitization and reprocessing: Implications for behavior therapy. *Behavior Therapy, 29,* 123–156.

Lonigan, C., Elbert, J. C., & Johnson, S. B. (1998). Empirically supported psychosocial interventions for children: An overview. *Journal of Clinical Child Psychology, 27*(2), 138–145.

Lubar, J. F., & Shouse, M. N. (1977). Use of biofeedback in the treatment of seizure disorders and hyperactivity. In B. B. Lahey & A. E. Kazdin (Eds.), *Advances in clinical child psychology* (Vol. 1, pp. 203–265). New York: Plenum Press.

Mattes, J. A. (1983). The Feingold diet: A current reappraisal. *Journal of Learning Disabilities, 16,* 319–323.

Mattes, J. A., & Gittleman-Klein, R. (1978). A crossover study of artificial food colorings in a hyperkinetic child. *American Journal of Psychiatry, 135,* 987–988.

Meichenbaum, D., & Goodman, J. (1971). Training impulsive children to talk to themselves: A means of developing self-control. *Journal of Abnormal Psychology, 77,* 115–126.

Milich, R., Wolraich, M., & Lindgren, S. (1986). Sugar and hyperactivity: A critical review of empirical findings. *Clinical Psychology Review, 6,* 493–513.

MTA Cooperative Group. (1999a). A 14–month randomized clinical trial of treatment strategies for attention-deficit/hyperactivity disorder. *Archives of General Psychiatry, 56,* 1073–1086.

MTA Cooperative Group. (1999b). Moderators and mediators of treatment response for children with attention-deficit/hyperactivity disorder. *Archives of General Psychiatry, 56,* 1088–1096.

National Institute of Mental Health (1996). *Unpublished findings from conference on Alternative Pharmacology of ADHD.* Washington, DC: Author.

Nemzer, E., Arnold, L. E., Votolato, N. A., & McConnell, H. (1986). Amino acid supplementation as therapy for attention deficit disorder (ADD). *Journal of the American Academy of Child Psychiatry, 25,* 509–513.

Nichols, S. G., & Waschbusch, D. A. (2002). *Ecological validity of laboratory mea sures of attention-deficit/hyperactivity disorder: What have we learned in the last decade?* Manuscript submitted for publication.

O'Leary, K. D., Pelham, W. E., Rosenbaum, A., & Price, G. H. (1976). Behavioral treatment of hyperkinetic children: An experimental evaluation of its useful-ness. *Clinical Pediatrics, 15*(6), 510–515.

Pelham, W. E. (1993). Pharmacotherapy for children with attention-deficit hyperac-tivity disorder. *School Psychology Review, 22*(2), 199–227.

Pelham, W. E. (1999). The NIMH multimodal treatment study for ADHD: Just say yes to drugs? *Clinical Child Psychology Newsletter, 14* (Summer), 1–6.

Pelham, W. E. (2000). Implications of the MTA study for behavioral and combined treatments. *ADHD Report,* 9–13, 16.

Pelham, W. E., Carlson, C., Sams, S. E., Vallano, G., Dixon, M. J., & Hoza, B. (1993). Separate and combined effects of methylphenidate and behavior modification on boys with attention-deficit hyperactivity disorder in the classroom. *Journal of Consulting and Clinical Psychology, 61,* 506–515.

Pelham, W. E., Gnagy, E. M., Greiner, A. R., Hoza, B., Hinshaw, S. P., Swanson, J. M., Simpson, S., Shapiro, C., Buckstein, O., & Baron-Mayak, C. (2000). Behavioral vs. behavioral and pharmacological treatment in ADHD children attending a summer treatment program. *Journal of Abnormal Child Psychology, 28,* 507–525.

Pelham, W. E., Greiner, A. R., Gnagy, E. M., Hoza, B., Martin, L., Sams, S. E., & Wil-son, T. (1996). Intensive treatment for ADHD: A model summer treatment pro-gram. In M. Roberts & A. LaGreca (Eds.), *Model programs for service delivery for child and family mental health* (pp. 193–212). Hillsdale, NJ: Erlbaum.

Pelham, W. E., & Hoza, B. (1996). Intensive treatment: A summer treatment program for children with ADHD. In E. Hibbs & P. Jensen (Eds.), *Psychosocial treat-ments for child and adolescent disorders: Empirically based strategies for clini-cal practice* (pp. 311–340). New York: APA Press.

Pelham, W. E., & Milich, R. (1991). Individualized differences in response to ritalin in classwork and social behavior. In L. L. Greenhill & B. B. Osman (Eds.), *Ritalin: Theory and patient management* (pp. 203–221). New York: Mary Ann Liebert.

Pelham, W. E., & Murphy, A. (1986). Attention deficit and conduct disorders. In M. Hersen (Ed.), *Pharmacological and behavioral treatment: An integrative ap-proach* (pp. 108–148). New York: Wiley .

Pelham, W. E., Schnedler, R. W., Bender, M. E., Nilsson, D. E., Miller, J., Budrow, M. S., Ronnei, J. Paluchoswki, C., & Marks, D. A. (1988). The combination of behavior therapy and methylphenidate in the treatment of attention deficit dis-orders: A therapy outcome study. In L. Bloomingdale (Ed.), *Attention deficit dis-orders III: New research in attention, treatment, and psychopharmacology* (pp. 29–48). London: Pergamon.

Pelham, W. E., & Waschbusch, D. A. (1999). Behavioral intervention in ADHD. In H. C. Quay & A. E. Hogan (Eds.), *Handbook of disruptive behavior disorders* (pp. 255– 278). New York: Plenum Press.

Pelham, W. E., Wheeler, T., & Chronis, A. (1998). Empirically supported psycho-social treatment for attention deficit hyperactivity disorder. *Journal of Clinical Child Psychology, 27*(2), 190–205.

Rapp, D. J. (1978). Does diet affect hyperactivity? *Journal of Learning Disabilities, 11,* 56–62.

Rapport, M., Carlson, G., Kelly, K., & Pataki, C. (1993). Methylphenidate and desipramine in hospitalized children: Separate and combined effects on cognitive function. *Journal of the American Academy of Child and Adolescent Psychiatry, 32,* 333–342.

Reichenberg-Ullman, J., & Ullman, R. (1996). *Ritalin free kids: Safe and effective homeopathic medicine for ADD and other learning problems* [On-line]. Available: www.healthy.net/othersites/Rbullman/books.htm

Reuter Media News. (2000). *Supplement marketer made false claims about treating ADHD* [On-line]. Available: www.medscape.com/reuters/prof/2000/08/08.17/20000817leg1004.html

Richters, J. E., Arnold, L. E., Jensen, P. S., Abikoff, H., Conners, C. K., Greenhill, L. L., Hechtman, L., Hinshaw, S. P., Pelham, W. E., & Swanson, J. M. (1995). NIMH collaborative multisite multimodal treatment study of children with ADHD: I. Background and rationale. *Journal of the American Academy of Child and Adolescent Psychiatry, 34,* 987–1000.

Rimland, B. (1983). The Feingold diet: An assessment of the reviews by Mattes, by Kavale and Forness and others. *Journal of Learning Disabilities, 16,* 331–333.

Robins, J. (1998, May/June). Wired for miracles? *Psychology Today, 31,* 41–44.

Rossiter, T. R., & LaVaque, T. J. (1995). A comparison of EEG biofeedback and psychostimulants in treating attention deficit/hyperactivity disorders. *Journal of Neurotherapy, 1,* 48–59.

Rowe, K. S. (1988). Synthetic food colorings and hyperactivity: A double-blind crossover study. *Australian Pediatric Journal, 24,* 143–147.

Rowe, K. S., & Rowe, K. J. (1994). Synthetic food coloring and behavior: A dose–response effect in a double-blind, placebo-controlled, repeated-measures study. *Journal of Pediatrics, 125,* 691–698.

Safer, D. J., & Krager, J. M. (1988). A survey of medication treatment for hyperactive/inattentive students. *Journal of the American Medical Association, 260,* 2256–2258.

Safer, D. J., & Krager, J. M. (1994). The increased rate of stimulant treatment for hyperactive/inattentive students in secondary schools. *Pediatrics, 94*(4), 462–464.

Seay, B. (1999). *A choreographed campaign of misinformation* [On-line]. Available: http://add.about.com/health/add/library/weekly/aa062299.htm

Shapiro, F. (1989). Eye movement desensitization: A new treatment for post-traumatic stress disorder. *Journal of Behavior Therapy and Experimental Psychiatry, 20,* 211–217.

Shapiro, F. (1995). *Eye movement desensitization and reprocessing: Basic principles, protocols, and procedures.* New York: Guilford Press.

Shaywitz, B. A., Sullivan, C. M., Anderson, G. M., Gillespie, S. M., Sullivan, B., & Shaywitz, S. E. (1994). Aspartame, behavior, and cognitive function in children with attention deficit disorder. *Pediatrics, 93,* 70–75.

Smith, L. (1975). *Your child's behavior chemistry.* New York: Random House.

Spencer, T. J., Biederman, J., & Wilens, T. (1998). Pharmacotherapy of ADHD with antidepressants. In R. A. Barkley (Ed.), *Attention-deficit hyperactivity disorder: A handbook for diagnosis and treatment* (2nd ed., pp. 552–563). New York: Guilford Press.

Stein, T. P., & Sammaritano, A. M. (1984). Nitrogen metabolism in normal and hyperkinetic boys. *American Journal of Clinical Nutrition, 39,* 520–524.

Sternberg, E. M. (1996). Pathogenesis of L-tryptophan eosinophilia-myalgia syndrome. *Advances in Experimental Medicine and Biology, 398,* 325–330.

Stine, J. J. (1976). Symptom alleviation in the hyperactive child by dietary modification: A report of two cases. *American Journal of Orthopsychiatry, 46,* 637–647.

Swanson, J. M. (1992). *School based assessments and interventions for ADD students.* Irvine, CA: K. C. Publishing.

Swanson, J. M., McBurnett, K., Christian, D. L., & Wigal, T. (1995). Stimulant medications and the treatment of children with ADHD. In T. H. Ollendick & J. R. Prinz (Eds.), *Advances in clinical child psychology* (Vol. 17, pp. 265–322). New York: Plenum Press.

Tinker, R. H., & Wilson, S. A. (1999). *Through the eyes of a child: EMDR with children.* New York: Norton.

Wadhwani, S., Radvanski, D. C., & Carmody, D. P. (1998). Neurofeedback training in a case of attention deficit hyperactivity disorder. *Journal of Neurotherapy, 3,* 42–49.

Waschbusch, D. A. (2002). A meta-analytic examination of comorbid hyperactive-impulsive-inattention problems and conduct problems. *Psychological Bulletin, 128,* 118–150.

Waschbusch, D. A., Kipp, H. L., & Pelham, W. E. (1998). Generalization of behavioral and psychostimulant treatment of attention deficit/hyperactivity disorder (ADHD): Discussion and case study examples. *Behavior Research and Therapy, 36,* 675–694.

Weiss, B. (1982). Food additives and environmental chemicals as sources of childhood behavior disorders. *Journal of the American Academy of Child Psychiatry, 21,* 144–152.

Weiss, G., & Hechtman, L. T. (1993). *Hyperactive children grown up: ADHD in children, adolescents, and adults.* New York: Guilford Press.

Weisz, J. R. (2000). Lab-clinic differences and what we can do about them: II. Linking research and practice to enhance public impact. *Clinical Child Psychology Newsletter, 15,* 1–4, 9.

Werry, J. (1980). Imipramine and methylphenidate in hyperactive children. *Journal of Child Psychology and Psychiatry, 21,* 27–35.

Wolraich, M. L. (1988). Aspartame and behavior in children. In R. J. Wurtman & E. Ritter-Walker (Eds.), *Dietary phenylalanine and brain function* (pp. 201–206). Boston: Birkhauser.

Wolraich, M. L., Lindgren, S. D., Stumbo, P. J., Stegnik, L. D., Applebaum, M. I., & Kiritsy, M. C. (1994). Effects of diets high in sucrose or aspartame on the behavior and cognitive performance of children. *New England Journal of Medicine, 330,* 301–307.

Wood, D. R., Reimherr, F. W., & Wender, P. H. (1985). Amino acid precursors for the treatment of attention-deficit disorder, residual type. *Psychopharmacology Bulletin, 21,* 146–149.

Zametkin, A. J., Karoum, F., & Rapaport, J. (1987). Treatment of hyperactive children with d-phenylalanine. *American Journal of Psychiatry, 144,* 792–794.

Zentall, S. (1993). Research on the educational implications of attention deficit hyperactivity disorder. *Exceptional Children, 60*(2), 143–153.

13

The Myriad of Controversial Treatments for Autism

A Critical Evaluation of Efficacy

RAYMOND G. ROMANCZYK
LAURA ARNSTEIN
LATHA V. SOORYA
JENNIFER GILLIS

CHARACTERISTICS OF AUTISM

Autism is a severe developmental disorder that affects many areas of functioning. It has received remarkable levels of research, clinical, and public attention for over 50 years, yet remains a controversial disorder (Berkell Zager, 1999; Cohen & Volkmar, 1997; Matson, 1994; Romanczyk, 1994; Schopler & Mesibov, 1988). Currently there are no medical diagnostic tests for autism. Diagnosis is made using the *Diagnostic and Statistical Manual of Mental Disorders*, fourth edition (DSM-IV), of the American Psychiatric Association (1994), which classifies autism as a pervasive developmental disorder (PDD). DSM-IV lists five disorders under the broad category of PDD, including autism and Asberger's disorder. The diagnosis of autism is based on qualitative impairment in three major domains of functioning: (1) communication, (2) social interaction, and (3) restricted behavior patterns.

Because of the qualitative nature of current diagnostic procedures, the diagnosis of autism encompasses a wide range of individual differences. Thus, an individual diagnosed with autism may or may not have verbal communication skills, may display limited or no social interaction, and may or may not display stereotyped self-stimulatory behavior and repetitive ritualistic behavior. Furthermore, IQ range is very broad, from severe degree of mental retardation to normal IQ. However this distribution is skewed, so that the majority of individuals with autism display significant mental retardation.

There are two other general characteristics that are important with respect to this chapter and the theme of this book. First, as a group, individuals with autism often display wide variation in their behavior such that measurement of change must incorporate multiple sampling procedures. Second, individuals with autism typically display uneven skill development such that there are typically areas of relative strength as well as relative weakness. The selection of assessment instruments and procedures to evaluate change or improvement must be both broad-based and specific (Cohen, Schmidt-Lackner, Romanczyk, & Sudhalter, in press).

There are numerous assessment and diagnostic instruments that are commonly used for diagnosis and progress evaluation. Most lack suitable sensitivity and specificity, and there are no generally accepted standards for what specific instruments should or should not be included in an evaluation battery (Esteban, Cochran, Valluripalli, Arnstein, & Romanczyk, 1999). There is, however, general consensus that an evaluation should include attention to the three major functioning areas that are affected by autism: communication, social interaction, and restricted behavior (New York State Department of Health, Early Intervention Program, 1999b). Thus, great care needs to be exercised in evaluating anecdotal reports, as well as research reports, with respect to the specific diagnostic procedures utilized and the specific assessment instruments used. Obtaining an accurate differential diagnosis for young children, as well as the critical process of obtaining a functional assessment of the child's development, remains a difficult and complex process (Harris & Handleman, 2000; New York State Health Department, 1999a; Powers & Handleman, 1984; Romanczyk, Lockshin, & Navalta, 1994; Schopler & Mesibov, 1988).

The prevalence of autism is highly controversial. Autism has historically been viewed as a rare disorder, occurring in approximately 4.5 per 10,000 children. There has been a trend for several years toward increasing prevalence rates. Most recently, much higher rates have been proposed, in some cases as high as 20–40 in 10,000 children (e.g., California Department of Developmental Services, 1999). Given that diagnostic criteria have changed over time, that there is increased vigilance for early detection and diagnosis through early intervention programs, and that access to services often requires a diagnosis, it is difficult to interpret the apparent increase in prevalence (Chakrabarti & Fombonne, 2001; Fombonne, 1999; Powell et al., 2000). This interpretational difficulty is compounded by the lack a national reporting system of prevalence, especially for young children.

REVIEW OF COMMON TREATMENT APPROACHES

Educational/Experiential Approaches

Facilitated Communication

For persons diagnosed with autism, a core characteristic is that social and communicative processes are severely impaired. In this context of dual impairment, facilitated communication (FC) rapidly became a nationwide phenomenon in autism treatment, with features on such television shows as *ABC Prime Time Live* and *PBS Frontline* (Kaplan, 1992; Palfreman, 1993). Adoption by mainstream clinicians and programs occurred with great speed. In response to the tremendous increase of interest in FC, a special institute for FC at Syracuse University was created, seminars were conducted across the country to train thousands of facilitators, and extravagant and unwarranted claims of FC's success were reported by the media. Although still currently popular and widely used, it is a controversial treatment for persons with autism (Delmolino & Romanczyk, 1995; Green, 1996; Herbert, Sharp, & Gaudiano, 2002; T. Smith, 1996). Based upon Rosemary Crossley's FC program in Australia, FC was introduced to the United States and Canada in 1990 by Douglas Biklen (Biklen, 1990a). Central to the theory behind FC is the assumption that individuals with autism have movement disorders that limit their communication abilities. Proponents claim that FC is a method that enables individuals with autism to reveal their ability to express themselves and form relationships.

In his seminal article on FC, *Communication Unbound: Autism and Apraxia*, Biklen (1990a), described how Crossley first applied FC to individuals with cerebral palsy to guide their hand/finger movements when using a picture board to communicate. Encouraged by clients' apparent successes at communicating, Crossley introduced FC to children with autism. FC has since been extended for use with populations that have an array of other communication disorders.

FC is presented as a means of facilitating language expression for those with absent or limited communicative abilities. Its proponents assert that by assisting children to control their motor movements, hidden language abilities will change suddenly and dramatically. The following is a description of FC in a memo from Biklen for teachers, speech pathologists, and others interested in autism and FC: "The method involves initial hand-over-hand and/or arm support, pulling the hand back after each selection, slowing down the movements, assistance in isolating the index finger, verbal reassurances, and encouragement. Over time, the physical support can be faded back completely or to just a hand on the shoulder" (1990b, p. 1).

According to proponents of FC, children can use a variety of communicative devices including electronic typewriters, handheld computers, keyboards, and letter and picture boards (Biklen, 1990a). FC purportedly enables a child with autism to communicate independently with an augmentative communication device, as the stated goal is to eventually allow the child to type or point independently of the facilitator (Biklen, 1990b).

It may sometimes be difficult to distinguish augmentative communication from facilitated communication. Augmentative communication is an empirically demonstrated method of aiding a person with communication, sometimes using devices similar to those used in FC. However, in augmentative communication, devices are modified to allow direct voluntary control, using even the most subtle muscle movements. This permits independent communication (Cummins & Prior, 1992). In contrast, FC uses the facilitator as an "intermediary" for communication purposes. Thus, what distinguishes FC from augmentative communication is the procedure, not the devices and labels given to the procedure. This is important because some portrayals of "augmentative communication" actually use facilitated communication procedures even though the term FC is not used.

Cummins and Prior (1992) described one such system that uses a pointer attached to a headband to point to a letter board, which is held in front of the individual. An examination of a video of this procedure indicated that the facilitator was moving the letter board, rather than the individual moving the pointer (Palfreman, 1993). Another example involves a child with severe impairments who is credited with being a gifted author (Olsen, 1999). The system used for communication is not referred to as FC, but resembles FC in many ways. Primarily, the child is provided hand-over-hand assistance to point to a letter board. As in FC, the adult focused visually on the letter board, but the child did not (Olsen, 1999).

Biklen (1990a) emphasized the role of apraxia in autism. Apraxia is a disorder of movement or gesture. The treatment of apraxia usually involves improving visuomotor control and substantial motor learning. However, FC does not seem to produce visuomotor control. In fact, it has been noted that there are many instances of individuals receiving facilitation who do not look at the keyboard while typing (Palfreman, 1993).

Jacobson and Mulick (1992) noted that the demonstration of FC requires evidence that the individual is communicating independently, and not being influenced by the facilitator. One method used to remove potential influence from the facilitator is to pose questions to the individual but not the facilitator (Dayan & Minnes, 1995). Results have shown that when facilitators are unable to hear the questions, or hear conflicting information, the individual consistently responds incorrectly (Bebko, Perry, & Bryson, 1996).

Another methodology presents the individual with questions or information in the absence of a facilitator. Later, the facilitator joins the individual in order to answer questions about the events prior to the presence of the facilitator. Using this method, Regal, Rooney, and Wandas (1994) reported that no correct responses were made, even though the facilitator was confident that the individual performed well.

Wheeler, Jacobson, Paglieri, and Schwartz (1992) assessed differences in performance when the facilitator was able to see or not see what was being presented. This study used a table with a divider in the middle that permitted the facilitator and child to see different views, while allowing the facilitator to provide FC for the child. The results of this study revealed no support for FC and suggested a strong facilitator influence on the children's responses.

M. D. Smith, Haas, and Belcher (1994) investigated the effects of facilitator knowledge and level of assistance with amount of facilitator influence. In half of the trials the facilitator was aware of the stimulus that the child had seen. Three levels of facilitator support were examined. They were no help, hand-over-hand assistance without prevention of errors, and hand-over-hand with preventing errors. The authors found that correct responses occurred only when the facilitator was aware of the stimulus and full support was given.

Edelson, Rimland, Berger, and Billings (1998) provided a hand-support device that removed the possible facilitator influence from FC. In this study, individuals with autism were taught to type using three methods: a human-facilitated condition, a mechanical-facilitated condition, and a nonfacilitated condition (i.e., the individual received no form of assistance when typing). After 8 weeks, a nonfacilitated maintenance test of performance showed no evidence of learning based on the facilitated condition.

Kezuka (1997) described a technique similar to FC. The individual communicated using a computer-controlled word and sound processor with physical support from assistants. The technique used was similar to FC, even though the author stated that the assistants had no knowledge of FC. Kezuka designed a strain gauge, which measured pressure. The strain gauge information was used to objectively measure the physical influence of facilitation on an individual. A greater amount of strain was recorded when the individual's finger was in the vicinity of the correct answer. Results from Kezuka's study suggest that the facilitators exercised control of motor movements of the individual by directing the individual's movements with pressure cues.

Proponents of FC claim that the experimental studies conducted are inappropriately designed and do not accurately measure performance. Silliman (1995) asserted that the studies were conducted out of the subjects' normal social context, creating an unfamiliar environment that hinders performance. Duchan (1995) states that, "The context of interaction is not a naturally occurring one, but one that is tampered with in a variety of ways" (p. 208).

To address such criticisms, Kerrin, Murdock, Sharpton, and Jones (1998) conducted a well-designed study in children's typical classroom settings, thus addressing the concern about unfamiliar environments. The study was conducted by the classroom teacher and speech pathologist. The two subjects in this study were diagnosed with autism and were familiar with both instructors. For 1 week prior to the study, the speech pathologist wore sunglasses. When the study began she continued to wear the sunglasses in the classroom and while facilitating with both subjects. Throughout the day, children received a picture/written word labeling task that required them to point to the correct picture or word after a verbal request (e.g., "Point to . . . "). The two facilitator conditions, blind (i.e., the facilitator wore the sunglasses with cardboard on the lenses to prevent sight) or sighted (i.e., the facilitator wore sunglasses only, enabling sight) were conducted on alternating days. The results from this study show that the subjects' responses were significantly influenced by the facilitator's ability to see the stimuli. Even though the facilitator did not believe she was intentionally influencing subjects' responses, results indicate that when the facilitator was able to see the stimuli, these responses were significantly more accurate.

Perry, Bryson, and Bebko (1998) administered questionnaires to 16 facilitators, first a few weeks prior to FC training, then after FC training. They found that after the FC training there was a significant increase in positive attitude toward FC and that the more positive the attitude, the more influence by the facilitator on subjects' responses in controlled studies.

Given this complete lack of any supportive evidence for FC, several ethical implications arise concerning the use of FC in applied settings. One implication is the determination of educational placement. Because FC provides false evaluations of the individual's intellectual and achievement level, incorrect educational placement can result. Children communicating with FC have been placed in grades inconsistent with their ability level (Beck & Pirovano, 1996; Jacobson & Mulick, 1992). This can lead to false hopes and expectations of parents and facilitators, as well as denial of appropriate educational services.

Another important ethical issue concerning FC is its use in determining allegations of sexual and physical abuse by a parent or relative. Siegel (1995) assessed allegations of sexual molestation of two adolescents made through FC. In an assessment with two trained facilitators who were unaware of the allegations, both adolescents showed random responses to both open-ended questions and objective information. Neither adolescent showed negative affect toward fathers.

No empirical evidence for the use of FC with autistic children has been found (Bebko et al., 1996; Delmolino & Romanczyk, 1995; Green, 1996; Herbert et al., 2002; Mostert, 2001; Regal et al., 1994; M. D. Smith et al., 1994). The most consistent conclusion is that authorship belongs to the facilitator, not the individual. A recent review of FC studies published since 1995 examines the methodologies and claims of studies showing the efficacy of FC (Mostert, 2001). This review supports the conclusions of previous reviews; when methodologically sound control procedures are used, no positive results for the use of FC are found.

Sensory Integration Therapy

Sensory integration (SI) therapy is based on the sensory integration theory developed by Jane Ayres in the 1970. The therapy has been applied to a wide variety of populations, including children with learning disabilities, attention-deficit/hyperactivity disorder (ADHD; see also Chapter 12 for a discussion of the use of SI with children with ADHD), and autism. Ayres (1972) offered the following definition of SI: "Information from the environment is organized and interpreted for the planning and execution of interaction with the environment, particularly the tangible, three dimensional, gravity-bound world" (p. 26). It follows that a child with a sensory integration dysfunction has difficulty integrating this type of information from the outside world and may therefore fail to learn and develop in a typical manner. The symptoms of sensory integrative dysfunction can include hyperactivity, distractibility, behavior problems, poor speech development, poor muscle tone and coordination, and learning problems (Ayres, 1979). The therapy is purported to help children with sensory integration dysfunction to change how the brain processes and organizes sensations by providing sensory stimulation (Ayres, 1979).

SI is a widely used treatment for children with autism. Some researchers believe that children with autism and other developmental disorders are hypersensitive or hyposensitive to sensory input (Cook, 1990). Many symptoms associated with autism are conceptualized by SI proponents as behaviors that are caused by sensory abnormalities. For example, a child who insists on wearing only specific clothing is thought to be overly sensitive to certain types of fabrics. Sensory problems are also thought by some to be at the root of such stereotyped behaviors as hand-flapping, rocking, and light gazing.

The goal of SI is not to teach specific behaviors or skills. Instead, SI is intended to remediate perceived sensory difficulties in order to allow the child to interact with the world in a more adaptive fashion. According to Cook (1990), "The primary goal when using a sensory integrative approach with children with autism is to facilitate interaction with a variety of environments and people in a functional, more satisfying way" (p. 5). According to proponents of this theory, children with autism may experience problems integrating information from the vestibular, tactile, and proprioceptive systems. The olfactory, auditory, gustatory, and visual systems may also be affected, but are less typically the focus of SI. The treatment uses a variety of techniques in order to stimulate the use of sensory systems and facilitate reorganization of the following systems:

- *Vestibular.* The vestibular system is composed of inner-ear structures that detect head movement. Dysfunction in the vestibular system may lead to difficulty with balance or locomotion. SI therapists provide vestibular stimulation through movement on such equipment as large balls, suspended nets, and swings (Arendt, MacLean, & Bandmaster, 1988).
- *Tactile.* The tactile sensory system is composed of nerves located under the skin that send information about touch to the brain. A child with tactile difficulties may be over- or undersensitive to touch and pain. Ayres (1979) coined the term "tactually defensive" to refer to children who react to tactile stimulation, particularly light touch, with extreme negative emotional reactions. For example, SI provides tactile stimulation by brushing the child on various parts of the body using brushes or textured fabrics or by rolling the child between two mats (Ayres, 1972, 1979).
- *Proprioceptive.* The proprioceptive system uses information from muscles and joints to provide the brain with information about the body's position. Proprioceptive abnormalities may lead to difficulties in performing simple motor tasks such as using silverware or sitting in a chair. SI therapists may have students navigate on scooter boards while riding on their stomachs, a task requiring the use of proprioceptive information (Ayres, 1972, 1979).

Sensory stimulation is typically provided through the use of games played with the aforementioned equipment. An assessment such as the Sensory Integration and Praxis Test (SIPT; Ayres, 1989) is used to diagnose the child's deficits and to determine the focus of therapy. Ayres (1972, 1979) promoted a "self-directed" therapeutic atmosphere in which children choose their own activities. According to Ayres (1972), children typically seek out activities that are needed to remediate their own deficits.

It is important to note that sensory integration theory itself lacks empirical support. Sensory integration is a broad concept that cannot be measured directly; instead, it must be inferred from a variety of behaviors and deficits that are used as indicators of sensory integration dysfunction. However, this range of "symptoms" is wide and encompasses almost any type of maladaptive responding and/or skill deficit: hyperactivity, behavior problems, speech delays, coordination problems, and learning problems (Ayres, 1972). Logically, this leads to the false conclusion that maladaptive responding is evidence of poor sensory integration and adaptive responding is the result of good sensory integration. Arendt and colleagues (1988) provided an excellent overview of the problems with the validity of the construct of sensory integration and focused on nonspecificity of terms, lack of correspondence to known central nervous system research, and definitional circularity.

A second problem with sensory integration theory arises from Ayres's (1979) assertion that sensory integration dysfunction is caused by "irregular activity in the brain," even though she admitted that neurologists are typically unable to find evidence of this irregular activity in children with purported sensory integration deficits (p. 52). Ayres, who specifically targets children with autism as a population needing SI, also asserted that "(a)utistic children represent a heterogeneous group with certain symptoms in common, one of which is disturbance in sensory processing" (Ayres & Tickle, 1980, p. 375). However, disturbance in sensory processing is not one of the diagnostic criteria for autism in the DSM-IV.

Volumes of information have been written about sensory integration theory, SI techniques, and the use of SI with a variety of populations. Unfortunately, publications regarding the use of SI with children with autism are composed entirely of theoretical explanations, descriptive accounts, or case studies. The experimental studies that have been conducted on the efficacy of SI with other populations (e.g., children with learning disabilities and mental retardation) are often confounded by such variables as maturation and changes in the child's routine. Additionally, the outcome measures used are often indirect and subject to observer bias. Such limitations such as sample sizes, failure to follow a consistent definition of SI, and failure to employ appropriate control groups render many findings difficult to interpret.

Our review of the literature failed to find a single well-controlled clinical study supporting the use of SI with children with autism. According to a review conducted by the New York State Department of Health, 29 articles regarding the use of SI with children with autism met the criteria to be reviewed (New York State Health Department, 1999a). After carefully reviewing each of these articles, the committee concluded that none used experimentally sound scientific methodology and could not be used to demonstrate SI's efficacy.

SI is not designed specifically for children with autism. However, reviews of the evidence of the efficacy of SI with broader populations have also produced largely negative results. Review articles on the use of SI with children with mental retardation (Arendt et al., 1988), learning disabilities (Hoehn & Bandmaster, 1994), and language disorders (Griffer, 1999) all found insufficient evidence to support the use of SI (see also Chapter 12). Specifically, Arendt and colleagues (1988) concluded that for mental retardation "there exists no convincing empirical or theoretical support for the continued use of sensory integration therapy with that population outside of a research context" (p. 410).

In summary, there are no experimentally sound studies supporting the use of sensory integration in the treatment of children with autism (see also Herbert et al., 2002). This raises the question of competition for limited resources, such as time and money, that could be spent on empirically supported treatments. Because the number of hours per week spent on SI and the length of the actual therapy differ greatly from case to case, the magnitude of this expenditure is difficult to estimate.

Auditory Integration Training

Although not part of the diagnostic criteria for autism, abnormalities in hearing have commonly been reported in individuals with autism or PDD. Presumed abnormalities range from "deafness" to hypersensitivity to everyday sounds (e.g., microwave, vacuum cleaner). One survey of parents of individuals with autism (Rimland & Edelson, 1995) reported that up to 40% of individuals with autism may experience some level of oversensitivity to sound. However, it appears that there may be significant false positives in identifying "hearing sensitivity" (Valluripalli & Gillis, 2000).

Although auditory integration training (AIT) was originally proposed to treat such hearing disorders as hearing loss, the treatment later was applied to children with various learning and language problems, including autism. The perceived prevalence of hypersensitive hearing ("hyperacusis") in autism, coupled with the media attention focused on AIT as a "cure for autism," has increased both parent and professional interest in AIT. Interest in AIT increased following the publication of *The Sound of a Miracle: A Child's Triumph over Autism* written by Annabel Stehli, the mother of an 11-year-old girl with autism. The book describes the family's experience with AIT, in which her daughter "recovered" from autism after a relatively brief (10-hour) intervention (Stehli, 1991). While the initial popularity of AIT spread through parent circles, researchers took interest in scientifically evaluating the procedure.

The original AIT procedure was developed by otolaryngologist Guy Berard in the 1960s to treat such auditory disorders as hearing loss or hearing distortion. The treatment procedure involves electronically filtering sounds to which an individual previously demonstrated hypersensitivity in an audiogram. Repeated presentation of the modified sounds is believed to desensitize and retrain individuals' auditory systems to the sounds they previously found distressing. From the early 1980s, Berard began publishing his views on the integral role of disorders of auditory processing on learning and behavior. Berard held that hypersensitivity, distortions, and delays in auditory signals contribute to inefficient learning and may cause persons with these problems to exhibit maladaptive behaviors. Berard later modified his original procedure with the intention of using AIT to improve communication skills by focusing the latter half of treatment on the right ear, which sends auditory input to the left hemisphere of the brain. Berard hypothesized that stimulation of the left hemisphere will increase language perception (*http://www.autism.org/ait2.html*).

A handful of outcome studies have been published on the use of AIT with individuals with autism (Bettison, 1996; Edelson et al., 1999; Gill-berg, Johansson, & Steffenberg, 1997; Mudford et al., 2000; Rimland & Edelson, 1995; Zollweg, Vance, & Palm, 1997). Of the available research, two studies are supportive of the use of AIT and three are not. Only one supportive study and three nonsupportive studies used a double-blind, placebo-control methodology. The standard methodology employed in a placebo-controlled AIT study involves the treatment group undergoing the typical AIT procedure and the placebo group listening to unfiltered music for the same time intervals as the treatment group.

The one well-controlled supportive study of AIT by Rimland and Edelson (1995) contained flaws that limit interpretation of the data. The flaws include the presence of statistically significant differences between treatment and control groups prior to the intervention and questionable clinical significance of the results (Howlin, 1997; Zollweg et al. 1997). Rimland and Edelson found statistically significant differences between the eight children in the experimental group and nine children in the control group on both the Autism Behavior Checklist (ABC) and Fisher's Auditory Problems Checklist (FAPC). For the ABC, the authors used summary scores across the varied subscales of the ABC rather than the conventional use of mean scores. Zollweg and colleagues (1997) extrapolated the data from Rimland and Edelson and found an ABC mean pre- to post-AIT difference score of only .33. Other researchers (Howlin, 1997; Zollweg et al., 1997) have argued that the difference found in mean scores on the ABC lacks clinical significance. Finally, given the a priori differences between treatment and control groups, interpretation of the results of Rimland and Edelson are further complicated.

Edelson and colleagues (1999) conducted a double-blind study that remedied the methodological flaws of Rimland and Edelson (1995). The authors used multiple methods to assess change, including two measures of behavior change and one measure of change in auditory sensitivity. Significant change was observed in only one measure of behavior, the ABC, at only the last of three measurement intervals. Although the authors regarded their findings as supportive of the use of AIT with individuals with autism, their conclusions should be interpreted with caution. Many factors, including the small sample size, lack of replicability across similar measures of behavior, lack of replication by other laboratories, and the questionable clinical significance of their single positive finding limit the generalizability of their findings.

Studies that do not support the use of AIT with individuals with autism include Bettison (1996), Zollweg and colleagues (1997), Gillberg and colleagues (1997), and Mudford and colleagues (2000). Gillberg and colleagues conducted an open, nonblind pilot study that found no significant changes on the two measures of autism-related behavior employed. Both Bettison, Zollweg and colleagues, and Mudford and colleagues conducted double-blind, placebo-controlled studies in which no difference was found between treatment and control groups. These studies found improvement in autism-related behavior as measured by the ABC in both the treatment and placebo-control groups. In fact, Mudford and colleagues found that parents of children in their control group rated their children as better on measures of hyperactivity and ear-occlusion than parents of children who received AIT. Bettison was the only study that investigated Berard's hypothesis regarding the effects of AIT on cognition and learning. Bettison found improvements in both groups on the Peabody Picture Vocabulary Test (PPVT) and the Leiter International Performance Scale (LIPS).

The findings of improvement in both the treatment and control groups in Bettison (1996), Mudford and colleagues (2000), and Zollweg and colleagues (1997) raise important concerns regarding the use of AIT with individuals with autism. First, the majority of studies of AIT use subjective measures of behavior change. The findings of improvement on subjective measures may reflect an increased expectancy on the part of parents and clinicians for improvement given the start of an intervention (i.e., a self-fulfilling prophecy) (Zollweg et al., 1997). The one consistent measure of direct behavioral change employed in all the studies involved the audiogram, a test administered by a trained audiologist. However, only one of the reviewed studies (Bettison, 1996) found significant changes in audiogram results, but these changes were evident for both the treatment and placebo groups. Bettison also used another measure of directly observable change in the standardized measures of verbal and performance intelligence (Peabody Picture Vocabulary Test [PPVT] and Leiter International Performance Scales [LIPS], respectively). Again, improvement was observed on these measures for both treatment and placebo groups. The results on direct measures of behavior in Bettison suggest an effect of listening to music rather than a direct effect of auditory integration training. However, these findings remain to be replicated.

Beyond the limitations of the research findings, reports of negative side effects of the treatment raise ethical questions concerning the use of this procedure with individuals with autism. The side effects have been largely based on parent and teacher reports and have been found in both treatment and control groups (Bettison, 1996). The reported side effects of AIT include an increase in behavior problems (e.g., aggression and hyperactivity), sleep disturbances, eating disturbances, earaches, headaches, and stomachaches (Bettison, 1996; Edelson et al., 1999). The reported side effects have in part influenced the New York State Education Department (1993; in Berkell, Malgeri, & Streit, 1996) to classify AIT as an invasive procedure that could cause harm if not properly administered or monitored.

Given the numerous issues surrounding the use of AIT with individuals with autism, the popular acceptance of this expensive procedure is disconcerting. Research in this area must incorporate measures of directly observed behavior (e.g., Bettison, 1996). Additionally, given that sound sensitivity has not been found to differ pre- or post- AIT treatment, the mechanism underlying supposed behavioral change should be more clearly explicated. If validation of the treatment finds it to be effective for some individuals, the field faces the challenge of standardizing the delivery and practice of AIT. The nonstandardized and unregulated manner in which AIT is currently practiced may place individuals seeking this treatment at risk. The aforementioned issues, compounded with reported negative side effects, point to yet another popular, but unsubstantiated, treatment for autism.

Developmental, Individual-Difference, Relationship-Based Model

According to Dr. Stanley Greenspan, the developer and primary proponent of the Developmental, Individual-Difference, Relationship-Based Model (DIR), the DIR model is a "functional developmental approach" that "examines how children integrate their capacities (motor, cognitive, language, spatial, sensory) to carry out emotionally meaningful goals" (Greenspan & Wieder, 1999, p. 148). The DIR model is used to conceptualize the problems of children with varying developmental challenges, including, but not exclusive to, autism. Interventions based on this approach, sometimes referred to as "floor-time," have become popular in recent years with families of children with autism and PDD through publications, seminars, and internet sites.

Greenspan and Wieder (1998) outlined their conceptual model of the causes, assessment, and treatment of children with autism and PDD in the book *The Child with Special Needs*. The model is based on Greenspan and Wieder's (1999) affect-diathesis hypothesis, which has clear roots in psychoanalytic theory (Greenspan, 2001). According to this hypothesis, children with symptoms of autism may have a "unique biologically based processing deficit involving the connection of affect, motor planning, and sequencing capacities, and symbol formation" (p. 150). According to the authors, the ability to connect affect to motor function and symbolic representation is a critical skill that develops in the second year of life.

The affect-diathesis hypothesis assumes that affect is central to emotional and cognitive development. Emotional development is considered a core developmental process that is the basis for all skills. For example, a child may learn cause and effect through a noninteractional means (e.g., accidentally dropping a spoon and hearing a "clang") or through an "emotional" means (e.g., smiling at mom and having mom return the smile). Greenspan and Wieder (1998) hypothesized that a child who learns cause and effect in an emotional context will have a stronger foundation in cause-and-effect learning than other children.

The complex DIR model presumes that children with autism or PDD have underlying sensory processing and/or motor planning difficulties that hinder their cognitive and affective development. The fit of a family's inter-actional pattern with the child's specific deficits also is considered a critical component of the model. For example, if a father has a loud, expressive style with a child who displays auditory hypersensitivity, the child is likely to have more trouble overcoming his or her sensory difficulties. According to the model, the child in this example would retreat further into a world of isolation to escape the overstimulation of the family environment. The goal of techniques based on the DIR model is to identify the child's biologi-cal weaknesses (e.g., sensory-processing difficulties, motor planning and sequencing problems) and the family's interactional patterns. This infor-mation is then used to design an individualized treatment plan for the child with special needs (Greenspan & Wieder, 1998).

The remediation of the child's biological and developmental needs is conducted through the floor-time technique. Floor-time is a child-directed, daily playtime. The goals of floor-time are to establish and stabilize the six fundamental developmental milestones outlined by the authors: (1) self-regulation and interest in the world, (2) intimacy, (3) two-way communica-tion, (4) complex communication, (5) emotional ideas; and (6) emotional thinking. Attainment of each of these milestones occurs in a stage-like pro-gression, according to the authors. Children with autism or PDD may pos-sess splinter skills in each of the different milestones, but mastery of each of the milestones is considered necessary for typical development. The floor-time technique teaches parents how to help their children sequentially master the milestones through relationship-building play. The floor-time technique is believed to help some children be "more trusting," "intimately related to parents," and "joyful" (Greenspan & Wieder, 1998, p. 463).

Although the model contains elements of quality generic clinical deci-sion making including individualized approaches to assessment and treat-ment, focus on motivational variables, and focus on typical developmental progression, the theory proposed by Greenspan and Wieder (1998) lacks scientific foundation. Many aspects of the theory appear to be based on personal clinical experience and anecdotal evidence. The assumptions re-garding the purported powerful role of emotion in cognitive development are not supported by developmental, learning, or cognitive research. As as-serted by Greenspan and Wieder: "That the emotional lesson comes first and is the basis for the cognitive lesson is opposite to the traditional view of cognition and learning" (p. 123).

A chart-review of 200 children with autism or PDD by Greenspan and Wieder (1997; in Greenspan & Wieder, 1998) has been used as support for the DIR model. Besides lacking experimental control, the study contained many of the classic flaws of such reviews, including a biased sample, use of unvalidated outcome measures, and use of a single clinician who was not blind to the hypotheses to review progress on the charts.

This study also compared the results of children in the chart review with a pseudo-control group. The pseudo-control group consisted of children who were receiving other traditional interventions. Despite the lack of experimental control to conduct such a comparison, the authors presented data comparing the outcomes of children enrolled in their program with the children not enrolled in their program. The statistical analysis of this comparison is clearly inappropriate given the flaws and limitations of the methodology employed.

The DIR approach appears attractive to parents because of its focus on the atypical emotional reciprocity characteristic of autism. The model provides hope to parents that "normal" social interactions can be obtained, but only with an approach that focuses on emotional development. By accusing behavioral interventions, albeit falsely, of not focusing on emotional development, the DIR model is incorrectly presented as unique in its ability to bring about a "warm, loving, empathetic relationship" with an autistic child (*http://www.interactivemetronome.com/GreenspanArticle. htm*). However, to date, no controlled studies support the use of the DIR model.

Dolphin-Assisted Therapy

Dolphin-assisted therapy (DAT) has attracted many parents of children with autism. DAT received significant attention after it was presented on Cable News Network (CNN, March 28, 1998; *http://www.cnn.com/ HEALTH/9803/28/dolphin.therapy/index.html#op*). The basic procedure of DAT was depicted, with the child completing a one-to-one teaching session with a therapist and then being given the opportunity to swim with a dolphin. The child's interaction with the dolphins was described as motivating the child to participate in therapy sessions (*http://www.nextstep.com*). Dolphins are currently the only nondomesticated animals used regularly as treatment partners with children with autism.

The website of the Human Dolphin Therapy Center in Miami reports a success rate of 97%, which is not defined with respect to the assessment instruments and measurements utilized (*http://www.cnn.com/HEALTH/ 9803/28/dolphin.therapy/index.html#op*). The average cost for dolphin therapy is $2,600 per week (*http://www.nextstep.com/stepback/cycle9/ 109/dolphin_therapy.html*). Families have reported raising over $10,000 for the small number of sessions. This cost excludes airfare and lodging (*http://www.cnn.com/HEALTH/9803/28/dolphin.therapy/index.html#op*). The time and cost of this treatment may foster an expectation of positive results.

According to Christopher Peknic, founder and executive director of the Dolphin Institute, the use of dolphins as treatment partners for autism and other childhood disorders is a natural and positive therapeutic technique (*http://www.dolphininstitute.org/text/cp.htm*). He believes that "dolphins have a very special bond," and are "attracted to young children" (*http://www.dolphininstititute.org/text.cp.htm*). In addition, supporters of DAT suggest that dolphins possess an uncanny ability to "understand and respond to the needs of special people" (*http://www.dolphininstitute.org/isc/text/e_smith.htm*).

Some of assumptions of DAT are closely related to the concept of peak experiences. As defined by DeMares and Krcyko (*http://www.dolphins intitute.org*), a peak experience is a strong positive emotional response to a particular event. It is asserted by some that there is a certain "connectedness" that is perceived during a peak experience. That is, "for the human, there is a feeling of being permanently changed or enlightened by the experience" (*http://www.dolphininstitute.org*).

David Cole, a strong proponent of DAT, suggested that "one hypothesis that's beginning to kind of emerge from this is that the dolphin's echolocation can change cellular metabolism in the human body, which would happen at such a core level that it would explain all of the phenomena that we are observing." Others assert that a dolphin's sonar helps children relax and encourages learning (*http://www.nextstep.com/stepback/cycle9/109/dolphin_therapy.html*).

Drawing on data collected on children who underwent a 1–2 week program of DAT, Nathanson (1998) reported that DAT yields long-lasting improvements in areas of speech, gross and fine motor skills, and attention. Nevertheless, a methodological analysis of his report by Marino and Lilienfeld (1998) reveals several serious flaws. The authors found that Nathanson's research contained several threats to internal validity including (1) the lack of a control group, rendering it impossible to determine whether the effects found were solely due to DAT and not other factors, and (2) a failure to address maturation as an explanation for changes in participant characteristics. In addition, Nathanson's questionnaire assessing parents' subjective reports of their child's change over time was vulnerable to demand characteristics and expectation bias. For example, Nathanson stated that "each behavioral item was preceded by the statement, 'As a result of Dolphin Human Therapy, my child has maintained or improved in his/her ability to . . . '." Moreover, independent evaluation of Nathanson's conclusions is difficult because the data reported are overall means for combined samples rather than individual statistics.

To date, there have been no independent, well-controlled research studies to support claims of DAT's effectiveness. There is also no empirical support for the claim that dolphin echolocation produces beneficial cellular metabolic changes.

Biological Approaches

Secretin

Historically, a variety of drugs have been touted as breakthrough cures for autism. The most recent "miracle drug" comes in the form of the hormone secretin. Secretin was publicized widely as a treatment for autism after a 3-year-old boy with autism was reported to have shown improvement after receiving secretin during an assessment of his digestive functioning. According to a report presented by *Dateline* (Larson, 1998), the child showed dramatic changes after the assessment, including the disappearance of his digestive problems, improved sleep, and improved language.

Secretin is a polypeptide hormone involved in the regulation of gastric function. The hormone causes the pancreas to secrete digestive enzymes that help to process food in the small intestines. A single injection or infusion of secretin has been approved by the Food and Drug Administration (FDA) for use in tests of digestive functioning to diagnose gastrointestinal illnesses. It can be used alone or in conjunction with pancreozymin or cholecystokinetic agents as a test for exocrine pancreatic function and in the diagnosis of biliary-tract disorders. Secretin can be derived from the duodenum of pigs, and is called purified porcine secretin in this form. Pure human secretin can also be synthesized and manufactured (Sandler et al., 1999).

Proponents of secretin do not agree on the rationale supporting its use with children with autism. Horvath, Papadimitriou, Rabsztyn, Drachenberg, and Tildon (1999) presented one hypothesis to support the use of secretin. They found that children with autism who have gastrointestinal symptoms show a greater gastrointestinal response to secretin than do typically developing children matched on age and gastrointestinal symptoms. The authors suggested that a possible absence of typical secretin stimulation in the autistic group may result in an upregulation of secretin receptors in the pancreas.

Starting in early October of 1998, secretin began to receive extensive media attention. By the end of that month, the demand for secretin was so enormous that physicians and parents wishing to experiment with the hormone had difficulty locating it. The use of secretin as a treatment for autism was supported by Horvath and colleagues (1998) in an uncontrolled, published report of three children with autistic spectrum disorders who underwent upper gastrointestinal endoscopy including the intravenous administration of secretin. The authors reported decreases in the severity of the children's gastrointestinal symptoms as well as subjective behavioral improvements. For example, the children reportedly showed improvements in eye contact, alertness, and language.

Despite the reported success of secretin, the results of the experimental studies are negative. Sandler and colleagues (1999) conducted a double-blind, placebo-controlled trial of a single intravenous dose of synthetic human secretin in 60 children with autism or PDD. Outcome assessments were completed by the child's parents and teachers, and by clinicians associated with the study. All parents, teachers, and clinicians were blind to the child's group assignment. The results showed that 9 out of the 27 children in the secretin group and 7 out of the 25 in the placebo group showed a significant response following treatment. Scores on the Autism Behavior Checklist decreased significantly (a decrease in scores indicates improvement in functioning) in both the secretin and placebo groups, but the groups did not differ significantly. In fact, the placebo group's scores decreased slightly more than those of the secretin group. In addition, scores were not significantly better with secretin treatment than with placebo for overall severity of autistic symptoms, communication skills, specific diagnostic features of autism, or nonspecific features of autism.

One of the most interesting findings of Sandler and colleagues (1999) is that after parents in both groups were made aware of their own child's group assignment and progress as well as the overall results of the study, 63% of the parents in the secretin group and 76% of the parents in the control group indicated a desire to continue or start secretin treatment with their children. Such choice to pursue a treatment when measured results are negative perhaps offers insight into the decision-making process used by parents to evaluate a drug's efficacy, and reflects the extent to which parental evaluation may be influenced by factors other than the child's actual behavior.

Chez and colleagues (2000) also conducted an outcome study on secretin that yielded negative results. During the first phase of the study, 56 children with autism were administered an open-label trial of secretin. Parent-report measures revealed statistically significant improvement in gastrointestinal symptoms, language, and social behavior. The second phase of the study consisted of a double-blind trial with 25 children. Half of the children received a dose of secretin followed 4 weeks later by a placebo injection; the remainder of the children received the doses in the reverse order. Results from this double-blind portion of the study did not reveal significant differences in outcome between the placebo and secretin treatments. The authors were also unable to identify a subclass of responders based on such factors as age, gender, gastrointestinal symptoms, and medical history. These results suggest that reported improvements following treatment with secretin may be the result of adult expectations and not of a true drug effect.

Several researchers have replicated the findings of Sandler and colleagues (1999) and Chez and colleagues (2000). Corbett and colleagues (2001) and Owley and colleagues (2001) both conducted double-blind, placebo-controlled crossover studies to investigate secretin's effects. Both studies used widely accepted standardized measures, including the Autism

Diagnostic Observation Schedule (ADOS). Neither study demonstrated a treatment effect of secretin over the placebo.

Thus far, all of the evidence supporting the use of secretin is anecdotal and consists mostly of parental and physician report (see also Herbert et al., 2002). Aman and Armstrong (2000) conducted a survey of parents whose children had received secretin. In striking contrast to the results of numerous objective studies of secretin, many survey respondents reported observing improvements in gastrointestinal functioning, eye contact, communication, and intellectual functioning. The *Autism Research Review International* (December 1999) estimated that several thousand children with autism have received infusions of secretin, despite the lack of evidence for its efficacy. The safety of secretin, particularly repeated administrations of the hormone, is unclear. There have been at least two reports of seizures occurring after the administration of secretin and at least one report of a child who stopped breathing after receiving the hormone (Rimland, 1999), although the extent to which these side effects were attributable to the drug is unclear. Secretin is not approved by the FDA as a treatment for autism.

Diet Therapies

Parents, dietitians, and physicians have explored "therapeutic diets" in an effort to treat children with autism (see also Chapter 12, this volume, for a review of diet therapies for ADHD). The most popular are "elimination diets," in which either gluten (found in wheat products) or casein (found in milk products), or both, are eliminated from the child's diet. In addition, a skin prick test to determine food allergies is used to select other food items to be eliminated from the diet.

Gluten and casein both produce peptides that affect opiate receptors in the brain (Shaw, 1998). According to proponents of gluten- and casein-free diets, the peptides can cause a neurotransmitter imbalance that produces the symptoms of autism. Currently, there is no evidence to support this hypothesis.

A recent issue of the popular magazine *Parents* contained an article by a mother who claims that she "cured" her son's autism with a gluten- and casein-free diet (Seroussi, 2000). Despite the popularity of gluten- and casein-free diets, very little research has been conducted on the diets' effects. In a study by Lucarelli and colleagues (1995), 36 children with autism were placed on a cow's milk–free diet. In addition, all foods that yielded a positive result on a skin-prick test were eliminated for 8 weeks. Results were measured using the Behavior Summarized Evaluation scale, which consists of 20 items grouped into seven categories related to autistic symptoms. The authors reported that children with autism improved on five out of seven scales on the autism behavior scale while on the elimination diet.

In addition, children who improved on the diet were given a challenge test in which either a milk protein or a placebo was introduced in a randomized, double-blind procedure. There was some worsening on three of the seven scales following this challenge test. However, the authors did not report the number of children showing improvement on the diet, or the number that worsened after the challenge test; they reported only means. The authors also did not report the qualifications of the evaluators or whether they were blind to the hypotheses of the study.

Reichelt, Ekrem, and Scott (1990) tested the effects of either a gluten-free and milk-reduced diet or a milk-free and gluten-reduced diet on children with autism. Children were assigned to groups based on the reported onset of autism (late onset, neonatal onset, or early onset with late worsening), and the diet was followed for 1 year. Parental and teacher reports were used to document behavioral changes. This type of evaluation is susceptible to observer bias and placebo effects. Such improvements as better sleep, increased verbalizations, decreased behavioral difficulties, and decreased seizure activity were reported in some children. However, because the investigators did not include a control group, it is impossible to know whether these effects (regardless of the validity of the parent/teacher reports) can be attributed to dietary changes. In summary, no well-controlled double-blind studies have been conducted on elimination diets, and there is no evidence to suggest that these diets are effective.

A second type of "therapeutic diet" is the anti-yeast diet. This diet is based on the hypothesis that autism can be linked to an overgrowth of yeast in the digestive system. A special diet is sometimes used in combination with the anti-yeast drug nystatin (Semon, 1998), which is used to treat yeast problems. The anti-yeast diet often includes the elimination of many foods, in addition to gluten and casein, described previously. Like gluten and casein elimination diets, anti-yeast diets are intended to be continued indefinitely. The literature on anti-yeast diets consists primarily of anecdotal reports by parents. No controlled studies have been conducted to support the use of such a diet.

Despite the fact that very little research has been done on the effects of elimination diets, they remain popular. Unfortunately, they are not without risk. Some children may experience severe withdrawal reactions when gluten and casein are removed from the diet (Shaw, 1988). Many children with autism are selective eaters who insist on eating a narrow range of foods. The elimination of stock favorite foods may trigger tantrums and refusals to eat. In addition, any elimination diet can place a child at risk for malnutrition if the child's nutritional intake is not monitored carefully. Special diets can also be problematic for parents. Elimination diets, particularly those that aim to eliminate multiple food groups, can be costly and time-consuming for parents.

Vitamin B Treatment

The concept that mental illness can be treated by vitamins and minerals, also known as orthomolecular psychiatry, was introduced by Pauling (1968). According to Pauling, mental illness can result from inadequate concentrations of vitamins and minerals. Consequently, mentally disordered individuals may not show abnormally low levels of a nutrient in standard evaluations, but may nevertheless benefit from vitamin supplements. Pauling's hypotheses have been used to support the use of vitamin treatments for a variety of mental illnesses, including autism. As in the case with individuals with Down's syndrome, fragile X syndrome, and attention-deficit/hyperactivity disorder, the use of vitamins with individuals with autism has not demonstrated effects in well-designed studies (Kozlowski, 1992).

Vitamin B_6 is the most studied and controversial vitamin treatment for individuals with autism. According to a relatively recent survey, vitamins were the fifth most commonly used medication/psychotropic agent used with children with autism (Aman, Van Bourgondien, Wolford, Sarphare, 1995). Vitamin B_6 is a collective term for three naturally occurring pyridines: pyridoxine, pyridoxal, and pyridoxamine. Within autism research, vitamin B_6 is referred to as pyridoxine and is typically administered with magnesium. A study by Martineau, Barthelemy, Garreau, and Lelord (1985) revealed that the B_6-magnesium treatment resulted in more significant clinical improvement than B_6 alone or magnesium alone. However, the findings of Martineau and colleagues are limited due to the measurement problems discussed later in this chapter.

Two laboratories are largely responsible for the early research on the behavioral and physical effects of Vitamin B_6. The laboratories of Bernard Rimland and Gilbert Lelord and colleagues have typically reported improvements in individuals with autism after Vitamin B_6 treatment. However, the majority of studies from these laboratories are marked by methodological shortcomings. A review of the literature identified such shortcomings as parent report questionnaires with questionable reliability and validity, infrequent measurement, and questionable clinical significance of findings (Pfeiffer, Norton, Neison, & Shott, 1995).

Rimland and colleagues have published few studies on the effects of B_6 treatment on autism (Rimland, Callaway, & Dreyfus, 1978, in Rimland, 1987). Rimland and colleagues (1978) conducted a double-blind, placebo-controlled trial of vitamin B_6 with magnesium and reported positive effects for 30–40% of the subjects placed on the treatment (Rimland, 1998). Behavioral changes were measured by an unstandardized "target symptom checklist." It is unclear which behaviors were targeted on the symptom checklist, how the checklist was devised, and whether each subject received the same checklist. Furthermore, the clinical significance and effect sizes of the observed changes were unclear. Rimland (1987) noted that parents reported improvements in eye contact, speech, and "interest in the world." According to Rimland (1998), the children in the B_6 plus magnesium study "became more normal, although they were not completely cured" (p. 178).

A series of French studies conducted by Gilbert Lelord and colleagues also reported positive results of vitamin B_6-magnesium treatment with individuals with autism. These studies varied in methodology, ranging from use of double-blind, placebo-controlled trials to open trials. The strength of the French studies rests in their use of multiple measures to assess change. However, as discussed by Pfieffer and colleagues (1995), many problems with the design, measurement, and interpretation of the results preclude confidence in their validity. Although some studies used a double-blind, placebo-group design, the validity of some of these studies is compromised due to the use of the same subjects across studies. For example, Lelord and colleagues (1981) used the subjects from the open trial in a subsequent double-blind, placebo-controlled trial. Although the authors reported using this methodology to identify treatment responders and nonresponders, the results of the double-blind, placebo-controlled trial are limited. According to Pfeiffer and colleagues, it is possible that the same subjects were used across multiple publications.

The measurement problems in the French studies include use of unstandardized, infrequently used questionnaires and the unclear relationship between physiological findings and reported clinical improvement. The physiological measures employed by the French researchers included homovanillic acid (HVA) levels and evoked potentials (EP). Levels of HVA, a dopamine metabolite, were measured because these levels were previously found to be elevated in autistic children (Lelord, 1978; cited in Martineau et al., 1985). A number of the French studies found HVA levels to decrease significantly after pyridoxine treatment (Martineau, Garreau, Barthelemy, Callaway, & Lelord, 1981; Martineau et al., 1985). Researchers have hypothesized that changes in HVA levels indicate that B_6-magnesium treatment may induce changes in dopamine metabolism. However, this hypothesis has neither been supported nor refuted. Alternative hypotheses, such as changes in HVA levels indicating changes in the excretion, rather than the metabolism, of dopamine, have not been ruled out (Pfeiffer et al., 1995). As noted, some French studies also used EP or averaged evoked potentials (AEP) and reported significant changes (Martineau et al., 1985; Martineau, Barthelemy, Callaway, Garreau, & Lelord, 1981; Martineau, Barthelemy, Roux, Garreau, & Lelord, 1989). However, given the wide individual variability in EP readings, the validity of "improved" EPs is questionable. Furthermore, the small number of subjects in the studies of EP or AEP readings limits the generalizability of these findings to the heterogeneous population of individuals with autism. Finally, the lack of correlation between the physiological changes and the reported clinical/behavioral changes call into question the clinical utility of the physiological measures.

Two studies from independent laboratories found no significant improvements after B_6-magnesium treatment. However, these studies contained methodological flaws that complicate the interpretation of their findings (Findling et al., 1997; Tolbert, Haigler, Waits, & Dennis, 1993). Tolbert and colleagues (1993) conducted an open trial and administered lower doses of B_6-magnesium combinations than typically used. The authors found no difference in behavioral ratings using unstandardized measures. Findling and colleagues (1997) conducted a double-blind, placebo-controlled trial but did not use standardized measures. They found no difference between experimental and control groups, but did find evidence for a placebo effect in vitamin treatments. The largest change on the Childhood Psychiatric Rating Scale (CPRS) occurred in the first 2 weeks, when all subjects were placed on placebo pills.

The lack of support for the use of vitamin treatments for individuals with autism is worrisome considering the relatively widespread use of this treatment and the known side effects of megadoses of many vitamins, including B_6. Although B_6 has not been shown to have direct toxicity, as have megadoses of vitamin C and B_3, side effects have been reported. The negative side effects of vitamin B_6 megadoses alone include possible physical dependency and withdrawal symptoms (e.g., seizures) when B_6 is removed. Rimland (1987) reported that some subjects experienced behavior problems after B_6 treatment in an earlier study, leading to the termination of this treatment after the completion of the study. The researchers, however, interpreted the withdrawal symptoms as indication of the efficacy of vitamin B_6 in improving behavioral skills rather than a standard side effect of megadoses of the vitamin. Some researchers have also found evidence for vitamin B_6 toxicity, including peptic ulcer disease (Gualtieri, Evans, & Patterson, 1987).

EFFECTIVE TREATMENTS FOR AUTISM

To address the effectiveness of treatment approaches and procedures, it is necessary to carefully specify the dependent variables that will be used to assess progress (Dawson & Osterling, 1997). Because autism is a pervasive developmental disorder, it manifests itself in multiple symptoms that reflect a complex constellation of problems. In a review of the literature concerning the choice and type of assessment instruments used in research publications to diagnose and assess individuals with autism, no clear consensus was found (Cochran, Esteban, & Romanczyk, 1998).

To compound this problem, autism is characterized by an uneven skill presentation and unstable behavior over time. Such fluctuations within the context of symptom variability and the heterogeneous population of individuals with autism clearly limit the use of simple assessment tools. In this regard, the most common form of "outcome evaluation" is the use of interviews or checklists that are completed by parents and other caregivers. Such instruments are susceptible to unintended bias and reactivity, and may not assess actual child behavior change that is clinically significant or stable. If one uses a broad base of assessment procedures, particular those incorporating direct observation with appropriate reliability, this problem can be attenuated.

In various sections of this chapter, many references were made to the weak measurement methodologies utilized to assess behavior change. In contrast, Applied Behavior Analysis (ABA), which has strong historical ties to behavior therapy and behavior modification, features the direct and objective measurement of performance and behavior. ABA refers to an approach for educational and treatment intervention that derives primarily from research in basic learning principles from experimental psychology (Anderson & Romanczyk, 2000). It requires the precise quantification and analysis of behavior and learning patterns and the conditions that serve to elicit and maintain them. This approach, which is known as functional analysis, focuses on the "ABCs" (antecedents, behaviors, consequences) as well as the individual's learning history. ABA is characterized by use of single-subject research methodology (Hersen & Barlow, 1981) to determine intervention effectiveness.

There are approximately 500 published reports on the use of ABA with autism (Matson, Benavidez, Compton, Paclawskyj, & Baglio, 1996). These studies form a very impressive, conceptually consistent line of research that consistently replicates the effectiveness of this approach for individuals with autism. Moreover, several controlled studies have addressed the efficacy of ABA with autistic children; six of these have evaluated intensive (minimum of 1 year) ABA using an array of developmental measures (e.g., intellectual functioning, language, social interactions, adaptive functioning, and personality development). These studies (Anderson, Avery, DiPietro, Edwards, & Christian, 1987; Birnbrauer & Leach, 1993; Lovaas, 1987; McEachin, Smith, & Lovaas, 1993; Sheinkopf & Siegel, 1998; T. Smith, Eikeseth, Klevstrand, & Lovaas 1997) provide clear support for intensive, comprehensive intervention using ABA. Furthermore, many efficacious program models for autism incorporate key features of ABA (e.g., Anderson, Campbell, & O'Malley, 1994; Handleman & Harris, 2000; McClanahan & Krantz, 2000; Romanczyk, Matey, & Lockshin, 2000).

Independent reviews (e.g., Delmolino & Romanczyk, 1994; Green, 1996; Olley & Gutentag, 1999; Smith, 1996) have consistently concluded that the popular "mainstream" treatments for autism are ineffective. Several important government sources have reached the same conclusion. The New York State Department of Health conducted an extensive 2-year review of the literature concerning young children with autism as part of best practices guidelines (New York State Department of Health, 1999a, 1999b). Based on long-term treatment studies with adequate methodology, the NYSDOH concluded that ABA possessed the strongest research support. In particular, they reviewed long-term treatment outcome studies that utilized appropriate methodology with which to draw conclusions from the results. Furthermore, in a scientific review concerning the status of mental health in the United States commissioned by the Surgeon General (Satcher, 1999), ABA in the context of a structured setting was the recommended treatment for autism. A recent report (National Research Council, 2001) commissioned by the U.S. Department of Education, after a comprehensive review of the scientific literature, reached similar conclusions: There is substantial evidence for efficacy of ABA, but evidence remains lacking for other popular therapies such as those presented here.

Despite the convergence of the scientific evidence, many nonvalidated treatment procedures remain popular (see also Herbert et al., 2002, for a review). There appears to be a substantial gap between empirical validation and clinical practice. The central factor contributing to this gap is the inadequacy of assessment instruments used to gauge change. Many instruments and evaluation methods are subject to bias on the part of respondents, which is compounded by the extensive variability in the behavior of many individuals with autism. This naturally occurring variability may be misinterpreted by observers as evidence of positive treatment effects. Treatments that promise to produce substantial changes in short periods of time with little effort are understandably attractive to parents and professionals. But because of expectation and measurement bias, a positive outcome can be a self-fulfilling prophecy.

GLOSSARY

Applied behavior analysis: The scientific study of behavior that uses a specific conceptual and methodological approach for direct quantification and analysis of behavior. It historically derives primarily from research in psychology on basic learning processes. Applied Behavior Analysis refers to the precise measurement and analysis of behavior and learning patterns and the conditions that serve to elicit and maintain these behaviors and patterns.

Auditory-integration training: Repeated presentation of modified sounds hypothesized to alleviate atypical responses to sound in children with learning and developmental disabilities.

Elimination diet: Any eating plan that eliminates a specific food group from the diet. In autism, foods commonly eliminated include those containing gluten (found in wheat products) or casein (found in milk products).

Facilitated communication: A technique that involves providing physical assistance with the use of a communicative device (e.g., computer keyboard, letter board) to aid persons with autism to control motor movements to permit nonverbal communication.

Floor-time: Child-directed playtime used to teach the six fundamental milestones that are the basis of Stanley Greenspan's Developmental-Individual Difference, Relationship-Based model.

Hyperacusis: The term used in auditory-integration training to describe hypersensitive hearing to environmental sounds (e.g., vacuum cleaner, microwave). Hyperacusis can lead to negative reactions to sounds of a particular frequency. Hyperacusis for common environmental stimuli is associated with individuals with autism.

Secretin: A polypeptide hormone that causes the pancreas to secrete digestive enzymes which help to process food in the small intestines.

Sensory Integration Therapy: Client-directed therapy whose stated goal is to enable the child to better process and organize information from the sensory world using a variety of equipment designed to stimulate various sensory systems (e.g., balls, scooter boards, nets).

Splinter skills: Markedly above-average skills in one domain, a phenomenon observed in approximately 10% of children with infantile autism.

Vitamin B_6 treatment: A vitamin (B_6) that is typically administered in combination with magnesium and is presumed to reduce problem behaviors in individuals with autism.

REFERENCES

Aman, M. G., & Armstrong, S. A. (2000). Regarding secretin for treating autistic disorder. *Journal of Autism and Developmental Disorders, 30,* 71–72.

Aman, M. G., Van Bourgondien, M. E., Wolford, P. L., & Sarphare, G. (1995). Psychotropic and anticonvulsant drugs in subjects with autism: Prevalence and patterns of use. *Journal of the American Academy for Child and Adolescent Psychiatry, 34*(12), 1672–1681.

American Psychiatric Association. (1994). *Diagnostic and statistical manual of mental disorders* (4th ed.). Washington, DC: Author.

Anderson, S., & Romanczyk, R. G. (2000). Early intervention for young children with autism: Continuum based behavioral models. *Journal of the Association for Persons with Severe Handicaps, 24*(3), 162–173.

Anderson, S. R., Avery, D. L., DiPietro, E. K., Edwards, G. L., & Christian, W. P.

(1987). Intensive home-based early intervention with autistic children. *Education and Treatment of Children, 10,* 352–366.

Anderson, S. R., Campbell, S., & O'Malley Cannon, B. (1994). The May Center for Early Childhood Education. In S. L. Harris & J. S. Handleman (Eds.), *Preschool education programs for children with autism* (pp. 15–36). Austin, TX: Pro-Ed.

Arendt, R. E., MacLean, W. E., & Bandmaster, A. A. (1988). Critique of sensory integration therapy and its application in mental illness. *American Journal on Mental Retardation, 92,* 401–411.

Ayres, A. J. (1972). *Sensory integration and learning disorders.* Los Angeles, CA: Western Psychological Services.

Ayres, A. J. (1979). *Sensory integration and the child.* Los Angeles, CA: Western Psychological Services.

Ayres, A. J. (1989). *Sensory integration and praxis tests.* Los Angeles, CA: Western Psychological Services.

Ayres, A. J., & Tickle, L. S. (1980). Hyper-responsivity to touch and vestibular stimuli as a predictor of positive response to sensory integration procedures by autistic children. *American Journal of Occupational Therapy, 34,* 375–381.

Bebko, J. M., Perry, A., & Bryson, S. (1996). Multiple method validation study of facilitated communication: II. Individual differences and subgroup results. *Journal of Autism and Developmental Disorders, 26*(1), 19–42.

Beck, A. R., & Pirovano, C. M. (1996). Facilitated communicators' performance on a task of receptive language. *Journal of Autism and Developmental Disorders, 26*(5), 497–512.

Berkell, D., Malgeri, S., & Streit, M. K. (1996). Auditory integration training for individuals with autism. *Education and Training in Mental Retardation and Developmental Disabilities, 31*(1), 66–70.

Berkell Zager, D. (Ed.). (1999). *Autism: Identification, education, and treatment* (2nd ed.). Hillsdale, NJ: Erlbaum.

Bettison, S. (1996). The long-term effects of auditory integration training on children with autism. *Journal of Autism and Developmental Disorders, 26*(3), 361–374.

Biklen, D. (1990a). Communication unbound: Autism and praxis. *Harvard Educational Review, 60*(3), 291–314.

Biklen, D. (1990b). *Information packet on facilitated communication.* Syracuse, NY: Syracuse University.

Birnbrauer, J. S., & Leach, D. J. (1993). The Murdock Early Intervention Program after 2 years. *Behaviour Change, 10,* 63–74.

California Department of Developmental Services. (1999). *A report to the legislature: Changes in the population of persons with autism and pervasive developmental disorders in California's Developmental Services system: 1987 through 1998.* Sacramento: California Health and Human Services Agency.

Chakrabarti, S., & Fombonne, E. (2001). Pervasive developmental disorders in preschool children. *Journal of the American Medical Association, 285,* 3093–3099.

Chez, M. G., Buchanan, C. P., Bagan, B. T., Hammer, M. S., McCarthy, K. S., Ovrutskaya, I., Nowinski, C. V., & Cohen, Z. S. (2000). Secretin and autism: A two-part clinical investigation. *Journal of Autism and Developmental Disorders, 30,* 87–94.

Cochran, M., Esteban, S., & Romanczyk, R. (1998). *Diagnostic and assessment instruments for autism: A review of recent journal publications.* Paper presented at the 24th Annual Convention of the Association for Behavior Analysis, Orlando, FL.

Cohen, D. J., & Volkmar, F. R. (Eds.). (1997). *Handbook of autism and pervasive developmental disorders* (2nd ed.). New York: Wiley.

Cohen, I. R., Schmidt-Lackner, S., Romanczyk, R. G., & Sudhalter, V. (in press). The PDD Behavior Inventory: A rating scale for assessing response to intervention in children with PDD. *Journal of Autism and Developmental Disabilities*.

Cook, D. A. (1990). A sensory approach to the treatment and management of children with autism. *Focus on Autistic Behavior, 5,* 1–19.

Corbett, B., Khan, K., Czapansky-Beilman, D., Brady, N., Dropik, P., Zelinsky-Goldman, D., Delaney, K., Sharp, H., Mueller, I., Shapiro, E., & Ziegler, R. (2001). A double-blind, placebo-controlled crossover study investigating the effect of porcine secretin in children with autism. *Clinical Pediatrics, 40,* 327–333.

Cummins, R. A., & Prior, M. P. (1992). Autism and assisted communication: A response to Biklen. *Harvard Educational Review, 62*(2), 228–241.

Dawson, G., & Osterling, J. (1997). Early intervention in autism: Effectiveness and common elements of current approaches. In M. J. Guralnick (Eds.), *The effectiveness of early intervention: Second generation research* (pp. 307–326). Baltimore: Paul H. Brookes.

Dayan, J., & Minnes, P. (1995). Ethical issues related to the use of facilitated communication techniques with persons with autism. *Canadian Psychology, 36,* 183–189.

Delmolino, L. M., & Romanczyk, R. G. (1995). Facilitated communication: A critical review. *Behavior Therapist, 18*(2),27–30.

Duchan, J. F. (1995). The role of experimental research in validating facilitated communication: A reply. *Journal of Speech and Hearing Research, 38,* 206–210.

Edelson, S., Arin, D., Bauman, M., Lukas, S., Rudy, J., Sholar, M., & Rimland, B. (1999). Auditory integration training: A double-blind study of behavioral and electrophysiological effects in people with autism. *Focus on Autism and Other Developmental Disabilities, 14*(2), 73–81.

Edelson, S. M., Rimland, B., Berger, C. L., & Billings, D. (1998). Evaluation of a mechanical hand-support for facilitated communication. *Journal of Autism and Developmental Disorders, 28*(2), 153–157.

Esteban, S. E., Cochran, M. L., Valluripalli, L., Arnstein, L., & Romanczyk, R. G. (1999, May). *Assessment instruments used with children with autism: Recommendations for research and practice.* Paper presented at the 25th Annual Convention of the Association for Behavior Analysis, Chicago.

Findling, R. L., Maxwell, K., Scotese-Wojtila, L., Huang, J., Yamashita, T., & Wiznitzer, M. (1997). High-dose pyridoxine and magnesium administration in children with autistic disorder: An absence of salutary effects in a double-blind, placebo-controlled study. *Journal of Autism and Developmental Disorders, 27*(4), 467–478.

Fombonne, E. (1999). The epidemiology of autism: A review. *Psychological Medicine, 29,* 769–786.

Gillberg, C., Johansson, M., & Steffenberg, S. (1997). Auditory integration training in children with autism: Brief report of an open pilot study. *Autism, 1,* 97–100.

Green, G. (1996). Evaluating claims about treatments for autism. In C. Maurice, G.

Greene, & S. C. Luce (Eds.), *Behavioral intervention for young children with autism* (pp. 15–28). Austin, TX: Pro-Ed.

Greenspan, S., & Wieder, S. (1997). Developmental patterns and outcomes in infants and children with disorders in relating and communicating: A chart review of 200 cases of children with autistic spectrum disorder. *The Journal of Developmental and Learning Disorders, 1,* 87–141.

Greenspan, S., & Wieder, S. (1998). *The child with special needs: Encouraging intellectual and emotional growth.* Reading, MA: Addison Wesley Longman.

Greenspan, S., & Wieder, S. (1999). A functional developmental approach to autism spectrum disorders. *Journal of the Association for Persons with Severe Handicaps, 24*(3), 147–161.

Greenspan, S. I. (2001). Children with autistic spectrum disorders: Individual differences, affect, interaction, and outcomes. *Psychoanalytic Inquiry, 20,* 675–703.

Griffer, M. R. (1999). Is sensory integration effective for children with language-learning disorders? A critical review of the evidence. *Language, Speech, and Hearing Services in Schools, 20,* 393–400.

Gualtieri, T., Evans, R. W., & Patterson, D. R. (1987). The medical treatment of autistic people: Problems and side effects. In E. Shopler & G. B. Mesibov (Eds.), *Neurobiological issues in autism* (pp. 373–388). New York: Plenum Press.

Handleman, J. S., & Harris, S. L. (2000). The Douglass Developmental Disabilities Center. In S. L. Harris & J. S. Handleman (Eds.), *Preschool education programs for children with autism* (2nd ed., pp. 71–86). Austin, TX: Pro-Ed.

Harris, S. L., & Handleman, J. S. (2000). *Preschool education programs for children with autism* (2nd ed.). Austin, TX: Pro-Ed.

Herbert, J. D., Sharp, I. R., & Gaudiano, B. A. (2002). Separating fact from fiction in the etiology and treatment of autism: A scientific review of the evidence. *Scientific Review of Mental Health Practice, 1,* 23–43.

Hersen, M., & Barlow, D. (1981). *Single case experimental designs.* New York: Pergamon.

Hoehn, T. P., & Bandmaster, A. A. (1994). A critique of the application of sensory integration therapy to children with learning disabilities. *Journal of Learning Disabilities, 27,* 338–350.

Horvath, K., Papadimitriou, J. C., Rabsztyn, A., Drachenberg, C., & Tildon, J. T. (1999). Gastrointestinal abnormalities in children with autistic disorder. *Journal of Pediatrics, 135,* 559–563.

Horvath, K., Stefanatos, G., Sokolski, K. N., Wachtel, R., Nabors, L., & Tildon, J. T. (1998). Improved social and language skills after secretin administration in patients with autistic spectrum disorders. *Journal of the Association for Academic Minority Physicians, 9*(1), 9–15.

Howlin, P. (1997). When is a significant change not significant? [Letter to the editor]. *Journal of Autism and Developmental Disorders, 27*(3), 347–348.

Jacobson, J. W., & Mulick, J. A. (1992). Speak for yourself, or . . . I can't quite put my finger on it! *Psychology in Mental Retardation and Developmental Disabilities, 17*(3), 3–7.

Kaplan, R. (Producer). (1992, February). Free from silence. In *Prime time live.* New York: ABC News.

Kerrin, R. G., Murdock, J. Y., Sharpton, W. R., & Jones, N. (1998). Who's doing the pointing? Investigating facilitated communication in a classroom setting with students with autism. *Focus on Autism and Other Developmental Disabilities,* *13*(2), 73–79.

Kezuka, E. (1997). The role of touch in facilitated communication. *Journal of Autism and Developmental Disorders, 27*(5), 571–593.

Kozlowski, B. W. (1992). Megavitamin treatment of mental retardation in children: A review of effects on behavior and cognition. *Journal of Child and Adolescent Psychopharmacology, 2*(4), 307–320.

Larson, J. (Producer). (1998, October 7). Autism: A new cure? A report on a possible new cure for autism. In *Dateline.* New York: NBC.

Lelord, G., Muh, J. P., Barthelemy, C., Martineau, J., Garreau, B., & Callaway, E. (1981). Effects of pyridoxine and magnesium on autistic symptoms: Initial observations. *Journal of Autism and Developmental Disorders, 11*(2), 481–493.

Lovaas, O. I. (1987). Behavioral treatment and normal educational and intellectual functioning in young autistic children. *Journal of Consulting and Clinical Psychology, 55*, 3–9.

Lucarelli, S., Frediani, T., Singoni, A.M., Ferruzzi, F., Giardi, O., Quinteieri, F., Barbat, M., D'eufemia, P, & Cardi, E. (1995). Food allergy and infantile autism. *Panminerva Medica, 37*, 137–141.

Marino, L., & Lilienfeld, S. O. (1998). Dolphin-assisted therapy: Flawed data, flawed conclusions. *Anthrozoos, 11*(4), 194–200.

Martineau, J., Barthelemy, C., Callaway, E., Garreau, B., & Lelord, G. (1981). Effects of vitamin B_6 on averaged evoked potentials in infantile autism. *Biological Psychiatry, 7*, 627–641.

Martineau, J., Barthelemy, C., Garreau, B., & Lelord, G. (1985). Vitamin B_6, magnesium, and combined B_6-Mg: Therapeutic effects in childhood autism. *Biological Psychiatry, 20*, 467–478.

Martineau, J., Barthelemy, C., Roux, S., Garreau, B., & Lelord, G. (1989). Electrophysiological effects of fenfluramine or combined vitamin B_6 and magnesium on children with autistic behavior. *Developmental Medicine and Child Neurology, 31*, 721–727.

Matson, J. L. (Ed.). (1994). *Autism in children and adults.* Pacific Grove, CA: Brookes Cole.

Matson, J. L., Benavidez, D. A., Compton, L. S., Paclawskyj, T., & Baglio, C. (1996). Behavioral treatment of autistic persons: A review of research from 1980 to the present. *Research in Developmental Disabilities, 17*, 433–465.

McClanahan, L., & Krantz, P. (2000). The Princeton Child Development Institute. In S. L. Harris & J. S. Handleman (Eds.), *Preschool education programs for children with autism* (2nd ed., pp. 191–213). Austin, TX: Pro-Ed.

McEachin, J. J., Smith, T., & Lovaas, O. I. (1993). Long-term outcome for children with autism who received early intensive behavioral treatment. *American Journal on Mental Retardation, 97*(4),359–372.

Mostert, M. P. (2001). Facilitated communication since 1995: A review of published studies. *Journal of Autism and Developmental Disorders, 31*, 287–313.

Mudford, O. C., Cross, B. A., Breen, S., Cullen, C., Reeves, D., Gould, J., & Douglas, J. (2000). Auditory integration training for children with autism: No behavioral benefits detected. *American Journal of Mental Retardation, 105*, 118–129.

Nathanson, D. E. (1998). Long-term effectiveness of dolphin-assisted therapy for children with severe disabilities. *Anthrozoos, 11(1)*, 22–32.

National Research Council, Committee on Educational Interventions for Children with Autism, Division of Behavioral and Social Sciences and Education. (2001). *Educating children with autism.* Washington, DC: National Academies Press.

New York State Department of Health, Early Intervention Program. (1999a). *Clinical practice guideline: Report of the recommendations. Autism/PDD, assessment and intervention in young children (age 0–3 years)* (No. 4216). Albany, NY: Author.

New York State Department of Health, Early Intervention Program. (1999b). *Clinical practice guideline: Guideline technical report. Autism/pervasive developmental disorders, assessment and intervention for young children (ages 0–3 years)* (No. 4217). Albany, NY: Author.

Olley, G., & Gutentag, S. S. (1999). Autism: Historical overview, definition, and characteristics. In D. Berkell Zager (Ed.), *Autism: Identification, education, and treatment* (2nd ed., pp. 3–22). Hillsdale, NJ: Erlbaum.

Olsen, M. (Producer). (1999, December). A voice within. In *CNN and TIME.* Atlanta, GA: Cable News Network.

Owley, T., McMahon, W., Cook, E. H., Laulhere, T., South, M., Mays, L. Z., Shernoff, E., Lainhart, J., Modahl, C. B., Corsello, C., Ozonoff, S., Risi, S., Lord, C., Leventhal, B. L., & Filipek, P. A. (2001). Multisite, double-blind, placebo-controlled trial of porcine secretin in autism. *Journal of the American Academy of Child and Adolescent Psychiatry, 40,* 1293–1299.

Palfreman, J. (Producer). (1993, October). Prisoners of silence. In *Frontline.* Alexandria, VA: Public Broadcasting Services.

Pauling, L. (1968). On the orthomolecular environment of the mind: Orthomolecular theory. *American Journal of Psychiatry, 131,* 1251–1257.

Perry, A., Bryson, S., & Bebko, J. (1998). Brief report: Degree of facilitator influence in facilitated communication as a function of facilitator characteristics, attitudes, and beliefs. *Journal of Autism and Developmental Disorders, 28*(1), 87–90.

Pfeiffer, S. I., Norton, J., Nelson, L., & Shott, S. (1995). Efficacy of Vitamin B_6 and magnesium in the treatment of autism: A methodology review and summary of outcomes. *Journal of Autism and Developmental Disorders, 25*(5), 481–493.

Powell, J. E., Edwards, A., Edwards, M., Pandit, B. S., Sungum-Paliwal, S. R., & Whitehouse, W. (2000). Changes in the incidence of childhood autism and other autistic spectrum disorders in preschool children from two areas of the West Midlands, UK. *Developmental Medicine and Child Neurology, 42,* 624–628.

Powers, M. D., & Handleman, J. S. (1984). *Behavioral assessment of severe developmental disabilities.* Rockville, MD: Aspen Systems.

Regal, R. A., Rooney, J. R., & Wandas, T. (1994). Facilitated communication: An experimental evaluation. *Journal of Autism and Developmental Disorders, 24*(3), 345–355.

Reichelt, K. L., Ekrem, J., & Scott, H. (1990). Gluten, milk proteins and autism: Dietary intervention effects on behavior and peptide secretion. *Journal of Applied Nutrition, 42,* 1–9.

Rimland, B. (1987). Megavitamin B_6 and magnesium in the treatment of autistic children and adults. In E. Shopler & G. B. Mesibov (Eds.), *Neurobiological issues in autism* (pp. 389–405). New York: Plenum Press.

Rimland, B. (1998). The use of vitamin B_6, magnesium, and DMG in the treatment of autistic children and adults. In W. Shaw (Ed.), *Biological treatments for autism and PDD: What's going on? What can you do about it?* (pp. 176–195). Manhattan, KS: Sunflower Publications.

Rimland, B. (1999). Secretin update: The safety issue. *Autism Research Review International, 13*, 1–2.

Rimland, B., Callaway, E., & Dryfus, P. (1978). The effects of high doses of vitamin B6 on autistic children. *American Journal of Psychiatry, 135*, 472–475.

Rimland, B., & Edelson, S. (1995). Brief report: A pilot study of auditory integration training in autism. *Journal of Autism and Developmental Disorders, 25*(1), 61–70.

Romanczyk, R. G. (1994). Autism. In V. S. Ramachandran (Ed.), *The encyclopedia of human behavior* (Vol. 1, pp. 327–336). San Diego, CA: Academic Press.

Romanczyk, R. G., Lockshin, S., & Navalta, C. (1994). Differential diagnosis of autism. In J. Matson (Ed.), *Autism in children and adults: Etiology, assessment, and intervention* (pp. 99–126). Pacific Grove, CA: Brookes/Cole.

Romanczyk, R. G., Matey, L., & Lockshin, S. B. (2000). The Children's Unit for Treatment and Evaluation. In S. L. Harris & J. S. Handleman (Eds.), *Preschool education programs for children with autism* (2nd ed., pp. 49–94). Austin, TX: Pro-Ed.

Sandler, A. D., Sutton, K. A., DeWeese, J. D., Giardi, M. A., Sheppard, V., & Bodfish, J. W. (1999). Lack of benefit of a single dose of synthetic human secretin in the treatment of autism and pervasive developmental disorder. *New England Journal of Medicine, 341*, 1801–1806.

Satcher, D. (1999). *Mental health: A report of the Surgeon General, 1999* [Online]. Available: http://www.surgeongeneral.gov/library/mentalhealth/chapter3/sec6.html#autism

Schopler E., & Mesibov, G. M. (Eds.). (1988). *Diagnosis and assessment in autism.* New York: Plenum Press.

Seroussi, K. (2000, February). We cured our son's autism. *Parents*, pp. 118–125.

Shaw, W. (1998). Abnormalities of the digestive system. In W. Shaw (Ed.), *Biological treatments for autism and PDD: What's going on? What can you do about it?* (pp. 124–138). Manhattan, KS: Sunflower Publications.

Sheinkopf, S. J., & Siegel, B. (1998). Home-based behavioral treatment of young children with autism. *Journal of Autism and Developmental Disorders, 38*, 15–23.

Siegel, B. (1995). Brief report: Assessing allegations of sexual molestation made through facilitated communication. *Journal of Autism and Developmental Disorders, 25*(3), 319–326.

Silliman, E. R. (1995). Issues raised by facilitated communication for theorizing and research on autism: Comments on Duchan's (1993) Tutorial. *Journal of Speech and Hearing Research, 38*, 200–206.

Smith, M. D., Hass, P. J., & Belcher, R. G. (1994). Facilitated communication: The effects of facilitator knowledge and level of assistance on output. *Journal of Autism and Developmental Disorders, 24*(3), 357–367.

Smith, T. (1996). Are other treatments effective? In C. Maurice, G. Greene, & S. C. Luce (Eds.), *Behavioral intervention for young children with autism* (pp. 45–62). Austin, TX: Pro-Ed.

Smith, T., Eikeseth, S., Klevstrand, M., & Lovaas, O. I. (1997). Intensive behavioral treatment for preschoolers with severe mental retardation and pervasive developmental disorder. *American Journal on Mental Retardation, 102*, 238–249.

Stehli, A. (1991). *The sound of a miracle*. New York: Doubleday.

Stokes, T. F., & Osnes, P. G. (1988). The developing applied technology of generalization and maintenance. In R. Horner, G. Dunlap, & R. L. Koegel (Eds.), *Generalization and maintenance: Life-style changes in applied settings*. Baltimore: Paul H. Brookes.

Tolbert, L., Haigler, T., Waits, M. M., & Dennis, T. (1993). Brief report: Lack of response in an autistic population to a low dose clinical trial of pyridoxine plus magnesium. *Journal of Autism and Developmental Disorder, 23*(1), 193–199.

Valluripalli, L., & Gillis, J. (2000, May). *Communication and language acquisition*. Paper presented at the meeting of the Association for Behavior Analysis, Washington, DC.

Wheeler, D. L., Jacobson, J. W., Paglieri, R. A., & Schwartz, A. A. (1992). *An experimental assessment of facilitated communication* (TR #92 – TA1). Schenectady, NY: OD Heck/ER DDSO.

Woolf, S. H. (1991). *AHCPR interim manual for clinical practice guideline development* (Agency for Health Care Policy and Research, Public Health Service; AHCPR Publication No. 91–00018). Rockville, MD: U.S. Department of Health and Human Services.

Zollweg, W., Vance, V., & Palm, D. (1997). The efficacy of auditory integration training: A double blind study. *American Journal of Audiology, 6*, 39–47.

PART V

CONTROVERSIES REGARDING SELF-HELP AND THE MEDIA

14

Self-Help Therapy

The Science and Business of Giving Psychology Away

GERALD M. ROSEN
RUSSELL E. GLASGOW
TIMOTHY E. MOORE

The notion that people can overcome problems through their own efforts was the basis of a social and philosophical movement long before modern book stores had "Self-Help" sections. In its earliest form, "self-help" referred to the coming together of peers who would assist each other independent of professional assistance. Katz and Bender (1976) traced the beginnings of these self-help peer efforts to 19th-century England. The phenomenon of peer self-help groups continues to the present day (Jacobs & Goodman, 1989), with Gartner and Riessman (1977) estimating at least 500 self-help organizations active in the United States two decades ago, a figure that is now dwarfed by hundreds of "chat" groups on the World Wide Web. (See also Chapter 15, for a discussion of the commercialization of self-help through the media.)

Self-help treatment books represent another early form of guidance, available to the public without the involvement of psychologists. Ellis (1977) suggested that the oldest and best-selling self-help text was the Bible, a document that developed without the assistance of mental health professionals. In more recent times, best-selling self-help books continue to be written by authors outside the health professions. Norman Vincent Peale's (1952) *The Power of Positive Thinking* was a best-seller through much of the second half of the 19th century. Peale was a minister, not a psychologist. At the time of the writing of this chapter, the *Wall Street Journal* (Best selling books, 2000) listed as number 10 on their Nonfiction Best Sellers List *The Art of Happiness* by the Dalai Lama.

Also coincidental to writing this chapter was an article in the January 10, 2000, edition of *Newsweek* titled "Self Help U.S.A." The article observed:

> Since Colonial times, Americans have devoured "success literature," those pragmatic guides to a better life from authors including Ben Franklin, Dale Carnegie. . . . Today they're called self-help books, and they constitute a $563 million-a-year publishing juggernaut. Books are just one avenue to a brand-new you. From seminars to CDs to "personal coaching," the self-improvement industry rakes in $2.48 billion a year, according to the research firm Marketdata Enterprises, which predicts double-digit annual growth through 2003.

Given the enormous popularity of self-help materials and their goal of helping people to help themselves, it is not surprising that psychologists and other health care professionals have provided their share of advice. A text by the physician Samuel Smiles (1881) titled *Self-Help* is an early example. Dr. Smiles (1886) also wrote *Happy Homes and the Hearts That Make Them*, a delightful text that contained chapters on "The Art of Living," "Influence of Character," and "Helping One's Self." Another self-help book more widely known to psychologists is Edmund Jacobsen's (1934) *You Must Relax*. A full accounting of the history of self-help books and influential authors has been provided by Starker (1989).

The explosive growth of do-it-yourself books that dominated the industry in the 1970s was nearly equaled by the development of self-help audiocassettes and videotape programs in the 1980s. A 1988 New York Times article reported that one company, Mind Communications, Inc., sold more than $6 million worth of subliminal tapes in that year, a tenfold increase in sales in just 2 years (Lofflin, 1988). The American Psychological Association also entered the business of developing, marketing, and promoting self-help audiocassettes during this time period, an issue discussed later in this chapter. In the 1990s yet another expansion occurred in the self-help industry as computer programs for self-change were developed (Newman, Consoli, & Taylor, 1997). Self-help over the Internet is the most recently developed avenue for delivering self-administered treatments to the public (Jerome & Zaylor, 2000; Strom, Pettersson, & Andersson, 2000).

The self-help industry has also grown by increasing the scope of issues it addresses. For example, in the area of parenting skills, there used to be general books of advice by authors such as Dr. Benjamin Spock. By the 1980s there were individualized audiotapes that parents could play to children before bedtime for the more specific purposes of eliminating fears or bed-wetting problems, or improving self-esteem. There was a book specifically targeted to help infants with colic (Ayllon & Freed, 1989) and another program directed at issues with toilet training (Azrin & Foxx, 1974). This trend toward greater specificity of focus, coupled with multiple modalities for delivering instructional programs, helps to explain how the self-help movement has become such big business (Lofflin, 1988; Self-help U.S.A., 2000).

PSYCHOLOGY'S CONTRIBUTION
TO SELF-HELP DURING THE 1970S

Although the history of self-help spans centuries, it was not until the 1970s that leading academic psychologists became involved to any serious extent in writing and promoting these programs. Lewinsohn wrote on depression (Lewinsohn, Munoz, Zeiss, & Youngren, 1979), Mahoney and Brownell on weight loss (Brownell, 1980; Mahoney & Mahoney, 1976), Heiman and LoPiccolo on sexual dysfunction (Heiman, LoPiccolo, & LoPiccolo, 1976), Coates and Thoresen on insomnia (1977), Lichtenstein on smoking cessation (Danaher & Lichtenstein, 1978), Zimbardo on shyness (1977), and Azrin on habit control (Azrin & Foxx, 1974; Azrin & Nunn, 1977). These individuals and other prominent psychologists contributed to what remains an unprecedented push by academicians to develop self-help therapies (Rosen, 1976a).

At first glance, the involvement of psychologists in the development of self-help materials would seem beneficial. Psychologists who provided advice to the public appeared to be following George Miller's (1969) urgings to "give psychology away" (p. 1074). Miller had used this phrase in his 1969 Presidential Address to the American Psychological Association to clarify what he saw as the major social responsibility of his profession—*to learn how to help people help themselves.* Certainly, this was the spirit of self-help or "do-it-yourself" treatment books in the 1970s—a theme of social consciousness that fit the times.

In line with Miller's urgings, psychologists appeared to be in a unique position to contribute to the self-help movement. By virtue of their training, psychologists were equipped to develop and evaluate the effectiveness of self-help instructional programs. Systematic work in the area had the potential to make available tested self-help therapies that consumers could self-administer or therapists could employ as adjuncts to their office-based interventions. No other professional group combined the skills and expertise that psychologists could bring to bear on the development of these programs. In the most utopian fantasy, psychology would bring a new dawn to the self-help movement, one in which empirically supported materials were available for specific targeted goals. At an American Psychological Association symposium in 1977, Albert Ellis invited psychologists to imagine the great potential for improved human functioning a set of scientifically researched, written, and periodically revised do-it-yourself manuals could have (Ellis, 1977). This was the enthusiasm that permeated the 1970s when psychologists rushed head-long into the self-help movement.

In addition to numerous self-help programs developed by prominent psychologists, a considerable amount of research was conducted in the 1970s. Glasgow and Rosen (1978, 1982) located 117 studies or case reports from this time period that evaluated behaviorally oriented self-help instructional materials. This constituted a sizeable body of research, for which psychologists are to be commended. Nevertheless, consideration of findings from these studies suggests a number of sobering conclusions, and demonstrates that the task of "giving psychology away" is more complex than initially thought.

THE LIMITS OF SELF-HELP

One important finding that emerged from research in the 1970s was that techniques applied successfully by a therapist were not always self-administered successfully. For example, a study by Matson and Ollendick (1977) evaluated a book titled *Toilet Training in Less Than a Day* (Azrin & Foxx, 1974). The study found that four of five mothers in a therapist-administered condition successfully toilet trained their children, whereas only one of five mothers who used the book in a self-administered condition was successful. This study also revealed that unsuccessful self-administered interventions were associated with an increase in children's problem behaviors and negative emotional side effects between mothers and children. In other words, highly successful interventions based in a clinic or supervised by a therapist did not necessarily translate into a helpful do-it-yourself program. The implications of this finding are apparent. If, for example, 100,000 copies of *Toilet Training in Less Than a Day* were sold and Matson's and Ollendick's (1977) findings applied, then 20,000 children might be expected to benefit from the self-instructional program, an impressive result at extremely low cost. Unfortunately, this seemingly positive outcome would say nothing about the 80,000 parents who might be frustrated, if not angry, because their children were among the 80% who did not respond to the program.

Matson and Ollendick's findings were not unique. Zeiss (1978) conducted a controlled outcome study on the treatment of premature ejaculation. Couples were assigned, on a random basis, to receive either self-administered treatment, minimal therapist contact, or therapist-directed treatment. As in earlier reports by Zeiss (1977) and Lowe and Mikulas

(1975), treatment with only minimal therapist contact was effective. But of six couples who self-administered their treatment in Zeiss's (1978) study, none successfully completed the program.

Yet another demonstration that well-intentioned instructional materials are not necessarily effective was provided in the 1970s. Rosen, Glasgow, and Barrera (1976) found that subjects who were highly fearful of snakes, and able to totally self-administer a written desensitization program, significantly reduced their anxiety reactions. This positive and encouraging outcome was tempered by the additional finding that 50% of subjects in the self-administered condition failed to comply with their program and carry out instructional assignments. Other studies on self-administered fear reduction programs had shown similar problems with compliance. For example, 14 of 29 eligible subjects dropped out in Clark (1973), 5 of 11 dropped out in Marshall, Press and Andrews (1976), and two thirds of subjects failed to complete their program in Phillips, Johnson, and Geyer (1972). Because the compliance/follow-through issue was a major impediment to helping people help themselves, an attempt to increase compliance was attempted by Barrera and Rosen (1977). In this study, phobic subjects were randomly assigned to the original self-administered program used in the 1976 study, or to a revised program with self-reward contracting. The addition of a self-reward contracting module to self-administered desensitization was consistent with self-management efforts promoted at the time (Mahoney & Thoresen, 1974). The results of the study were totally unexpected. As in the 1976 outcome study, 50% of subjects completed the original program and substantially reduced their fears. However, in the revised program, in which self-contracting had been added, the number of subjects who followed the instructions dropped from 50% to 0%. In other words, no subject completed the new and "improved" program. The importance of this unanticipated finding cannot be overemphasized for it clearly demonstrates that *well-intentioned changes in instructional materials can have a significant and negative impact on treatment outcome.* An important corollary to this point is that *the value of a self-help program can only be known by testing the specific content and instructions of that program under the conditions for which it is intended* (Glasgow & Rosen, 1978).

A RUSH TO PUBLISH

How did research findings from the 1970s impact the behavior of psychologists and the marketing of self-help products? Recall that this research supported several conclusions with clear implications for the clinical efficacy of self-help materials. First, the effectiveness of a treatment program under one set of conditions cannot be assumed to generalize to all conditions. Therefore, effective treatments based in a clinic may not yield proce dures that can be effectively self-administered. Second, ineffective programs can actually lead to the worsening of a problem. Third, well-intentioned instructional changes can lead to ineffective programs, such that the effect of *any* change in instructional content must be assessed, not assumed.

In the context of these cautionary conclusions drawn from research at the time, Zeiss published an untested revision of his program for premature ejaculators (Zeiss & Zeiss, 1978) despite the finding that no couple successfully administered an earlier draft. Azrin and Foxx (1974), in the face of ample evidence that toilet training was not accomplished in less than a day, contracted with a manufacturer of musical toilet seats and produced a combination program titled *Less Than a Day Toilet Trainer.* Azrin also published a new and untested book under the title *Habit Control in a Day* (Azrin & Nunn, 1977). Rosen, despite findings from well-controlled studies showing follow-through rates as low as 0%, revised his desensitization program yet another time and published *Don't Be Afraid* (Rosen, 1976b).

To appreciate fully these findings within a historical perspective, it can be noted that an earlier text titled *Don't Be Afraid* was published by Edward Cowles in 1941. This older *Don't Be Afraid* differed in content from the *Don't Be Afraid* of 1976, promoting nerve fatigue theories rather than "modern" desensitization. However, without appropriate research, psychologists and consumers cannot know if any advance in the self-treatment of phobic disorders occurred during a quarter of a century. For all we know, the 1941 *Don't Be Afraid* is just as effective, or more effective, compared to any of the well-intentioned drafts developed by Rosen in the 1970s. A similar historical example pertains to the self-help book *Mind-Power* by Zilbergeld and Lazarus (1987). As it turns out, Olston (1903) and Atkinson (1912) published advice books under the same *Mind Power* title. Because all three of these books lack empirical support, it is unknown whether the 1987 publication is any more helpful to readers than its predecessors published eight decades earlier.

In addition to rushing untested programs to market in an effort to "give psychology away," some psychologists (perhaps unwittingly) allowed their programs to be accompanied by unsubstantiated claims. This observation may provide the most dramatic demonstration that commercial factors, rather than professional standards, dominate the marketing of self-help books. Take for example, the 1976 *Don't Be Afraid*, which stated on its book jacket: "In as little as six to eight weeks, without the expense of professional counseling, and in the privacy of your own home, you can learn to master those situations that now make you nervous or afraid" (Rosen, 1976b). Note that research findings are not mentioned to clarify that, at best, 50% of people succeeded at self-administered treatment.

Other examples of claims made by publishers demonstrate the absence of constraint. Consider claims provided on the back cover of *In the Mind's Eye* (Lazarus, 1977), a book that presented cognitive-behavioral strategies that were touted to help the reader "enhance your creative powers, stop smoking, drinking or overeating, overcome sadness and despondence, build self-confidence and skill, overcome fears and anxiety." Lazarus (1977) personally intervened and was able to have the publisher drop these claims at the next printing of the text. But, three years later, Jerome Singer, then the Director of the Clinical program at Yale University, published *Mind Play: The Creative Uses of Fantasy* (Singer & Switzer, 1980), another book presenting cognitive-behavioral techniques. This time, according to the book jacket, a reader could "relax, overcome fears and bad habits, cope with pain, improve your decision-making and planning, perfect your skill at sports and enhance your sex life."

PSYCHOLOGY AND SELF-HELP IN THE 1980s AND 1990s

If the 1970s represented a decade during which psychologists tried to "give psychology away," unencumbered by concerns over the therapeutic value of their gifts, then the following two decades represented a time when marketing strategies were refined, programs proliferated, and data remained sparse (Rosen, 1987, 1993). We found support for this appraisal by logging on to the Web, at *www.amazon.com*, where 137 self-help books were listed for just the letter "A." Among the titles listed by *www.amazon.com* were *A.D.D. and Success*, *Access Your Brain's Joy Center: The Free Soul Method*, *Amazing Results of Positive Thinking*, and *The Anxiety Cure: An Eight-Step Program for Getting Well*. There also were many titles with the word "Art," as in *The Art of Letting Go*, *The Art of Making Sex Sacred*, and *The Art of Midlife*. Findings were similar for the letters B through Z.

We next visited PsychInfo, a search engine on the Web that the American Psychological Association maintains to archive articles from major peer-reviewed journals. In response to the key words "Self-Help Books," we found only 83 references listed for three entire decades, spanning 1970 through 1999. A somewhat more optimistic picture initially presented itself when we used the single key word "bibliotherapy." Here we found 60 records listed for the decade of the 1970s, 207 records listed for the 1980s, and 205 records listed for the 1990s. Such findings suggest a continuing and active interest in self-help materials, with psychologists productively studying and advancing the development of these programs.

Unfortunately, a more detailed inspection of the records was not encouraging. Take, for example, the bibliotherapy references for the time frame of 1990 through 1999. If one *excludes* from the 205 listed references all dissertations, chapters, commentaries, and review articles on the use of bibliotherapy, and *includes* only controlled studies that actually assessed a self-help book, then the number of references for the entire decade of the 1990s dwindles to 15. This represents a very small number of studies that bear on the thousands of self-help books available at *www.amazon.com* and other retailers. This state of affairs should not come as a surprise. The presence of limited empirical findings on the efficacy of current self-help books extends a finding obtained many years ago by Glasgow and Rosen (1978, 1982). These authors conducted two reviews of the literature on behavioral self-help programs in the late 1970s, and noted that the overall ratio of studies to books dropped from .86 to .59 from the time of the first review to the writing of the second.

At the same time that empirical findings have diminished, statements extolling the virtues of self-help therapies have been on the rise (Ganzer, 1995; Johnson & Johnson, 1998; Lanza, 1996; Quackenbush, 1992; Warner, 1992). In fact, of the 205 references that constituted the 1990s professional literature on bibliotherapy, there were more position papers urging psychologists to use these programs than there were controlled studies on their effectiveness. One author alone contributed 14 such references (Pardeck, 1990a, 1990b, 1990c, 1991a, 1991b, 1992a, 1992b, 1993, 1994, 1996, 1997; Pardeck & Markward, 1995; Pardeck & Pardeck, 1993, 1999).

At the same time that general position papers were arguing for the use of self-help books, several meta-analytic studies demonstrated the general effectiveness of tested programs (Gould & Clum, 1993; Kurtzweil, Scogin, & Rosen, 1996; Marrs, 1995; Scogin, Bynum, Stephens, & Calhoon, 1990). Nevertheless, these publications have added little to the advancement of empirically based self-help interventions. The general conclusion that self-help books can be effective has been known for some time (Glasgow & Rosen, 1978), along with the caution that the value of a particular program can only be known by testing that specific program. Grouping a limited number of extant studies into a meta-analysis provides no empirical basis for evaluating the vast majority of untested programs.

There also came into existence in the 1990s general reviews of self-help books, in the form of consumer guides for the public. The *Authoritative Guide to Self-Help Resources in Mental Health* (Norcross et al., 2000) is the most recent example of this genre. Such reviews are not based on actual outcome studies: Instead, their recommendations are based on personal preferences and/or surveys that poll psychologists on the materials they like to use. Popularity polls among psychologists who use self-help materials in therapist-assisted contexts provide no useful information on the public's ability to self-administer a program at home. This critical point was demonstrated back in the 1970s and was discussed earlier in this chapter. A "1–5 star" rating system provided by opinion surveys falls short of good science, and does not provide a sound basis for consumer confidence.

A FEW POSITIVE DEVELOPMENTS

The Debunking of Subliminal Self-Help Tapes

Despite the failure of psychologists to provide an empirical foundation on which to advance the bulk of self-help materials, there have been several positive developments for which psychologists are to be credited. One area in which psychologists have clarified important issues through the conduct of systematic research concerns subliminal self-help programs. These programs started to appear in bookstores in the form of self-help audiotapes in the early 1980s. They shared a common format in that the only consciously perceivable sounds on the tapes consisted of music, ocean waves, and the occasional bird cry. The intended therapeutic effects were purportedly brought about by the unconscious (i.e., subliminal) perception of specific affirmations contained on the tapes. The range of problems that subliminal tapes claimed to alleviate was extensive and included weight loss, memory enhancement, breast enlargement, improvement of sexual function, and relief from constipation.

The notion of technological mind control has always been a popular topic with journalists and the general public (Pratkanis, 1992). Without empirical support, claims of the sort made on behalf of subliminal self-help programs are no better and no different than similar declarations made on behalf of snake-oil over 100 years ago (Young, 1961). Moreover, subliminal self-help tapes are often manufactured in "Research Institutes" owned or staffed by self-proclaimed experts, "doctors," or hypnotists with little or no background in psychology. Not only are the marketing strategies of the subliminal tape industry similar to those of the snake-oil salesmen of yesteryear, the nature of the purported "cure" is similar in that regardless of the problem, there is ostensibly a single, common solution. Subliminal tapes supposedly send a therapeutic message directly to the unconscious, where it quickly transforms the listener's psyche. Similarly, snake-oil could supposedly cure anything from diphtheria to a toothache.

As Koshland (1991) noted, however, the ultimate criterion for resolving a scientific controversy must be the data in a well-run experiment. To the credit of psychologists, it did not take long for researchers to demonstrate that claims of subliminal therapeutic influence were unfounded (cf. British Psychological Society, 1992; Eich & Hyman,1991; Greenwald, Spangenberg, Pratkanis, & Eskenazi, 1991; Merikle, 1988; Merikle & Skanes, 1992; Moore, 1992; 1995; Pratkanis, Eskenazi, & Greenwald, 1994; Russell, Rowe, & Smouse, 1991).

Nevertheless, as with yesterday's critics of snake-oil, today's skeptics of subliminal self-help tapes have not generally been well received. One of us (Moore) was referred to as an "intellectual terrorist" in an advertising brochure by a Michigan manufacturer of subliminal self-help tapes (Mind Communications, 1990). Other critics within the scientific community have been subjected to personal attacks and insults by defenders of the subliminal tape industry.

Two methods have been used for testing the efficacy of subliminal tapes. As the tapes are designed to bring about improvements of various kinds, the most obvious means of appraising effectiveness would be to look for evidence of improved functioning or enhanced performance. In an innovative study by Pratkanis and colleagues (1994), participants listened daily for 5 weeks to tapes designed to improve either self-esteem or memory. Unbeknownst to the subjects, half of them received tapes that were mislabeled. That is, half the subjects with self-esteem tapes actually listened to tapes designed to improve memory. Similarly half the subjects who thought they had memory tapes were really listening to self-esteem tapes. Pre- and posttest measures of both self-esteem and memory revealed that no improvements in either domain of functioning were brought about by the use of the tapes. Interestingly, participants *believed* that they had benefited from the tapes in a manner consistent with the tapes' labels (and with the manufacturers' claims), even though objective measures showed no such improvements. The investigators thus obtained what they called an *illusory placebo effect*. Participants' expectations of improvement appear to have created the illusion of improvement, even though no improvement actually occurred.

Merikle and Skanes (1992) evaluated subliminal weight loss tapes by recruiting overweight subjects who had a desire to lose weight and who also believed that such tapes could help. Some participants were assigned to a placebo condition in which tapes identical to those in the weight loss condition were used, with the exception that the subliminal affirmations pertained to dental anxiety as opposed to weight loss. The appearance, packaging, and supraliminal materials on the placebo tapes were otherwise indistinguishable from the weight loss tapes. Another group of subjects was assigned to a "wait-list control" condition. All subjects were weighed once a week for 5 weeks. Subjects in all three groups lost about a pound over the 5 weeks, with no evidence of subliminal influences or of placebo effects. It seems likely that simply participating in the study may have made subjects more conscious of weight-related issues. Other investigators have found no evidence that subliminal tapes can improve study skills (Russell et al., 1991) or reduce anxiety (Auday, Mellett, & Williams, 1991).

Another evaluation approach has been to assess the nature of the subliminal auditory signal contained on the subliminal tapes. Although subliminal perception is a valid phenomenon, past research has shown that it occurs only under certain carefully controlled conditions. Subliminal perception is most appropriately defined as a situation in which there is a discrepancy between the viewer's phenomenal experience and his or her ability to discriminate between different stimulus states. Participants are often sensitive to stimuli they claim not to have seen. When required to distinguish between two or more stimuli, subjects can do so with some success, even while professing to be guessing (Holender, 1986). On the other hand, there is little reliable evidence of semantic processing of stimuli that cannot be discriminated (Cheesman & Merikle, 1986). Because stimulus discriminability is a necessary condition for semantic activation and attendant higher-level decision processes (Greenwald, 1992), a failure to demonstrate such discrimination would preclude any effects attributable to the semantic content of a word or message. With respect to subliminal tapes, Merikle (1988) showed that listeners were unable to distinguish a subliminal tape from a placebo control in a forced-choice task. This presence/absence discrimination required a "placebo" tape that was identical to its companion subliminal tape but without any subliminal message. Similarly, Moore (1995) used matched pairs of audiotapes from three different manufacturers and found that subjects could not discriminate between tapes containing ostensibly different subliminal messages. Merikle's and Moore's data are important, for they strongly suggest that no perceptual activity is triggered by the subliminal content of the tapes tested. It should not, therefore, surprise us that no therapeutic benefits have been obtained by any of the evaluation studies mentioned. The signal detection data show that there could never be any therapeutic benefits from such devices because they do not appear to contain a signal that is capable of triggering any perceptual activity—conscious or otherwise.

Of course, research findings have not led to the demise of subliminal audiocassettes, and many can be purchased along with self-help books at *amazon.com*. Nevertheless, the scientific community can take some credit for placing unfounded claims concerning these tapes in proper perspective.

The Evaluation of Self-Help Books

In addition to sound research evaluating the unfounded claims for subliminal self-help tapes, two systematic research programs have demonstrated how self-help books can be evaluated. Scogin and his colleagues (Scogin, Jamison, & Davis, 1990; Scogin, Jamison, & Gochneaur, 1989) have shown that a book on depression (Burns, 1980) can assist older adults with mood problems. Clum and his associates (Gould & Clum, 1995; Gould, Clum, & Shapiro, 1993; Lidran, Watkins, Gould, & Clum, 1995) have assessed a self-help book for the treatment of panic (Clum, 1990) and found support in controlled studies. At the same time, a recent study by Febbraro, Clum, Roodman, and Wright (1999) found that a totally self-administered application of the program was *not* effective, thereby casting "doubt on the efficacy of bibliotherapy and self-monitoring interventions when utilized absent from contact with a professional who conducts the assessment and monitors treatment compliance" (p. 209). This finding is consistent with previously cited research from the 1970s (Mattson & Ollendick, 1977; Zeiss, 1978), in which effects associated with therapist-assisted programs did not generalize to self-administered conditions, and more recent findings from a meta-analysis (Marrs, 1995), in which the amount of therapist contact was found to moderate outcome for individuals with anxiety problems.

It is highly significant that recent findings have replicated one of the most critical points derived from early research in the 1970s. Once again, it has been demonstrated that *the only way to know the effectiveness of well-intentioned instructional materials, when they are entirely self-administered, is to test those specific materials in the specific context of their intended usage. Psychologists who write self-help materials based on methods they find effective in office settings have no assurance that the public can successfully apply these procedures on their own.*

THE AMERICAN PSYCHOLOGICAL ASSOCIATION AND SELF-HELP

In spite of a few positive developments arising from systematic research efforts, and a better understanding of the potential benefits and limitations of self-help instructional materials, the overall landscape of self-help therapies has not improved over the years. Research findings have not led to the demise of subliminal audiocassettes, and the "Self-Help" section of any local bookstore convincingly demonstrates that untested books of advice flourish. Furthermore, psychologists have contributed to the glut of untested programs more than they have advanced the empirical foundations of self-help.

When Miller (1969), more than 30 years ago, urged psychologists to "give psychology away," his admonition was to promote "human welfare" and encourage the systematic development and assessment of effective self-help methods. Miller was not encouraging the headlong rush to market untested materials that has characterized the behavior of most authors over a 30-year period. In one sense, of course, there is nothing wrong with selling programs of advice. Certainly, everyone has the right to market whatever wisdom or guidance they wish to tell the public. On the other hand, psychologists who publish untested programs with misleading titles and unwarranted claims are not meeting professional standards, nor are these individuals applying the science of psychology for the advancement of self-care.

Psychologists who use the status of their profession to promote untested self-help programs provide justification for the public to be skeptical of science (Rosen, 1987, 1993). Robitscher (1980) expressed this concern while addressing a psychiatric audience:

> Every commercial exploitation of psychiatry, large or small, detracts from an integrity that psychiatry needs if it is to have meaning . . . when it becomes commercial, psychiatry dwindles down to a treatment of symptoms and an exploitation of techniques, a pretense of helping another that helps only the self. Many psychiatrists do not approve of the commercialism of psychiatry . . . but almost no psychiatrist speaks out against it. They turn their eyes away to avoid the sight of the money tree being shaken. . . . In the absence of psychiatrists who do not exploit psychiatry, those who do flourish.

There is little indication that the present situation is changing. In the 1970s and 1980s, interested groups within the American Psychological Association (APA) formed Task Forces on Self-Help Therapies. The Task Forces issued recommendations in 1978 and 1990 that suggested the following actions on the part of the APA:

1. Develop a set of guidelines for psychologists similar to the standards that guide developers of psychological test materials. Such guidelines could clarify methodological and outcome evaluation issues pertinent to the adequate development of self-help therapies.
2. Provide to psychologists a list of informational points that should be included in a commercially available self-help program. For example, books would contain a front page that discussed the extent to which the program was evaluated, recommended uses of the program, and reading level of the written instructions.
3. Provide a set of guidelines to aid psychologists who negotiate with publishers. The publication of sample contract clauses could significantly improve the position of psychologists who wish to set limits on claims or other promotional efforts.
4. Develop a short pamphlet to educate the public in the use of self-help therapies. The public could be informed as to how self-help therapies are used as adjuncts to therapist-assisted treatment, or by themselves. The issue of developing realistic expectancies in light of sensationalized claims could be addressed.
5. Consider working in concert with other professional or consumer-advocate groups in an effort to educate the consumer public and possibly develop a review process to review current evidence on self-help programs. In time, it was suggested, standards for establishing a formal "approval seal" might be possible.

The sponsoring groups who originated the Task Forces on Self-Help Therapies did not endorse any of these listed recommendations (Rosen, 1993, 1994). More significantly, the membership of APA was itself, perhaps unwittingly, involved in the development, marketing, and promotion of untested self-help materials. This came about through APA's 1983 purchase of *Psychology Today* and the companion *Psychology Today* Tape Series. By 1985, psychologists on the staff of *Psychology Today* were contracting for new audiotapes to be added to the series. A consumer could order *Personal Impact*, in which "clinical psychologist Cooper helps listeners become aware of and enhance their self-presentation to improve the impact they make on others." Under the catalog section "Becoming More Self-Reliant," the potential consumer was told, "You [can] become a more attractive, appealing person." About *Mental Imagery*, developed by Lazarus, the consumer was told: "Harness the powers of your mind! A noted psychologist explains how to use mental imagery to increase self-confidence, develop more energy and stamina, improve performance and proficiency, cope more effectively, overcome fears, and lose weight." The consumer who ordered one of these untested tapes also received a brochure with the name of the American Psychological Association on the front cover. On the back of this brochure, it stated, "Backed by the expert resources of the 87,000 members of the American Psychological Association, the *Psychology Today* Tape Series provides a vital link between psychology and you." By 1988, the APA Board of Directors had disengaged from *Psychology Today* and sold the magazine to another publisher. Thus, for at least 3 years, the most prominent professional organization representing psychologists actively sought, produced, and promoted untested self-help materials accompanied by unsubstantiated claims that were purportedly backed (without membership approval) by the then 87,000 members. By engaging in these activities, APA not only turned its eyes away from the "money tree" noted by Robitscher (1980), but, for a period of time, APA was itself harvesting the tree's fruits. Further, by developing and marketing untested self-help tapes, APA failed to provide a model or higher standard for its members, some of whom were publishing their own untested programs.

THE FUTURE OF SELF-HELP

In looking to the future, it appears that earlier recommendations to advance psychology's contributions to self-help require modification. These recommendations focused on programs that were likely to be developed by individual psychologists who worked in a specialized area of clinical expertise. The general notion was that the psychologist would assume responsibility for the proper development and assessment of self-help instructional materials, and that such professional organizations as APA would assist psychologists by providing guidelines for negotiating with publishers, and assist consumers by providing guidelines for how best to choose among available programs. This model for promoting empirically supported self-help materials has failed over the past three decades. An alternative model is needed.

In contrast to an "individualistic" approach to the development and evaluation of self-help materials, a "public health" approach is more likely to advance the efficacy of these programs. Such an approach would employ three of the key characteristics of public health: (1) "transdisciplinarity," (2) an emphasis on the reach and breadth of treatment effects, and (3) attention to the social-environmental context (Abrams et al., 1996; Brownson, Remington, & Davis, 1998; Winett, King, & Altman, 1989). The first of these characteristics, "transdisciplinarity," involves a team of professionals from diverse professions who collaborate to develop a program whose origins are in the project itself, rather than any one individual. Transdisciplinary approaches to self-help are needed because there are multiple factors, in addition to program content, that influence the availability, use, and results of these materials. These factors include marketing considerations, the framing of health messages, literacy and readability, and the family and sociomedical context in which a book is used. Consequently, there is room in the development of self-help programs for contributions from professionals in health communications, marketing, cultural diversity, and other health professions. Consider, for example, the topic of weight loss, one of the single most popular self-help topics. We have learned over the past decades that eating behavior and metabolic outcomes have numerous genetic, physiological, nutritional, exercise, physiology, and social determinants in addition to the core psychological and behavioral processes addressed by psychologists. Research programs that have continuity and address these issues within a broad multidisciplinary perspective stand the best chance of systematically advancing the development of an empirically based self-help weight loss program, as compared to programs developed by individual "leading figure" psychologists who write their well-intentioned but untested books of advice, only to be replaced by the next and most current "authority."

Instead of placing the possibly unreasonable burden on a single author for evaluation of a self-help program, the empirical basis for effective self-help programs will be advanced more rapidly by having programs tested by a variety of individuals, in a variety of settings, and under a variety of conditions. For example, if a national group of educators, family physicians, or researchers were to decide that a given health topic was appropriate for self-help intervention, then members of related professional organizations, clinics, HMOs, or health care systems could coordinate multiple site studies and pool their results. Examples of such multidisciplinary collaboration are available from the interactions among multiple scientists, including several psychologists, in formulation of the evidence-based guidelines on smoking cessation (Fiore, Jorenby, & Baker, 1997) and development of implementation guidelines by the Agency for Health Care Quality Research (*www.ahqr.gov*).

The second key feature of a public health approach is focus on the breadth and reach of an intervention program (Glasgow, Vogt, & Boles, 1999; Oldenberg, Hardcastle, & Kok, 1997). This perspective is focused on the consumer and can be contrasted with current self-help programs that generally have been developed without thorough consumer input. Self-help programs are more likely to attract and maintain the involvement of users to the extent that the program addresses the concerns and needs of a given group of consumers, and can present information and strategies in a way that makes sense from their worldview, personal model, or illness representation (Hampson, 1996; Leventhal & Diefenbach, 1991). In particular, there is concern regarding whether an intervention reaches those most in need—or only the relatively healthy, affluent individuals who have sufficient time and resources to devote to a program (Conrad, 1987; Glasgow, Eakin, & Toobert, 1996). This concern translates into suggestions for design and distribution of self-help books, and also evaluation criteria. Glasgow and colleagues (1999) suggested that health promotion researchers need to "RE-AIM" their evaluations to explicitly consider the issues of *Reach, Efficacy, Adoption* (within different settings and professionals), *Implementation*, and *Maintenance* of intervention effects. These criteria apply equally well to self-help psychology programs.

The third important characteristic of a public health approach is attention to the social-environmental context. As applied to self-help programs, social context issues include whether instructional materials are used as a stand-alone intervention or are supplemented by therapist or peer contact. We noted previously that some self-help books proved effective when used with therapist support, but not when used alone. It may also be that a book given to patients by their physician or therapist, whom patients understand will check on their progress, may be more effective than one they pick up at a bookstore. Other contextual factors include adjunctive therapeutic modalities such as proactive or reactive telephone support (e.g., Lichtenstein et al., 1996), the use of computer technology or "expert systems" to personalize or tailor intervention (Abrams, Mills, & Bulger, 1999), and an ever-increasing array of other modalities such as the Internet, videotape or CD-ROM materials, and World Wide Web chat rooms. Specification of the conditions under which a self-help program is effective, or not effective, will advance the development of empirically based self-help approaches and lead to development of a more sophisticated "stepped care, matched intervention approach" (Abrams et al., 1996; Brownell & Wadden, 1992) in which an initial assessment recommends conditions of administration likely to be most cost-effective for a given individual.

GUIDELINES FOR PSYCHOLOGISTS AND CONSUMERS

Authors of good will, religious leaders, and health professionals will continue to write books of advice just as they always have done. Nowadays, well-intentioned authors can also expand their advice-giving efforts to audio- and videotapes, and computerized programs. Publishers also will likely continue to promote these instructional materials, as they have done for many years, often accompanying their products with unwarranted titles and claims. Of course, "business as usual" in the self-help industry does not assure us that this year's book of advice will be more effective than last year's best-seller.

In the 1970s, there was a sense of great optimism that the science of psychology was in a unique position to contribute to the advancement of self-help therapies. Recommendations were made to encourage psychologists to use their unique research and clinical skills to develop and promote empirically supported self-help programs. With the wisdom of hindsight and 30 years of experience, we now see that earlier recommendations made to psychologists who wanted to "give psychology away" were overly optimistic. The notion that individual psychologists would carry the burden of assessing and improving their programs, while a professional organization such as the American Psychological Association would assist with supportive guidelines, has not been realized.

It is clear that self-help has not advanced substantially over the past three decades and it is unlikely to advance over the next 30 years if prevailing models are maintained. Unless a new direction is taken, there is no reason to expect that the next *Don't Be Afraid*, published perhaps in the year 2010, will be any more effective than the *Don't Be Afraid*s of 1976 and 1941, or that the next *Mind-Power* will be anymore effective than the *Mind Power*s of 1987, 1912, or 1903. It is in this context that we provide guidelines for psychologists who hold an interest in advancing the empirical status of self-help therapies, and recommend a new, broader, and more inclusive approach to the development, use, and evaluation of self-help therapies. Rather than focusing all the responsibility on an individual author of a self-help program, a public health approach to self-help is strongly encouraged. This broader based approach involves the coordinated efforts of health organizations, clinician groups, government agencies, and professional societies. Based upon this approach and the consideration of "who benefits under what conditions," we have developed a checklist of questions (see Table 14.1) to help developers of self-help programs address key issues *before* marketing their programs. This table uses the RE-AIM framework previously discussed to organize questions under the headings of Reach, Efficacy, Adoption, Implementation, and Maintenance.

The checklist provided in Table 14.1 can also help consumers who are considering adoption of a particular program and want to consider the full range of issues that may affect their selection. However, since the vast majority of current self-help products remain untested, a consumer interested in self-change must follow a few very simple rules. First, the consumer can take comfort in the notion that most self-help products are inexpensive, and, in that regard, there is little harm in buying the product. Next, the consumer should appreciate that claims made for the product are not to be taken seriously unless there is independent empirical evidence in support of the claims. This point is true even when the author of a program is a noted authority within a professional group, such as psychology or psychiatry. Third, the consumer should not feel bad or experience any self-blame if the instructional materials are difficult to apply, or not helpful when applied. Like the 80% of mothers who could not use on their own a toilet training procedure for their children (Matson & Ollendick, 1977), the 100% of males who could not successfully self-administer a program for sexual dysfunction (Zeiss, 1978), the 100% of snake phobics who failed to implement a self-administered desensitization procedure with self-reward contracting (Barrera & Rosen, 1977), and the panic disorder patients who failed to benefit from their self-administered program (Febbraro et al., 1999), the consumer may be dealing with an untested product that simply is not written in a manner that people can use.

In closing, we want to recall the 1977 symposium on Self-Help Therapies that was mentioned earlier in this chapter. At that event, Albert Ellis invited psychologists to imagine the great potential a set of scientifically based do-it-yourself manuals could have. Ellis and others in the 1970s held out a great deal of hope that psychologists would contribute to the development of effective and empirically based self-help programs, thereby fulfilling Miller's (1969) directive to promote human welfare by "giving psychology away." More than three decades later, we continue to support the idealism of the 1970s, and continue to believe that psychologists will play an important role in the development of effective self-help materials. Imagine if you will, to paraphrase Ellis, that a multidisciplinary group of professionals develops self-help programs, educates consumers in their proper use, and continually evaluates and improves these programs in the context of long-term public health projects. It is in this vision of "program-based" methods, rather than "individually authored" products, that the future of an empirically sound self-help movement lies. With a touch of irony for individual authors and their economically motivated publishers, it will be these organizationally based programs that move to the top of best-seller lists.

TABLE 14.1. Guidelines for Developing, Selecting, or Evaluating a Self-Help Program: Questions to Ask

REACH (How broadly applicable is the program?)

1. What percentage of the population having the particular problem, goal, or diagnosis is this program designed to address? Are there subgroups that are more or less likely to participate in this type of program?
2. Are there data on the percentage of individuals who were offered this program who tried it?
   a. If yes, what percentage participated and were they different from those who declined?

EFFICACY (How effective is this program?)

1. Has this program been evaluated? If yes:
   a. Did it do better than a randomized or other type of control condition?
   b. Did the program produce improvements on objective measures of outcome?
   c. Were results reported for all persons who began the program—or only those who liked it and finished?
2. Has the program been evaluated for possible negative or unwanted side effects? If so, what were these?
3. Under what conditions has the program been administered? (Do NOT assume that results will be the same under different conditions.)
   a. Completely self-administered; minimal therapist contact; as a supplement to regular counseling.
   b. What modalities has the program been tested under (e.g., written form; audio- or videotape; computer administered, etc.)?
4. What is the cost of the program—both for purchase and amount of time required relative to other alternative programs?
5. Does the evidence for the program appear to match the claims that are made of it?

ADOPTION (How broadly has the program been used by groups other than the authors—and have the results of these other groups been equally positive?)

1. Is there any information on the range of groups of clinicians, health systems, or researchers who have used or tested the program?
2. Is there any information on the types of professionals or organizations that are likely to use versus not use this program?

IMPLEMENTATION (How easy to use is the program?)

1. What percentage of the initial users of this program complete the program, and how are they different from those who do not?
2. Are there any patient, setting, or procedural considerations for which this program seems to work best?
3. Is there any way to get consultation or technical assistance with the program, if needed?

MAINTENANCE (Does the program produce long-term or lasting results?)

1. What are the longest follow-up assessments that have been conducted, and does the program still seem effective at longer-term follow-ups?
2. Have the organizations or clinicians that have used the program continued to use it?

GLOSSARY

Adoption: The percentage and representativeness of professionals (or medical groups, clinics, health systems, and so on) who will use a given intervention or self-help program.

Bibliotherapy: The use of written materials (e.g., books, manuals) to further a personal goal or therapeutic objective.

Breadth: The range of applicability of a program. In this case, how broad a cross-section of patients and providers will use and benefit from the program.

Compliance: The extent to which a patient follows professional advice. This term has largely been superseded by alternatives such as "self-management," which suggests a more central role for the patient in behavior change (Glasgow & Anderson, 1999).

Program Completion: The percentage and representativeness of persons beginning a program who complete the intervention and follow its recommendations. This term, like "self-management," is preferred to the term "compliance."

Reach: The percentage of persons with a given condition or problem who try a given approach or intervention, and the representativeness of this group of the entire population exhibiting this problem.

Self-Help: The efforts of an individual to achieve behavior change or other personal goals without professional assistance.

Social-Environmental context: The setting in which persons live (their family, neighborhood, cultural group, income level) and in which a program is used (e.g., purchased at a bookstore, used as part of therapy with a professional).

Subliminal: Commonly thought of as referring to the presentation of a stimulus below a threshold of conscious awareness, this term is best defined as a discrepancy between viewers' phenomenal experience and their ability to discriminate among different stimulus states.

Transdisciplinarity: Professionals from a variety of disciplines working together to address a problem.

REFERENCES

Abrams, D. B., Mills, S., & Bulger, D. (1999). Challenges and future directions for tailored communications research. *Annals of Behavioral Medicine*, 21, 299–306.

Abrams, D. B., Orleans, C. T., Niaura, R. S., Goldstein, M. G., Prochaska, J. O., & Velicer, W. (1996). Integrating individual and public health perspectives for treatment of tobacco dependence under managed care: A combined stepped care and matching model. *Annals of Behavioral Medicine*, 18, 290–304.

Atkinson, W. W. (1912). *Mind-Power: The secret of mental magic.* Chicago: Yogi Publication Society.

Auday, B. C., Mellett, J. L., & Williams, P. M. (1991, April). *Self-improvement using subliminal self-help audiotapes: Consumer benefit or consumer fraud?* Paper presented at the annual meeting of the Western Psychological Association, San Francisco.

Ayllon, T., & Freed, M. (1989). *Stopping baby's colic.* New York: Putnam.

Azrin, N. H., & Foxx, R. M. (1974). *Toilet training in less than a day.* New York: Simon & Schuster.

Azrin, N. H., & Nunn, R. G. (1977). *Habit control in a day.* New York: Simon & Schuster.

Barrera, M., Jr., & Rosen, G. M. (1977). Detrimental effects of a self-reward contracting program on subjects' involvement in self-administered desensitization. *Journal of Consulting and Clinical Psychology, 45*, 1180–1181.

Best selling books. (2000, January 7). *Wall Street Journal*, p. W4.

British Psychological Society. (1992). *Subliminal messages in recorded auditory tapes, and other "unconscious learning" phenomena.* Leicester, England: Author.

Brownell, K. D. (1980). *The partnership diet program.* New York: Rawson.

Brownell, K. D., & Wadden, T. A. (1992). Etiology and treatment of obesity: Understanding a serious, prevalent, and refractory disorder. *Journal of Consulting and Clinical Psychology, 60*, 505–517.

Brownson, R. C., Remington, P. L., & Davis, J. R. (1998). *Chronic disease epidemiology and control* (2nd ed.). Washington, DC: American Public Health Association.

Burns, D. D. (1980). *Feeling good: The new mood therapy.* New York: Morrow.

Cheesman, J., & Merikle, P. M. (1986). Distinguishing conscious from unconscious perceptual processes. *Canadian Journal of Psychology, 40*, 343–367.

Clark, F. (1973). Self-administered desensitization. *Behaviour Research and Therapy, 11*, 335–338.

Clum, G. A. (1990). *Coping with panic.* Pacific Grove, CA: Brooks/Cole.

Coates, T., & Thoresen, C. E. (1977). *How to sleep better: A drug-free program for overcoming insomnia.* Englewood Cliffs, NJ: Prentice-Hall.

Conrad, P. (1987). Who comes to worksite wellness programs? A preliminary review. *Journal of Occupational Medicine, 29*, 317–320.

Cowles, E. S. (1941). *Don't be afraid!* New York: McGraw-Hill.

Danaher, B. G., & Lichtenstein, E. (1978). *Become an ex-smoker.* Englewood Cliffs, NJ: Prentice-Hall.

Eich, E., & Hyman, R. (1991). Subliminal self-help. In D. Druckman & R. Bjork (Eds.), *In the mind's eye: Enhancing human performance* (pp. 107–119). Washington, DC: National Academy Press.

Ellis, A. (1977, August). Rational-emotive therapy and self-help therapy. In G. M. Rosen (Chair), *Non-prescription psychotherapies: A symposium on do-it-yourself treatments.* Symposium conducted at the meeting of the American Psychological Association, San Francisco.

Febbraro, G. A. R., Clum, G. A., Roodman, A. A., & Wright, J. H. (1999). The limits of bibliotherapy: A study of the differential effectiveness of self-administered interventions in individuals with panic attacks. *Behavior Therapy, 30,* 209–222.

Fiore, M. C., Jorenby, D. E., & Baker, T. B. (1997). Smoking cessation: Principles and practice based upon the AHCPR guidelines, 1996. *Annals of Behavioral Medicine, 19,* 213–219.

Ganzer, C. (1995). Using literature as an aid to practice. *Families in Society, 75,* 616–623.

Gartner, A., & Riessman, F. (1977). *Self-help in the human services.* San Francisco: Jossey-Bass.

Glasgow, R. E., Eakin, E. G., & Toobert, D. J. (1996). How generalizable are the results of diabetes self-management research? The impact of participation and attrition. *Diabetes Educator, 22,* 573–585.

Glasgow, R. E., & Rosen, G. M. (1978). Behavioral bibliotherapy: A review of self-help behavior therapy manuals. *Psychological Bulletin, 85,* 1–23.

Glasgow, R. E., & Rosen, G. M. (1982). Self-help behavior therapy manuals: Recent development and clinical usage. *Clinical Behavior Therapy Review, 1,* 1–20.

Glasgow, R. E., Vogt, T. M., & Boles, S. M. (1999). Evaluating the public health impact of health promotion interventions: The RE-AIM framework. *American Journal of Public Health, 89,* 1322–1327.

Gould, R. A., & Clum, G. A. (1993). A meta-analysis of self-help treatment approaches. *Clinical Psychology Review, 13,* 169–186.

Gould, R. A., & Clum, G. A. (1995). Self-help plus minimal therapist contact in the treatment of panic disorder: A replication and extension. *Behavior Therapy, 26,* 533–546.

Gould, R. A., Clum, G. A., & Shapiro, D. (1993). The use of bibliotherapy in the treatment of panic: A preliminary investigation. *Behavior Therapy, 24,* 241–252.

Greenwald, A. G. (1992). New look 3: Unconscious cognition reclaimed. *American Psychologist, 47,* 766–779.

Greenwald, A. G., Spangenberg, E. R., Pratkanis, A. R., & Eskenazi, J. (1991). Double-blind tests of subliminal self-help audiotapes. *Psychological Science, 2,* 119–122.

Hampson, S. E. (1996). Illness representations and self-management of diabetes. In J. Weinman & K. Petrie (Eds.), *Perceptions of illness and treatment: Current psychological research and applications* (pp. 323–347). Chur, Switzerland: Harwood Academic.

Heiman, J., LoPiccolo, L., & LoPiccolo, J. (1976). *Becoming orgasmic: A sexual growth program for women.* Englewood Cliffs, NJ: Prentice-Hall.

Holender, D. (1986). Semantic activation without conscious identification in dichotic listening, parafoveal vision, and visual masking: A survey and appraisal. *Behavioral and Brain Sciences, 9,* 1–23.

Jacobs, M. K., & Goodman, G. (1989). Psychology and self-help groups: Predictions on a partnership. *American Psychologist, 44,* 536–545.

Jacobson, E. (1934). *You must relax: A practical method of reducing the strains of modern living.* New York: McGraw-Hill.

Jerome, L. W., & Zaylor, C. (2000). Cyberspace: Creating a therapeutic environment for telehealth applications. *Professional Psychology: Research and Practice, 31,* 478–483.

Johnson, B. W., & Johnson, W. L. (1998). Self-help books used by religious practitioners. *Journal of Counseling and Development, 76,* 459–466.

Katz, A. H., & Bender, E. I. (Eds.). (1976). *The strength in us: Self-help groups in the modern world.* New York: New Viewpoints.

Koshland, D. (1991). Credibility in science and the press. *Science, 254,* 629.

Kurtzweil, P. L., Scogin, F., & Rosen, G. M. (1996). A test of the fail-safe N for self-help programs. *Professional Psychology: Research and Practice, 27,* 629–630.

Lanza, M. L. (1996). Bibliotherapy and beyond. *Perspective in Psychiatric Care, 32,* 12–14.

Lazarus, A. (1977). *In the mind's eye.* New York: Rawson.

Leventhal, H., & Diefenbach, M. (1991). The active side of illness cognition. In J. A. Skelton & R. T. Croyle (Eds.), *Mental representation in health and illness* (pp. 246–272). New York: Springer-Verlag.

Lewinsohn, P., Munoz, R. F., Zeiss, A., & Youngren, M. A. (1979). *Control your depression.* Englewood Cliffs, NJ: Prentice-Hall.

Lichtenstein, E., Glasgow, R. E., Lando, H. A., Ossip-Klein, D. J., & Boles, S. M. (1996). Telephone counseling for smoking cessation: Rationales and review of evidence. *Health Education Research, 11,* 243–257.

Lidran, D. M., Watkins, P. L., Gould, R. A., & Clum, G. A. (1995). A comparison of bibliotherapy and group therapy in the treatment of panic disorder. *Journal of Consulting and Clinical Psychology, 62,* 865–869.

Lofflin, J. (1988, March 20). Help from the hidden persuaders. *New York Times.*

Lowe, J. C., & Mikulas, W. L. (1975). Use of written material in learning self-control of premature ejaculation. *Psychological Reports, 37,* 295–298.

Mahoney, M. J., & Mahoney, K. (1976). *Permanent weight control.* New York: Norton.

Mahoney, M. J., & Thoresen, C. E. (1974). *Self-control: Power to the person.* Monterey, CA: Brooks-Cole.

Marrs, R. W. (1995). A meta-analysis of bibliotherapy studies. *American Journal of Community Psychology, 23,* 843–870.

Marshall, W. L., Presse, L., & Andrews, W. R. (1976). A self-administered program for public speaking anxiety. *Behaviour Research and Therapy, 14,* 33–40.

Matson, J. L., & Ollendick, T. H. (1977). Issues in toilet training normal children. *Behavior Therapy, 8,* 549–553.

Merikle, P. M. (1988). Subliminal auditory tapes: An evaluation. *Psychology and Marketing, 46,* 355–372.

Merikle, P. M., & Skanes, H. (1992). Subliminal self-help audiotapes: A search for placebo effects. *Journal of Applied Psychology, 77,* 772–776.

Miller, G. A. (1969). Psychology as a means of promoting human welfare. *American Psychologist, 24,* 1063–1075.

Mind Communications. (1990). *Dr. Paul Tuthill's subliminal success: Subliminal tapes and accessories for effortless self-improvement.* Grand Rapids, MI: Author.

Moore, T. E. (1992). Subliminal perception: Facts and fallacies. *Skeptical Inquirer, 16,* 273–281.

Moore, T. E. (1995). Subliminal self-help auditory tapes: An empirical test of perceptual consequences. *Canadian Journal of Behavioral Science, 27*, 9–20.

Newman, M. G., Consoli, A., & Talor, C. B. (1997). Computers in assessment and cognitive behavioral treatment of clinical disorders: Anxiety as a case in point. *Behavior Therapy, 28*, 211–235.

Norcross, J. C., Santrock, J. W., Campbell, L. F., Smith, T. P., Sommer, R., & Zuckerman, E. L. (2000). *Authoritative guide to self-help resources in mental health*. New York: Guilford Press.

Oldenburg, B., Hardcastle, D. M., & Kok, G. (1997). Diffusion of innovations. In K. Glanz, F. M. Lewis, & B. Rimer (Eds.), *Health behavior and education research: Theory, research and practice* (pp. 270–286). San Francisco: Jossey-Bass.

Olston, A. R. (1903). *Mind power and privileges*. Boston: Rockwell and Churchill Press.

Pardeck, J. T. (1990a). Bibliotherapy with abused children. *Families in Society, 71*, 229–235.

Pardeck, J. T. (1990b). Children's literature and child abuse. *Child Welfare, 69*, 83–88.

Pardeck, J. T. (1990c). Using bibliotherapy in clinical practice with children. *Psychological Reports, 67*, 1043–1049.

Pardeck, J. T. (1991a). Bibliotherapy and clinical social work. *Journal of Independent Social Work, 5*, 53–63.

Pardeck, J. T. (1991b). Using books to prevent and treat adolescent chemical dependency. *Adolescence, 26*, 201–208.

Pardeck, J. T. (1992a). Using books in clinical practice. *Psychotherapy in Private Practice, 9*, 105–119.

Pardeck, J. T. (1992b). Using reading materials with childhood problems. *Psychology: A Journal of Human Behavior, 28*, 58–65.

Pardeck, J. T. (1993). *Using bibliotherapy in clinical practice: A guide to self-help books*. Westport, CT: Greenwood Press.

Pardeck, J. T. (1994). Using literature to help adolescents cope with problems. *Adolescence, 29*, 421–427.

Pardeck, J. T. (1996). Bibliotherapy: An innovative approach for helping children. *Early Child Development and Care, 110*, 83–88.

Pardeck, J. T. (1997). Recommended self-help books for families experiencing divorce: A specialized form of bibliotherapy. *Psychotherapy in Private Practice, 15*, 45–58.

Pardeck, J. T., & Markward, M. J. (1995). Bibliotherapy: Using books to help children deal with problems. *Early Child Development and Care, 106*, 75–90.

Pardeck, J. T., & Pardeck, J. A. (1993). *Bibliotherapy: A clinical approach for helping children*. Langhorne, PA: Gordon & Breach Science.

Pardeck, J. T., & Pardeck, J. A. (1999). An exploration of the uses of children's books as an approach for enhancing cultural diversity. *Early Child Development and Care, 147*, 25–31.

Peale, N. V. (1952). *The power of positive thinking*. Englewood Cliffs, NJ: Prentice-Hall.

Phillips, R. E., Johnson, G. D., & Geyer, A. (1972). Self-administered systematic desensitization. *Behaviour Research and Therapy, 10*, 93–96.

Pratkanis, A. (1992). The cargo cult science of subliminal persuasion. *Skeptical Inquirer, 16*, 260–272.

Pratkanis, A. R., Eskanazi, J., & Greenwald, A. G. (1994). What you expect is what you believe (but not necessarily what you get): A test of the effectiveness of subliminal self-help audiotapes. *Basic and Applied Social Psychology, 15*, 251–276.

Quackenbush, R. L. (1992). The prescription of self-help books by psychologists: A bibliography of selected bibliotherapy resources. *Psychotherapy, 28*, 671–677.

Robitscher, J. (1980). *The powers of psychiatry.* Boston: Houghton-Mifflin.

Rosen, G. M. (1976a). The development and use of nonprescription behavior therapies. *American Psychologist, 31*, 139–141.

Rosen, G. M. (1976b). *Don't be afraid.* Englewood Cliffs, NJ: Prentice-Hall.

Rosen, G. M. (1987). Self-help treatment books and the commercialization of psychotherapy. *American Psychologist, 42*, 46–51.

Rosen, G. M. (1993). Self-help or hype? Comments on psychology's failure to advance self-care. *Professional Psychology: Research and Practice, 24*, 340–345.

Rosen, G. M. (1994). Self-Help Task Forces revisited: A reply to Dr. Lowman. *Professional Psychology: Research and Practice, 25*, 100–101.

Rosen, G. M., Glasgow, R. E., & Barrera, M., Jr. (1976). A controlled study to assess the clinical efficacy of totally self-administered systematic desensitization. *Journal of Consulting and Clinical Psychology, 44*, 208–217.

Russell, T. G., Rowe, W., & Smouse, A. (1991). Subliminal self-help tapes and academic achievement: An evaluation. *Journal of Counseling and Development, 69*, 359–362.

Scogin, F., Bynum, J., Stephens, G., & Calhoon, S (1990). Efficacy of self-administered treatment programs: Meta-analytic review. *Professional Psychology: Research and Practice, 21*, 42–47.

Scogin, F., Jamison, C., & Davis, N. (1990). Two-year follow-up of bibliotherapy for depression in older adults. *Journal of Consulting and Clinical Psychology, 58*, 665–667.

Scogin, F., Jamison, C, & Gochneaur, K. (1989). Comparative efficacy of cognitive and behavioral bibliotherapy for mildly and moderately depressed older adults. *Journal of Consulting and Clinical Psychology, 57*, 403–407.

Self-help U. S. A. (2000, January 10). *Newsweek,* pp. 43–47.

Singer, J. L., & Switzer, E. (1980). *Mind play: The creative uses of fantasy.* Englewood Cliffs, NJ: Prentice-Hall.

Smiles, S. (1881). *Self-help: With illustrations of character, conduct, and perseverance.* Chicago: Belford, Clarke.

Smiles, S. (1886). *Happy homes and the hearts that make them.* Chicago: U. S. Publishing House.

Strom, L., Pettersson, R., & Andersson, G. (2000). A controlled trial of self-help treatment of recurrent headache conducted via the Internet. *Journal of Consulting and Clinical Psychology, 68*, 722–727.

Warner, R. E. (1992). Bibliotherapy: A comparison of the prescription practices of Canadian and American psychologists. *Canadian Psychology, 32*, 529–530.

Winett, R. A., King, A. C., & Altman, D. G. (1989). *Health psychology and public health: An integrative approach.* New York: Pergamon.

Young, J. H. (1961). *The toadstool millionaires: A social history of patent medi-*

cines in America before federal regulation. Princeton, NJ: Princeton University Press.

Zeiss, R. A. (1977). Self-directed treatment for premature ejaculation: Preliminary case reports. *Journal of Behavior Therapy and Experimental Psychiatry, 8,* 87–91.

Zeiss, R. A. (1978). Self-directed treatment for premature ejaculation. *Journal of Consulting and clinical Psychology, 46,* 1234–1241.

Zeiss, R. A., & Zeiss, A. (1978). *Prolong your pleasure.* New York: Pocket Books.

Zilbergeld, B., & Lazarus, A. A. (1987). *Mind power.* Boston: Little, Brown.

Zimbardo, P. G. (1977). *Shyness.* New York: Jove.

15

Commercializing Mental Health Issues

Entertainment, Advertising, and Psychological Advice

NONA WILSON

For many mental health professionals—clinicians, researchers, and professors—the world of television talk shows and mass market self-help handbooks might seem easily dismissed as having little or no relevance to their field of study, in terms of either its current practice or its future direction. Having worked hard to complete academic training, attain professional credentials, and practice within established ethical guidelines, many mental health professionals may be tempted to view the popular "advice industry"—that is, the mass market, commercialized version of professional, psychological expertise—as merely an annoying doppelgänger that is best ignored. Although there certainly are professional grounds for regretting the existence of this shadow presence, ignoring it, I will argue, is much like ignoring a sizable and growing tumor. Not only has the advice industry used the mental health profession as a host to sustain it, but it has metastasized in ways that threaten to displace the profession itself.

The thesis of this chapter is that when psychological expertise and services enter the mass market, they become beholden to marketplace values and strategies. Moreover, as commercialized forms of mental health expertise and services succeed in the mass market, they not only degrade, but ultimately displace, the original upon which they are based. The chapter will consider the convergence of two dominant cultural movements—

entertainment and advertising—over the course of the last two centuries that underlie the current success of the "advice industry." By tapping into the persuasive devices of those movements, the commercial advice industry significantly enhances its power to alter public opinions about the mental health profession, and to substitute itself for professional expertise and services. Before beginning our historical explication, let us first quickly preview where it will lead us: the talk shows and self-help products of the last two decades.

THE CONTEMPORARY ADVICE INDUSTRY

Talk TV: 1985–2002

By the late 1980s and 1990s, daytime television talk shows were at once enormously popular and highly controversial, with both characteristics in large part resulting from the shows' often sensational and tawdry content. Bringing viewers a mix of shows as shocking as "Abducted by a Serial Killer," "Women Who Marry the Men Who Rape Them," "Satanists," "Killer Kids," or "Sexually Assaulted under Hypnosis" alongside more mundane programs such as "Prom Makeovers" and "Perpetual Dieters"—and presenting all of them with the same degree of fanfare and urgency—talk TV earned almost equal measures of public fascination and disdain. Both fans and detractors held strong convictions. The critics decried the "lows" to which the shows were sinking and issued warnings about how the programs not only reflected, but contributed to, contemporary social ills and a frightening loss of public decency. Some critics focused on the guests, labeling them "sleazy," "aberrant" "trailer trash" looking for their 15 minutes of fame and willing to do anything to get it. Some critics blamed the audiences and called attention to the public's unchecked voyeurism and prurient interest in other people's suffering. Still others saw the producers, hosts, and experts as parasitic, with interests only in making money while feigning concern for the guests.

Such criticism resonated with many who saw the entire enterprise as "tasteless," but it also provoked equally vigorous—and disparate—defense of the shows. Some fans dismissed outright any preachy, moralistic examinations and defended their "right" to be entertained by guests willing to make their private lives public. Such hosts as Jerry Springer endorsed that position by maintaining that the shows were about creating spectacles and should be understood as such. Others argued that the shows provided a public service. Some hosts vehemently maintained their interest in helping people to help themselves, and claimed that guests or topics were selected to educate viewers and to give voice to a segment of the population in need of a public venue to air its concerns. This position was supported by some academics and cultural critics who maintained that the shows, though in some ways problematic, actually embodied both the country's long-standing democratic ideals and its contemporary diversity (Munson, 1993; Rapping, 1996). Those more positively inclined proposed that by bringing to the fore in an open and participatory format the full range of American experiences, particularly those of historically marginalized groups, the shows advanced feminist and multicultural principles.

Although the debate went on about whether the shows entertained, enlightened, or degraded their audiences, one thing was clear: The shows were hugely popular. By the mid-1990s, their heyday, there were at least 30 daytime talk shows in syndication, giving viewers at least 150 shows to choose from each week (Heaton & Wilson, 1995). Even with such shows as those of Oprah, Donahue, Geraldo, Ricki Lake, Montel Williams, Sally, Jenny Jones, Jerry Springer, and Leeza capturing substantial market shares, producers were confident that there was room for more. *America's Talking*, a cable station airing only talk shows 24 hours a day, was introduced in 1994 (Heaton & Wilson, 1995).

With the shows' popularity came profits. By 1994, each talk show episode was costing only about $50,000 to produce, yet earning about $400,000 in profits (Williams, 1993). The launching in 2000 of *O: The Oprah Magazine*, Oprah's monthly publication, was identified as the most successful in the history of magazine publishing, and the average paid circulation reached 2 million within just 6 months ("Oprah on Oprah," 2001). All told, Oprah's fortune is now estimated at about 800 million dollars (Gonser, 2001). Although the frenzy over the shows has calmed down and their numbers have diminished, the shows that remain continue to attract huge audiences and loyal fans.

What has happened—and continues to happen—on talk shows, and the public's response to it, should be of considerable interest to the mental health profession. Through the shows millions of people have obtained their understanding not only of mental health problems and their symptoms, but also of "professional" intervention and treatment. During the 1980s and 1990s, about 70% of the shows included guests identified as "experts" (Timney, 1991). On many of those shows, the standard procedure was to spend a considerable portion of the allotted time elaborating and demonstrating the guests' problems and then, in the final moments of the show, to involve the "expert" whose job it was to offer solutions and neatly sum up the show.

Heaton and Wilson (1995) discussed in detail the myriad difficulties arising from that formula. Because of the repeated blurring of distinctions between credentialed mental health professionals and unregulated, pseudo-experts (the so-called relationship therapists, life-style advisers, communication experts), the public has been at a disadvantage in attempting to sort out what constitutes standard practice within the field. Beyond that, even when qualified professionals participate, their ability to fairly represent current knowledge or practice within the field is severely impaired because of the shows' format and goals, which hinge on capturing and maintaining the audience's attention. The overarching point is that because of their enormous popularity, their repeated use of mental health issues, and the involvement of "experts," the shows have become the leading source of mental health information for the general public—whether or not that information is accurate or useful. The difficulties are only further exacerbated by the willing participation of professionals. A similar circumstance exists with a closely related branch of the advice industry, self-help publications and products (see Chapter 14), which talk shows have both drawn from and promoted.

"Self-Help" in the 1980s and Beyond

As millions of viewers tuned in to their favorite talk shows, they not only learned about guests' problems and the experts' advice, they also "learned" that the problems were both common and underrecognized. Moreover, they were urged to seek help, conveniently available through self-help publications, groups, workshops, and seminars promoted during the shows. Reviews of the self-help movement (Kaminer, 1993; Rapping, 1996; see also Chapter 14) have demonstrated that the most popular trend during the 1980s was the "recovery" movement. The prevailing recovery "programs" were modeled after the 12-step approach of Alcoholics Anonymous (see Chapter 10) and were applied to a loose constellation of problems ranging from drug abuse to codependency (see Chapter 4), eating disorders, gambling, compulsive shopping, and even child abuse (Kaminer, 1993). Talk shows, along with primetime docudramas and made-for-TV movies, brought the names of "Bradshaw, Beattie, Norwood, and Schaef—the gurus of the recovery movement—and words like 'inner child,' 'dysfunctional families,' 'working your program,' 'recovering abuser' " into common parlance and public consciousness (Rapping, 1996, pp. 16–17). As the public became steeped in the recovery model through television, they bought the accompanying publications *en masse*. Kaminer (1993) reported that by 1991, Harper's listed *Codependent No More* by Melody Beattie as one of its top sellers, having achieved over 100 weeks on the *New York Times* best sellers list and having sold over 2 million copies. Likewise, Anne Wilson Schaef's 1990 publication *Meditations for Women Who Do Too Much* is reported to have sold over 400,000 copies in one year, while John Bradshaw's *Bradshaw On: The Family and Healing the Shame That Binds You* doubled that number (Kaminer, 1993).

But by the mid-1990s, amid increasing skepticism about ever-widening definitions of abuse, increasingly sensational claims of childhood traumas (see Chapter 8), and growing intolerance of the preoccupation with victimization (Kaminer, 1993), the direction of the self-help tide was turning. In doing so, the movement successfully deflected the backlash it had provoked and responded to the public's irritation—or boredom—with victims by creating a new breed of self-help leaders. Perhaps the best example of how this worked is revealed by the evolution of "Dr. Laura" Schlessinger's career. In 1993, as an outsider to the recovery movement, she derided it and its followers. Putting an especially sharp point on growing public sentiment, she labeled the books as "apologetic" and their leaders as "rationalizing their self-destructive behaviors by identifying themselves as 'sick' " (Klinghoffer, 1999, p. 56). Such views were met with quick success—and contempt—and the resulting controversy helped her to ride to the top of a new wave of "self-help" experts advocating personal responsibility. In 1995, Schlessinger published *Ten Stupid Things Women Do to Mess up Their Lives* and in 1996 a companion version for men, along with *How Could You Do That?!: The Abdication of Character, Courage, and Conscience*. Several more books followed, the titles of which leave no doubt that there is a market for self-help that scolds and goads, including her 2000 release *Cope with It*!

A slightly more palatable version of the personal responsibility creed reaches millions of people via Oprah's current "lifestyle expert," Dr. Phil McGraw. Dubbing him "Tell-It-Like-It-Is-Phil," Oprah openly delights in the "no-nonsense" oneliners he fires at deserving guests. Dr. McGraw, who holds a PhD in psychology (emphasis in neuropsychology), has a substantial background in civil court consultation, having cofounded Courtroom Sciences, Inc., a legal consulting business (Tarrant, 1999). He met Oprah Winfrey, in fact, when he served as a consultant to her much-publicized "Mad Cow" trial.[1] She reportedly appreciated his help and encouraged him to write an advice book. His brand of self-help not only stresses responsibility but seeks to minimize ambiguity in personal matters by applying the clear-cut certitude that derives from law. That black-and-white approach is the hallmark of his first book, *Life Strategies, Doing What Works, Doing What Matters* (1999). The recommended strategies are based on his "laws of life," and the text sold more than 500,000 copies in less than 3 months (Tarrant, 1999).

Undoubtedly, McGraw's connection with Oprah has helped fuel his success, but her selection of him also reflects her savvy in knowing how to yet again ride the current trend of popular sentiments to its maximum success. She opened her 13th season in 1998 with yet another "renewed mis-

---

[1]During a 1998 interview on her show with rancher Howard Lyman, Oprah stated that she would never eat another hamburger because of the risk of "mad cow" disease (bovine spongiform encephalopathy, or BSE). Beef prices in the United States quickly fell to the lowest in years and Oprah was named in a $12 million, widely publicized libel suit. Oprah won the case.

sion to enlighten, educate and entertain" her viewers. Promising that television can "do something it's never done before," that is, "change people's lives," Oprah introduced "Change Your Life TV" and a panel of experts, each with their own elixir ("Oprah begins 13th season," 1998).

"Dr. Phil" is chief among those experts, and his second book, *Relationship Rescue*, is also a best seller and is regularly promoted, as are his Relationship Rescue seminars, on the show. He is featured prominently on Oprah's Webpage, where "visitors" can call up his preformulated advice to a wide range of topics, participate in online "chats" with him, or send e-mail questions to him. His advice is also a feature of *O: The Oprah Magazine*, which is also advertised during her show.

Leaning perhaps even further to the business side of the self-help market is Stephen Covey, who has attracted a legion of followers. With approximately 12,000 "licensed client facilitators," Covey brings his "seven habits of highly effective people" to nearly 750,000 people each year through workshops (Klinghoffer, 1999). Undergirding his approach is the idea that "effective" people "do not blame circumstances, conditions, or conditioning for their behavior" (Klinghoffer, 1999). Covey's strategy, like Dr. Phil's, is a crossover approach that encourages people to view their personal lives as they would business transactions and to seek a similar degree of efficiency.

Pitching life in that direction appealed to a public that (especially during a time when the United States had been enjoying unprecedented economic growth) apparently no longer wanted to be—or to tolerate—victims. The self-help movement of the 1990s emphasized success. Tony Robbins, perhaps the reigning guru of self-help, urges his followers to train themselves to go to "an exalted state" (McGinn, 2000). Robbins came to fame in the early 1990s on late-night television and through "infomercials" for a product whose name heralds the new self-help's credo: "Personal Power." With such works as *Awaken the Giant Within: How to Take Immediate Control of Your Mental, Emotional, Physical and Financial Destiny* (1991); *Unlimited Power* (1997); *Giant Steps* (1994); and *The Driving Force* (2002), Robbins's message is all about grand ambitions and taking charge. Whether the subject is love or money, the same advice applies. His push of "Unlimited Success" (attainable in only 30 days) has been exactly that for him. He now has a cult-like following, advising everyone from average citizens to pro athletes to former President Bill Clinton. He earns about $60,000 per appearance: In 1993, his seminars alone grossed approximately $22 million, with another $30 million from infomercial sales (Stanton, 1994). The stock value of his new venture, a self-improvement Website, is estimated at $300 million (McGinn, 2000).

No survey of the contemporary self-help market would be complete without some discussion of John Gray, who epitomizes several of the movement's central controversies. Although the greeting on his Website may seem grandiose—"Welcome to John Gray's universe"—his doctrine is certainly far-reaching. His seminal first book, *Men Are from Mars, Women Are from Venus* (1992) has reportedly sold at least 10 million copies and has been translated into 43 languages ("Club Med teams," 2000; "Los Angeles Times," 1998). Gray has appeared on dozens of television shows, from Oprah to Larry King, and has been featured in *Time*, *Newsweek*, and *People* magazine. He pens a nationally syndicated column that reaches approximately 30 million readers through such newspapers as the *Los Angeles Times*, the *New York Daily News*, and the *Chicago Sun-Times* ("All about John Gray," 2001). He contributes to *Redbook* and *Parents* magazines, both of which have sizeable readerships. There are also a half-dozen other books, as well as tapes, CDs, videos, workshops (including an exclusive deal with ClubMed), radio and television "Mars and Venus" talk shows, and much more ("Club Med teams," 2000; "Dr. John Gray," 1999; Glieck, 1997).

Unlike the self-help advisors who came on the market in the early and mid-1990s, Gray is less scolding, more "supportive," and he found his niche by smoothing out gender conflicts. His bromide is that conflicts between men and women arise from their inherent differences, which should be honored. This more acceptance-based doctrine links him to earlier, more "therapeutic" incarnations of the self-help movement. This therapeutic slant (along with its remarkable simplicity and spiffed-up sexism) is the source of much of the controversy surrounding his popularity. In *Mars and Venus in the Bedroom* (1995), for example, Gray gave advice about what he believes to be effective communication skills: To "give feedback in sex, it is best for women to make little noises and not use complete sentences" because "when a woman uses complete sentences, it can be a turn off" (p. 57). Additionally, he instructed readers about the meaning of women's underwear. He explained that when "she wears silky pink or lace, she is ready to surrender to sex as a romantic expression of loving vulnerability" (p. 106) and that a "cotton T-shirt with matching panties . . . may mean she doesn't need a lot of foreplay" (p. 107). Moreover, according to Gray such clothing indicates that the woman wearing it "may not be in the mood for an orgasm" but rather might be "happy and satisfied" by feeling her partner's "orgasm inside her" (p. 107). Offering such opinions is part of what Gray states he does "best," which he believes is to "save marriages, create romance and passions and relationships" (Adler, 1995, p. 96).

"Dr." Gray's professional credentials have been strongly contested. He received a doctorate in human sexuality and psychology from Columbia Pacific University (CPU) in California, a correspondence school with a questionable accreditation (Gleick, 1997; Rebuttal from Uranus, n.d.). He holds no professional license, yet is repeatedly identified (often by himself) as a "leading authority in communication and relationships" ("Welcome to John Gray's Universe," 2001). The self-anointed nature of his credentials makes his juggernaut of Mars/Venus Couples counseling centers, with their attendant "certification" process for therapists, especially controversial (Marano, 1997).

As with talk TV, the self-help vanguard has amassed enormous profit (see Chapter 14). The books alone are a $563 million-a-year business (McGinn, 2000). In fact, sales of "advice" books were substantial enough by 1983 to warrant their own category in the *New York Times* best sellers listings. An announcement made by the *Times* explaining the additional category stated that it was added because biographies, memoirs, and essays of contemporary and historical interest were potentially being "crowded off the General list by books concerned mainly with self-improvement" ("Times Book Review," 1983). There are also workshops and seminars. When conducted by the masters themselves, those events can draw thousands of participants. A recent Tony Robbins seminar attracted 10,000 people at $49 per head—a substantial bargain per person compared with the $6,995 per ticket price to his week-long "Life Mastery" course (McGinn, 2000). That kind of revenue makes speaker fees such as the $50,000 John Gray commands seem modest and begins to account for Gray's estimated $10 million annual income. Further, Robbins, Covey, and Gray each oversee a cadre of acolytes who are sanctioned to provide additional workshops (as many as 500 a month for Gray) or other services and who share in the profits (McGinn, 2000). There are also the tapes, CDs, and Websites with additional "related" products for sale. All told, the business generates an estimated at $2.43 billion a year (McGinn, 2000).

Contemporary popular culture is riddled with commercialized versions of professional psychological expertise and services. Commercialization can be understood as consisting of two processes: (1) commodification, which involves transforming an item into an object of purchase and which renders vendability as its primary value, and (2) marketing, which involves inserting the object into a network of exchanges of goods (Guelzo, 1995). Through TV talk shows and self-help books, mental health expertise and services have been commodified and reduced to their most vendable component—advice. Despite the fact that advice giving is controversial among professionals and has traditionally been discouraged, it is highly marketable and yields large profits for an industry of assorted products and services which then form a commercial nexus.

The commercialized advice industry works as follows. The talk shows feature experts who have written books that are promoted on the shows. The shows become popular for offering such help (and for entertaining audiences). Because they are popular, the shows serve to endorse the experts and their products, aiding sales. The experts become well known and are then invited to more shows because of their popularity. The experts expand their product-line to include more books, tapes or CDs, and workshops that are then marketed as products seen on the popular shows. The workshops then become a vehicle for selling even more products. The success of all of this encourages more "experts" to participate, increasing competition and often necessitating a second rung of sanctioned representatives who can assist in carrying forward the message and the products. The increased competition encourages grander claims about the products' results, which in turn increase sales, and the commercialization process continues in a seemingly ever-widening loop.

The resulting thicket of commercialized advice has overgrown its professional base. The advice industry's reach now far exceeds that of any profession newsletter, journal, or public education campaign. Although mass market, commercialized advice constitutes a very large and thriving industry, within that industry self-help methods with empirical support are sorely underrepresented (see also Chapter 14). Likewise, the power of popular talk show hosts or "advice experts" to shepherd public perceptions outstrips that of any professional organization or representative. One of the main reasons is that legitimate professionals do not make public claims about instant cures or unfailing success.

To understand the significance of the current commercialization of advice, mental health professionals must look beyond the borders of their own profession—or even the latest trends in the advice market. In fact, the basis of any critical understanding of this topic is a historical examination of its cultural antecedents. Let us then consider two of those antecedents: entertainment and advertising. These industries are instructive for at least two reasons: (1) First arising in the context of the relatively new and competitive mass market of the late 1800s, each adapted itself to that marketplace, and (2) as a result, over time each has helped to anchor that marketplace and the values that now buttress the commercialization of mental health expertise and services.

MARKETPLACE VALUES

Entertainment

The advice industry products that have attained widespread popularity and that form the cornerstone of mass market psychological materials draw extensively upon entertainment values to capture their intended audiences' attention and secure their purchases. The connection is so well recognized that some refer to this blending of psychological materials and entertainment as "psychotainment" (Marano, 1997). Let us consider just a few examples of this new brand of mass amusement. Workshops offered by Tony Robbins, creator of the "Personal Power" programs and leading self-help guru, provide an excellent starting point.

Before his arrival, a crowd of thousands is likely to be already in the auditorium or convention center, having pushed their way in, and chanting for "Tony" to appear. He takes the stage and, larger-than-life (literally, as his image may be broadcast on multiple 22-foot screen TVs), he commands the crowd's attention (Greenberg, 1998). Throughout his performances, the lighting changes, rock music blares, or he squirts audience members with huge water-guns—all to keep them attentive and energized (Greenberg, 1998). TONY ROBBINS t-shirts are thrown periodically to the crowd, and dozens of times he invites the audience to mimic his actions or speech. He also is known to get the crowd collectively moaning and groaning, making the noises of "sexual ecstasy" in order to link public speaking (ostensibly a needed skill for achieving Personal Power) to orgasm (Levine, 1997).

But the real spectacle, the hallmark of many Tony Robbins workshops, is the firewalk or "Mind Revolution." Imitating a former mentor (a practice Robbins strongly promotes), he persuades his overwrought crowds to walk across 12-foot-long beds of red-hot, burning logs. Advertisements for the workshops promise that participants will learn to "overcome lifelong fears . . . addictions . . . impotence . . . chronic depression" and learn to know, instantly, the most effective ways to communicate with and persuade people" (Leikind & McCarthy, 1991, p.185). The walk serves as both a climax to some of Robbins's workshops and as alleged evidence for their success. The walks are often accompanied by much "weeping and jubilation" (Griffin & Goldsmith, 1985, p. 41) and participants celebrate having overcome their fears by accessing what they have been told are their previously "untapped" mental powers (Leikind & McCarthy, 1991, p. 186). Then, in their exhausted, exhilarated state, participants are prompted to buy more products or sign up for a weekend's worth of training: "I guarantee it will be the most important weekend of your life. Put it on Mastercard or Visa—however you have to pay for it" (Griffin & Goldsmith, 1985, p. 48).

Although the firewalks generate a great amount of interest and awe, firewalkers succeed in traversing red-hot embers without burning their feet not because of special mental powers, but because of the laws of thermal physics (Leikind & McCarthy, 1991). Despite what our "common sense" tells us, red-hot wood actually has a low heat capacity and poor thermal conductivity, and participants' feet are not likely to be on the logs long enough to get hot enough to burn. Additionally, by exhausting participants beforehand, creating a noisy, distracting environment, and teaching them distraction techniques to use while walking, Robbins diminishes participants' likelihood of feeling (that is, noticing) pain (Leikind & McCarthy, 1991).

Encouraging the public to believe that firewalking is evidence of improved life skills and that firewalking will somehow help people to unleash their personal power is all part of the package of products that Robbins considers "psychology made practical" (Levine, 1997). His description not only promotes his products while misleading the public, but also obscures the truth and implies that scientifically based psychology is impractical or of little use to the public.

Robbins is not alone, however, in his use of entertainment strategies to market psychological materials. John Gray's entire oeuvre was inspired by the entertainment industry; Gray reports that he stumbled upon the Mars portion of his Mars/Venus analogy after watching the movie ET (Marano, 1997). Gray has since continued to use entertainment to promote his products, which are so wide-ranging and entertainment-oriented as to be considered "an almost Disneylike multimedia empire" (Weber, 1997, p. B6). Gray's recent CD features a Mars and Venus song he helped to write. Alternating female and male vocalists sing such lyrics as "Everytime I try to tell you something, you get mad and run off to your cave" and "You're so up and down with your emotions" (quoted in Gleick, 1997, p. 69). Gray even secured a deal with Mattell to produce a board game for adults under the Mars/Venus moniker ("All about John Gray," 2001). He launched a one-man Mars/Venus Broadway show that opens with a 1½-hour monologue, unaided by notes or a prompter. Gray explained his ability to pull off the lengthy soliloquy by noting that prior to writing his first book, he had already learned "which stories, which examples entertain people and validate them" (Marano, 1997). His presentations have been described as involving "splashy verbal theatrics—including tears, lots of humor, a good bit of insight, personal anecdotes and his obvious eagerness to please" (Peterson, 1994, p. 3C).

Often, as with Gray's work, the advice industry's use of entertainment to sell products seems humorous and, as a consequence, harmless. But in fact, amusement is one of entertainment's most insidious qualities (Postman, 1985). Such critics of mass media as Marshall McLuhan (1964; McLuhan & Fiore, 1967) and Mark Crispin Miller (1988) have argued that the mass media's adoption of a perpetually "hip" and irreverent stance lulls us into a bemused state, disengages our critical impulses, and effectively installs illusion in place of reality. This bait-and-switch routine brings with it serious implications for the mental health profession. Daytime television talk shows provide an excellent example of how the advice industry has applied theatrical techniques to mental health issues and then downgraded those issues to sources of mass audience amusement, thereby effectively replacing the reality of the guests' lives, their difficulties, and the real-life mental health interventions that might help them, with satisfying illusions (Heaton & Wilson, 1995).

The power of mass entertainments to distort reality and to turn everything into a source of amusement was meticulously examined by Neal Gabler in *Life: The Movie, How Entertainment Conquered Reality* (1998). Gabler elucidated two issues that are especially useful in considering the commercialization of mental health issues: (1) the triumph of sensation over intellect, and (2) the mass market's preference for provoking a common response, not a unique experience.

The Triumph of Sensation over Intellect

Gabler (1998) maintained that entertainment is "first and foremost about the triumph of sensation over reason" (p. 31). As mass market entertainment became available to the general public in the mid-1800s, a wide range of highly sensational forms proliferated: dime novels, caustic humor almanacs, erotic and pornographic literature, crime pamphlets, dance crazes, loud bands, and renderings of more temperate plays that featured bawdy, melodramatic acting and that larded the scenes with magicians, acrobats, and dancers where originally there were none (Gabler, 1998). In essence, the early mass entertainments established a circus-style standard, to which subsequent mass entertainments and their audiences have remained true.

Early popular entertainments were also criticized as uncultured, immoral, and base. Although such entertainments might then tip their hat to more refined sensibilities, they primarily catered to physical, that is, sensational, responses rather than attempting to edify their audiences. The link between the early circus-style standard and the tactics employed today by Robbins, the daytime talk shows, and others in the commercialized advice industry is clear. Another legacy of the triumph of sensation over intellect, however, which may not be as apparent, is the privileging of emotion over reason—an inheritance that is far from inconsequential for the mental health profession.

The commercialized advice industry trades in emotion. Tony Robbins, for example, defined success as living "your life in a way that causes you to feel tons of pleasure and very little pain" (Stanton, 1994, p. 106). John Gray maintained that "everyone wants lasting happiness" and that his goal is to "share with millions of readers some simple solutions" to help them attain it ("Los Angeles Times," 1998). For all practical purposes, the industry's survival depends upon appeals to emotion. Provoking strong emotions—whether they be joy, sorrow, anger, or compassion—generates thrills. On any daytime television talk, viewers can witness not only the entertainment value of watching others experience intense emotion, but also the contagious nature of strong emotion. The guests unleash their emotions through tearful confessions, angry outbursts, or loving embraces, and soon enough the audience members are doing the same.

Especially useful to the advice leaders is that the emotion they stir up can short-circuit thinking. The advice industry strongly advocates the misleading notion that all emotions are valid and, therefore, can reliably guide decision making. When paired with the injunction to "follow your heart" or to "listen to your inner voice," emotional responses take on a glorified, or in Robbins's language, an "exalted" state. A kind of "I feel it, so it must be true" logic takes hold. Cognitive therapists label this "emotional reasoning" and recognize it as a common, problematic approach to decision making that can easily distort information (Beck, 1995).

The advice industry fosters "emotional reasoning" by provoking strong emotion and then suggesting that such emotion confirms a proposition's veracity. Emotional response is the standard by which the industry and its followers evaluate all sorts of issues, from the validity of a concept or testimony to the effectiveness of an intervention. In fact, the advice industry encourages the public to entertain any idea that elicits emotions, no matter how far-fetched. Because its primary objective is profit, the commercial advice industry is served well by fostering the notion that "anything goes" in psychology (Stanovich, 2001, p. 219). It is particularly cunning, however, that commercialized advice is articulated in the language of emotion and personal experience, which stress individuality, given that one of its dominant goals is to ensure a common response.

Targeting a Common Response

Some of the criticisms of early popular entertainments emphasized their failure to achieve the status of "art"—whose goal, unlike entertainment, is to transport the observer/participant from the physical realities of the moment toward a reputedly more worthy, eternal world of the mind and spirit (Gabler, 1998). Inherent in this difference between art and entertainment are their divergent stances toward their intended audiences. Art fosters individual, unique, and inventive responses. Entertainment not only expects, but depends upon a collective, generic, and formulaic response. That is, to appeal to the greatest possible audience—and that is the market goal of entertainment—entertainment must target a common response.

Of importance to mental health professionals is not whether art is better than entertainment, but what the consequences are for mental health expertise and services entering a marketplace dominated by entertainment values. One consequence, among many, is a tilt toward the generic. A hallmark of professional mental health services, regardless of theoretical orientation, has been to respect the uniqueness of individuals and, even when using established interventions, to fit the treatment to the individual, not the individual to the treatment.

Commercialized advice, however, like mass market entertainment, cannot lucratively accommodate idiosyncratic approaches. Unshared concerns and their solutions have little mass appeal. Nor are advice-industry products well-suited to sustained exploration of unique life experiences that may bring many people to the same problem, but for widely differing reasons. Ferreting out unique aspects of an issue, understanding the sources that contribute to and maintain an individual's difficulties, and then collaboratively identifying potential solutions that might work for that individual—that is, doing the work of therapy—can be a laborious process with little entertainment value. Thus, a more general prescription is called for, and that is what the advice industry delivers.

In an examination of advice giving on call-in radio shows, Hutchby (1995) identified a set of communication techniques for "doing expertise" that reshape the more typically private dialogue of advice giving into an exchange that will interest the listening public (p. 226). Among those techniques is what he terms a "generalizing orientation" by which the expert appears to respond to an individual's concern, but is in fact targeting the wider listening audience. This is in keeping with Scannell's (1991) observation that "all broadcast output is knowingly, wittingly public" (p. 11). As a result, even when advice is putatively designed for a particular person, it is in reality contrived for the benefit of a wider audience (Hutchby, 1995). "Doing expertise," then, replaces personal response with public retail. What is at once interesting and regrettable about this tendency is the contradiction that inheres: That is, the ultimate outcome of all the commercial clamor about personal growth may be depersonalization, a generic conceptualization of psychological concerns and their resolution.

A generic approach is the most predictable outcome because what sells to a mass audience is a kind of one-size-fits-all method of mental health evaluation and service provision. Problems are prepackaged and labeled—anger, jealousy, spousal arguments, infidelity—and stripped of idiosyncratic details. Likewise, their solutions are fashioned in a ready-to-wear style, often delineated in "steps." Although the "steps," ostensibly, are intended to make the advice user-friendly, they are typically articulated in language that is so generic as to be of no practical use, but that seems specific.

On Oprah's Website, one simply needs to click on Dr. Phil's list of "topics for advice" to see this phenomenon in action. The "topics" are organized into three categories—Marriage and Couplehood, Family, and Life Strategies. Moreover, there are separate pages devoted to "Dr. Phil's Relationship Advice," his "Relationship Rescue Online," as well as his "Getting Real Video Seminar" through which visitors to the site are encouraged to "experience Dr. Phil's life-transforming message from your very own computer!" (*www.oprah.com*). The elaborate organization and the process of having to click into separate pages to access the advice suggest that one is about to obtain something fairly significant. What one obtains are such items as "Dr. Phil's Anger Management Plan" outlined in seven steps, including such "transformative" advice as "Have the courage to change your life," or "Realize you don't have to get mad," and "Choose a different reaction."

Although such recommendations as "Have courage" or "Don't get mad" are unlikely to be harmful, they in no way represent specialized, professional knowledge. They reflect what Stanovich (2001) termed "personal psychologies" that are "often unfalsifiable" and represent "a mixture of platitudes and clichés, often mutually contradictory, that are used on the appropriate occasion" (p. 213). McGraw offered a dozen other such "plans" on his site. What they lack in specificity, they make up for in certitude.

McGraw's "Formula for Success" includes such steps as identifying "the bad spirits that contaminated" previous relationships, embracing the "Personal Relationship Values that will configure" one for success, and committing to "tapping into" one's "core of consciousness" (McGraw, n.d.). Dr. Phil's "Ten Steps to Positive Communication and Rescuing Your Relationship" instruct visitors to the site that "if something is wrong with your relationship it's because you set it up that way" and that they must "teach people how to treat" them (McGraw, n.d.). Likewise, his "Claiming Responsibility" advice states authoritatively that "partners in a relationship either contribute or contaminate to [sic] what's happening between them. There's no middle ground. If one partner is unhappy, they [sic] begin to contaminate the relationship with their [sic] negative feelings" (McGraw, n.d.). His "Seven Step Strategy for Reconnecting with Your Partner" and his "Life Laws" (McGraw, n.d.) are similarly constructed with injunctions to "define and diagnose your relationship" and to "take personal responsibility," and are replete with such mottos as "you either get it or you don't" and "life is managed, not cured."

Such pronouncements are popular, in part, because they reassure people that the world is as they already wish it to be. The success that McGraw and other advice leaders enjoy by selling what the public already accepts can largely be accounted for by a few well-established phenomena. First, psychologists (Dickson & Kelly, 1985) have demonstrated that most people will endorse generic personality analyses as specific to themselves. The tendency has been termed the P. T. Barnum effect, a label that reflects the circus-act quality of eliciting the response (see also Chapter 2). Thus, when McGraw and others in the commercialized advice industry put forth generalized recommendations, recipients of the information are likely to experience it erroneously as having unique relevance to them. Ofshe and Walters (1994) described the desire to accept even dubious explanations as "an effort after meaning" (p. 45). That is, when people seek help they are predisposed to believe in it—and belief alone is often sufficient to effect change. The power of that phenomenon is so well documented that in scientific studies researchers must account for placebo effects to accurately determine an intervention's true therapeutic quality (see Chapters 6 and 11). Moreover, even if the recommendations offered are Barnum-like and the results are placebo-induced, many of those who experience benefit will be willing to attest that the benefit resulted from the recommendations (Gilovich, 1991; Hines, 1998; Medawar, 1967), thus rendering testimonials largely useless as dispositive evidence.

Understanding the mechanisms by which commercialized advice achieves its results does not mean, however, that those mechanisms are always harmless. The vast majority of people watching Oprah, buying her magazine, or seeking Dr. Phil's assistance are women. Because of that, baldly declaring that if something is wrong with a relationship the person set it up that way and has the responsibility to "teach people" how to be better partners is problematic. Such statements ignore the power differences (economic, social, and physical) between women and their male partners; in doing so they suggest that solutions to difficult problems are much more easily achieved than they actually are. If, for example, we consider only the very frequent and dangerous incidents of domestic violence leveled against women, such directives, even if intended to be liberating, are not especially helpful. They may even prove risky if not carefully tailored to the individual and pursued in the context of real support.

Dr. Phil, of course, is not alone in marketing generalized advice. John Gray considers his work a "fantastic opportunity . . . to share with millions of readers some simple solutions for some of life's most important, most persistent problems" ("Los Angeles Times," 1998). Apparently, Gray sees no contradiction in proposing "simple solutions" for complex, long-standing problems. But then, as noted earlier, the commercialized advice industry depends on the notion that anything goes and, in order to sell products without empirical support, has a "vested interest in obscuring the fact that there are mechanisms for testing behavioral claims" (Stanovich, 2001, p. 219).

Thus, within the commercialized advice paradigm, the only interesting problems are common ones and profound solutions—we are to believe—reside in the catchy phrase or pithy slogan. But as oversimplified as this approach to mental health may be, it is far from benign. Commercialized advice is troublingly reductive. First, the industry depersonalizes private concerns by compressing widely varying and nuanced issues into a single problem. Then, having defined the problem, it offers up a single, simple solution. By pressing upon society a uniform approach to mental health problems and their solutions, the commercialized advice industry promotes conformity. As standardized advice pours forth from commercial radio and television, popular press books, and mass-audience seminars, the public is flooded with ideas and products that are safely mainstream—conventional, conservative, and consumerist—not because those are necessarily the ideas or products that are most useful to the public, but because they succeed in the mass market.

Ultimately, the commercialized advice industry becomes a tool for discouraging real change or enhanced psychological understanding by inculcating mainstream values and perspectives. Although commercialized mental health products and services purport to offer some fresh and innovative way to a better life, they actually promote conventional wisdom—only repackaged to sound new and improved—whose most likely net effect is to fuel the desire for a better life. Anyone remotely familiar with popular culture will instantly recognize this circular strategy as the apotheosis of the mass market's most ubiquitous enterprise: advertising. Furthermore, the similarity in strategy is no coincidence. Entertainment and advertising are not just related mass market endeavors; they work in tandem to promote sales. So that just as any enterprise that enters the mass market becomes beholden to entertainment values, so too does it become subject to advertising's imperatives. For that reason, advertising—and its ability to overrun both public enterprises and private aspirations—is relevant to our understanding of the commercialized advice industry.

ADVERTISING

Advertising pervades modern life. It is the zeitgeist of the 20th, and now the 21st, centuries, upon which the mass market depends. The histories of the mass market and of advertising are inextricably entwined. As the mass market in the late 1890s generated a surplus of material goods in need of consumers, modern advertising evolved to deliver those consumers (Leach, 1993; Lears, 1994; Mazur, 1996). The essential goal of all modern advertising is to persuade consumers that products will satisfy their deepest desires because believing that they will—when they cannot—serves to intensify longing and increase consumption. Earlier, 19th-century ads had promised the high quality of their product lines. In contrast, advertising campaigns of the 20th and 21st centuries suggest that the products can promise high-quality personal lives. To supply sufficient consumers to meet the demands of new products, advertisers could no longer merely promise that products would satisfy an existing desire, such as for clean hair, fresh breath, or a hearty meal. Instead, advertisers would need first to arouse new desires (or awaken latent ones) that they would then promise to fulfill (Leach, 1993; Lears, 1994). Moreover, modern advertisers realized that the most fruitful desires were not practical, but psychological—such as desires for emotional security, sexual fulfillment, and even spiritual transcendence (Kilbourne, 1999; Leach, 1993; Marchand, 1983).

The shift in strategy incalculably altered modern life and allowed advertisers to become the arbiters of our collective sense of "the good life." Numerous scholars have meticulously traced the ascendence of advertising, its machinations, and its influence on public sensibilities (Bordo, 1993; Kilbourne, 1999; Leach, 1993; Lears, 1994; Marchand, 1983). Such scholarship reveals how, over the course of the 20th century, advertisers perfected strategies designed to trigger feelings of insecurity and inadequacy in their targeted audiences and then salved the resulting discomfort with products. As advertising persuaded the public that they could buy a better future, the resulting consumerist culture "confused the good life with goods" (Leach, 1993, p. xiii). Thus, by the start of the 21st century, advertising could quite successfully offer "us products, both as solace and as substitutes for the intimate human connections we all long for and need" but that have been displaced by corporate culture (Kilbourne, 1999, p. 26).

In modern society, our deepest, most personal desires are increasingly brokered by advertisers who are relentless in their task. From magazines, newspapers, billboards, television, the Internet, movies, and radio, the public is beset by advertisements that simultaneously inflate the number and significance of personal deficiencies and exaggerate the ease with which they can be corrected. By the mid-1990s, the average American was exposed to an estimated 1,500 advertisements every day, with a cumulative lifetime exposure to television commercials totaling 1½ years (Kilbourne, 1994). Near the end of the 20th century, advertising had become a $200 billion a year endeavor (Kilbourne, 1994). Advertising's ubiquity allows it not only to shape desires but to dictate increasingly the content of public information.

Advertising supports "more than 60 percent of magazine and newspaper production and almost 100 percent of electronic media" affording advertisers a great deal of influence (Kilbourne, 1999, p. 34). The point is that as advertising has wormed its way into virtually every aspect of modern life, modern life has been required to yield up more and more of itself in service to this hungry guest.

Mass market products and services are now not merely made possible by advertisements, but rather they exist for advertisements. Just as that is true for television programming, newspapers, and magazines, and essentially every other component of the mass market, it also holds true for the advice industry. Not surprisingly, a populace that has been bedeviled for 100 years by advertisers' promises of radical transformations easily achieved, of life-altering consequences realized through trivial changes, of immediate and profound reversals of fortune, is especially susceptible to the claims of the advice industry. In essence, advertising and the advice industry make the same promises. In fact, when psychological expertise and services enter the mass market and are reduced to their most vendable component—advice—they become almost indistinguishable from advertisements.

Advice as Advertisement

Unlike most television programming or popular print materials, for the advice industry there is no clear-cut demarcation between program and commercial, or content and ad copy. Commercialized advice is more often like the derided "infomercial," where what presents itself as a substantive program is actually a corporate-paid commercial. Made possible by former President Ronald Reagan's deregulation of the FCC (which previously limited advertisers to 12 minutes per broadcast hour), infomercials allow for 30 minutes of uninterrupted commercial time (Stanton, 1994). Although they are self-serving, infomercials have adopted the conventions of more objective investigative programming, such as tests of the product, reviews from purchasers, and "expert" commentary, and have enjoyed tremendous success.

It was through late-night infomercials that reigning advice-guru Tony Robbins's career skyrocketed. In the 5 years between 1989 and 1994, Robbins sold $120 million worth of self-help tapes through infomercials (Stanton, 1994). In part from that success, Robbins signed in 1991 a $3 million contract with Simon and Schuster (Stanton, 1994). By 1997, his infomercial had been running for 8 years and Robbins had sold 25 million copies of his Personal Power program (Levine, 1997). Though Robbins is the advice industry leader associated with informercials officially, all contemporary advice leaders oversee "informercials" of a sort. That is, the most successful advice materials collapse the product and its advertisements into one product-promoting package.

Dr. Phil McGraw's appearances on Oprah are especially infomercial-esque. Beginning in 2000, Oprah began a series of shows called "Relationship Rescue," featuring Dr. Phil and adopting the title of one of his books. Borrowing heavily from the infomercial format, the shows feature Oprah excitedly informing her audience about a wonderful new product (Dr. Phil's advice) and how it has been transforming people's lives. A series of "product demonstrations" are conducted with "real-life" couples in front of a live audience. Invariably, whatever the guests' relationship problem, Dr. Phil's advice, if properly applied, quickly resolves it. Throughout the program, as on the infomercial, the host raises questions, asks for clarification, or underscores important features—all to highlight the product's versatility for the viewing audience.

The August 8, 2000, show, "Dr. Phil's Best Relationship Advice," illustrates well these elements. The show begins with several very short clips of Dr. Phil's responses to guests, after which Oprah reminds her audience that she has "been doing these seminars around the country, like Phil has." She notes that whenever she mentions him, people "go 'Whoo-ooh, ooh, aah' " which she understands to mean that "that bald head of yours is getting to be very popular." Oprah then goes on to explain that the show is a great one to watch and is based on McGraw's book, which has been so helpful to her. Her endorsement confirms for viewers that not only do ordinary people find the product useful, celebrities do as well. The remainder of the show entails a series of excerpts from some of Dr. Phil's previous appearances, during which he offers intuitive maxims and easy wisecracks—

but his commonplace comments earn Oprah's emphatic praise. The cumulative effect of the program is an hour-long exercise in self-promotion. For example, the program brings viewers the following exchanges:

- In response to an excerpt about a loss of sexual interest in marriage, Oprah states, "Wow. You know, this is such a big issue that in O *Magazine* this month, which is on newsstands now available . . . (*McGraw interrupts to draw attention to the fact that he is on the cover*) . . . we . . . do . . . a big series of articles on this. . . . "
- Oprah prepares the audience for a clip by stating, "Well, Dr. Phil next faces off with cheating spouses. Ooh! You'll want to hear his no-nonsense advice on how to get over an affair. But first, we call them Philisms. Throughout the show, Dr. Phil's best oneliners that sometimes crack me up." A clip is then shown in which a man asks, "Doctor, can you help me?" and McGraw replies, "Yeah, I can help you. You just need to shut up and go with the flow."
- Dr. Phil informs guests and audience that if they ask themselves "What if?" about a troubling situation, they need to answer with "I'll get through it again. Because I believe in me, and I'm betting on me, not them." Oprah responds: "Damn, that's good, Phil! Good gracious, that's good. . . . Tarnation, that was good. That really was an ephiphanal [sic] moment for me."
- Dr. Phil states that in relationships a person should "never invest more than you can afford to lose." Oprah exclaims, "Ooh, ooh, that was good too."

Any sensible accounting of this show would be hard-pressed not to conclude that it is an infomercial. If Dr. Phil's interventions were evaluated based on what is commonly understood as effective practice within the professional mental health community, they clearly would not warrant the astonished enthusiasm they receive. The guests take a backseat to Dr. Phil and his "advice" and serve merely as a launching pad for his performance—which is to pronounce upon their lives. His comments fall largely into two categories: telling people what they are doing wrong and what they must do to correct it.

From time to time, McGraw borrows from a counseling technique that involves having two people talk directly to each other, rather than to the therapist about each other, except that on the show, Dr. Phil provides their script. On "Dr. Phil Helps Jealous People," a couple discloses that the husband has a serious problem with jealousy and has had an affair—which the wife found out about only when she talked with one of the show's producers. McGraw asks some questions, and tells them what their problems are and why they are happening. He then has them sit face to face on the stage. First telling the husband to "look her in the eye. . . . You did it, you deal with it," McGraw instructs the wife to "start talking and don't stop till I tell you." As she speaks, McGraw directs her with statements such as "You tell him, 'You hurt me and here is how' " and " . . . you tell him right now, 'This won't continue. I will not live with you this way ever again.' " Apparently it is inconsequential whether the wife truly understands what the statement entails or if she would be capable of carrying through with such a plan.

If the husband were unsure how to respond, that would have been no problem, because McGraw knew his lines for him: "Can you tell her, 'The jealousy—that's about me. It's not about you. It's about me.' " The husband does so, and McGraw continues, "You ask her for a second chance, and you promise her you'll get whatever you need to turn the corner." The husband again delivers his lines as he is told to. Then after confirming with the wife her willingness to work on this problem with her husband, McGraw tells her, "Then I want you to say one last thing to him for me. I want you to say, 'Jimmy, we're not getting a divorce and we're not staying married like this anymore, either.' " She does, the discussion closes, and McGraw informs the couple that "we're going to watch both of you like a hawk." Again, confirming the guests' understanding or their ability to follow through carries little import. What matters is a dramatic enactment of how the product supposedly works.

The segment demonstrates well how entertainment and advertising work in tandem to create mass market success. The situation on the show is staged, the viewers can see it being staged, and everyone knows McGraw appears on the show to promote his merchandise and that Oprah wants viewers. One can hardly imagine any other promotional program actually showing the sponsors telling guests what to say right on camera, but here it works. It works because the show is selling Dr. Phil's advice and the sale hinges on igniting the right emotions—anxiety, insecurity, and then relief—in the audience. In quick succession, Dr. Phil's advice takes the couple from suffering to salvation, and then the show moves swiftly on to the next demonstration before anyone has time to reflect on what has occurred. The formula has great entertainment value, and all along the way the entertainment serves to advertise the product.

Professional psychological literature warns therapists against routinely giving advice because it "spares the patient a laborious adjustment to reality" (Abraham, 1925/1955, p. 326). That is, even if people follow advice they are given—and often they do not—they come away with little or no new understanding of how they got into their difficulties or why doing as prescribed would make a difference. Advice, in essence, divests them of their circumstances. That result counters the goal of psychotherapy, but aligns with advertising's mission. Advertising courts magical thinking, promising consumers that they can escape life's limitations and be spared a laborious adjustment to reality if they buy the right products. Advertising does not hesitate to make grand claims about its goods or to link our deepest desires to commercial products. Neither does the advice industry.

Tony Robbins tells his listeners that if they use the right strategies—obtainable through his products—they can "make someone fall in love with you in 5 minutes" and that he can "cure any psychological problem in a session" (Griffin & Goldsmith, 1985, p. 41). He has also claimed that through neurolinguistic programming (NLP), clinicians can "cure people of tumors and long-standing psychological problems in a fraction of the time required by conventional treatments (Leikind & McCarthy, 1991, p. 186). NLP is a scientifically unsubstantiated therapeutic method that purports to "program" brain functioning using a variety of techniques, including mirroring the postures and nonverbal behaviors of clients. Robbins claimed that NLP has allowed him to "read people's motives like an open book." It also has allowed him to "make a woman have an orgasm without touching her," and even "bring a person who was brain-dead back to life" (p. 186). Moreover, he cautions that if therapists see their clients for more than two sessions, they have "no integrity" (Griffin & Goldsmith, 1985, p. 41).

Within the commercialized advice industry, little effort is made to marshal sound research evidence to support strong claims. Testimonials, endorsements, and more advertising are profitable substitutes. For instance, in his books John Gray replaces the standard reference list that appears at the end of professional psychology texts with a list of phone numbers for contacting his counseling centers and advertisements of his products. No references are provided for the material in *How to Get What You Want and Want What You Have*. Instead, the final pages of the text inform readers that "if you like what you just read and want to learn more . . . call our representatives, Mars–Venus Institute, twenty-four hours a day, seven days a week, toll free." Advertisements for Gray's products follow. What is important to Gray is not scientific substantiation, but sales.

Expanding Markets

John Gray and those associated with his work aggressively promote his products and seem to find no end to their potential market. On January 19, 1999, Gray launched *How To Get What You Want and Want What You Have*, through a 1-hour, primetime appearance on the home-shopping channel QVC. The program was estimated to reach 68 million homes across the United States and it advertised Gray's library and video sets, his audiotapes, and his board game ("Dr. John Gray," 1999). Press releases before the event provided details for placing advance orders by phone or through the QVC Website.

A pyramid approach, whereby others can become sanctioned to sell the products, extends the reach of advice industry leaders beyond what they could manage on their own and yields substantial profits. By 1994, Tony Robbins had franchised himself to approximately 45 entrepreneurs, each of whom paid at least $36,000 for the opportunity to earn money by presenting their own versions of Robbins's workshops (Stanton, 1994). Gray oversees a franchise of Mars/Venus counseling centers, wherein therapists first pay approximately $2,500 for training in Gray's "technique," followed by a "licensing" fee of $1,900 for the right to use his logo and identify themselves with him, and then continue to make monthly payments to Gray of $300 (Gleick, 1997).

Another way of widening the market is to increase the range of products. The advice industry has discovered that it need not limit its market to items directly related to advice. The leaders themselves become associated with "the good life" and as a result, virtually anything they promote becomes a symbol of that idealized, illusive state and therefore is alluring. John Gray plans to offer such "romantic accessories" as candles, flowers, and even lingerie on his Website (McGinn, 2000). His products have been so successful that his work can now attract customers for other businesses.

In 1997, HarperCollins—Gray's publisher—worked with bookstores across the country to set up *Mars and Venus on a Date* social events (Maryles, 1997). With invitations and catered food, and a special video-taped appearance by Gray himself, the events were especially clever. In conjunction with the events, Barnes and Noble hosted a "cyberevent" for the book and was able to reach approximately 2,000 people who logged on to their Website (Maryles, 1997). Hallmark also participated by partnering with Gray to produce an exclusive edition of Gray's work titled *Mars and Venus in Touch: Enhancing the Passion with Great Communication* (Guest, 2000). The book was available at Hallmark stores for under $3 with the purchase of any Hallmark card.

Such events and the products and services discussed thus far support the first of this chapter's twofold thesis. That is, as professional psychological expertise and services enter the commercial domain, we should expect them to become beholden to marketplace values: entertainment and advertising. Let us now consider the second component of the thesis, which is that as commercialized versions of psychological expertise and services succeed in the marketplace, we should expect them to exert influence on the profession itself. Specifically, we should see evidence that marketplace imperatives—entertainment and advertising—are encroaching on the profession.

THE INCURSION OF MARKETPLACE VALUES

The American Psychological Association (APA) officially recognized the significant influence of the mass media by forming Division 46, Media Psychology, which "focuses on the roles psychologists play in various aspects of the media, including, but not limited to, radio, television, film, video, newsprint, magazines, and newer technologies" (Division 46-Media Psychology, n.d.). Division 46 has been in existence for approximately 20 years, and its Website identifies four objectives, the first of which is to "assist psychologists to use the media more effectively for informing the public about the science and profession of psychology." Thus, Division 46 aims to help professionals use mass media as a way of reaching the public. Educating the public is a laudable goal and, in fact, by the mid-1980s almost all candidates for APA president were declaring "support for disseminating the fruits of the discipline to the public" (McCall, 1988, p. 87). Not surprisingly, the emphasis on public communication began increasing within APA during a time when mental health issues were receiving more public attention through the rapidly expanding commercialized advice industry, especially TV talk shows and self-help materials (see Chapter 14). But as professionals have attempted to harness the power of the media, they have encountered the same dilemma that faced their 19th-century predecessors: the choice to cater to popular tastes for entertainment or become obsolete.

Entertainment and Professional Psychology

As early as 1983, some professionals were linking future professional viability to effective use of mass media, while stressing the importance of maintaining professional standards—and noting the difficulty of attempting to do both. The "Suggestions for Media Mental Health Professionals" prepared by the Guidelines Committee of the Association for Media indicated that professionals must "walk the thin line between being entertaining enough to attract the broad audiences needed for survival, and remaining professional" (Broder, 1983; cited in Heaton & Wilson, 1995, p. 220).

In Tuning in Trouble: Talk TV's Destructive Impact on Mental Health, Heaton and Wilson (1995) documented how that goal is rarely achieved. Many of the professionals they interviewed reported being pressured to make their appearances entertaining, even if doing so would compromise professional ethics, and often having little control over the final outcome. Nancy Steele, a professional psychologist, was pushed by producers of Sally Jesse Raphael to arrive for the show "Wives of Rapists" within 3 days, bringing with her both the wives and the rapists (Heaton & Wilson, 1995). She realized later that such a request should have alerted her to the show's interest in her ability to provide entertainment, not sound psychological information. Likewise, Laurel Richardson, author of *The New Other Woman* (1985), had hoped to discuss how getting involved in affairs with married men keeps women in traditional roles. The producers and host of the Sally Jesse Raphael show were more interested in instigating fights among the guests and audience members—and even suggested that Richardson was organizing an "Other Woman's" movement (Heaton & Wilson, 1995).

Stuart Fischoff, former president of Division 46, noted that such talk show experiences have left some professionals feeling "extremely mistrusting and cynical" (p. 104) but that others are "so thrilled by the idea of being on TV they tend to suspend good judgment and good taste" (Fischoff, 1994, cited in Heaton & Wilson, 1995, p. 118). Charlotte Kasl, author of *Women, Sex, and Addiction* (1989), was not especially pleased when Donahue's producers suggested titling the show she was to appear on "Women Who Love Sex," but she stated that "Hey, I wanted to be on Donahue. . . . This is a way to get to people 4 to 10 million at time" (p. 118). That kind of commercial incentive, coupled with the current professional push to bring mental health information to larger audiences through the media, may make professionals susceptible to media pressures. Producers typically interview several potential experts before selecting the ones who will be featured, and their decisions often hinge on the professionals' ability to present information in exciting ways. Other things being equal, the entertaining professional gets the exposure. Thus, entertainment value becomes the gatekeeper for professional information in the mass media, which supports the argument that when entertainment becomes a factor, it becomes the deciding factor.

Furthermore, when professionals do not comply with the media's desire for entertainment, they simply are replaced by those who do, whether or not their replacements' credentials and presentations are equally valid (Kelly, Rotton, & Culver, 1985). That management strategy on the part of media has prompted a wide range of media-focused activity within the profession designed to remedy professionals' media "deficiencies." When the entertainment industry's standards for skillful speaking become the standard by which professionals are evaluated, more traditional scientific conventions are devalued. Fischoff, for example, noted that it is "hard to find a psychologist who can speak on camera and be other than stunningly boring" (quoted in Heaton & Wilson, 1995, p. 102). Individuals and organizations within the profession have addressed the perceived problem with how-to books and training seminars.

Recent issues of *The Amplifier*, the newsletter for Division 46, provide examples of how popular interests have begun to commingle with professional goals. The Fall 2000 issue contained a piece by Doe Lang titled "How to Be a Smash Hit on TV," in which Lang offered tips on "learning to be the center of attention" as well as "increasing on-camera charisma." She encouraged readers to practice "one-minute free for alls" and to realize that "total deadpans (that some psychologists equate with objectivity) are BORING and hard to watch" (Lang, 2000). Additionally, Lang instructed readers to "practice keeping your breathing slow, steady, smooth. . . . Breathing seven breaths or less a minute keeps you calm; with lots of oxygen going to the brain . . . the right thing to say—great ad libs—will just naturally flash into your brain." The recipe-like instruction and the implied absolute success of the strategies is akin to the kind of material found in mass market, advice industry products. Thus, it is not completely surprising that the article identified Lang as president of a consulting firm, *Charismedia*, and informed readers that "more helpful hints can be found" in Lang's book, *The New Secrets of Charisma* (1999).

What is especially disturbing about Lang's article is that the professional organization that is ostensibly devoted to fostering effective, professional use of the media would publish it. Division 46 should be at the forefront of educating professionals and the public about why Lang's approach to advice giving and to interacting with the media do not represent the "science of psychology," rather than encouraging professionals to make use of such approaches when they want to represent the profession in public.

Lang's priority is the commercial consideration of "how to be a smash hit," not the protection of professional standards. A similar emphasis characterizes "Breaking into TV Production," which appeared in the Summer 2000 issue of *The Amplifier*. Jeff Guardalabene, who was identified as having been a television producer for 15 years, offered advice to mental health professionals who want TV producers to consider their proposals for stories. Section headings included "tell a story . . . make it visual," and readers were instructed to weave into their stories, if they can, "some fascinating characters" to increase the chances it will get noticed (Guardalabene, 2000). To make his point, Guardalabene (2000) asked readers directly: "Which show about depression recovery would you rather watch: one with an expert spouting research results, or one following a friend or neighbor as they [sic] recover from a major depressive episode?"

The language Guardalabene used to pose his question reflects the mass media's typical lack of interest in research evidence, and presupposes that this lack of interest is commonly shared—or at least that mental health professionals would be willing to stop "spouting research results" if doing so would get them on television. Furthermore, by suggesting that professionals replace data with case studies, testimonials, or descriptions of personal experiences, Guardalabene's article encourages professionals to offer the public information that the science of psychology considers inadequate evidence to support a theory or a therapy (Stanovich, 2001). Following his instruction would lend support to the kind of "personal psychologies" that are not verifiable, but nonetheless dominate the commercial advice industry, and that confuse the public about what constitutes professional psychological expertise (Stanovich, 2001). That approach is not new to the mass market.

Somewhat new is the promotion by professionals of mass market films as useful instructional tools in professional training programs. Between 1997 and 2001, at least five articles whose primary topic advocated such use were published in professional journals; there were likely others that did so secondarily to another topic. In "The Use of Film in Marriage and Family Counselor Education," Higgins and Dermer (2001) "introduce an innovative technique that can be included in marriage and family counselor education curricula" to develop "perceptual, conceptual, and executive counseling skills" (p. 182). They also outlined "the advantages for using film" in instruction. Likewise in "Cinemeducation: Teaching Family Systems through Movies," Alexander and Waxman (2000) reported that movie clips are "powerful and entertaining ways to expose learners to such family therapy concepts as the family life cycle, differentiation, coalition and homeostasis" (p. 455). The authors also provided a "practical guide to movie scenes on video that can be readily incorporated into family systems training" (p. 455). Fredrick Miller (1999) maintained that although most movies offer bad examples of psychotherapy, "Ordinary People" is "so accurate and well done" that it "can be used, like process notes, to teach psychiatric residents and other students the major principles and techniques of psychodynamic psychotherapy" (p. 174).

Unlike Miller, who argued that only a few films could be useful, Hyler and Schanzer (1997) provided a list of "33 films depicting various aspects" of borderline personality disorder that they believe could be useful for "teaching medical students, residents, and other mental health trainees" about the disorder, as well as "other various topics in psychiatry" (p. 458). Hudock and Warden (2001), who presented a "movie-based assignment" for introductory level family therapy, were the only authors to note in their Abstract that they would address the disadvantages of using movies. The absence of such cautions in the other abstracts is disconcerting, given the well-known tendency of Hollywood to distort reality and to perpetuate race, class, and sex stereotypes.

Social and cognitive psychologists have demonstrated that when making decisions people are more likely to retrieve from memory and use information that is more accessible (the availability heuristic; Nisbett & Ross, 1980; see also Chapter 2). In accessing information, vividness matters more than its reliability. That is, when faced with clinical decision making, students trained with a combination of Hollywood films and empirically supported lectures would be more likely to retrieve and use the "knowledge" they gained from the films.

Specifically informing the students of the limitations or atypical nature of the films' depictions would likely have no influence on the impressions they develop as a result of watching the films. Hamill, Wilson, and Nisbett (1980) demonstrated that even when more accurate information is available, a single, vivid example is likely to dominate people's judgments. Furthermore, once the films have been shown in classes and thereby validated by faculty members, students would be unlikely to recall later which aspects were considered "true" and useful and which were not. Graduate students, and their faculty, are no more immune to the "errors of sampling, perception, recording, retention, retrieval, and inference to which the human mind is subject" than is the general public (Meehl, 1993, p. 728). Thus, the profession should be especially cautious in using entertainment industry products to train those who represent the future of the profession.

It is interesting to note that during the 1990s, when there was an increased emphasis on media skills and use of entertainment films for instruction, a number of sensational, unscientific treatments arose within clinical psychology: unvalidated treatments for trauma (see Chapter 9), suggestive techniques for recalling repressed memories of childhood abuse (see Chapter 8), subliminal self-help tapes (see Chapter 14), and facilitated communication for autism (see Chapter 13; Lilienfeld, 1998). Such treatments align with the demands of entertainment industry far better than they do with scientific standards. They often promise dramatic, quick-fix "cures" supported largely by "clinical experience" or testimonials. That kind of support lends little research evidence, but a great deal of effective advertising.

ADVERTISING AND PROFESSIONAL PSYCHOLOGY

After appearing on the Sally Jesse Raphael show, Laurel Richardson concluded that the show was "dreadful, disempowering, and divisive. But my publicist thought it was great—and that I was great—because I handled the conflict in a way which would generate interest in the book" (Richardson, 1987, cited in Heaton & Wilson, 1995). The publicist, no doubt, recognized that the conflict generated on the show would captivate and entertain its audience, and that with entertainment comes an enhanced opportunity for sales. As discussed earlier in this chapter, the mass market imperative of entertainment frequently works in tandem with advertising. Thus, we should expect that an increased emphasis on meeting media standards (thus, on entertainment) would be linked to an increased emphasis on advertising. In fact, it is.

Professionals who have written books know well the vital link between sales and the media. Publicity increases sales, and currently almost nothing creates more publicity for mental health professionals than an appearance on a daytime talk show. Even better for sales has been to have a book selected for Oprah's Book Club. Writing for *People*, Chin and Cheakalos (1999) stated that a "Pulitzer Prize is nice. A Nobel even nicer. But to hit the literary jackpot . . . what an author wants is an Oprah" (p. 112). Each book selected for the her book club has gone quickly to the top of the best seller lists. Although the kinds of materials typically promoted by talk shows—McGraw's *Life Strategies*, Gray's *Mars and Venus* series, Robbins's "Personal Power"—have been commercialized advice, the potential financial benefits of mass market exposure have not gone unnoticed within the profession. If professionals cannot secure them through appearances on commercial television, the Internet offers another avenue for reaching the public.

Professionals are increasingly encouraged to develop their own Websites, and assistance in doing so is now promoted as a "member service" by some professional organizations. The American Mental Health Counselors Association, for example, identified five "great benefits" of membership on its Website ("Member services," n.d.). Three of these benefits concern financial or promotional issues, the other two professional information. More specifically, members are offered the chance to have "their own personal Website" at a low, discounted price. They are also offered the chance to communicate "practice information to consumers" including contact information and specialties. They are reminded, however, that AMHCA "does not examine, determine or warrant the competence of any professional listed on the Registry." Both of these professional "member services" support commercial interests over and above professional standards.

They do so in the following ways. Members are not offered assistance in accessing databases of the latest empirically supported treatments for the common psychological concerns they are likely to encounter in their practices, nor to the Websites of well-established treatment centers to which they could refer clients. Either of these would support professional interests. Rather, they are encouraged to develop their own Websites. Moreover, they are encouraged to join a cohort of "professionals" whose claimed competencies remain unverified, but are already being promoted to the public. That invitation sounds a good deal like what television talk shows offer: the chance to compete in a mass market that accords little attention to professional standards. It also indirectly encourages professionals to hone their "presentation" skills and to advertise themselves in ways that will set them apart from others. Elbert Hubbard, a magazine editor in the early days of modern advertising, warned that "everyone should advertise while they are alive. The man who does not advertise is a dead one, whether he knows it or not" (quoted in Lapham, 1993, p. 10). Hubbard's assertion has a disturbing relevance for the contemporary mental health profession. Increasingly, professional attention is directed toward successful marketing and promotion. No doubt mass market livelihood depends upon such skills. More disturbingly, exceptional advertising has allowed one form of commercialized advice a place within the profession: John Gray's work.

As noted earlier, John Gray received a doctorate in human sexuality and psychology from Columbia Pacific University in California, a correspondence school with questionable accreditation, and he holds no professional license (Gleick, 1997; "Rebuttal from Uranus," n.d.). He openly acknowledges that he does not engage in research in the "academic way" such as double-blind studies. Instead, Gray explains his research as follows: "For 10 years I sat with a group of 30 people, and I got women talking about their issues, men talking about their issues" and "found generalizations that were true" (Marano, 1997, p. 28). In order to arrive at those generalizations, he drew upon his "own intuitive sense and practice" (Carlson & Nieponski, 2001, p. 7).

In fact, Gray has described his ideas and the methods he uses to both obtain and confirm them in ways that others would consider the essence of psychological pseudoscience (Stanovich, 2001). What is remarkable is that he provided much of that description through a special "phone bridge" interview for *The Family Journal: Counseling and Therapy for Couples and Families*, the official journal of the International Association of Marriage and Family Counselors (IAMFC), which it published as their lead article. Not once was Gray confronted about the unscientific nature of his ideas or pressed to verify his claims. The article does, however, provide an editor's note: " For more information about John Gray's clinical training, call 800-Mars-Venus or visit the Web site at www.mars-venus-counselors.com" (Carlson & Nieponski, 2001, p. 7).

Gray also serves on IAMFC's Distinguished Advisory Board for their journal, in addition to being one of its four consulting editors. Furthermore, Gray was invited in 2000 to present at the American Counseling Association convention by the IAMFC board as part of the convention's Distinguished Presenters venue. IAMFC also presented Gray with their Media Award in "recognition of his impact" through his book *Men are from Mars, Women are from Venus*, which the IAMFC president described as having let couples worldwide "know that their relationship can be different" (P. Stevens, personal communication, March 6, 2001). Gray's ability to achieve, through commercial success, professional distinctions otherwise reserved for those with substantial professional achievements captures the essence of the issues presented in this chapter.

CONCLUDING THOUGHTS

The thesis of this chapter is that when psychological expertise and services enter the mass market, they become beholden to marketplace values and strategies. That thesis involved the notion that as commercialized forms of professional expertise succeed in the mass market, they not only degrade, but ultimately displace, the original on which they are based.

If the profession hopes to not be displaced by commercialized forms of itself, then it needs to be careful to not invite them in. Additionally, the profession should resist the encroachment of entertainment and advertising into the profession. Although those imperatives promote commerce, they erode science. In the long run, science, not profit, will advance the profession.

GLOSSARY

Advice industry: The mass market, commercialized version of professional and psychological expertise.

Availability heuristic: The tendency for an individual's judgments to be influenced by the ease of recall. Rather than being solely an indicator of accuracy, easy recall can result from several factors (e.g., the strength of verbal associative connections among events may influence how well one "remembers" the co-occurrence of those events).

Commodification: The process of transforming an item into an object of purchase and that renders vendability (salability) its key value.

Effort after meaning: The desire to seek and accept even dubious causal explanations for one's current life problems.

Firewalking: The technique, popular among many self-help and motivational leaders, of walking on burning embers to demonstrate the power of purportedly untapped mental powers. In fact, firewalking is entirely consistent with the laws of physics and involves no special psychological or physical powers.

Neurolinguistic programming: Unvalidated therapeutic method that purports to "program" brain functioning through a variety of techniques, including mirroring the postures and nonverbal behaviors of clients. Some proponents of neurolinguistic programming have claimed to be able to cure phobias in a matter of minutes.

P. T. Barnum effect: The tendency of individuals to accept vague and highly generalized, but nonobvious, personality descriptors (e.g., "You have a great deal of unused potential that you have not turned to your advantage") as highly self-descriptive (see also Chapter 2).

REFERENCES

Abraham, K. (1955). Psychoanalytic notes on Cove's system of self-mastery. In H. Abraham (Ed.), *Clinical papers and essays on psycho-analysis* (H. Abraham & D. R. Ellison, Trans.) (pp. 306–327). New York: Basic Books. (Original work published 1925)

Adler, J. (1995, October 2). The guru from Mars. *Newsweek, 126*(14), 96.

Alexander, M., & Waxman, D. (2000). Cimemeducation. Teaching family systems through movies. *Families, Systems and Health, 18*(4), 455–466.

All about John Gray [Online]. (2001). Retrieved March 10 2001, from http:www.mars venus.com /cgi-bin/link/johngray/bio.html

Beck, J. S. (1995). *Cognitive therapy: Basics and beyond.* New York: Guilford Press.

Bordo, S. (1993). *Unbearable weight: Feminism, Western culture, and the body.* Berkeley: University of California Press.

Carlson, J., & Nieponski, M. K. (2001). John Gray—A man from earth: *The Family Journal* phone bridge. *The Family Journal: Counseling and Therapy for Couples and Families, 9*(1), 7–10.

Chin, P., & Cheakalos, C. (1999, December 20). Touched by an Oprah. *People,* p. 112.

Club Med teams with "Men are from Mars, women are from Venus" author to host first-ever Mars–Venus parenting skills workshop. (2000, February 10). *PR Newswire* [Online]. Retrieved March 11, 2001 from InfoTrac Onefile database.

Convention Highlights. (2000, Fall). *The Amplifier* [Online]. Retrieved September 2, 2001 from http://www.apa.org/.divisions/div46/NLFall2K.html

Dickson, D. H., & Kelly, I. W. (1985). The "Barnum effect" in personality assessment: A review of the literature. *Psychological Reports, 57,* 367–382.

Division46–Media psychology [Online]. (n.d.). Retrieved June 26, 2001, from http:// www.apa. org/ about/division/div46.html

Dr. John Gray, author of the number-one international bestseller "Men are from Mars, women are from Venus," launches his new personal success book on QVC. (1999, January 13). *PR Newswire* [Online]. Retrieved March 11, 2001, from InfoTrac Onefile database.

Gabler, N. (1998). *Life: The movie, how entertainment conquered reality.* New York: Vintage Books.

Gilovich, T. (1991). *How we know what isn't so: The fallibility of human reason in everyday life.* New York: Free Press.

Gleick, E. (1997, June 16). Tower of psychobabble. *Time, 149*(24), 68–71.

Gonser, S. (2001, February). The incredible, sellable O. *Folio: The Magazine for Magazine Management, 30*(3), 26–30.

Gray, J. (1992). *Men are from Mars, women are from Venus: A practical guide for improving communication and getting what you want in your relationship.* New York: HarperCollins.

Gray, J. (1995). *Mars and Venus in the bedroom: A guide to lasting romance and passion.* New York: HarperCollins.

Greenberg, D. (1998, April). Tony Robbins live! *Success, 45*(4), 68–773.

Griffin, N., & Goldsmith, L. (1985, March). The charismatic kid: Tony Robbins, 25, gets rich peddling a hot self-help program. *Life, 8,* 41–46.

Guardalabene, (2000, Summer). Breaking into TV Production [Online]. *The Amplifier.* Retrieved September 2, 2001, from http://www.apa.org/divisions/div46/ NLSum2K.html

Guelzo, A. C. (1995, April 24). Selling God in America. *Christianity Today, 39*(5), 27–30.

Guest, C. (2000, February 11). Hallmark links Mars, Venus. *The Kansas City Business Journal* [Online]. Retrieved October 30, 2001 from InfoTrack Onefile database.

Hamill, R., Wilson, T. D., & Nisbett, R. E. (1980). Insensitivity to sample bias: Generalizing from atypical cases. *Journal of Personality and Social Psychology, 39*, 578–589.

Heaton, J., & Wilson, N. (1995). *Tuning in trouble: Talk TV's destructive impact on mental health.* San Francisco: Jossey-Bass.

Higgins, J. A., & Dermer, S. (2001). The use of film in marriage and family counselor education. *Counselor Education and Supervision, 40*, 182–192.

Hines, T. M. (1998). *Einstein, history and other passions: The rebellion against science at the end of the Twentieth Century.* Reading, MA: Addison-Wesley.

Hudock, A. M., Jr., & Warden, S. A. G. (2001). Using movies to teach family systems concepts. *Family Journal: Counseling and Therapy for Couples and Families, 9*(2), 116–121.

Hutchby, I. (1995). Aspects of recipient design in expert advice-giving on call-in radio. *Discourse Processes, 19*, 219–238.

Hyler, S. E., & Schanzer, B. (1997). Using commercially available films to teach about borderline personality disorder. *Bulletin of the Menninger Clinic, 61*, 458–468.

Kaminer, W. (1993). *I'm dysfunctional, you're dysfunctional: The recovery movement and other self-help fashions.* New York: Vintage Books.

Kasl, C. D. (1989). *Women, sex, and addiction: A search for love and power.* New York: Ticknor & Fields.

Kelly, I., Rotton, J., & Culver, R. (1985). The moon was full and nothing happened: A review of studies on the moon and human behavior and lunar beliefs. *Skeptical Inquirer, 10*, 129–143.

Kilbourne, J. (1994). Still killing us softly: Advertising and the obsession with thinness. In P. Fallon, M. A. Katzman, & S. C. Wooley (Eds.), *Feminist perspectives on eating disorders* (pp. 395–418). New York: Guilford Press.

Kilbourne, J. (1999). *Deadly persuasion.* New York: Free Press.

Klinghoffer, D. (1999, February 8). Publishing: Helping yourself. *National Review,* pp. 56–58.

Lang, D. (1999). *The new secrets of charisma: How to discover and unleash your hidden powers.* Chicago: Contemporary Books.

Lang, D. (2000, Fall). How to be a smash hit on TV [Online]. *The Amplifier.* Retrieved September 2, 2001, from http://www.apa.org/divisions/div46/NLFall2K.html

Lapham, L. H. (1993, November). Yellow brick road [Editorial]. *Harper's Magazine, 287*(1722), 10–13.

Leach, W. (1993). *Land of desire: Merchants, power, and the rise of new American culture.* New York: Vintage Books.

Lears, J. T. (1994). *Fables of abundance: A cultural history of advertising in America.* New York: Basic Books.

Leikind, B. J., & McCarthy, W. J. (1991). An investigation of firewalking. In K. Frazier (Ed.)., *The hundredth monkey and other paradigms of the paranormal* (pp.182–193). Buffalo, NY: Prometheus.

Levine, A. (1997, February 24). Peak performance is tiring: A reporter reaches for success with Tony Robbins. *U.S. News and World Report*, pp. 53–55.

Lilienfeld, S. O. (1998). Pseudoscience in contemporary clinical psychology: What it is and what we can do about it. *Clinical Psychologist, 51*(4), 3–9.

Los Angeles Times Syndicate launches John Gray's "Men are from Mars, Women are from Venus" syndicated advice column. (1998, November 2). *PR Newswire* [Online]. Retrieved March 11, 2001 from InfoTrac Onefile database.

Marano, H. E. (1997, May–June). When planets collide. *Psychology Today, 30*(3), 28–33.

Marchand, R. (1983). *Advertising the American dream: Making way for modernity, 1920–1940.* Berkeley: University of California Press.

Maryles, D. (1997, July 7). Behind the bestsellers [News about John Gray's "Mars and Venus on a Date" and other books]. *Publishers Weekly, 244*(27), 16.

Mazur, L. A. (1996, May–June). Marketing madness. *E Magazine*, pp. 36–41.

McCall, R. (1988). Science and the press: Like oil and water? *American Psychologist, 43*, 87–94.

McGinn, D. (2000, January 10). Self-help U.S.A. *Newsweek*, pp. 43–47.

McGraw, P. C. (1999). *Life strategies, doing what works, doing what matters.* New York: Hyperion Books.

McGraw, P. C. (n.d.). *Claiming responsibility* [Online]. Retrieved April 1, 2001 from http://www.oprah.com/phil/advice/phil_advice_responsibility.html

McGraw, P. C. (n.d.). *Dr. Phil's ten steps to positive communication and rescuing your relationship* [Online]. Retrieved April 1, 2001 from http://www.oprah.com/phil/advice/phil_ advice_poscom.html

McGraw, P. C. (n.d.). *The formula for success* [Online]. Retrieved April 1, 2001 from http://www.oprah.com/tows/pastshows/tows_2000/tows_past_ 2000 0307_e.html

McGraw, P. C. (n.d.). *The life laws—and what they mean* [Online]. Retrieved April 1, 2001 from http://www/oprah.com/phil/advice/phil_advice_lawmeaning.html

McGraw, P. C. (n.d.). *The seven step strategy for reconnecting with your partner* [Online]. Retrieved April 1, 2001 from http://www.oprah.com/phil/rescue/phhil_rescue_ 20000404 _c.html

McLuhan, M. (1964). *Understanding media: The extensions of man.* New York: McGraw Hill.

McLuhan, M., & Fiore, Q. (1967). *The medium is the massage.* New York: Random House.

Medawar, P. B. (1967). *The art of the soluble.* London: Methuen.

Meehl, P. E. (1993). Philosophy of science: Help or hindrance? *Psychological Reports, 72*, 707–733.

Member services [Online]. (n.d.) Retrieved June 26, 2001 from http://www.amhca.org/member services.html

Miller, F. C. (1999). Using the movie *Ordinary People* to teach psychodynamic psychotherapy with adolescents. *Academic Psychiatry, 23*(3), 174–179.

Miller, M. C. (1988). *Boxed in: The culture of TV.* Evanston, IL: Northwestern University Press.

Munson, W. (1993). *All Talk: The talkshow in media culture.* Philadelphia: Temple University Press.

Nisbett, R. E., & Ross, L. (1980). *Human interference: Strategies and shortcomings of social judgments.* Englewood Cliffs, NJ: Prentice-Hall.

Ofshe, R., & Walters, E. (1994). *Making monsters: False memories, psychotherapy, and sexual hysteria.* New York: Scribner's.

Oprah begins 13th season with "renewed mission." (1998, September 21). *Jet, 94*(17) [Online], 65. Retrieved October 30, 2001 from InfoTrac Onefile database.

Oprah on Oprah: Perfectionist. Optimist. Diva. The woman behind the most successful magazine launch ever still cries when she thinks of her failed project "Be-
loved." (2001, January 8). *Newsweek* [Online]. Retrieved March 11, 2001 from
InfoTrac Onefile database.

Peterson, K. S. (1994, May 4). Advice from outer space. *Detroit News*, p. 3C.

Postman, N. (1985). *Amusing ourselves to death: Public discourse in the age of show
business*. New York: Penguin Books.

Rapping, E. (1996). *The culture of recovery: Making sense of the self-help movement
in women's lives*. Boston: Beacon Press.

Rebuttal from Uranus, The. (n.d.). *Ph.D.? Where did John Gray get his Ph.D.?* [On-
line]. Retrieved June 26, 2001 from http://ourworld.compuserve.com/home
pages/women_rebuttal_from_uranus

Richardson, L. W. (1985). *The new other woman: Contemporary single women in affairs with married men*. New York: Free Press.

Robbins, A. (1991). *Awaken the giant within: How to take immediate control of your
mental, emotional, physical and financial destiny*. New York: Summit Books.

Robbins, A. (1994). *Giant steps: Small changes to make a difference, daily lessons in
self-mastery*. New York: Fireside Books.

Robbins, A. (1997). *Unlimited power: The new science of personal achievement*.
New York: Simon & Schuster.

Robbins, A. (2002). *The driving force*. New York: Simon & Schuster.

Scannell, P. (Ed.). (1991). *Broadcast talk*. London: Sage.

Schlessinger, L. (1995). *Ten stupid things women do to mess up their lives*. New York:
HarperPerennial.

Schlessinger, L. (1996). *How could you do that?!: The abdication of character, courage and conscience*. New York: HarperCollins.

Schlessinger, L. (2000). *Cope with it!* New York: Kensington Books.

Stanovich, K. E. (2001). *How to think straight about psychology* (6th ed.). Boston:
Allyn & Bacon.

Stanton, D. (1994, April). Aren't you glad you're Tony Robbins? *Esquire*, *121*(4),
100–107.

Tarrant, D. (1999, April 4). Phillip McGraw: With a book and boost from Oprah,
trial psychologist is flying high. *The Dallas Morning News* [Online]. Retrieved
March 8, 2001, from http://www.philmcgraw.com/news.asp

Times Book Review plans expanded best seller lists. (1983, December 12). *New York
Times*, p. 16.

Timney, M. C. (1991). *The discussion of social and moral issues on daytime talk
shows: Who's really doing all the talking?* Unpublished master's thesis, Department of Communications, Ohio University.

Weber, B. (1997, January 27). Taking the stage to help Mars and Venus kiss and make
up. *New York Times*, p. B6.

Welcome to John Gray's Universe [Online]. (2001). Retrieved March 10, 2001, from
http://www.marsvenus.com

Williams, M. (1993, May 10). Voices of 30–plus exclaim: Can we talk? *Advertising
Age*, *64*(10), S-6.

Weber, B. (1997, January 27). Taking the stage to help Mars and Venus kiss and make
up. *The New York Times*, p. B6.

16

Science and Pseudoscience in Clinical Psychology

Concluding Thoughts and Constructive Remedies

SCOTT O. LILIENFELD
STEVEN JAY LYNN
JEFFREY M. LOHR

We very much hope that this volume has provided readers with at least a taste of the breadth and depth of the problem of pseudoscience and otherwise questionable science in clinical psychology, and offered helpful guideposts for distinguishing mental health claims with and without adequate empirical support. In our closing comments, we wish to propose several remedies to combat the continuing spread of potentially pseudoscientific claims in clinical psychology.

We believe that the preceding chapters have made clear that the scientific underpinnings of the field of clinical psychology are threatened by the increasing proliferation of unsubstantiated and untested psychotherapeutic, assessment, and diagnostic techniques. Indeed, much of the book up to this point reads like a jeremiad. Readers who have made their way through most or all of the chapters in this book may be experiencing an understandable sense of pessimism concerning the long-term future of clinical psychology.

We believe that such nihilism may be unwarranted. In this concluding section of the book, we propose five remedies that we believe will go a sub-

461

stantial way toward healing the ills presently afflicting the field of clinical psychology. Despite the serious problems that this book has highlighted, we are reasonably confident that if these remedies are followed, the problem of pseudoscience in clinical psychology may ultimately prove amenable to a cure.

Here is our five point prescription for the field of clinical psychology:

1. All clinical psychology training programs must require formal training in critical thinking skills, particularly those needed to distinguish scientific from pseudoscientific methods of inquiry (see Lilienfeld, Lohr, & Morier, 2001, for helpful resources). In particular, clinical training programs must emphasize such issues as (1) clinical judgment and prediction, and the factors (e.g., confirmatory bias, overconfidence, illusory correlation; Garb, 1998; see also Chapter 2) that can lead clinicians astray when evaluating assessment information (see Grove, 2000, for similar recommendations); (2) fundamental issues in the philosophy of science, particularly the distinctions between scientific and nonscientific epistemologies (see Chapter 1); (3) research methodologies required to evaluate the validity of assessment instruments (see Chapter 3) and the efficacy and effectiveness of psychotherapies (see Chapter 6); and (4) issues in the psychology of human memory, particularly the reconstructive nature of memory and the impact of suggestive therapeutic procedures on memory (see Chapter 8). Moreover, the American Psychological Association (APA) must be willing to withhold accreditation from clinical PhD and PsyD programs that do not place substantial emphasis on these and related topics, which should be mandatory in the education and training of all clinical psychologists.

2. The field of clinical psychology must focus on identifying not only empirically supported treatments (ESTs; see Chambless & Ollendick, 2001), but also treatments that are clearly devoid of empirical support. In contrast to Garske and Anderson (Chapter 6), we regard the effort to produce explicit lists of ESTs as laudable, although we share some of their concerns regarding the criteria used to identify these techniques.

Nevertheless, the battle against pseudoscience is too substantial to be waged on only a single front. Although the identification of efficacious therapeutic techniques is an important long-term goal, we must also work toward identifying techniques that are either clearly inefficacious or harmful. The development of a formal list of "psychotherapies to avoid" would be an important start in that direction, both for practitioners and would-be consumers of psychotherapy. We would suggest that such techniques as facilitated communication for infantile autism (Chapter 13), rebirthing and reparenting (Chapter 7), and critical incident stress debriefing (Chapter 9) be among the first entries on this list.

3. The APA and other psychological organizations must play a more

active role in ensuring that the continuing education of practitioners is grounded in solid scientific evidence. A perusal of recent editions of the *APA Monitor on Psychology*, an in-house publication of the APA that is sent to all of its members, reveals that the APA has been accepting advertisements for a plethora of unvalidated psychological treatments, including Thought Field Therapy (see Chapter 9) and Imago Relationship Therapy, two techniques for which essentially no published controlled research exists. Among the workshops for which the APA has recently provided continuing education (CE) credits to practicing clinicians are courses in calligraphy therapy, neurofeedback (see Chapter 12), Jungian sandplay therapy, and the use of psychological theater to "catalyze critical consciousness" (see Lilienfeld, 1998). The APA has also recently offered CE credits for critical incident stress debriefing, a technique that has been shown to be harmful in several controlled studies (see Chapter 9). Some state psychological associations have not done much better. Very recently, the Minnesota Board of Psychology approved workshops in rock climbing, canoeing, sandplay therapy, and drumming meditation for CE credits (Lilienfeld, 2001).

If professional organizations intend to assist practitioners in the critical task of distinguishing techniques with and without adequate scientific support, they must insist on providing continuing education that serves this goal. Moreover, academics and clinicians who possess expertise in the differences between scientifically supported and unsupported assessment and therapeutic techniques must play a more active role in the development and dissemination of CE courses and workshops. To facilitate this process, academic clinical psychology programs must encourage their faculty members to participate in the construction and design of scientifically oriented CE courses.

4. The APA and other psychological organizations must play a more visible public role in combating erroneous claims in the popular press and elsewhere (e.g., the Internet) regarding psychotherapeutic and assessment techniques. These organizations have traditionally been reluctant to play the role of media "watchdogs" in the battle against unsubstantiated mental health methods and claims. In an era in which unsubstantiated mental health techniques are thriving with unabated vigor, such reluctance is becoming increasingly difficult to defend. The airwaves are increasingly dominated by talk show and media psychologists who dispense advice and information that is often not supported by research evidence (see Chapter 15), rather than by scientifically informed mental health professionals with the expertise necessary to provide the public with scientifically based information. As George Miller reminded us many years ago, "popular" psychology need not be a nonscientific psychology (Lilienfeld, 1998).

We therefore strongly recommend that the APA and other psychological organizations, including the American Psychological Society (APS), create coordinated networks of media contacts (ideally consisting of experts who possess expertise regarding questionable or untested techniques in clinical psychology) who can respond to problematic or unsubstantiated mental health claims whenever they are presented in the media, as well as to media inquiries regarding such claims.

5. Finally, the APA and other psychological organizations must be willing to impose stiff sanctions on practitioners who engage in assessment and therapeutic practices that are not grounded in adequate science or that have been shown to be potentially harmful. The APA Ethics Code clearly indicates that the use of unsubstantiated assessment techniques constitutes ethically inappropriate behavior. For example, APA Ethics Code Rule 2.01(b) mandates that "Psychologists' assessments, recommendations, reports, and psychological diagnostic or evaluative statements are based on information and techniques (including personal interviews of the individual when appropriate) sufficient to provide appropriate substantiation for their findings" and APA Ethics Code Rule 2.01(a) mandates that "Psychologists do not base their assessment or intervention decisions or recommendations on data or test results that are outdated for the current purpose." The APA Ethics Code (Rule 1.14) is similarly unambiguous in the case of potentially harmful psychotherapeutic methods: "Psychologists take reasonable steps to avoid harming their patients or clients, research participants, students, and others with whom they work, and to minimize harm where it is foreseeable and unavoidable."

Clinical psychologists who violate these codes of professional conduct must suffer appropriate consequences, and must be prevented from harming the general public. Appropriate sanctions on the part of the APA and other professional organizations are a prerequisite for safeguarding the integrity of the profession and ensuring the safety of clients. *Primum non nocere.*

We modestly believe that this book should be required reading for all clinical psychologists, as well as all clinical psychologists in training. Nevertheless, we also are hopeful that if our five prescriptions are followed, a future edition of this book may be able to safely drop the words "and pseudoscience" from its title.

ACKNOWLEDGMENTS

We thank James Herbert and Richard McNally for their helpful comments on an earlier version of this chapter.

REFERENCES

Chambless, D. L., & Ollendick, T. H. (2001). Empirically supported psychological interventions: Controversies and evidence. *Annual Review of Psychology, 52*, 685–716.

Garb, H. N. (1998). *Studying the clinician: Judgment research and psychological assessment*. Washington, DC: American Psychological Association.

Grove, W. M. (Chair). (2000). *APA Division 12 (Clinical) Presidential Task Force "Assessment for the year 2000": Report of the task force*. Washington, DC: American Psychological Association, Division 12 (Clinical Psychology).

Lilienfeld, S. O. (1998). Pseudoscience in contemporary clinical psychology: What it is and what we can do about it. *Clinical Psychologist, 51*, 3–9.

Lilienfeld, S. O. (2001, August 25). Fringe psychotherapies: Scientific and ethical implications for clinical psychology. In S. O. Lilienfeld (Chair), *Fringe psychotherapies: What lessons can we learn?* Presentation at invited symposium conducted at the Annual Meeting of the American Psychological Association, San Francisco.

Lilienfeld, S. O., Lohr, J. M., & Morier, D. (2001). The teaching of courses in the science and pseudoscience of psychology: Useful resources. *Teaching of Psychology, 28*, 182–191.

Index

Abuse, self-help therapy and, 428–429
Accountability
  defined, 201
  in New Age therapies, 188–194
Adderall, for ADHD, 335–336
ADHD. *See* Attention-deficit/hyperactivity disorder
Adinazolam, antidepressant effects of, 309
Admissibility, standards for, 83–84
Advice industry, 426–433, 455. *See also* Self-help therapy; TV talk shows
Age regression
  hypnotic, 218–219
  in memory recovery therapy, 216–218
Al-Anon, 278
Alcoholics Anonymous
  characteristics of, 295
  controversy over, 275–278
  format of, 275–276
  religious component of, 275
  as self-help model, 428
  studies of, 276–278
Alcoholism, 273–305
  treatment of
    with AA, 275–278
    with brief interventions, 293–294
    controversies over, 274–275
    with disulfiram, 279–281
    effective, 284–294
    history of, 273
    with Johnson intervention, 278–279
    with marital/family therapy, 291–293
    with moderation training/controlled drinking, 281–283
    with motivational enhancement therapy, 290–291

non-AA self-help groups for, 277–278
  with operant conditioning, 288–290
  with Project DARE, 293–294
  with relapse prevention, 287–288
  with social learning theory, 284–287
Aliens, therapy for encounters with, 196–197
Alters, 113–114
  defined, 135
American Psychological Association
  ethical standards of, 84–86
  forensic psychology guidelines of, 85
  Media Psychology division of, 447–448
  role as media watchdog, 463–464
  role in combatting pseudoscience, 462–463
  and sanctions against pseudoscience practitioners, 464
  self-help therapy and, 410–412
American Psychological Society, role as media watchdog, 464
Amino acid supplements, for ADHD, 347–348
Amnesia
  in dissociative identity disorder, 112
  infantile, 214–215, 232–233
Amphetamines, for ADHD, 335–336
Anatomically detailed dolls, 44, 57–61
  recommendations for, 65
  reliability and validity of, 58–61
  standardization and norms for, 57–58
  uses for, 59
Anecdotal evidence, 8
Antidepressant medications, 307–311
  for ADHD, 342
  controversy over, 306–307